Lipoplasty:
The Theory and Practice
of Blunt Suction Lipectomy

Lipoplasty
The Theory and Practice
of Blunt Suction Lipectomy

Edited by
Gregory P. Hetter, M.D.

Assistant Clinical Professor of Plastic Surgery,
University of Nevada School of Medicine, Reno;
Assistant Chief, Division of Plastic Surgery, Sunrise
Hospital, Las Vegas

Foreword by
Mario Gonzalez Ulloa, M.D.
Director, Dalinde Medical Center, Mexico City

Little, Brown and Company
Boston/Toronto

Library of Congress Catalog Card No. 84-81884
ISBN 0-316-35920-3
Printed in the United States of America
HAL

To Dr. Howard Lawrence of Phoenix, Arizona.
Dr. Lawrence was the first plastic surgeon in the
Southwest. He was first in the hearts of his
students because what others made complex he
made simple, what others made difficult he made
easy, and, above all, because he was not only one
of the most gifted of plastic surgeons but, most
unusually, also one of the finest of men.

Contents

Contributing Authors   xi
Foreword   xiii
Preface   xv

I. HISTORY AND BASIC THEORY

1. The Feminine Figure in Art, History, and Surgery   3
   Benito Vilar-Sancho

2. A History and Comparison of Suction Techniques Until Their Debut in North America   19
   Francis M. Otteni
   Pierre F. Fournier

3. The Origins of Lipolysis   25
   Yves-Gerard Illouz

4. Popularization of the Technique   33
   Pierre F. Fournier

5. Introduction of Lipolysis to the United States: A Three-Year Experience   37
   Norman Martin

6. Human Adipose Tissue Function, Development, and Metabolism   41
   Peter Arner

7. Body Image Disturbance and Eating Disorders   49
   James M. Ferguson

8. Harmony and Proportion in the Female Form   55
   Hale Tolleth

9. Nomenclature   65
   Gregory P. Hetter
   Carson M. Lewis
   Peter Arner

10. Photographic Documentation   77
    Gregory P. Hetter

11. Risk Management for Blunt Suction Lipectomy   87
    George Greenberg

12. Patient Selection: Psychological Aspects   91
    Carson M. Lewis

13. Physical Evaluation and Informed Consent   95
    Frank T. Herhahn

14. Anesthesia   105
    Michael C. Braunstein

15. The Use of Low-Concentration Epinephrine   115
    Gregory P. Hetter

16. Physics and Equipment   119
Gregory P. Hetter

17. Surgical Technique   137
Gregory P. Hetter

18. Alternative Patient Positioning and Pretunneling   155
Richard A. Mladick
Richard L. Morris

19. Dressings and Garments   163
Carson M. Lewis

20. Blood Chemistry Changes After Lipolysis   169
Frank T. Herbahn

21. Nutritional Support of Surgical Recovery   173
Patrick Quillin

22. Massage and Ultrasound   175
Carson M. Lewis
Margaret Pruitt

23. Convalescence   179
Gregory P. Hetter

II. CLINICAL APPLICATIONS

24. Adjunctive or Isolated Lipolysis of the Face and Neck   185
Gregory P. Hetter
Frank T. Herbahn

25. Lipolysis Combined with Facial Rhytidectomy   199
Richard A. Mladick

26. Lipolysis of the Arms   211
Boyd R. Burkhardt

27. Lipolysis as an Adjunctive Treatment for Gynecomastia   219
Carson M. Lewis

28. Lipolysis of the Female Breast   227
Adrien E. Aiache

29. Lipolysis and Lipoplasties of the Abdomen   233
Francis M. Otteni
Pierre F. Fournier

30. Lipolysis of the Flank   249
Paul L. Schnur

31. Lipolysis of the Iliac Crest   253
Gregory P. Hetter

32. Lipolysis of the Thigh and Knee   257
Gregory P. Hetter

33. Lipolysis of the Ankle and Calf   271
Adrien E. Aiache

34. Lipolysis Combined with Conventional Surgery 277
   Ricardo Baroudi

35. Lipolysis in Blacks, Including Treatment of Steatopygia 295
   Pierre F. Fournier
   Francis M. Otteni

36. Contour Deformities of the Upper Thigh 301
   Norman Martin

37. The Defatting of Flaps by Lipolysis 309
   James O. Stallings

38. The Use of Lipolysis for Unusual Diseases 323
   Gregory P. Hetter
   Carson M. Lewis
   Robert B. Winslow

Index 333

Contributing Authors

Adrien E. Aiache, M.D.
Instructor in Surgery, University of Southern California School of Medicine; Attending Surgeon, Cedars-Sinai Medical Center, Los Angeles

Peter Arner, M.D.
Associate Professor of Medicine, Karolinska Institute; Director of the Ward for Endocrine Disease, Huddinge Hospital, Stockholm

Ricardo Baroudi, M.D.
Attending Surgeon, Hospital Samaritano, Campinas City, Brazil

Michael C. Braunstein, M.D.
Assistant Clinical Professor of Anesthesiology, University of Nevada School of Medicine, Reno; Chief, Anesthesiology Department, Sunrise Hospital, Las Vegas

Boyd R. Burkhardt, M.D.
Attending Surgeon, Tucson Medical Center, Tucson

James M. Ferguson, M.D.
Associate Clinical Professor, University of California, San Diego, School of Medicine, La Jolla; Clinical Director, Eating Disorders Program, Alvarado Parkway Institute, La Mesa

Pierre F. Fournier, M.D.
Attending Plastic Surgeon, Clinique du Parc Monceau, Paris

George Greenberg, M.D.
Assistant Professor of Surgery, University of Nevada School of Medicine; Attending Surgeon, St. Mary's Hospital, Reno

Frank T. Herhahn, M.D.
Adjunct Clinical Professor of Surgery, University of New Mexico School of Medicine; Attending Surgeon, Presbyterian Hospital Center, Albuquerque

Gregory P. Hetter, M.D.
Assistant Clinical Professor of Plastic Surgery, University of Nevada School of Medicine, Reno; Assistant Chief, Division of Plastic Surgery, Sunrise Hospital, Las Vegas

Yves-Gerard Illouz, M.D.
Attending Surgeon, Clinique Spontini, Paris

Carson M. Lewis, M.D.
Associate Professor, Division of Plastic Surgery, University of California, San Diego, School of Medicine, La Jolla; Attending Surgeon, Hospital of the Scripps Clinic, La Jolla

Norman Martin, M.D.
Senior Attending Surgeon, Beverly Hills Medical Center, Los Angeles

Richard A. Mladick, M.D.
Chief of Surgery, Virginia Beach General Hospital, Virginia Beach, Virginia

Richard L. Morris, M.D.
Attending Surgeon, Virginia Beach General Hospital, Virginia Beach, Virginia

Francis M. Otteni, M.D.
Ancien Chef de Clinique des Hôpitaux de Strasbourg; Attending Surgeon, Clinique Toussaint, Strasbourg, France

Margaret Pruitt
Physical Therapist, Leucadia, California

Patrick Quillin, R.D., Ph.D.
Lecturer, Department of Family Studies, San Diego State University, San Diego; Nutritional Consultant, Hospital of the Scripps Clinic, La Jolla

Paul L. Schnur, M.D.
Clinical Associate in Surgery, University of Arizona College of Medicine; Attending Surgeon, Tucson Medical Center, Tucson

James O. Stallings, M.D.
Chairman, Department of Plastic and Reconstructive Surgery, Mercy Hospital Medical Center, Des Moines

Hale Tolleth, M.D.
Instructor in Plastic Surgery, University of California, Davis, School of Medicine, Davis; Attending Surgeon, St. Francis Hospital, San Francisco

Benito Vilar-Sancho, M.D.
Chief, Department of Plastic Surgery, Centro Especial Ramon y Cayal, Madrid; President, International Society for Aesthetic Plastic Surgery, 1983–1985

Robert B. Winslow, M.D.
Clinical Associate Professor, Division of Plastic and Reconstructive Surgery and Surgery of the Hand, University of North Carolina at Chapel Hill School of Medicine, Chapel Hill; Attending Staff Surgeon, Rex Hospital, Raleigh

Foreword

Our generation of plastic surgeons has lived through important advances in the techniques of aesthetic plastic surgery: augmentation in rhinoplasty, advances in rhytidectomies, in various forms of lipectomy leading to torsoplasty, and important discoveries in many inert substances useful in replacing volume deficiencies of the face and body. These favorable advances have been made use of by those in the medical profession who practice aesthetic plastic surgery. However, no technical advance has been so overwhelmingly interesting, invasive, and spectacular as the invention of the technique known as aspirative or suction lipoplasty.

Its history is relatively recent. Just a few articles have been published within the past couple of years; yet, it has now arrived at such a stage of excellence in the hands of its more skilled practitioners that the human face or body may be excavated and shaped, molding the adipose tissue into more harmonious contours. Lipoplasty clearly has new indications. The competent surgeon-artist must become well acquainted with the technique and must also possess the artistic talent and sensitivity to hollow out only until a defined and neat line of harmony is attained, leaving behind the prominences that are so important to the configuration of the body silhouette and the facial profile.

Lipoplasty is of great assistance to the aesthetic plastic surgeon who uses it as an addition to classical procedures in striving toward perfection in remodeling the profiles of the human figure. Many surgeons throughout the world are interested in finding new terms to describe the procedure, in determining all its indications, and in exploring when to combine it with classical surgery.

Body contouring by lipoplasty is a major intervention: It should be carried out in an operating theater with proper anesthesia attendance, cardiovascular monitoring, and strictly aseptic conditions. Of course, aspirative lipoplasty is not the solution to the problem of obesity—this is not the suggestion of the authors of this text. I believe that the treatment of obesity is being satisfactorily approached by the medical profession as an illness that alters metabolism or results from inadequate eating habits and exercise deficiency. However, through selective dermolipectomies, carried out surgically, prominent ptotic adipose tissue masses, lax skin, and striae may be simultaneously eliminated.

Aspirative lipoplasty, performed as a sole procedure, is indicated in large numbers of cases in which the adipose tissue masses are localized and require no surgical skin correction. Complications due to inadequate technique or to lack of anatomical knowledge or precautions can occur. The way in which to safely carry out the treatment of these patients to obtain highly satisfactory results is also known and is being made available to the plastic surgery community with this text.

I believe that this new procedure, used properly, with propedeutics well followed, and precise indications as to its use will become a great resource to the surgeon-artist in the pursuit of harmony and beauty. Observations from surgeons throughout the world are now ample. This is not an experimental procedure. The experience collected amounts to many, many thousands of operations. Physically, results are good. Patients consider it lenient and uncomplicated, and recovery and convalescence are relatively easy.

For the surgeon, lipoplasty has opened a field for further development and investigation. The technique appears easy but is highly sophisticated and demands wide and thorough anatomical knowledge and artistic experience. Thus, it should be performed only by highly experienced hands.

The mastery with which Gregory Hetter handles this technique, his finesse in dealing with tissues, his highly ethical reasoning, as well as his logical resume of exciting meditation, investigation, and experience have made this book possible. He has brought together 24 authors from plastic surgery and other disciplines to share with the reader the greatest expertise and experience available in lipoplasty. I think that *Lipoplasty: The Theory and Practice of Blunt Suction Lipectomy* is a must for the surgeon who desires to delve into this magnetic and novel field of surgery. The beauty and harmony disclosed in this book make it a classic and yet efficient guide.

Mario Gonzalez Ulloa, M.D.

In the fall of 1981, I accepted an invitation to speak at the Sacramento Otolaryngology Society's Symposium, which was held in February 1982 at Lake Tahoe. That invitation, casually accepted, later proved to have momentous impact. A French surgeon by the name of Pierre Fournier spoke at the symposium on a new technique by Yves-Gerard Illouz that was developed for fat extraction in the head and neck area. After the presentation I approached him in order to learn more. Later he showed me several carousels of pictures of body sculpture patients on whom this new technique, which he called lipolysis, had been performed with obvious startling results. I was eager to visit him to see firsthand the results of this new technique. Many surgeons were critical of the procedure without having any real knowledge of it. I wanted to see for myself.

After visiting France, I realized that lipolysis was by far the most important advance in body contouring that had been made during my professional lifetime (20 years). Whereas most previously written material concerned how to minimize the severe problems attendant on existing operations, this was a leap to an entirely different medium.

The Lipolysis Society of North America (an extension of, but independent from, the International Lipolysis Society formed by Illouz in Paris) was formed in February 1983 to teach the Illouz procedure to young, board-certified plastic surgeons. *Lipoplasty: The Theory and Practice of Blunt Suction Lipectomy* grew out of the meeting of the many talented and knowledgeable physicians who spoke at and attended the many symposiums that have been held around the world.

The text brings together the clinical experience of most of the American surgeons who began performing lipolysis in late 1982 and early 1983. The clinical experience with blacks described by Drs. Fournier and Otteni is exceeded by no one. Dr. Ricardo Baroudi's considerable experience with torso procedures has been modified by lipolysis to blend classic techniques with new. No surgeon has more experience in combined procedures. Dr. Norman Martin's careful review of more than three years' experience and over 2,000 procedures is exceeded by no North American surgeon. He has shared his knowledge about delayed sequelae with us.

The nomenclature for this new area is, of course, in flux. Different authors have used different terms to describe the Illouz technique: the extraction of subcutaneous fat from localized areas using blunt cannulas and high vacuum. The following terms are, therefore, used synonymously: lipolysis (Illouz), aspirative lipoplasty (generic), honeycombed lipectomy and collapsing surgery (Fournier), suction extraction of fat (generic), suction-assisted lipectomy (S.A.L.) (Grazier), blunt suction lipectomy (Hetter), liposuction (Newman and Dolsky), and fat sucking (colloquial). Curette techniques are not included in this text, and the reader must be aware that suction curettage is not synonymous with any of the above terms and should not be confused with them. Chapter 9 explains these and other new terms.

The guiding principle in this text has been to be uncompromisingly honest in recognizing all those who have played a role in this procedure's development, regardless of specialty, background, or society memberships. Because Dr. George Fischer of Rome and Drs. Illouz and Fournier of Paris are not members of their national plastic surgery organizations, the recognition of their innovations and ideas has been slow and is not as widespread as it should be.

The authors have made a sincere effort to expand the reader's understanding of the art, history, psychology, theory, and practice of aspirative lipoplasty. With the exception of Dr. Peter Arner, who is a professor and researcher, all of the authors are in private practice. The point of view is therefore practical and clinical and is related to the concerns of practicing plastic surgeons. I hope that readers find this text a revealing history, a thorough theoretical introduction, and an extensive guide to the dramatic aesthetic surgery of the 1980s: lipoplasty.

I would like to thank the following people for their help in the preparation of this book: Curt Abbott, for photographic processing; Susan Cuchiara, for manuscript processing; Mary Horton, for drawings; Ann Kahr, C.O.R.T., for photographic preparation; Alix Kerr, for idiomatic rendering of two French chapters; Priscilla Hurdle, for timely processing of the manuscript; and Curtis Vouwie, for having faith in the outcome.

G.P.H.

PART I

History and Basic Theory

CHAPTER 1

The Feminine Figure in Art, History, and Surgery

Benito Vilar-Sancho

Many of today's women subject themselves to a variety of torments. Many women undergo diets, medications, exhausting exercises, incredible massage routines, saunas, wraps, unknown injections, physiotherapies of all types, and even frightful surgical operations, at the cost of huge amounts of money and time, in an attempt to reduce their hips, buttocks, or thighs a few centimeters. "Why do they go to such lengths?" we might ask. In my opinion, there is but one answer: the "modern" concept of feminine beauty, particularly with respect to the shape of the gluteal and trochanteric regions. This concept is directly in line with the values of the so-called rhythmic cultures. In these cultures, men are dominant in one way or another, the sun is worshipped, and the straight line predominates over the curve.

The Egyptian civilization is the most ancient example of a rhythmic culture (Fig. 1-1). In this civilization, women's hips were straight (Fig. 1-2), almost masculine, with no sign of relief in the trochanteric regions (Fig. 1-3), which do not stand out at all from the "ilio-femoro-rotulian" line.*

This idealized artistic concept was maintained in classical Greece and Rome, although a little more femininity was perhaps added to the female shape, allowing a gentle curve in the ilio-femoro-rotulian line in consonance with the sensuality attributed to their mythological goddesses (Fig. 1-4). There was, however, no sign of relief in the trochanteric area (Fig. 1-5), which might break the purity of the line. The silhouettes of their amphoras, in which this line can be seen (Fig. 1-6), reproduce the female waist and hip.

This artistic representation of the female figure has come down to our day without any substantial variations in the shape of the trochanteric reliefs (i.e., the hip and thigh). This lack of variation can be observed in the paintings of the primitives and in those of the Renaissance (Fig. 1-7), even though their ideals of feminine beauty differed widely. Differences in ideals of feminine beauty can also be observed, for example, in works by Botticelli (Fig. 1-8), Durer (Fig. 1-9), Titian (Fig. 1-10), and Velázquez (Fig. 1-11). None of these artists, however, breaks the ilio-femoro-rotulian line with any more or less prominent reliefs. Not even Rubens with his obese, blond Flemish beauties (Fig. 1-12) does anything other than mark the abundance of fat in the gluteal region, never breaking the absolute purity of the line.

---

*Author's note: The ilio-femoro-rotulian line is an imaginary line that begins at the anterior iliac spine, is tangential to the tip of trochanter, and ends at the external femoral condyle.

Authorization for use of some of the illustrations in this chapter was given by Professor J. M. Gomez Tabanero, editor of the Spanish edition of *The Female Figure in Paleolithic Art.*

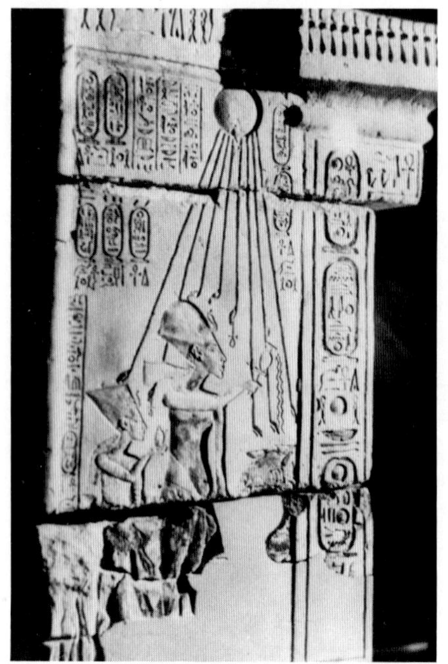

Fig. 1-1

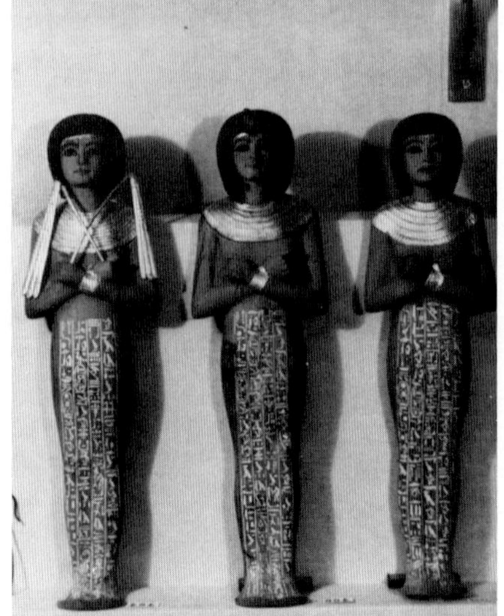

Fig. 1-2

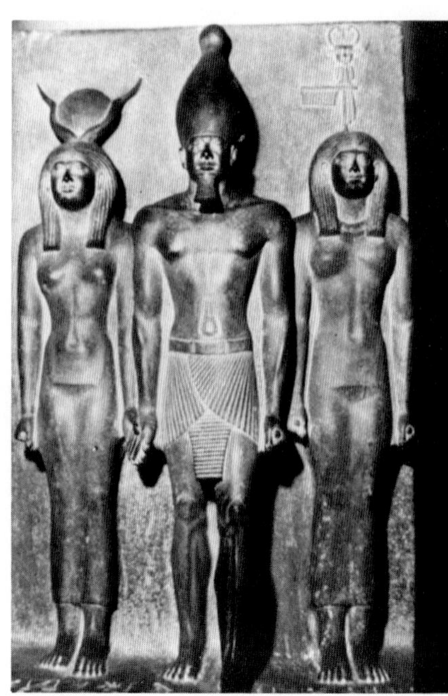

Fig. 1-3

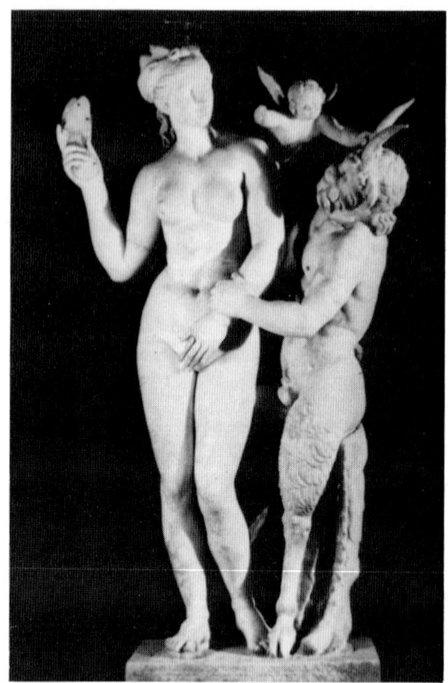

Fig. 1-4

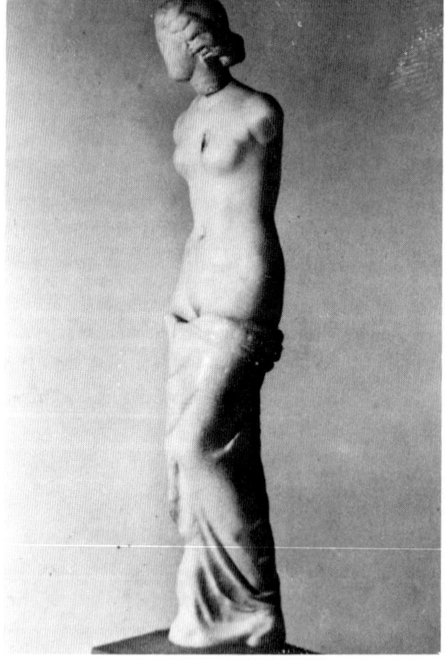

Fig. 1-5

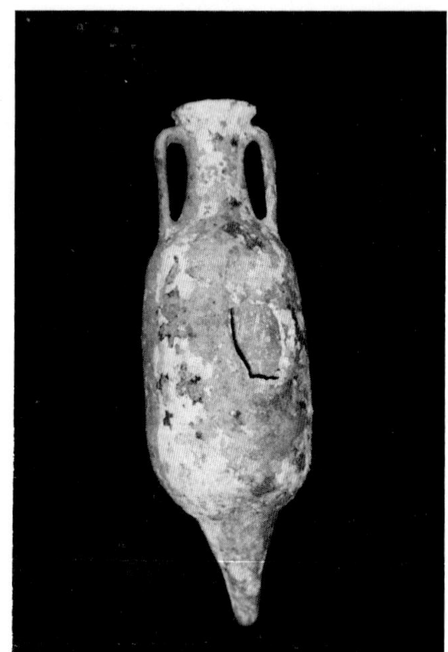

Fig. 1-6

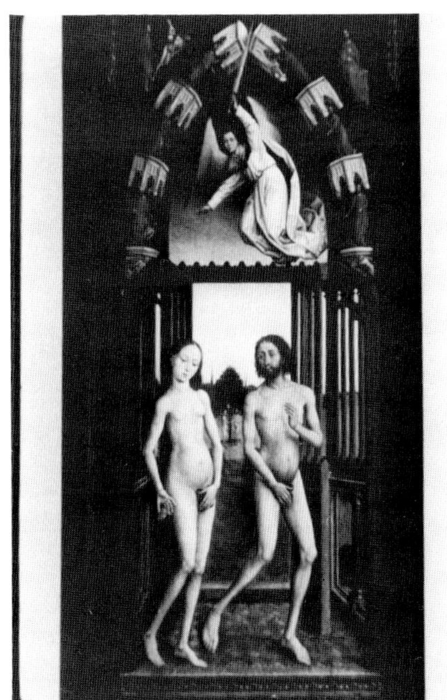

Fig. 1-7

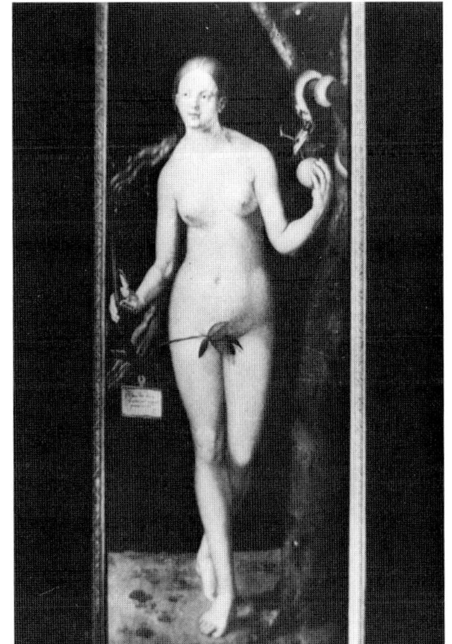

Fig. 1-9

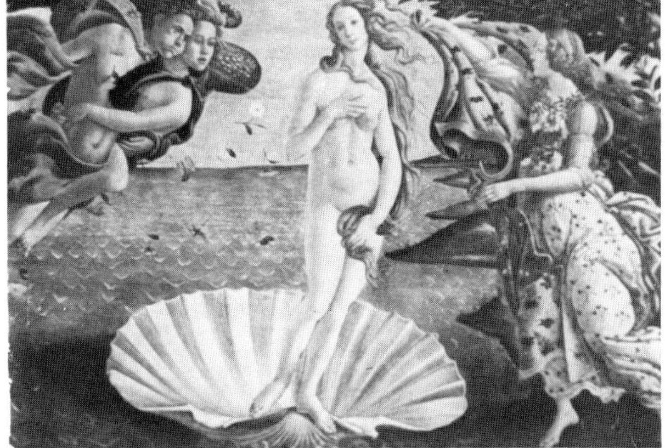

Fig. 1-8

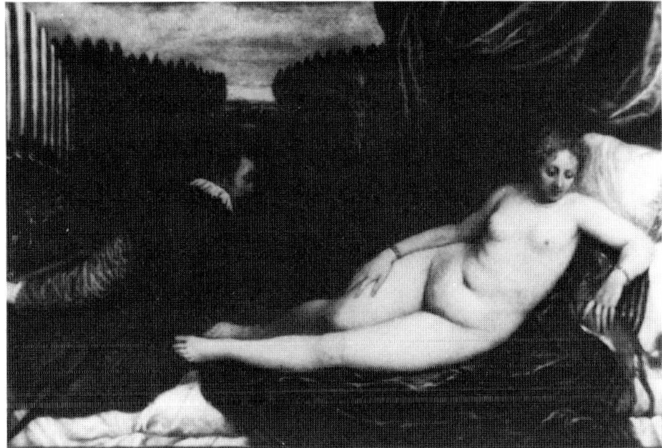

Fig. 1-10

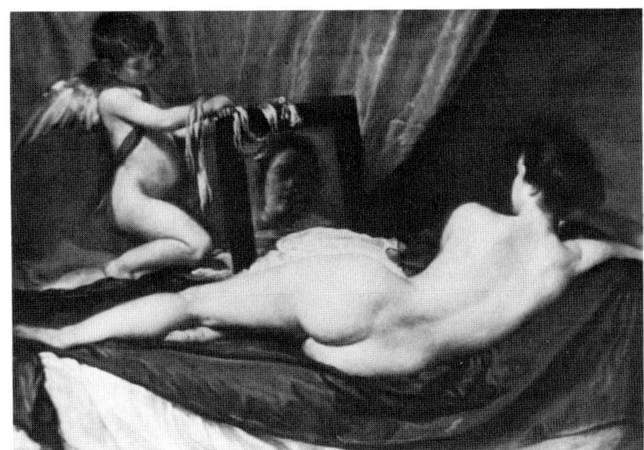

Fig. 1-11

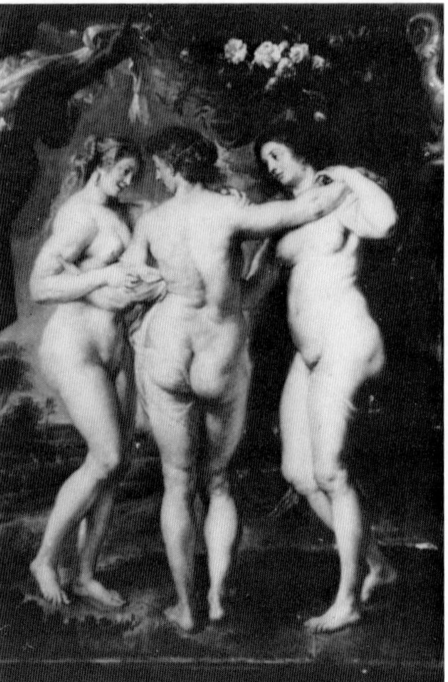

Fig. 1-12

Fig. 1-13

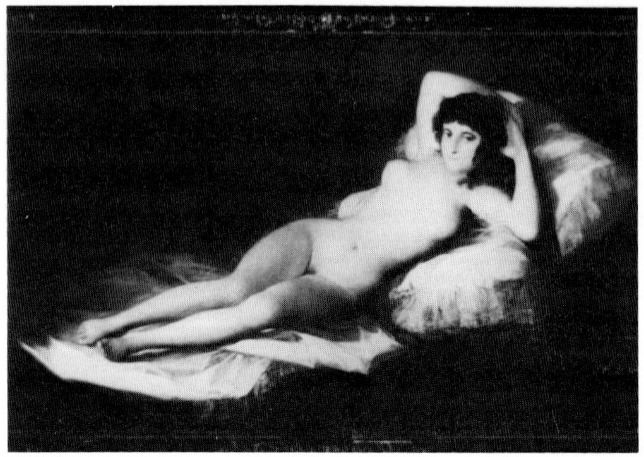

Fig. 1-14

This purity of the line is also seen in the works of the eighteenth- and nineteenth-century painters (Figs. 1-13 and 1-14). Not even the most realistic painters (Fig. 1-15), sculptors (Fig. 1-16), or photographers (Fig. 1-17) of our time dare to depict any other shapes of the feminine hip, remaining within what might be called the classical line of beauty.

Despite all the works of art of the rhythmic cultures, however, other shapes have existed and still exist in tangible reality (Fig. 1-18). Although these shapes have not been depicted in art for many thousands of years, they are clearly reflected in works of the remote cultures of the European Paleolithic Age, which dominated the world for an immensely longer period of time than our culture has prevailed up to now. These cultures are the melodic cultures, whose object of worship was the moon, real or symbolized. Here, women were predominant in some matriarchal way (despite what is, in my opinion, an ungrounded theory to the contrary held by certain archeologists), and the curve prevailed over the straight line. Their representation of women is now considered to be deformed (Fig. 1-19).

These ancient cultures flourished in Quaternary Europe at the end of the last Ice Age, concurrent with the appearance of the Cro-Magnon man *(Homo sapiens)*—the last link in human evolution between the tertiary hominids and the humans of today. Their cultural nuclei (communities) extended, geographically, from the Pyrenees to Russia and, chronologically, from the dawn of the Upper Paleolithic to the Neolithic, that is, a period of about 25,000 years, stretching from 35,000 BC to 10,000 BC. This period is five times longer than the historical existence of our most ancient civilization.

Throughout this extremely broad space of time, works that we now consider works of art were created; they astound us with their excellence and realism. These works of art include both cave paintings and the statuettes called Paleolithic Venuses or Venus figurines. The Venus figurines were a genuine expression of the men of those times. The best known, although perhaps not the most characteristic example of these works, is the *Willendorf Venus,* discovered in the Austrian village of that name (Fig. 1-19).

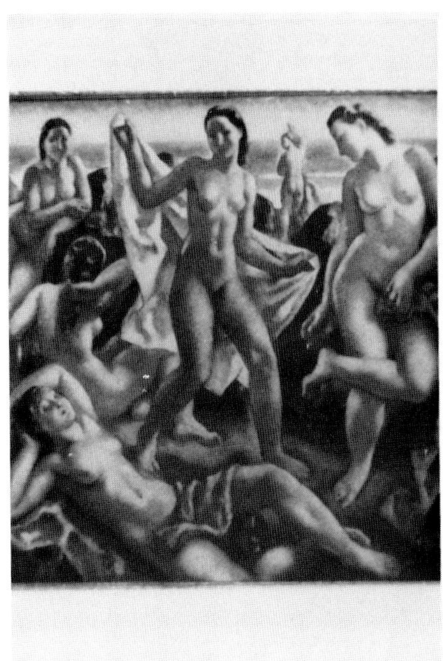

Fig. 1-15

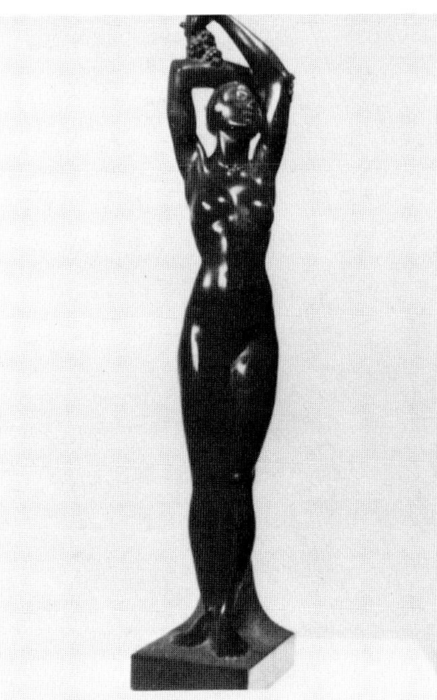

Fig. 1-16

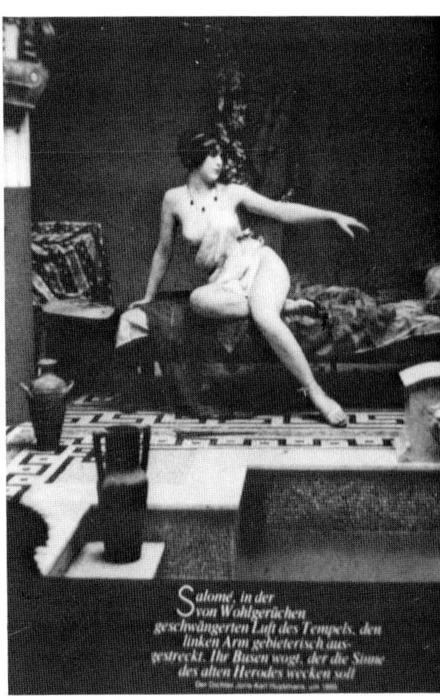

Fig. 1-17

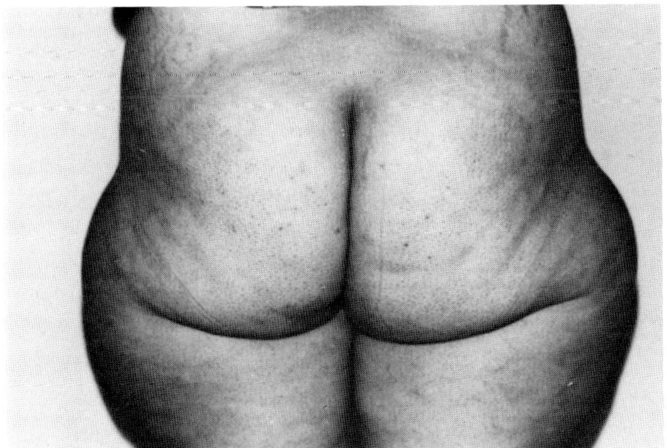

Fig. 1-18

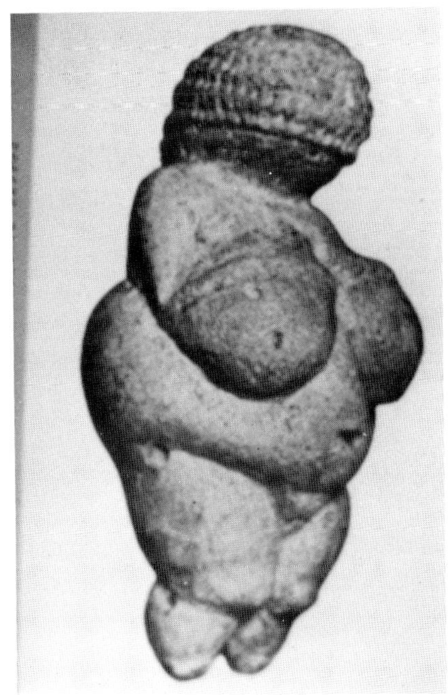

Fig. 1-19

The men whom we now call Paleolithic artists attempted to evoke or elicit something with the figures they fashioned, without concerning themselves with the creation of a work of art as such. Thus, I believe they were always realists just as when they strove to evoke the bison in their hunts through the exact representation of that animal. In the feminine figurines, they also strove to evoke femininity, motherhood, and sexuality.

These statuettes, which usually represent female figures, abound in all the nuclei of Paleolithic culture and are found in the settlements of different groups. No fewer than 300 figurines of this type have been found. A few of the most important figurines will be mentioned. They are of interest to us here since they present the

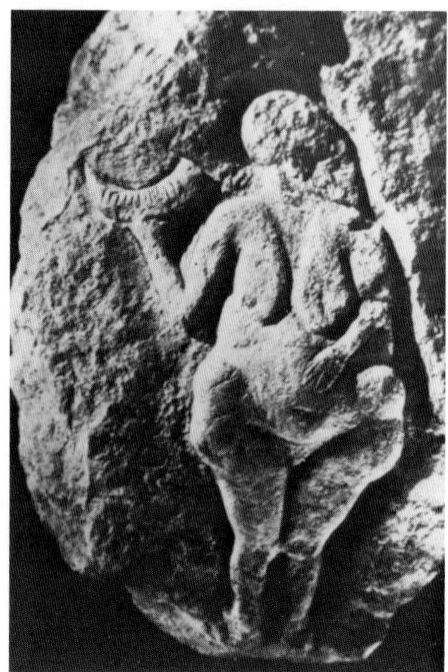

Fig. 1-20

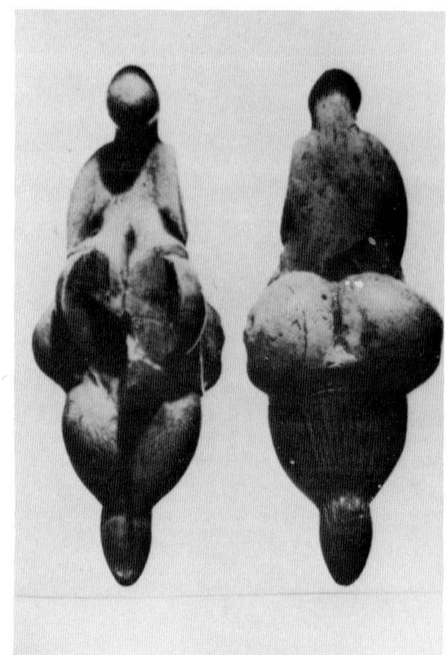

Fig. 1-21

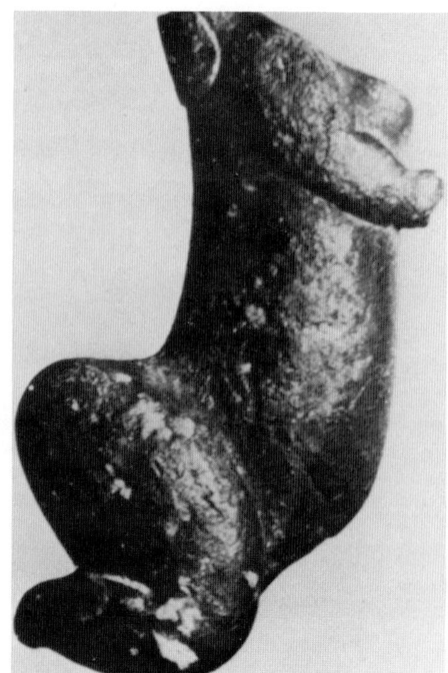

Fig. 1-22

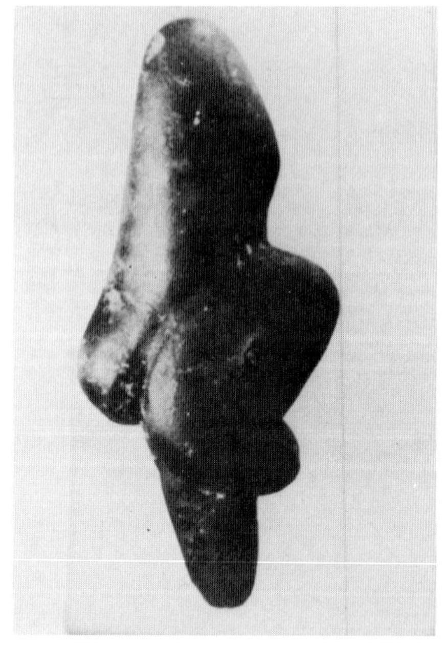

Fig. 1-23

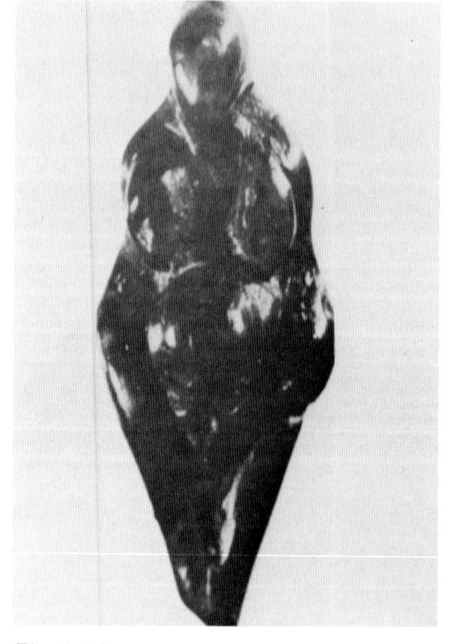

Fig. 1-24

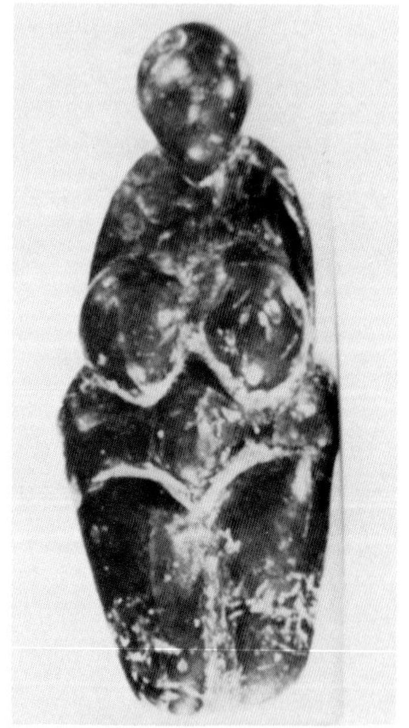

Fig. 1-25

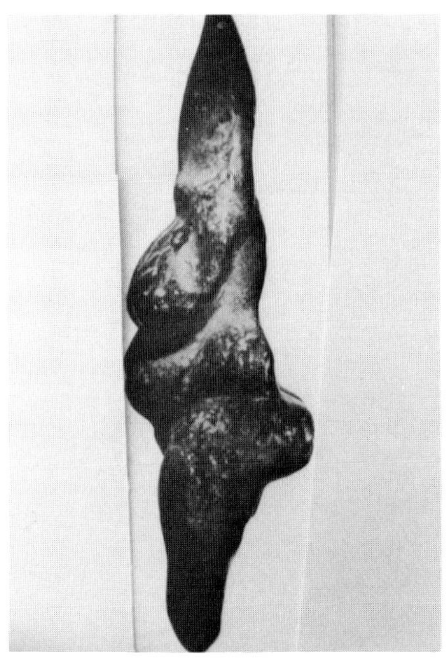

Fig. 1-26

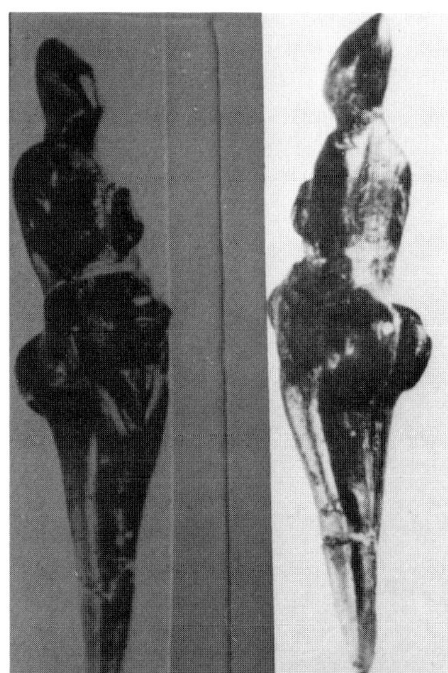

Fig. 1-27

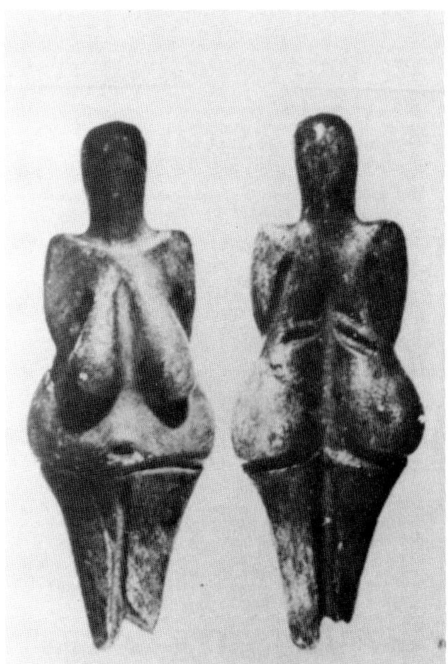

Fig. 1-28

shapes that now concern us. These objects have been found in the Pyrenean-Aquitanian, Italic, Rhenish-Danubian, and Russian cultural nuclei.

The figurines from the Pyrenean-Aquitanian group include the *Horn Venus* from the Lausell settlement (Fig. 1-20), and the *Lespugne Venus* (Fig. 1-21), the *Sireuil Venus* (Fig. 1-22), and the *Tursac Venus* (Fig. 1-23) from the settlements of the same names.

The Italic group includes such figurines as the so-called *Rhombus* (Fig. 1-24), the *Savignano Venus* (Fig. 1-25), the *Grimaldi Venus* (Fig. 1-26), and the *Policinella Venus* (Fig. 1-27) also from Grimaldi.

The Rhenish-Danubian group has provided the *Dolni Vestonice Venus* (Fig. 1-28), the previously mentioned *Willendorf Venus* (see Fig. 1-19), as well as others too numerous to mention here.

Within the Russian group, of particular interest for us, is the *Venus Number 3* of Koskenki (Fig. 1-29), which bears a striking resemblance to the *Lespugne Venus.* The Russian group includes the Gargarino settlement, which has produced *Venuses numbers 1, 2, and 4* (Fig.

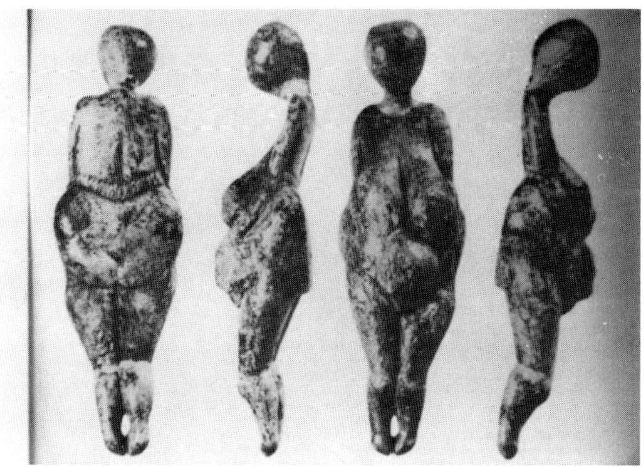

Fig. 1-29

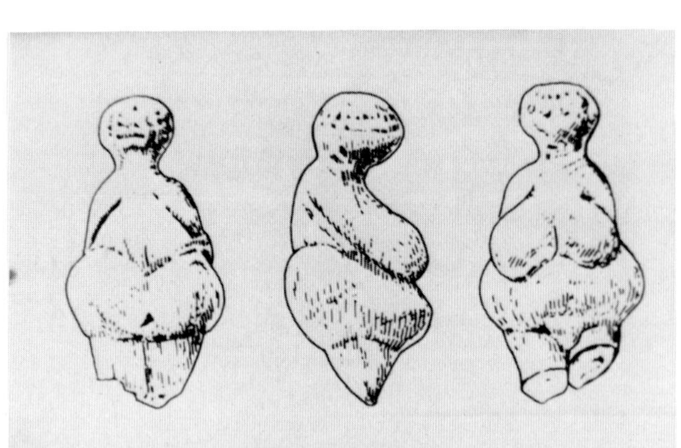

A

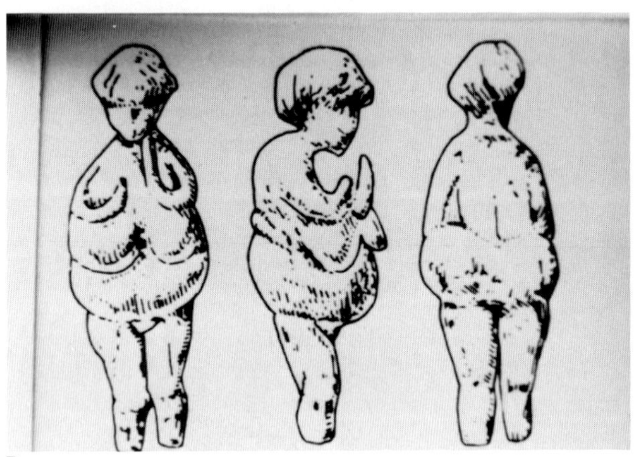

B

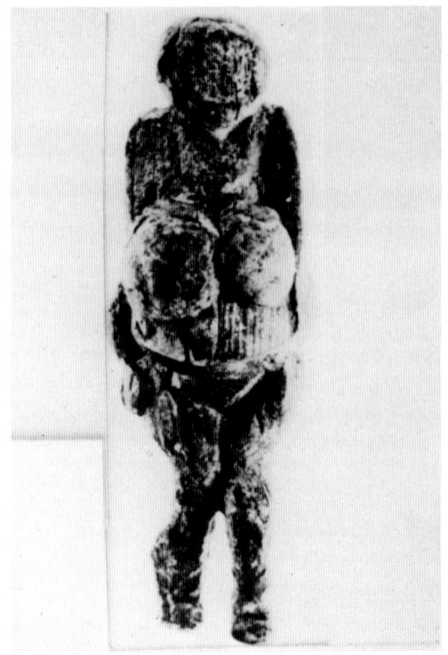

C
Fig. 1-30

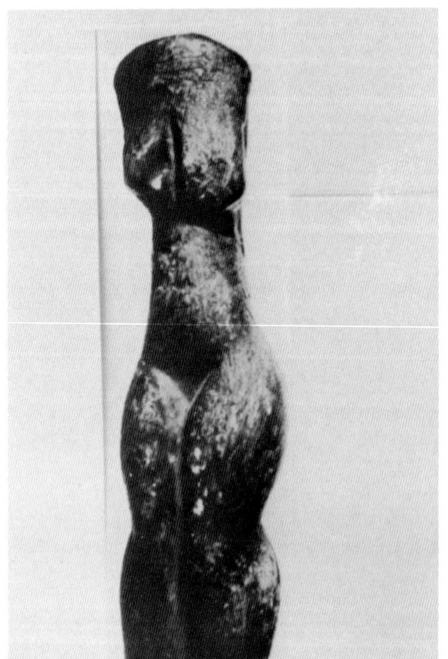

Fig. 1-31

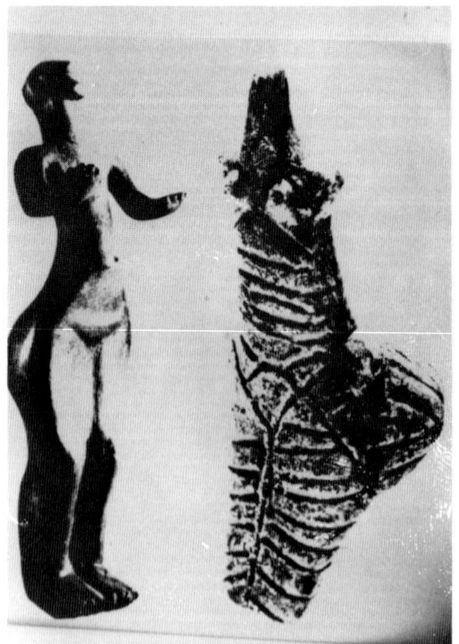

Fig. 1-32

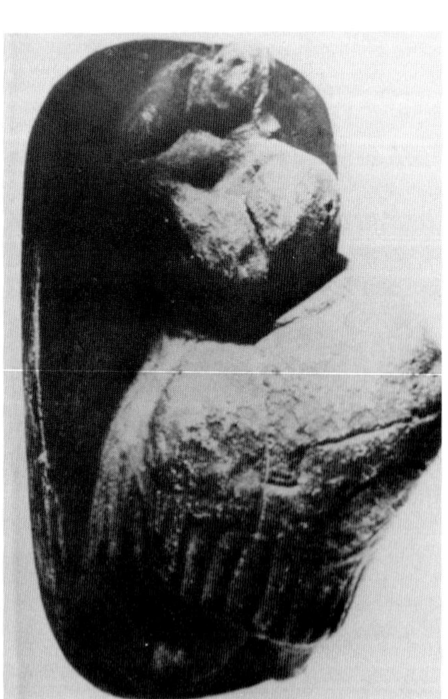

Fig. 1-33

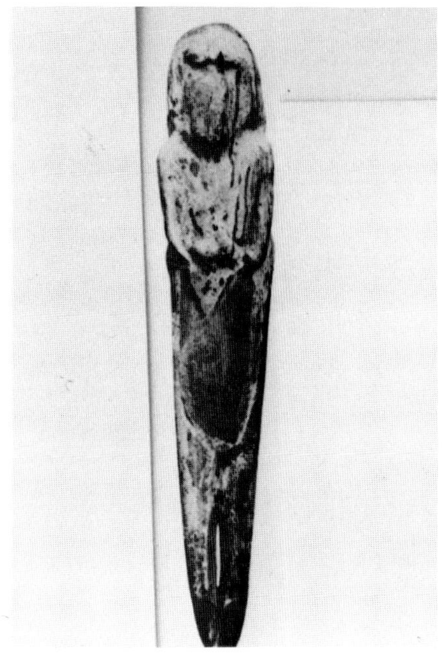

Fig. 1-34

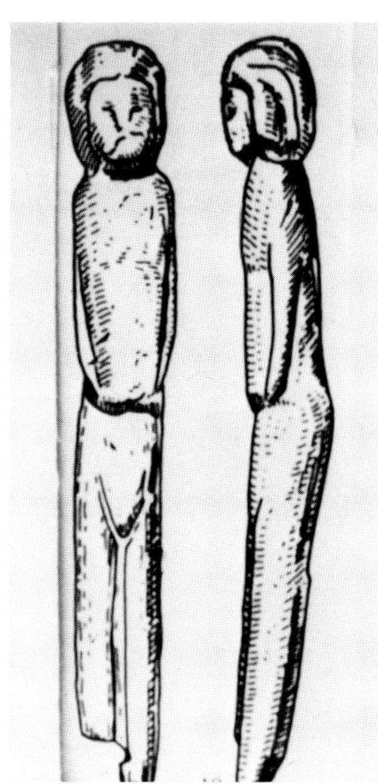

Fig. 1-35

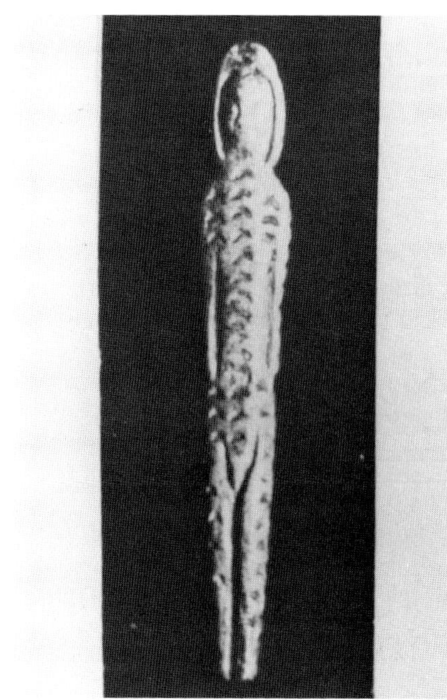

Fig. 1-36

1-30A,B,C) together with others of lesser importance. And lastly, within the Russian group, we have the *Eliseviche Torso* (Fig. 1-31). The purity of lines in this figurine makes it perhaps the most beautiful of all these figurines, bearing a great resemblance to the *Cacuteni Venus* (Fig. 1-32), which was made several thousand years later in the Neolithic period. Both statuettes present a perfectly carved and polished torso in which a steatomelia of the purest beauty is clearly represented.

The figurines from the island of Malta (Fig. 1-33), which might be called the last western Mediterranean link in the chain of Paleolithic Venuses, should also be included, even though they are actually from the Neolithic period.

Although the statuettes do not all have the same characteristics, they do follow a similar pattern of aesthetic taste that was widespread both over time and space. The representations of this type of figurine never showed rectilinear shapes but rather feminine figures with enormous buttocks, genuine steatomelias, and peritrochanteric lipodystrophies. Interestingly, many of these figurines present steatopygic characteristics: torsos with large breasts, often with small heads and thin arms and legs, that is, characteristics that are frequently observed today in many women of the Mediterranean basin, in several African tribes, and in the descendants of these peoples who now principally inhabit Central and South America.

In many cases, these cultural nuclei (communities) were separated from each other by thousands of kilometers and many thousands of years. It is very difficult to believe that these isolated communities could exert any direct influence on each other, considering the physical conditions that prevailed during Paleolithic times.

Not all the Paleolithic figurines, however, represented women who our modern world has come to consider deformed. In Siberia, near Lake Baikal, different settlements have been discovered in which slim figures (Fig. 1-34) without steatomeric or steatopygic accumulations have been unearthed. These figurines have broad shoulders and a larger head; they break with the rhomboidal shape characteristic of the European and Russian groups. The statuettes from the Malta settlement (Fig. 1-35) and the Buret settlement (Fig. 1-36) could be said to be the first works of art representing the figure sought by some women of today.

To understand the Paleolithic period and its art is a truly difficult, probably incomprehensible, task and goes beyond the scope of this study. To show how great the difficulty, we need only to mention the scarcity of data allowing chronological classifications with errors of less than one thousand years. In historical time, this would mean not knowing whether the Escorial was built in the times of Philip II or in those of Constantine the Great. And such relative accuracy would only be the most exact case, for it is still argued whether the figurines of the Siberian group are from the Magdalenian, about 12,000 BC, or the Paulian, about 26,000 BC, a difference of fully 14,000 years, which is the same time separating us from the Magdalenian period. To put this in perspective, it is like not knowing whether a Paleolithic man or Salvador Dali painted the Altamira caves. What is more, even though the artistic representations that have come down to us from those civilizations seem relatively abundant, they are extremely scarce if we consider the area of land and the amount of time involved.

For these reasons, plausible deductions can be made only when supported by specific facts, but irrefutable proof is highly unlikely. One has to choose among competitive suppositions on the basis of believability.

First, it is my belief that steatomelia and steatopygia had to exist in Paleolithic women, in the Perigordian and European Magdalenian. These shapes have persisted down to our day with little variation. Second, we can assume that this type of woman was, at least for the "artists," a source of inspiration and, as previously mentioned, evocation. What we cannot say, however, is whether this art was for religious, tribal, or sexual reasons. Or was it simply due to the fact, as is my belief, that all the women looked more or less like that, and the artists simply depicted them realistically as they did the bison?

Speculations on the Origins of Fatty Accumulations

What are the anatomical and physiological reasons for these "deformities," as they are called today? A categorical answer cannot be given because all is speculation in this respect. Precisely for this reason, I venture to give my personal opinion: steatopygia and steatomelia and the so-called peritrochanteric lipodystrophies were none other than fat reserves. These caloric storehouses allowed women to survive in the climatic rigors of the Ice Age when the prolonged winter isolated people and prevented them from obtaining the necessary food, especially for pregnant mothers. These shapes served the purpose of the hump of a camel (and I hope the reader will excuse this somewhat indelicate comparison).

In their origins, these fat reserves were secondary sexual attributes proper to the women of Europe. These people migrated along the great river routes of the Danube to the west and the Don to the north to settle the land from the Pyrenees to Russia.

The fact that the Siberian group presents slender feminine figurines I believe confirms my opinion that the art of this group was absolutely realistic. The Baikal sculptors carved their figurines the way their women looked: slim, with no signs of lipodystrophy, and in consonance with what might be called the artistic tastes of the times. For me, this is a clear sign that the Siberian communities belonged to a race with different anatomic characteristics than the European groups. Given the distance of more than 5,000 kilometers that separated them, this is not at all surprising.

Some speculations border on science fiction, although they are not much wilder than those of many archeologists. For example, suppose these Asiatic races, in their successive westward migrations, mixed with the indigenous inhabitants in their path and partly displaced them toward the Mediterranean basin. As the dominant race, the artistic tastes of the Asiatics prevailed over those of the Europeans without, of course, causing the genetic body type of the latter to disappear.

If this theory is accepted, all that remains to be explained to close the circle of thought is why the women of these Siberian races lacked steatomelia or steatopygia. I do not think it too risky to propose that, contrary to the fairly sedentary and matriarchal habits of the women of the European groups, which usually inhabited narrow valleys (thus enhancing the congenital tendency to accumulate fat in given areas), the Siberian groups were basically nomadic and patriarchal. This lifestyle obliged women, from childhood on, to make long marches burdened with all their belongings to leave the men's arms free for fighting. Thus, while natural selection inexorably caused the women least endowed with caloric reserves to disappear from among the sedentary races, the opposite occurred among the peoples who were constantly traveling. Here, the most obese female individuals gradually disappeared.

These speculations, by their very nature, will probably never be categorically answered, but one point is obviously true. At the present time, throughout Europe and especially in the area of the Mediterranean coast, two types of women are found. One type is slim, with straight hips, long thighs, legs, and arms, and relatively small breasts. The other is characterized by steatomelia, steatopygia and, specifically, peritrochanteric lipodystrophy, salient cheekbones, narrow shoulders, prominent clavicles, large breasts, and thin, short arms and legs. I believe these people to be just like their ancestors, as represented in the figurines from 20,000 to 30,000 years ago.

To this point I have attempted, hopefully with some degree of success, to show that there has not really been any change in the female figure, at least in the last 350 centuries. Moreover, the women with broad hips (Fig. 1-37), bulging buttocks, and fat accumulations in their thighs are not deformed in themselves. They are not a leap backward toward the dawn of man or living fossils; neither are the long-limbed women (Fig. 1-38) with straight hips who are our present models. Rather, both types are the logical genetic result of different races which, despite thousands of years of coexistence, frequently maintain the traits characteristic to each. Men also maintain their own characteristics although we lack such compelling evidence as for women, since representations of men in the Paleolithic cultures were quite scarce.

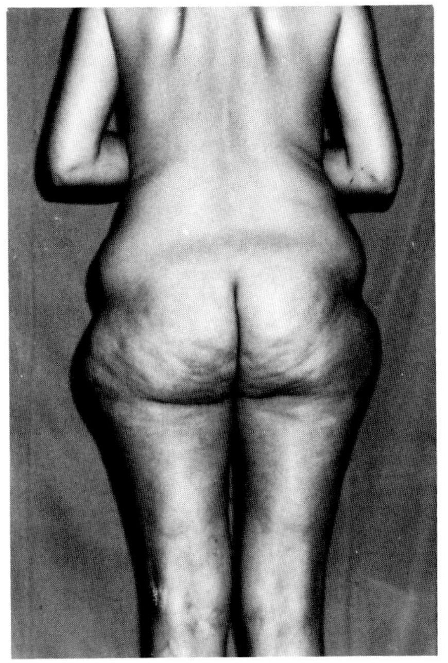

Fig. 1-37

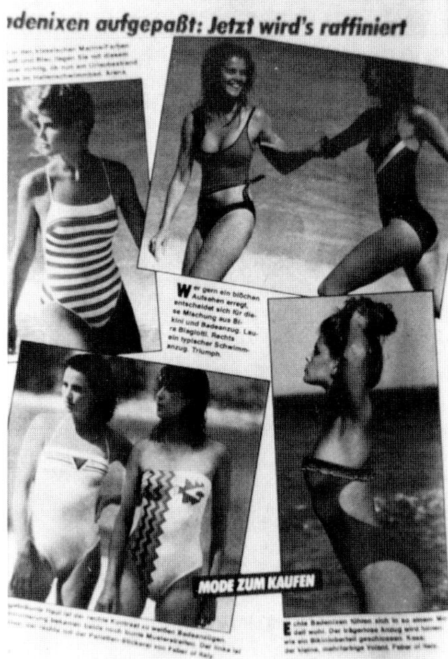

Fig. 1-38

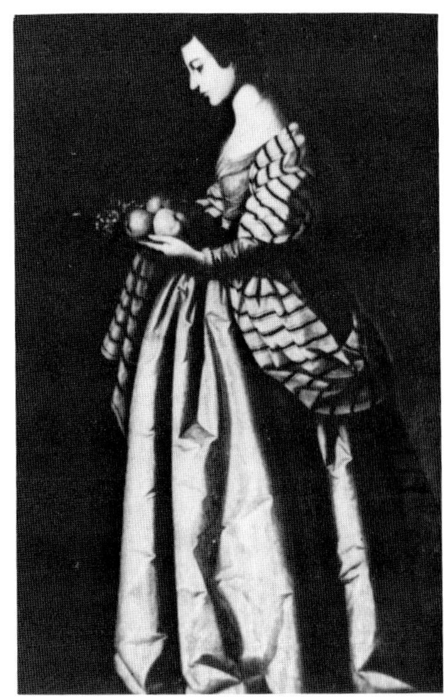

Fig. 1-39

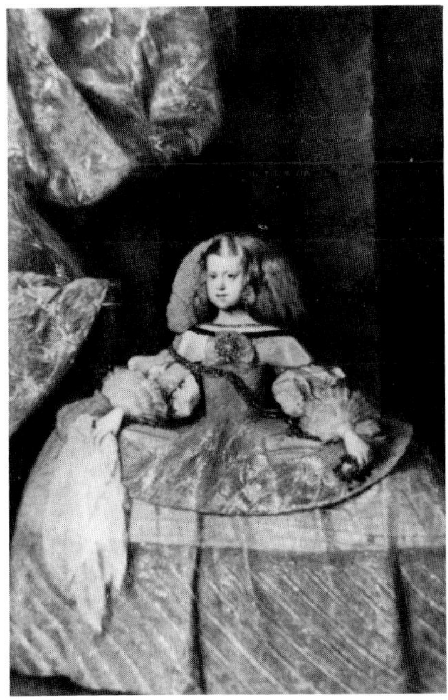

Fig. 1-40

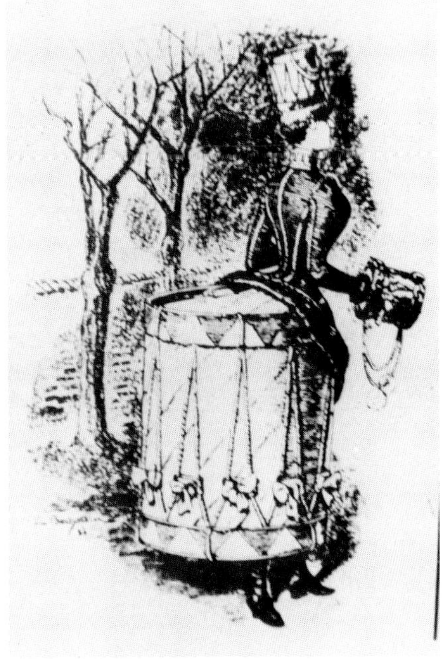

Fig. 1-41

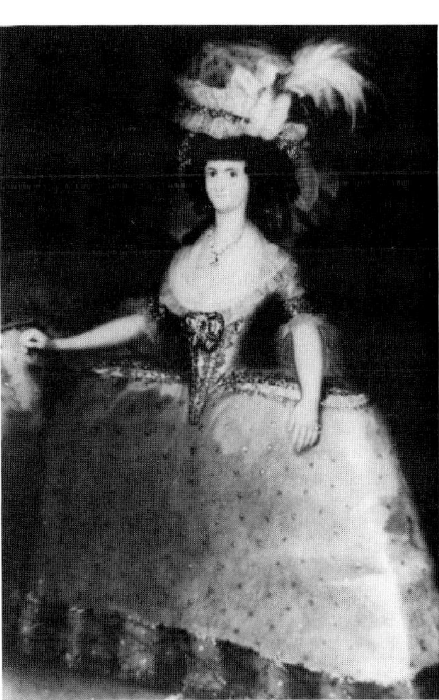

Fig. 1-42

For centuries, we might even say for thousands of years, the volume of women's hips, the prominence of their glutei, or the purity of their ilio-femoro-rotulian line posed no problems for them. Among other reasons, this was because the clothing they wore amply covered these areas of the body (Fig. 1-39) and because corpulence was practically synonymous with good health and well-being.

For many years the fashion of the hoop skirt (Fig. 1-40), and later that of the bustle (ridiculed in Fig. 1-41), used metal and whalebone stays to imitate the most monstrous hips and the most grotesque steatopygias. From these broad bases, a thin waist compressed by a corset—so thin that it seemed it might snap at the least movement—emerged like the stem of a flower from a vase (Fig. 1-42). These fashions concealed and even falsified women's true shapes, making them resemble the Paleolithic Venuses to a certain extent.

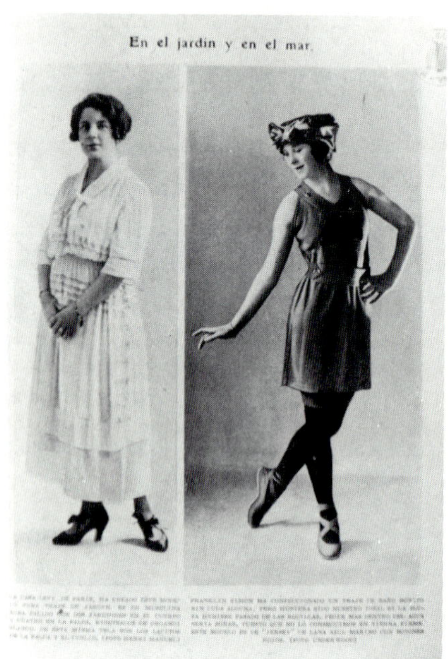

Fig. 1-43

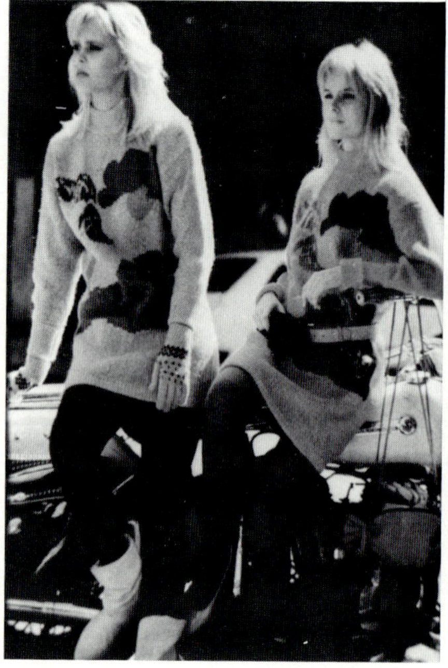

Fig. 1-44

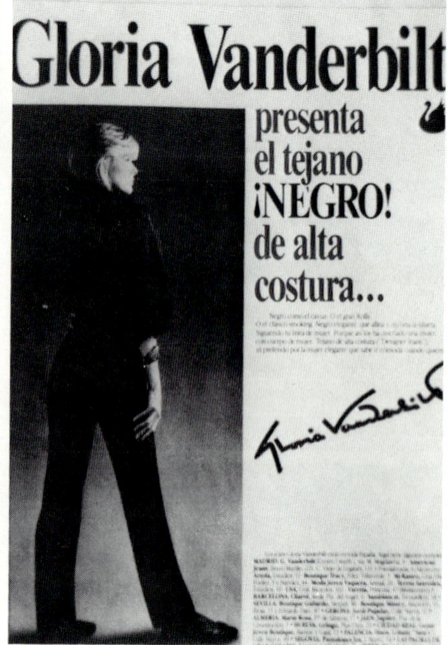

Fig. 1-45

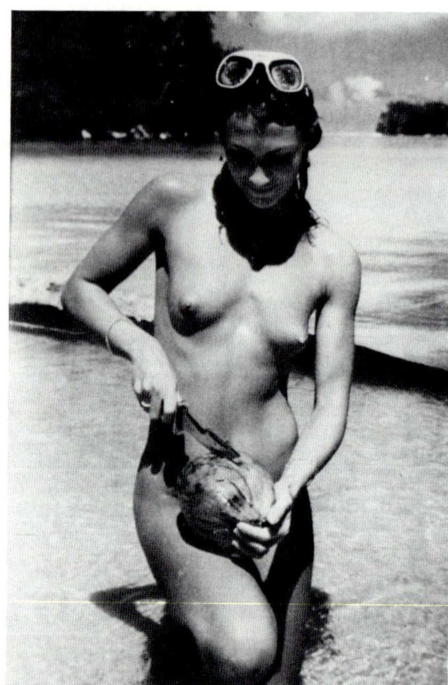

Fig. 1-46

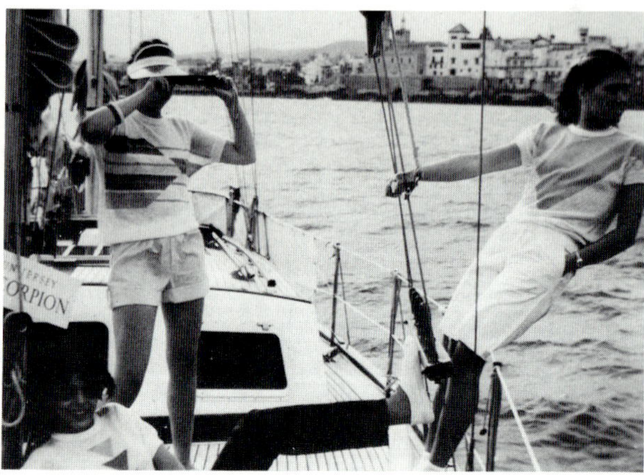

Fig. 1-47

Times and fashions change (Figs. 1-43 and 1-44). Many women now wear jeans (Fig. 1-45) rather than dresses. Some women display themselves practically or completely in the nude (Fig. 1-46) at the beach. Even when they dress in skirts or pants, these garments are frequently so short (Fig. 1-47) that, rather than covering their bodies from view, they serve to attract attention. Underwear, which was once abundant and jumbled (Fig. 1-48), is becoming scant or nonexistent (Fig. 1-49). Corsets and girdles are a thing of the past. Only the natural prevails. Under these conditions, a woman who does not have a slim, almost emaciated figure, whose thighs and buttocks accumulate fat, and whose ilio-

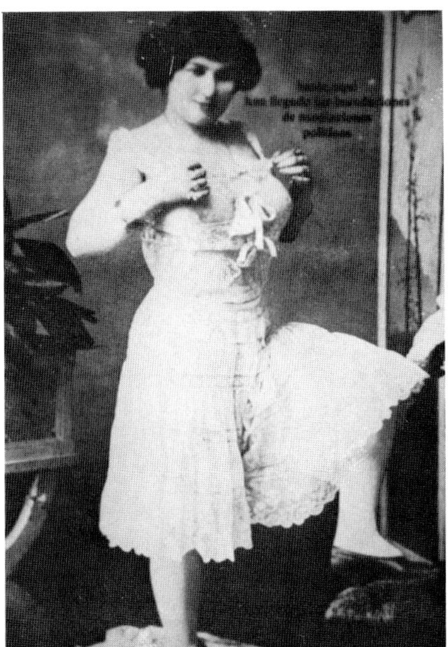

Fig. 1-48

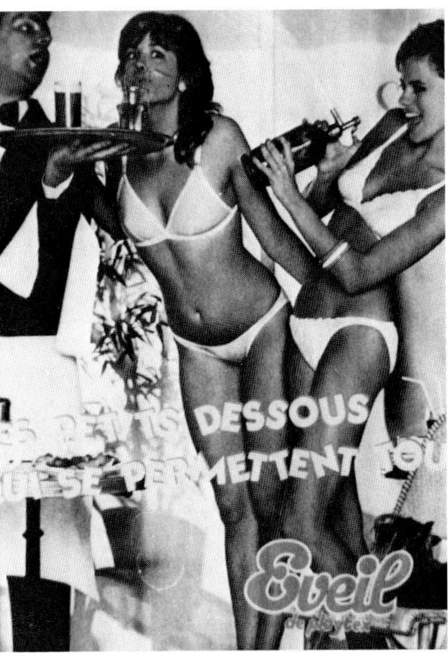

Fig. 1-49

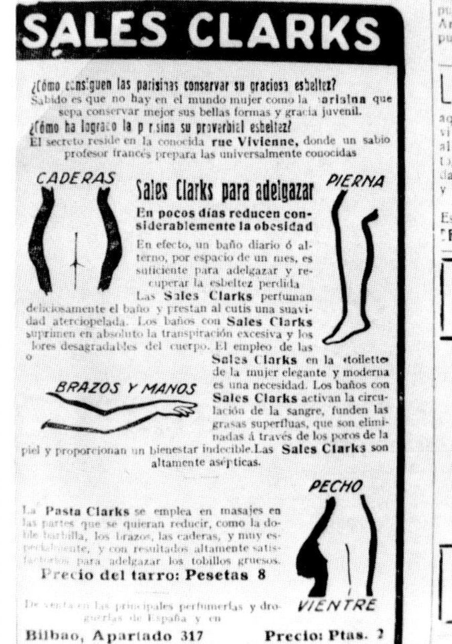

Fig. 1-50

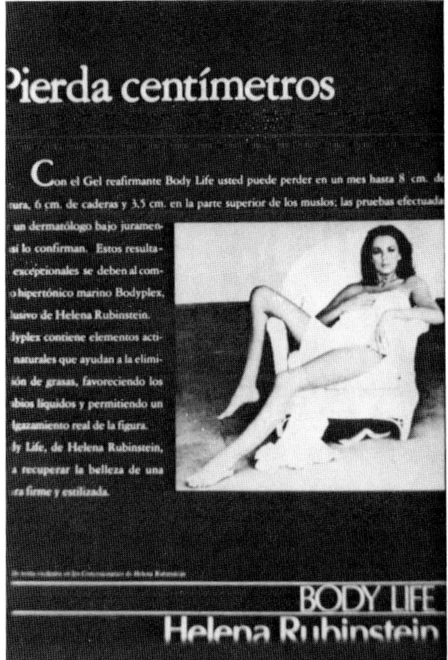

Fig. 1-51

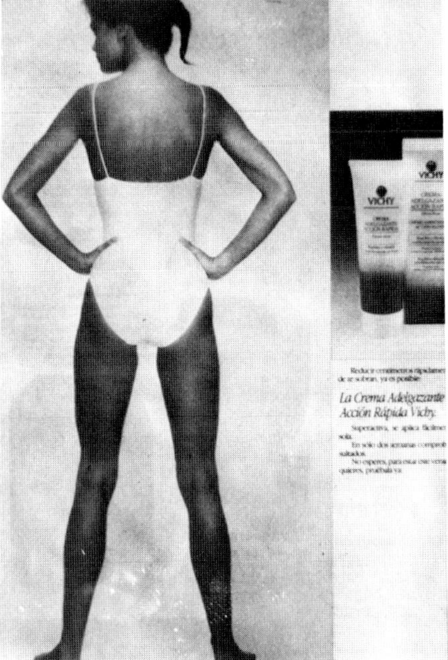

Fig. 1-52

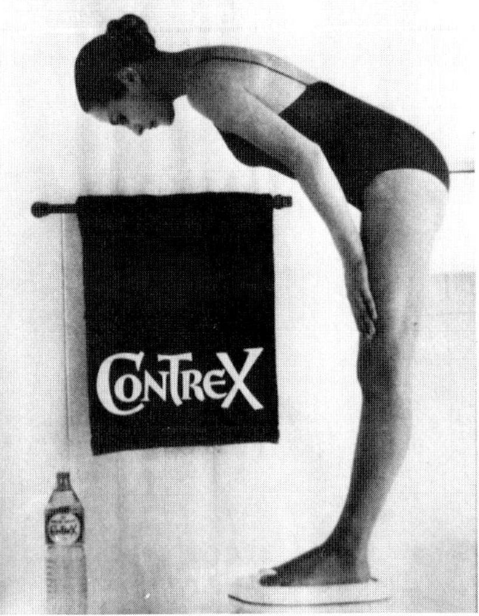

Fig. 1-53

femoro-rotulian line is broken by peritrochanteric fat feels miserable, humiliated, and self-conscious. Furthermore, she discriminates against herself by not dressing like the others, since the clothing in fashion is clearly not the type that would make her look most attractive. What such women do, of course, is attempt to make their shapes look more like those of the women of the other culture—the rhythmic culture—in which the straight line predominates over the curve, the sun is worshipped, and the world is ruled by men.

The beauty industry contributes toward making women who constitutionally accumulate fat in the lower half of the body feel unhappy and fall into their net like a fish. Promises are made to eliminate these imperfections with all sorts of products and methods (Figs. 1-50 and 1-51), none of which are really effective, of course. Also not effective for most women are reducing treatments (Figs. 1-52 and 1-53), physical exercise

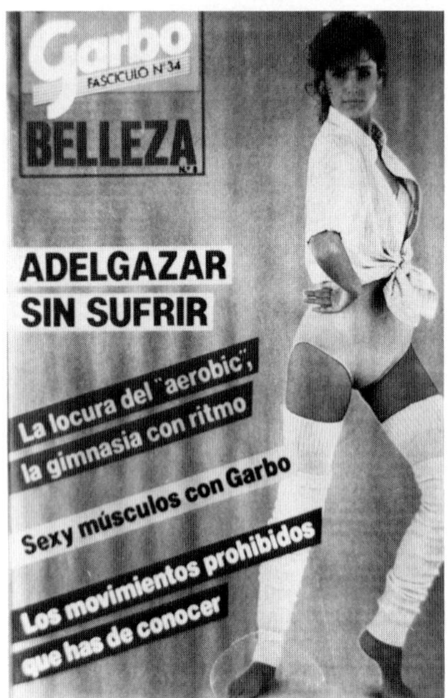

Fig. 1-54

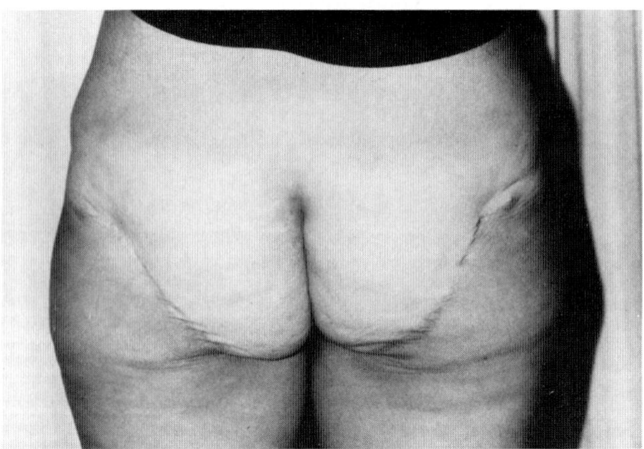

Fig. 1-55

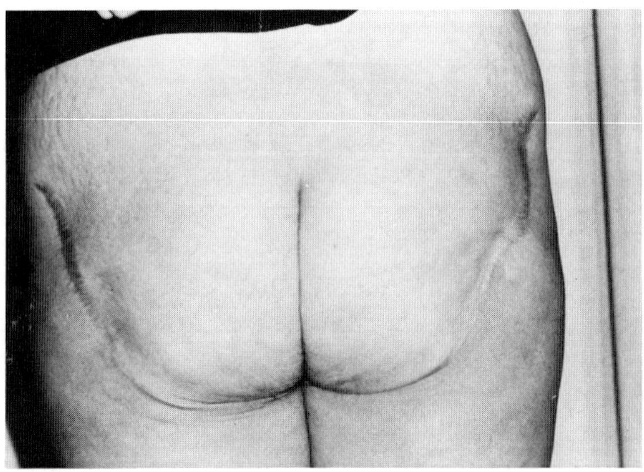

Fig. 1-56

(Fig. 1-54), massages, or physiotherapy because, for these women, selective weight loss is impossible using these methods.

In view of the failure of what might be called the conservative methods, some women have resorted to surgical procedures. They have willingly subjected themselves to operations of considerable scope that sometimes leave large scars (Figs. 1-55 and 1-56).

The Surgical Perspective

Since Pitanguy [1] first published what seems to be an original technique of Blair O. Rogers (Fig. 1-57) for the treatment of peritrochanteric lipodystrophy, the different methods directed toward the removal of this fat accumulation have multiplied. These operations have left a long list of mutilated women; in many, horrible scars were added to the unsolved original problem (Fig. 1-58).

I did no better in this respect than others. My own technique was added to those of the others, in an endeavor to solve this problem, but the solution was sought in the wrong direction (Fig. 1-59). Together with some qualified successes, always at the cost of substantial scarring, I had enough failures to relegate my own procedure to oblivion.

While the open methods of surgery were being developed, other techniques were also developed, which could be called closed or mixed. These methods were aimed at destroying the fat in situ through a small incision at a distance from the site of the problem. This was the case with Joseph Schrudde's "lipexeresis" technique [2], which was reported at the Rio de Janeiro Congress of the International Society of Aesthetic and Plastic Surgeons (ISAPS) in 1972 (although published several years previously).

Later, in Switzerland, Kesselring and Meyer [3] devised what was, to my knowledge,* the first aspirative procedure. They published a short note in the *American Journal of Plastic and Reconstructive Surgery*. In 1981 Teimourian and Fisher published a more extensive report in the same journal [4]. These reports discussed the pioneer experiences of a new treatment for the removal of fat accumulations that would leave only a small, in-

*Editor's note: See Chapter 4, where the work of Fischer (1976) is recognized as the first major effort in this respect.

conspicuous scar. Despite the successes of these procedures, however, the results often fell short of success because seromas (Fig. 1-60) were quite often produced and took months to disappear. The skin was also left in such condition that it could be compared to chesterfield upholstery.

These negative consequences explain why Kesselring's procedure did not become as popular as could have been expected. Although the guidelines and philosophy were at least partially correct, they did not work out in practice often enough. The current method of aspirative lipectomy, liposuction, lipolysis, or, better yet, aspirative lipoplasty, has origins that official plastic surgery would like to ignore.

In 1977 in France, a plastic surgeon, Dr. Yves-Gerard Illouz [5], began to use an aspiration method on lipodystrophies that differed from the technique up to that time. His method gave surprising results. It did not produce seromas and, correctly applied, it did not create skin depressions. This method soon came to the attention of other surgeons, especially Dr. Pierre Fournier, who helped to spread it quickly all over the world. It has

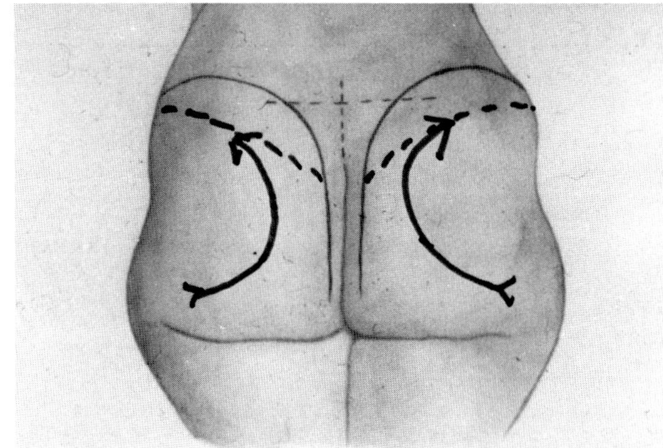

Fig. 1-59

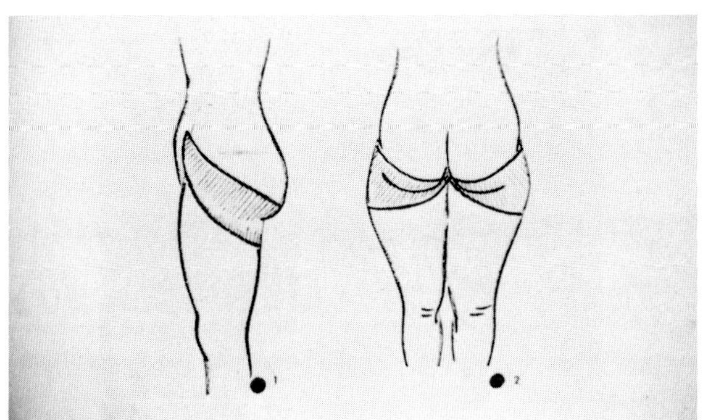

Fig. 1-57

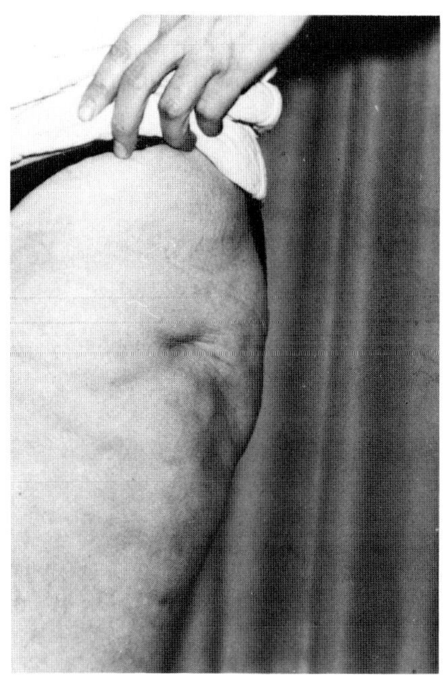

Fig. 1-60

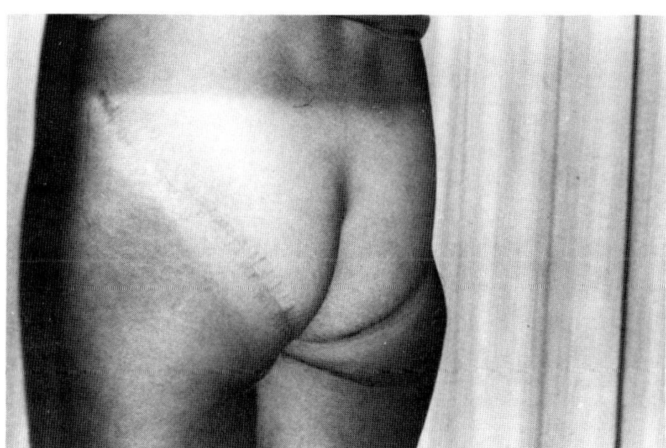

Fig. 1-58

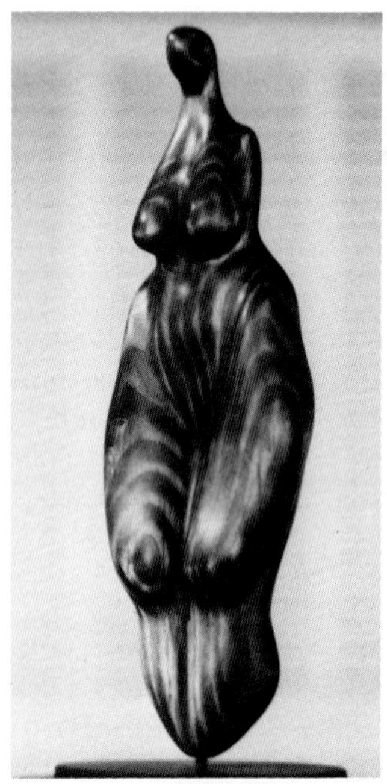

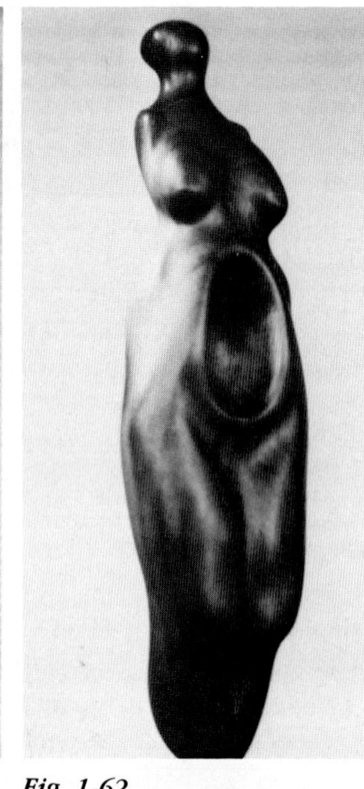

Fig. 1-61   *Fig. 1-62*

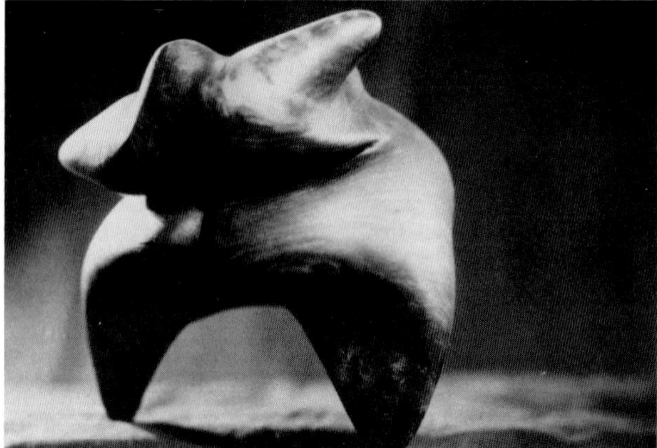

Fig. 1-63

now become the biggest boom in the field of plastic surgery, especially after its presentation to the American Society of Plastic and Reconstructive Surgery, the French Plastic Surgery Society, and, most recently, to the International Confederation for Plastic and Reconstructive Surgery meeting held in Montreal, where it made its official introduction.

Although far from considering this technique to be perfect, I can absolutely affirm that it is the best procedure that can be offered to some of our patients. The three beautiful sculptures (Figs. 1-61, 1-62, and 1-63), which I call *Venus 1, 2, and 3 of Port de's Torrent* (Ibiza, Spain), were created for me by the great Ibizan artist Antonio Hormigo as a homage to feminine beauty of a different type than the present ideal.

References

1. Pitanguy, I. Trochanteric lipodystrophy. *Plast. Reconstr. Surg.* 34:280, 1964.
2. Schrudde, J. Lipexeresis in the correction of local adiposity. First Congress of the International Society of Aesthetic and Plastic Surgeons. Rio de Janeiro, 1972. Abstract.
3. Kesselring, U. K., and Meyer, R. A suction curette for removal of excessive local deposits of subcutaneous fat. *Plast. Reconstr. Surg.* Aug., 1978.
4. Teimourian, B., and Fisher, J. D. Suction curettage to remove excess fat for body contouring. *Plast. Reconstr. Surg.* Jul., 1981.
5. Illouz, Y. G. Une nouvelle technique pour les lipodystrophies localisées. *Rev. Chir. Esth. Franc.* 6(19): Apr., 1980.

CHAPTER 2

A History and Comparison of Suction Techniques Until Their Debut in North America

Francis M. Otteni
Pierre F. Fournier

The aesthetic ideal of women in the 1980s is to have and keep a slim, athletic figure. A prime example is movie star Jane Fonda, who at 46 has the lithe body of a young woman of 20.

The influence of gender on the bodily distribution of fatty tissue was studied by Paul Richet [1]. He stressed that rounded feminine contours are fatty in nature and constitute secondary sexual characteristics. Some women, however, are obsessed by their figures and continuously fight every localized accumulation of excess fat. Most of the time the basic problem is not generalized weight excess but the presence of minimal or moderate areas of disproportionate fat, especially below the waist, on the abdomen, hips, or thighs.

To plastic surgeons, this battle against natural contours has posed an extraordinary challenge: developing new surgical procedures that remove localized fat deposits without leaving significant scars. For this reason, it is valuable to review the body-contouring techniques that have recently been tried and are in use today. As Frank McDowell, editor of *Plastic and Reconstructive Surgery* from September 1967 to January 1980, observed, "You have to learn what others have done, because you won't live long enough to make all the mistakes yourself."

Dermolipectomy

Until the 1970s, body contouring consisted mainly of traditional dermolipectomies. These open techniques combined a block lipectomy with skin resection. Closure of the wound edges took advantage of the stretchable properties of the skin. Two of the most common traditional procedures are abdominoplasty and Pitanguy's [2] operation. In addition to causing a significant morbidity, these operations result in two types of unaesthetic sequelae. The first is a long scar that often heals poorly and is difficult to hide. The second is subsequent recurrence of excessive fat on both sides of the scar. This bulging results from hypertrophy of the adipose tissue that was left untouched. Therefore, in many cases, dermolipectomies replace one deformity with another, besides producing a prominent scar. Because of the scarring, some areas of the body, such as the thighs, knees, or ankles, could not be treated by dermolipectomy and were regarded as taboo zones. For these reasons, a new operative approach—a "collapsing" or subcutaneous surgery—was investigated during the last decade.

Table 2-1. Chronology of closed techniques

Authors	First publication	Number of cases	First operation
Schrudde [3]	1972	?	1964
Fischer, A. and G. M. [4]	1977	245	1976
Kesselring and Meyer [5]	1978	?	?
Illouz [7]	1980	300	1977
Teimourian and Fisher [6]	1981	54	1977
Fournier and Otteni [8]	1981		
	Wet technique 1982	510	1979
	Dry technique	190	1981

"Collapsing" or Subcutaneous Surgery

Collapsing surgery uses only closed, or blind, lipectomy techniques that leave minimal scars of 1 cm or less. In contrast to open techniques, closed techniques use the shrinking properties of the skin to obtain good contouring of the operated area.

The dates of the first publications about closed techniques are summarized in Table 2-1. Sharp techniques were applied by Schrudde [3], the Fischers [4], Kesselring and Meyer [5], and Teimourian and Fisher [6]. The cannula, or blunt, technique was developed by Illouz [7] working independently.

CURETTE TECHNIQUES

Uterine Curette
The uterine curette, a sharp technique of subcutaneous surgery, was employed by many cosmetic surgeons, including Schrudde [3] in Cologne, Germany. Schrudde used the curette to remove fat from three areas: the outer lateral thighs, the inner side of the knees, and the calves and ankles. Through a small incision (2–3 cm), he undermined the subcutaneous tissue with long scissors and then removed adipose tissue with the curette. The approach resulted in many severe postoperative complications, such as persisting lymphorrhea, hematoma, skin necrosis, and localized skin excess. Because of its unreliability when used by other surgeons and its significant morbidity, the curette technique has not gained many adherents.

One cautionary anecdote is worth remembering. The first malpractice suit for aesthetic surgery in France was brought against Dujarrier in 1929 by a dancer who had to undergo a leg amputation, after injury to a major vessel following curette reduction of her calf.

Suction Curettage
The developers of the first suction curette technique appear to be Arpard and George Fischer [4] in Rome. They were the first to combine fat curettage and suction. Their techniques can be applied only to saddle bags.

The equipment used is a portable cellusuctiotome unit. A pocket is created after undermining the skin with a planotom. A very important point is to leave beneath the skin a 1-cm thick fat layer and also some fat over the aponeurosis in order to prevent adhesions. Fat is first crushed and then sucked out. The result is checked in two ways: manually by pinching the skin and visually in the vacuum jar. The dissection is extended 2 cm beyond the markings to prevent a step deformation. Suction drainage is continued for 15 days or more. The bandage consists of a first layer of paper strips and a second layer of elastic tape. The patient is advised to stay in bed for 5 to 6 days, alternately lying on the operated zones for periods of 15 to 20 minutes to facilitate readherence.

The suction curette technique resulted in numerous complications. In 10% of cases, the patient required further surgery. Continuous oozing in the cavity often produced a seroma with fibrous encapsulation and epithelialization, such as occurs after insertion of a mammary prosthesis. Other complications included hematomas and skin undulation. Because suction curettage proved to have so many complications, it was subsequently abandoned by the Fischers in favor of Illouz's technique.

Kesselring's original technique [5] differs somewhat from the Fischers' technique. Kesselring first undermined a large area with a scissors. Then, with a special sharp curette attached to a partial vacuum, he cut the adipose tissue so it could be easily sucked out. This technique was applied only to small trochanteric adiposities of young patients with good skin tone.

Teimourian's original technique [6], which is similar to Kesselring's, used only sharp instruments, such as a scissors, a modified fascia lata stripper, Kesselring's curette, and a uterine curette. More audacious than Kesselring, Teimourian applied the technique not only to trochanteric lipohypertrophies but also to the buttocks, knees, and ankles, as well as the arms or even the flanks. In addition, he sometimes used it in association with resection of excess skin or a dermolipectomy. It is important to note the high rate of seromas (30%) [6], which underlines the trauma of the dissection technique as originally performed.

All of the curette techniques essentially produce a cavity with the destruction of most of the septi between skin and fascia containing blood and lymphatic vessels. There is a consequent occurrence of much bleeding and lymphorrhea. Formation of a persistent seroma prevents scar contraction and facilitates development of secondary skin ptosis.

To summarize, suction curettage techniques have given good results in a few skilled surgeon's hands, but they do not do so consistently for most surgeons. The rate of complications is very high as is the necessity for secondary surgery. Therefore, few surgeons have used these techniques for very long.

CANNULA TECHNIQUES

Blunt cannula techniques differ from the preceding techniques in using very blunt instruments that spare most of the arcades of connective tissue and neurovascular elements. Multiple punch biopsies are performed that create tunnels, producing a selective partial lipectomy in a pattern resembling a sponge, a honeycomb, or a spider web. The originator of the cannula technique was Dr. Yves-Gerard Illouz [7,8,9]. The technique may be subdivided into three variants: the original wet technique of Illouz, the dry technique of Fournier, and the new wet technique of Hetter (see Chap. 17).

The Original Illouz Technique

The original Illouz technique uses the cannula to suck out normal or pathological adipose tissue after a mildly hypotonic saline solution containing hyaluronidase (Wydase) is injected throughout the area. According to his original idea, the hypotonic solution would help to emulsify the fat cells, making it easier to suck them out.

The Illouz technique has several major advantages. It can be applied to any part of the body where there is an excessive subcutaneous fatty tissue—normal or pathological. There are no taboo zones. Several areas can be treated simultaneously, for example, saddle bags and knees. The maximum amount of fat extracted may be as much as 3 kg in a patient with a huge deformity or with several deformities.

As is evident, the indications for the procedure are numerous. It not only solves many aesthetic problems but also corrects pathological conditions, such as single or multiple lipomas, fatty gynecomastia, adiposis dolorosa, and Launois-Bensaude syndrome. Moreover, the procedure may often be an adjunct to major dermolipectomies such as abdominoplasty, thigh plasty, or reduction mammoplasty, but also smaller problems such as face lifts, scar revisions, and flap defatting.

The Dry Technique

We used Dr. Illouz's original wet technique for approximately 2½ years. We then tried the procedure without fluid. An incident in the operating room occurred during anesthesia induction, and we wished to avoid the risk of any possible reaction to the hyaluronidase solution. We did the procedure without the usual solution and were amazed to observe that it seemed equally as easy. Since the results appeared the same, we decided to forego the solution and drew the conclusion that lipolysis was purely mechanical rather than chemical.

We believe trochanteric accumulations are the most difficult adiposity to treat accurately. In the wet technique, all elements combine to complicate the surgeon's task. The patient is in a prone position, which facilitates spreading of the deformity. Injection of the hypotonic solution adds to this distortion. The advantage of the dry technique seems obvious to us. There is no tissue distortion and thus a more accurate estimation of the fat to be suctioned can be made as the procedure is performed. Moreover, it saves some time and avoids any possible reaction to hyaluronidase, even if rare.

The disadvantages of the dry technique include the fact that suction is sometimes physically more difficult. There also may be more apparent bleeding (see Chap. 17), and thus blood pressure drop, if fluid replacement is not vigorous.

Whichever variant is used, wet or dry, we have been impressed by the excellence and consistency of the results achieved as well as the startling rarity of surgical complications. In fact, infections, seromas, and hematomas are rare even in cases of very large removals (up to 3000 g). Unaesthetic sequelae occur mostly in treated trochanteric accumulations. The major complication has been removal of too much fat, leaving a permanent depression in the tissue.

Remember that the most important element is not what you remove but what you leave behind and where you leave it. (Fournier's rule).

COMPARISON OF CLOSED TECHNIQUES

For clarification, it is interesting to compare the advantages and disadvantages of the different body contouring techniques.

First of all, it seems obvious that the advantages of the blunt cannula technique, compared with dermolipectomies, are considerable. We employ the cannula whenever possible. The only exceptions are cases of major deformities with skin laxity. In such situations, the surgeon either does a series of repetitive aspirations, which can be likened to repetitive excisions, or the surgeon first does suction lipectomy and later performs a skin resection, if necessary. Often a combined suction lipectomy with dermolipectomy can be performed in one stage.

Among the closed methods, our favorite is the cannula technique and, in particular, the dry variant. In Tables 2-2 through 2-5, we summarize the advantages of the cannula technique as we have seen them develop during the past 6 years.

Major reasons why the cannula technique is more useful are listed in Table 2-2. It is clear that if suction lipectomy has gained a worldwide following, the credit has to be given to its originator, Dr. Illouz. Within a few

Table 2-2. Major differences between closed techniques

	Curette technique	Cannula technique
Number of patients treated	Several hundred	Several thousand (many with multiple procedures)
Operative sites	Some taboo zones Principally, trochanteric lipodystrophy; seldom knees, ankles Only one site at a time	No taboo zones Everywhere in the body, head, or neck Multiple sites at the same time
Maximum weight of fat removed	A few hundred grams	Up to 2 or 3 kg

Table 2-3. Indications for closed techniques

	Curette technique	Cannula technique
Aesthetic indications; small and moderate lipodystrophies	Best indications	Best indications
Large lipodystrophies	Never	Possible
Combination with other procedures	Infrequent	Often
Combination with open techniques	Infrequent	Often
Pathological indications	Not published	Single or multiple lipoma, adiposis dolorosis, Launois-Bensaude syndrome, obesity with or without arthrosis

Table 2-4. Procedural differences between closed techniques

	Curette technique	Cannula technique
Instruments	Curette (sharp)	Cannula (blunt)
Operative process	Undermining Block lipectomy No peripheral undermining	No undermining Sponge lipectomy Peripheral mesh undermining
Drainage	$+++$	$+$

Table 2-5. Anatomical-pathological consequences of closed techniques

	Curette technique	Cannula technique
Fat resection method	Cavity	Honeycomb (tunnels)
Preservation of septi	None or few	Numerous
Nerve and vessel injury	Severe	Mild
Hemorrhage and/or lymphorrhea	Considerable	Negligible
Epithelialization	Highly possible	Highly improbable
Contraction of skin	Problematic	Considerable
Sagging of the skin	Likely	Unlikely except after age 35

years, his technique has spread to most countries where modern medicine is practiced. Surgeons in many countries obtain consistent results with his technique and equipment. Of course, caution is necessary because we do not as yet have the long-term follow-up of these procedures.

Indications for the closed techniques are compared in Table 2-3. We believe that cannula techniques are useful not only for aesthetic surgery but also for treating certain lipomatoses or gynecomastias. Although cannula techniques have not been considered a treatment for obesity, we do not know what the future holds in this regard. We have noticed spectacular weight losses in some cases following suction lipectomy. By changing an ugly figure into a more acceptable one, perhaps the procedure may favorably influence behavior.

Table 2-4 summarizes procedural differences. Both types of closed techniques may seem very easy to perform, but this is deceptive. They demand considerable training, judgment, and experience, since they deal with "sculpture in vivo" and the final result remains 6 months in the future. Suction lipectomy can be likened to the insertion of mammary prostheses: the operation looks easy, but troubles appear later.

The anatomical-pathological consequences of both techniques are compared in Table 2-5. Here, the blunt cannula technique has the clearest superiority, which has won it so many adherents: the postoperative course of the patient is much more problem-free.

Since the spread of the Illouz technique after his presentation at the annual meeting of the American Society of Plastic and Reconstructive Surgeons (ASPRS) in Hawaii in October 1982, the other techniques are now being presented in modified forms. Tunneling is now promoted instead of plane dissection; this acceptance by emulation confirms the superiority of the tunneling concept. This concept, with the sparing of the arcades and septi, has allowed suction lipectomy to become a resource in every plastic surgeon's armentarium for the 1980s.

References

1. Richet, P. Quoted in D. Duville, *L'Anatomie Artistique.* Editions H. Laurens. 1953. P. 15.
2. Pitanguy, I. Trochanteric lipodystrophy. *Plast. Reconstr. Surg.* 34:280, 1964.
3. Schrudde, J. Lipexeresis in the correction of local adiposity. First Congress of the International Society of Aesthetic and Plastic Surgeons, Rio de Janeiro, 1972. Abstract.
4. Fischer, A., and Fischer, G. M. Revised technique for cellulitis fat. Reduction in riding breeches deformity. *Bull. Int. Acad. Cosm. Surg.* Dec., 1977.
5. Kesselring, U. K., and Meyer, R. A suction curette for removal of excessive local deposits of subcutaneous fat. *Plast. Reconstr. Surg.* Aug., 1978.
6. Teimourian, B., and Fisher, J. D. Suction curettage to remove excess fat for body contouring. *Plast. Reconstr. Surg.* Jul., 1981.
7. Illouz, Y. G. Une nouvelle technique pour les lipodystrophies localisées. *Rev. Chir. Esth. Franc.* 6(19): Apr., 1980.
8. Illouz, Y. G. Reflexions après 4 ans et demi d'experience et 800 cas de ma technique de lipolyse. *Rev. Chir. Esth. Franc.* 6(24): Oct., 1981.
9. Illouz, Y. G. Body contouring by lipolysis: A 5-year experience with over 3000 cases. *Plast. Reconstr. Surg.* 72:591, 1983.

CHAPTER 3

The Origins of Lipolysis

Yves-Gerard Illouz

After finishing 7 years of residency in several Paris hospitals, I began private practice as a plastic surgeon in 1958. I was always interested in the problem of fat deposits. When Ivo Pitanguy [1] described his technique for removing riding breeches deformities, I attempted it several times.

The results, however, quickly disappointed me. The operation usually left a long, depressed scar, which sometimes was thick and red. Very often, the procedure produced a violin deformity (see Chap. 9), or the fat deposits recurred, forming new riding breeches.

Although I stopped using Pitanguy's technique, I kept thinking about the challenge of finding a technique that would remove fat and only fat, leave a minimal scar, and obviate recurrences. I had already been impressed by Björntorp's [2] theory that the body has a fixed number of adipose cells, which cannot multiply. This meant that when an adipose cell was removed from the body, it was gone forever.

I was sure the theory was correct because I had observed that excision of fat tissue was permanent. That is why careless removal of superficial fat results in a depressed scar. Also, it is the reason why, after an abdominoplasty, there is no recurrence in the lower part of the abdomen. We defat that part. We do not defat the upper part of the abdomen because it is dangerous; however, the upper part is where the defect recurs.

Another bit of evidence is that to get a good depression of the navel in abdominoplasty, it is necessary to defat the area around the navel. Finally, experience with trauma and burn patients proves that destruction of fat tissue is permanent.

Years later, at the International Meeting of Plastic and Aesthetic Surgeons in Mexico in April 1977, I heard a description of the new Italian technique for removing riding breeches developed by the Fischers [3] in Rome. It consisted of a 3-cm incision directly into the fat deposit, totally undermining the area, crushing all the adipose tissue, and suctioning out this "mud." The speaker said that the technique could result in terrible complications: hematomas, infections, frequent and persistent seromas that sometimes drained for months, skin slippage, and even skin slough.

Improvements to the Fischers' Technique

I found the Fischers' technique interesting, although conceptually wrong. It seemed to me that all of the complications came from the complete undermining done with a sharp instrument, which destroyed blood vessels and lymphatics. To avoid the undermining, I thought of creating tunnels with a blunt instrument that would preserve some septa and pass between major vessels, leaving them intact. But before trying the idea, I still had another problem to solve—the question of excess skin. Studying the way in which the subcutaneous tissues heal provided the answer. Fibroblasts quickly enter surgically created tunnels, producing fibrous tissue, and then healing results in retraction of both the subcutaneous tissue and skin.

Thus, my second idea was to take advantage of this healing retraction. Since creating well-placed, deep tunnels should lead to smooth retraction of the skin, the problem of excess skin might be solved, at least for moderate deformities. But the idea seemed revolutionary, even to me. I had been performing plastic surgery for a long time; whenever I had wanted to change a contour, it had always been necessary to undermine the tissue, resect skin, and make a big scar. Now I proposed to do the exact opposite with no undermining.

I spent considerable time thinking about how to proceed in perfecting the new concept. To be more secure, I decided to use hydrotomy. I had often used dissecting hydrotomy since learning it from Converse in New York in 1962, and I thought it would perfect the new concept. The hydrotomy helped give me the courage to start trying the new approach.

IMPLEMENTING MY TECHNIQUE

Since I obviously had to be cautious, I chose as my first case a young, pretty woman who had a big lipoma on her back and did not want a long scar. It was not a risky situation because, if my new technique did not succeed, I could immediately switch to the classical excision technique.

In this first operation, I used a 6-mm Karmen cannula with a standard vacuum motor. I decided not to use hydrotomy. When I saw the fat coming out, I was elated, but it was very hard and came out slowly. There was also some bleeding. In spite of these difficulties, the procedure worked. The lipoma was removed, the result after 3 weeks was good, and there was no excess skin.

Before doing a second lipoma, I tried to solve the technical problems encountered with the first patient. To minimize bleeding, I ordered a special cannula with a rounder tip and an absolutely blunt hole. I also thought that trauma could be reduced by suctioning the fat more quickly with fewer movements and with a cannula having a smaller diameter. I ordered the most powerful suction motor available; it turned out to be an industrial one.

I did the second case, a big polylobed lipoma of the arm, with preceding hydrotomy injections of normal saline. I was pleased to see that the fat came out more quickly and easily, almost without blood. I attributed this to the blunter cannula, stronger motor, and hydrotomy. The injected saline seemed to constrict vessels, expand the adipose cells, and make it easier to push the cannula.

I did a series of other lipomas, step by step working to perfect the technique. I thought a slightly hypotonic solution might rupture some adipose cell membranes and make it easier to advance the cannula. I tried many different concentrations, and the best seemed to be a slightly hypotonic solution (8 saline : 2 water) with some added hyaluronidase to aid diffusion.

Though the injection concept was reasonable, it did not work as well as I had hoped. Multiple biopsies showed that membranes of only a few fat cells were broken. Most of the cells were dilated but not ruptured because they pressed tightly against each other. Nevertheless, I felt hydrotomy made it easier to work, so I continued to use it.

The most remarkable observation from the early cases was the absence of complications: no hematomas, no seromas, no infections. As a rule, 3 weeks after surgery, bruising and swelling had disappeared. The skin retracted as if there had been no lipoma. The two premises were confirmed: (1) that tunnels could be used to remove fat without undermining, and (2) that skin retraction makes excision unnecessary.

TREATMENT FOR RIDING BREECHES
DEFORMITIES

After these successes, I did my first riding breeches case. Because I still wanted to be very cautious, it was a case in which the deformity recurred after I had performed a Pitanguy procedure 3 years earlier. The patient wanted the fat deposits reduced again and the scars revised. I used suction on the fat deposits. When I was revising the scar and had opened it along its length, I saw a spider web of vessels that were not bleeding. I tried cutting one septum and bleeding began immediately (Fig. 3-1).

This experience showed that my theory of using tunnels to preserve vessels was correct. If the big vessels are not damaged, major complications such as hematomas, seromas, and infection can be avoided. Results of the first case were very good. It had been a moderate deformity, and the skin retraction was good.

I realized that to avoid complications, the superficial fat must be respected and should *not* be removed. For one reason, it contains the major lymphatic vessels. Also, the adipose tissue between the skin and the fascia superficialis is normal fat* that is necessary for skin elasticity and for harmonious weight loss or gain. Therefore, the only fat I wished to remove was the fat between the

*Editor's note: We have as yet no evidence to substantiate this idea, although Dr. Arner is working on possible differences between the fat above and below the superficial fascia.

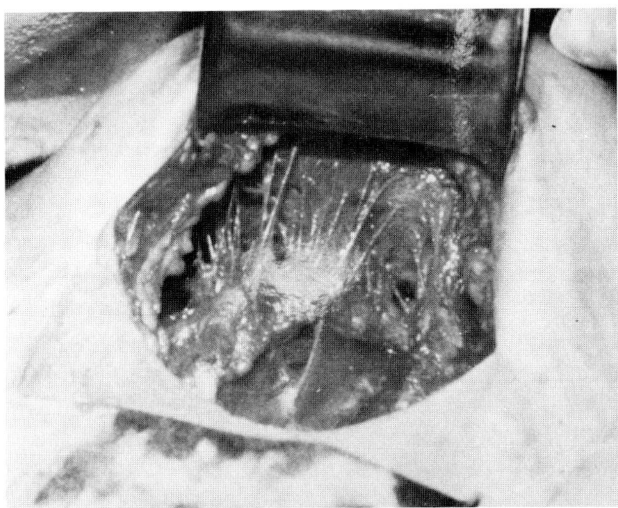

Fig. 3-1. An example of the spider web of vessels, nerves, and septa is seen in this figure in an abdominal case.

fascia superficialis and the aponeurosis of the deep muscles, but that is easier to say than to do.

Having discerned these principles, I proceeded to do only riding breeches. At first I did about 20 cases using supratrochanteric incisions. The most common complications I had (in 20 percent of the cases) were depressions, indentations, and lateral waves, which occur because of the skin lines even if you work sagittally. Yet there were no hematomas, seromas, or infections—just some ecchymosis and swelling that disappeared within a few weeks. As part of my caution in those days, I used suction drains for the first 2 postoperative days and gave patients antibiotics for 5 days.

After thinking about the cosmetic complications, I realized that almost all of them appeared when I worked too superficially. The waviness occurred when I came too close to the surface in some areas and when my tunneling was not in a regular pattern and caused irregular contraction. Depressions occurred when I did just single superficial tunnels. Indentations came about when the hole near the end of the cannula sucked out a glob of superficial fat. Some of the waviness, however, also resulted from operating on unsuitable candidates. A few patients were too old and had loose skin. The deformities of others were too big; after major removals, their skin did not retract well.

TECHNICAL MODIFICATIONS

I decided to make technical modifications to minimize these mishaps. First, I redesigned the cannula. The new design had a curved end, with the hole in the middle of the curve 2 cm from the tip. A guide mark was added to the cannula so the position of the hole could always be known. *The hole must be kept pointing down to remove only deep fat.* The cannula's curved end also helped to protect superficial fat, preventing indentations.

To ensure that the cannula was deep enough, I decided to pinch the fat deposit very hard with my left hand so I could feel exactly how deep the cannula was. I also started putting the patient in the prone position, which was more convenient and helped make my work more even. In addition, I worked with the pump factory to obtain a more effective motor. After many trials, we decided the best was a powerful motor that pulls close to 1 atmosphere (atm) at 100 L of air per minute. I learned later in the United States that this vacuum produces a special phenomenon—vaporization—which eases fat suction. I had observed this phenomenon in action at the time of my procedures. The tubing used is important, too. The best diameter is 1 cm. The tubing must be strong enough not to collapse under high vacuum and transparent enough to show exactly what is coming out.

From depressions that occurred as complications, I got the idea of deliberately making them to create folds. Many patients have buttocks with no folds; others have straight folds, which make a square bottom, or folds turning down, which make a "sad" bottom. I thought of creating folds that turn up, which make a "smiling" happy bottom. To do this symmetrically was another reason to put patients in a prone position.

To avoid producing waviness, I decided to refuse patients who had loose skin or were more than 35 years old. I now feel that this age limit is too low for skilled practitioners. We can do older patients. The important criterion is the skin tone, not the chronological age.

At this time, I also decided to remove very large deformities in two or three stages instead of one. I had noticed that when I removed more than 3 kg of fat tissue, patients sometimes went into shock and required blood transfusions. Thus, I limited my removals to no more than 3 kg of fat tissue in one operation. Now, with even greater experience, I am even more conservative. *I think removing 2 kg of fat at a time is enough,* and almost all localized deformities can be treated by removing that amount.

After making the above changes, I worked on riding breeches and buttock folds. The results were more and more gratifying. Then, a patient who was happy with the results of her riding breeches and fold surgery asked me to reduce her buttocks. This request frightened me because I was not sure I could make a good curve. I designed a new cannula, however, that had the ideal curve of a buttock, and I called it the Concorde after the French passenger plane.

So I attempted to reduce buttocks; after performing

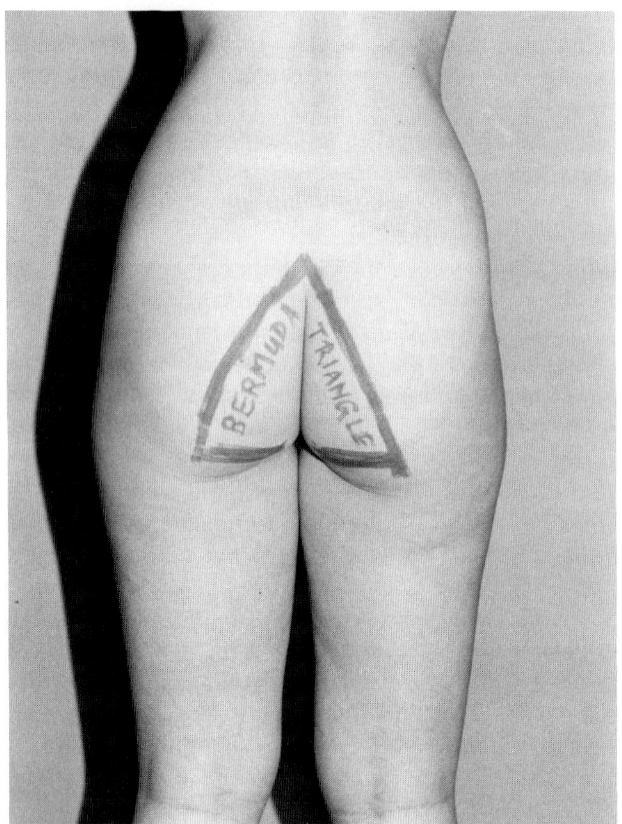

Fig. 3-2. The "Bermuda Triangle" marked on this model represents the internal triangle of fat that must be retained on the female buttocks.

several operations, I concluded that the buttock is a very forgiving area and that the only poor result is making buttocks too flat. After thoroughly studying the superficial anatomy of women and men, I found that, to remain round, female buttocks must retain an internal triangle of fat. This area, which I call the "Bermuda Triangle," must be respected (Fig. 3-2).

My technique became increasingly refined. I put patients in the prone position. Incisions were made in the infragluteal fold, just at the edge of the natural crease. Through these incisions, I could work on the riding breeches, buttocks, and fold. I had a good curved cannula for riding breeches, and I used my original one with a sharp profile to create folds. I had the Concorde cannula for buttocks, a good motor and tubing, and I felt I really had found a way to evenly remove deep fat.

In June 1978, after I had done 90 cases in the preceding year, I made my first report to the French Society of Aesthetic Surgery. The report was quite modest because I had only some recent results illustrated with bad Polaroid pictures. I said in my lecture that I needed another year to make sure the technique was safe and to

obtain more results, longer follow-up, and better photographs.

TREATMENT FOR OTHER AREAS OF THE BODY

From June 1978 to June 1979, I operated on just over 100 patients. Because I was confident that the approach would not cause major surgical complications, I decided to start treating other areas of the body. The first case involved only the knees. I performed the surgery under local anesthesia with xylocaine and epinephrine. I noted that there was no bleeding. The suction bottle contained pure fat.

After doing many other knee operations, I drew a number of conclusions. First, the knee can be defined as a concavity at the lower inner part of the thigh, along with a convexity of the condyle and another concavity of the upper part of the lower leg. Therefore, in treating a knee, we must work on the areas adjacent to the thigh and lower leg.

It is very easy to do knees with local anesthesia. The best incision site is the inner edge of the popliteal fold. The knee is a very forgiving area. We can work more superficially, as close to the surface as 1 cm, without problems. Older patients can have the surgery because the knee skin retracts very well. The best cannula to use is a straight one with a 6-mm diameter.

Postoperatively, the knees are a little more painful and swelling takes longer to disappear (2 to 3 months) than at other sites. Bruising is prominent. When the knee swelling subsides, patients tend to have ankle edema for a while.

The second problem I tackled in 1979 was the abdomen. The first case I tried was done in association with an abdominoplasty. The patient was a woman on whom I had done riding breeches and hips the year before with very satisfying results. She had a pendulous abdomen with an infraumbilical scar. Thus, my lipectomy technique was done through the navel scar like a culdoscopy. I made tunnels like the spokes on a wheel. Then I did a classical abdominoplasty with transposition of the navel. When I opened the lipectomy area, I found a spider web of intact vessels. The upper flap and lateral areas were defatted, and the abdominoplasty was much easier to do and gave a better result.

There are several reasons that the lipectomy plus abdominoplasty approach works better than abdominoplasty alone. First, the upper flap is defatted so that the fatty deposit cannot recur since the adipose cells have been removed. Only with great difficulty and with some dangers to the vasculatures can the upper flap be defatted in a classical abdominoplasty. Second, the upper flap has the same thickness as the lower one, so there is no disproportion and a better scar. Third, the scar can be shortened. By suctioning the lateral areas, "dog ears" are eliminated. Fourth, because the upper flap is defatted and the vessels are elastic, the upper flap does not have to be undermined as far as in a classical abdominoplasty. Less undermining minimizes bleeding since the most important lymphatics are in the supraumbilical part of the abdomen. Fifth, abdominoplasty can be associated with suction at the waist, giving better definition of the abdomen. Sixth, for the best definition of the abdomen, there should be a slight concavity above the navel and a slight convexity below it. That is why, when I previously did abdominoplasties, I defatted the medial area above the navel with a scissors for the new navel site. But this method led to bleeding and was dangerous. It is safer to defat this area with suction.

The first operation produced a good result with a minimal scar (like a Pfannenstiel). As a result of this experience, I began to do the abdomen with suction alone. At first, I selected only pot bellies on young patients. I soon observed that the abdomen is not a forgiving area, especially the supraumbilical area; therefore, the tunnels must be deep (2 cm) and regular. There is much more bleeding than in other parts of the body. Swelling is great, and significant bruising develops in the pubic area. Initially, waviness is very often present. It disappears slowly only after 6 months to 1 year.

The third area I tried at this time was the waist or hips. At first I used a direct approach that left two little scars on the sides of the spine, but patients said they did not like even these small scars to show when they wore bikinis at the beach. Next, I tried leaving only one medial scar; however, fibrous tissue in the medial area was hard to work through and there was considerable bleeding. I therefore invented a long cannula with an inverted curve that can go from the infragluteal fold directly to the hips. The special profile of this cannula transforms the convexity of the fat deposits on the hips to the concavity of the normal waist. With experience, I found that the hips are a very forgiving area. The results are seen as soon as you remove the bandages, and it is possible to do the hips of older patients with no risk of waviness or dimpling.

By this time, I had the necessary techniques to treat the most common deformity seen by plastic surgeons in Europe—what I call the "violin deformity." The violin deformity consists of convexity of the hips, with a depression below, and then riding breeches with an infragluteal fold that comes down, making a square or "sad" bottom. To correct this deformity, we must correct the hips, riding breeches, and fold to make a harmonious curve with a fold that goes up.

The fourth area I applied my technique to in this period was the ankle. After I had done a few cases, I realized that it was very difficult to create a good, symmetrical contour. Edema persists for a long time, sometimes even a year, and pain is intense. Because of the ankle's position on the lower part of the body, trophicity is not good. The fat is very hard and associated with a lot of collagen tissue. These characteristics increase the risk of waviness. Also, the ankle is the only part of the body where I have seen permanent postoperative deposition of residual pigment. The pigmentation comes from hemosiderin left by the bruises, which take a long time to disappear. Thus, the ankles are not a forgiving area, and fat removal must be close to the muscle fascia and regular.

After working on these four areas, I had the confidence to try my technique on submental fat. First, I operated on a young girl with a fat neck. I designed a short cannula for the purpose. It had an ideal curve for the submental area and a diameter of 5 mm. I used a 5-mm lateral incision. Since the results were good, I even used the lateral approach to remove submental fat during face lifts on older patients. This method made it easier to obtain very good results as compared with a classical submental approach.

ADDITIONAL IMPROVEMENTS TO MY TECHNIQUE

While trying these procedures, I also was thinking about doing big deformities in stages and experimenting to find the best postoperative bandaging method. I decided that a two- or three-stage approach for very large deformities would avoid shock, which tends to develop after excessive fat removal. This approach would permit progressive retraction of the skin. Testing the idea, I found that the best interval between the two stages was 6 months to minimize trouble with scar tissue.

As for bandaging, I tried a variety of dressing materials and experimented with keeping them on for different lengths of time. I found that using a very strong elastic bandage gave the best results. The best material was a French type of Elastoplast, applied to create a lift dressing and never circular. The ideal duration of bandaging proved to be 1 week. I tried 10 days and 2 weeks, but they obviously were too long. One week is the normal period for healing with properly applied dressings. Bandages left on too long can induce ridges and permanent adhesions.

Moreover, because patients often complained about postoperative bruising and swelling, I tried sending them to a physiotherapist. I was surprised at how much this therapy improved and hastened healing. With the physiotherapist, I tried a variety of postoperative treatments and found the best treatment involved alternating compression, ultrasound, drainage, massage, and low-frequency therapies.

Presentation of the Technique

After all this experience, in 1979 I made a 12-minute, 16-mm movie that I presented with a report to the French Society of Aesthetic Surgery. This paper, "A New Technique for Localized Lipodystrophies," was published in April 1980 [4]. The publication interested only a few people, so in 1980 I made other reports using the same material.

In May 1980, I described my technique in Osaka, Japan, at a meeting held at the Shirakabe Clinic. Drs. Shirakabe and Blair Rogers of New York were very interested. Dr. Rogers asked at the time for a reprint in English to publish in the United States. Then I lectured in Tokyo to the Japanese Society of Aesthetic Surgery; the audience was very interested and asked many questions. My report was published in the *Journal of the Japanese Society of Aesthetic Surgery* 19(2), 1980.

In June 1980, I was invited by Professor Vilain to attend a symposium on obesity. I gave him my first reprint and asked him for his opinion. In October, I was invited to Genoa, Italy, for the International Congress on Surgical Treatment of Obesity. The surgeons showed great interest and asked many questions. Almost all of them, however, were general surgeons doing ileal bypasses for obesity. They were not very concerned about correcting lipodystrophies.

In November 1980, I went to Brazil and gave a speech and surgical demonstration at the Hospital dos los Servitadores de Estados in Rio de Janeiro. Then in Fortaleza, I presented a report at the National Congress of the Brazilian Plastic Surgery Society. Here my technique caused a veritable sensation. I spoke for a long time with Dr. Ivo Pitanguy, who seemed quite interested but skeptical about the technique.

That same year I also wrote an article in French called "Reflections after four-and-one-half years of experience and 800 cases with the lipolysis technique." [5]. A few months later I wrote a long supplement for the same journal.

Dr. Clyde Litton, an old friend who had long before taught me the technique of face peeling, came from Washington, D.C., and Dr. Fischer came from Rome. Fischer was enthusiastic about my approach and said he had decided to give up his "crushing" technique.

For most of 1981, I worked on perfecting my technique and teaching it. In September, I went to Japan. In Osaka, I attended the Dalinde Symposium at the Shirakabe Clinic, where Dr. Clyde Litton presented my technique. It attracted a lot of interest and many surgeons asked me questions. Among them were Hinderer of Spain to whom I gave a cannula; Blair Rogers to whom I gave an English reprint and some pictures; Mario Gonzales-Ulloa; Trudy Vogt of Switzerland; and Vilar-Sancho of Spain, who came to Paris to learn my technique a few months later.

Next I went to Tokyo for the International Congress of Aesthetic and Plastic Surgery. I was not able to present my paper because there was not enough time, but I met a lot of friends, including Professor DaSuza Pinto, President of the Brazilian Plastic Surgery Society. He congratulated me because, after my speech at Fortaleza, he had tried my technique on a case of male fatty gynecomastia and had a very good result. After his remarks, I also used the technique for gynecomastia with success.

In October 1981, I went to New York to present my technique at Lenox Hill Hospital with Dr. Edgar P. Berry. My speech particularly interested Dr. Paula Moynahan, who came to see me in Paris. After presenting the aforementioned papers, some physicians began asking me if they could come to Paris to learn my technique. In the latter part of 1981, I had the pleasure of welcoming the following surgeons: Norman Martin of Los Angeles, Fournier of Paris, Cornelis of Belgium, Baroudi of Brazil, and Shirakabe and Professor Watanabe of Japan.

In November 1981, the annual meeting of the French Society of Aesthetic Surgery was devoted to fatty deposits. I gave a long lecture on my technique, and other reports were given by surgeons I had trained. These surgeons included Drs. Fournier of Paris, Otteni of Strasbourg, and Pechoux of Montpellier. These communications were published in the book *Chirurgie Esthetique 1981–1982* edited by Maloine of France. For this publication, I decided to name my technique "lipolysis," which comes from the Greek *lipo* (fat) and *lysis* (destroy). It seemed a good short name for the procedure.

Many of the surgeons I had trained during the year called to tell me they were having success using my technique on other areas of the body. Dr. Fevrier of France said it gave good results in the inner thighs of a fat young girl. I had been afraid to work there before, but then I started doing it, too. Dr. Fournier told me he successfully removed fat from the cheeks by suction during a face lift. In Belgium Dr. Cornelis said he was successful in removing fat deposits from the arms.

Thus, the year 1981 was very rich in ideas. As I continued working with the procedure, I discovered some useful little tricks. For example, I found a way to know in advance the results my technique would achieve on an abdomen. By asking patients to retract their abdomen, you can see exactly what the result will be and thus better select patients. Also, the way to know exactly what to remove on a buttock is to ask patients to stand on their toes; this makes it possible to differentiate muscle and fat.

That year (1981) I did many cases that were more and more difficult. I was amazed by the skin's great power of retraction, especially in two cases. A 64-year-old woman came to me with a huge double chin. It was so huge that I preferred using suction first under local anesthesia and then doing a face lift 2 months later to remove the excess skin. But the patient was so pleased after the first stage that she did not want the second operation. She honestly looked so much younger that it was not necessary.

The second case was the mother of a patient whose abdomen I had done with good results. The mother wanted a face lift and the same abdominal technique as used on her daughter. Since she had an abdomen with loose skin, however, I told her the results would be poor. She insisted, and I was surprised to see how well her skin retracted to give a good result.

In January 1982, I gave a lecture in Los Angeles to a group I had not known before, the Academy of Cosmetic Surgery. Again interest was high, and many questions were asked. In April, I went to Jakarta, Indonesia, to give a speech and operative demonstrations to the Plastic Surgery Society of Indonesia.

During 1982, I received so many requests for training that I decided to give a course in Paris on the twentieth and twenty-first of June. I did not imagine what would follow. It was a great success. I was happy to have four American plastic surgeons in the course: Adrian Aiache of Los Angeles; Frank Herhahn of Albuquerque, New Mexico; Gregory Hetter of Las Vegas; and Frederick Grazer of Newport Beach, California.

I did a number of surgical demonstrations and presented many patients. Some patients had been operated on recently; others had been operated on several years before. Everyone was enthusiastic.

Soon after, I was invited by Dr. Grazer to attend the American Society of Plastic and Reconstructive Surgery (ASPRS) Meeting in Honolulu, Hawaii, in October 1982. Dr. Grazer was to be the moderator of a course on classical lipectomy and he wanted to give me an hour to speak about my technique. He also asked me to give a 15-minute lecture as part of a panel.

Additional Lectures and Supervision of First Cases

At the beginning of October 1982, I went to Hospital Boucicaut to give a private lecture to Professor Vilain, who I had invited to my course in June but who did not come. He and his assistant, Dr. Mintz, attended the private lecture. Dr. Vilain was very enthusiastic and said he would come with me to Honolulu.

Before going to Hawaii, I had been invited by Dr. Hetter to Las Vegas to supervise his first cases and give him my advice. I helped him with the cases, and he made a videotape of our work. I mentioned to Dr. Hetter that I had just founded an International Society of Lipolysis to teach my technique. He then suggested starting an American branch. Thus was born the Lipolysis Society of North America. Our first effort was to plan a symposium to be given for ASPRS members for late January 1983 in Los Angeles with Drs. Aiache, Herhahn, and Hetter. My next stop was Los Angeles, where I gave similar coaching to Dr. Aiache.

At the annual meeting of ASPRS in Honolulu my course and lecture seemed to interest everyone. I was surprised to meet Dr. Kesselring of Switzerland, who lectured on a technique he had used on 36 cases of riding breeches deformity. It was a curette procedure with undermining that he did only on young patients with very small deformities. I was happy to have the opportunity to discuss our respective techniques.

At the meeting, several board members of ASPRS, including Drs. Simon Fredricks, Mark Gorney, and Rex Peterson, asked if it would be possible to come to Paris soon to evaluate my technique. I told them I was planning to give another course in Paris in December. They wanted to come before the course and have a separate exposure to my technique.

When I returned to Paris, I gave a lecture at the annual meeting of the French Plastic Surgery Society and was introduced by Dr. Vilain.

The American Society's task force grew from the appointed 5 to 14 members and came to Paris in December. I had the pleasure of greeting a group of very interested surgeons: Drs. Fredricks, Herhahn, Peterson, Cole, Kaye, Cohen, Hugo, Gradinger, Weiner, Baker, Belgram, Anastasia, Noone, and Davis. I showed them everything with lectures, surgical demonstrations, and recent and long-term case results.

A few days later, I gave my regular course, which was attended by Dr. Adamson of Norfolk, Virginia, Dr. Mladick of Virginia Beach, and Dr. Burkhardt of Tucson. Dr. Adamson invited me to stop on the way to Los Angeles for the Lipolysis Society Symposium and give a course at the Eastern Virginia Medical School in Norfolk, Virginia, in January 1983. I started the trip to the United States by stopping in New York, at the invitation of Drs. Hugo and James Smith, to give a lecture at Columbia University.

I then went to Norfolk to give a 3-day course, where I met Dr. Bahman Teimourian. It was the first time I became aware of his work. He spoke about interesting experiences using the Kesselring curette technique. Next I went to visit Dr. Fredricks to give a lecture to the

Plastic Surgery Society of Houston, Texas. At last I arrived in Los Angeles to give my course with the Lipolysis Society of North America.

From California, I went to Bogota, where the Colombian society had asked me to give a course. But I had to return to the USA at Dr. Fredricks' request to help him with his first cases in early February 1983. At last, I went back to Paris.

I was not home long, though. The University of California at Los Angeles and the Educational Foundation of ASPRS invited me to give a course in Los Angeles in April 1983. But first I went to San Francisco, where I was invited by Dr. Luis Vasconez. I gave a lecture and demonstrations at the University of California at San Francisco, followed by lectures and demonstrations in Los Angeles. Afterward, I went to Newport Beach, California, to participate in a meeting for the Orange County Medical Society arranged by Dr. Grazer. On the way home I stopped in New York to help Dr. Hugo with his first cases.

At the beginning of June, I was on the road again. I lectured to the Belgian Society of Plastic Surgery. At the end of the month, I gave another course in Paris, and after that I went to Chicago at the invitation of Dr. Richard C. Schultz of the University of Illinois. From Chicago, I traveled to Virginia Beach to participate in the second American symposium given by the Lipolysis Society of North America. Next, I went to New York to give a demonstration again at Columbia University, then to Montreal to present my results to the International Society of Plastic and Reconstructive Surgery Meeting and to participate in an instructional course. What a year!

In June 1983, it was exactly 6 years since I started doing my technique. After more than 6000 procedures on more than 2000 patients, I took stock of the progress. First, I noted that other surgeons were going further and further. Dr. Aiache in Los Angeles defatted the lateral part of the breast during reduction mammoplasty, giving a shorter scar. Dr. Alejandro in Venezuela used a 2-mm cannula to defat a thick flap in finger surgery. Dr. Grazer defatted a musculocutaneous flap. Dr. Herhahn defatted a vertical breast pedicle. Dr. Cornelis in Belgium successfully used defatting to treat arthrosis of the knees.

For my part, I applied my technique to very extreme fatty diseases. In August 1982, I had operated on a huge congenital deformity of the inner thighs of a young boy and removed 3 kg of fat. When I saw him recently, the result was spectacular. I also achieved very satisfying results for patients with Launois-Bensaude disease and generalized Dercum's disease.

Because I had noticed that patients lose weight after lipolysis, I did some reading on the subject. I found that the answer may lie in the theory of alpha-2 and beta-1 receptors developed by Drs. Lafontan and Berlan of Toulouse, France, and by Swedish researchers (see Chap. 6).

Summary

In conclusion, we can now say that under appropriate conditions a blunt cannula can be used to remove fat from almost any place in the body without danger. The only problem is to create a pleasing shape. Second, the tunnel technique can often be used instead of undermining, and this technique offers many advantages. Third, the relative elasticity of the skin and its harmonious response to the collapse of tunnels affords great possibilities in plastic surgery.

The three major ideas—subcutaneous suctioning of fat, the tunnel technique, and contraction of the skin—seem to constitute a new concept in plastic surgery that makes a bridge for the future. Surgeons should expand this new technique into all areas of aesthetic and reconstructive surgery.

References

1. Pitanguy, I. Trochanteric lipodystrophy. *Plast. Reconstr. Surg.* 34:280, 1964.
2. Björntorp, P., and Östman, J. Human adipose tissue. Dynamic and regulation. *Adv. Metab. Disord.* 5:277, 1971.
3. Fischer, A., and Fischer, G. M. Revised technique for cellulitis fat. Reduction in riding breeches deformity. *Bull. Int. Acad. Cosm. Surg.* 2(4): Dec., 1977.
4. Illouz, Y. G. Une nouvelle technique pour les lipodystrophies localisées. *Rev. Chir. Esth. Franc.* 6 (19): Apr., 1980.
5. Illouz, Y. G. Reflexions après 4 ans et demi d'experience et 800 cas de ma technique de lipolyse. *Rev. Chir. Esth. Franc.* 6(24): Oct., 1981.

CHAPTER 4

Popularization of the Technique

Pierre F. Fournier

To popularize any technique, one must first believe in it, that is, make it popular to oneself. The technique becomes popular when its results are confirmed by the test of time. As Sir Harold Gillies said, "Time is the plastic surgeon's greatest ally, but also his most trenchant critic."

Body sculpturing using suction-assisted extraction of subcutaneous fat has recently become very popular. I first became interested in this technique in 1977 and eventually became closely associated with it. I was fortunate to be in a position to observe the foundations being laid by its two foremost pioneers: Dr. George Fischer of Rome and Dr. Yves-Gerard Illouz of Paris. I observed its birth, development, and refinement. I participated in its dissemination and watched it reach its present great popularity.

Pioneer Developments

No surgeon knowledgeable in the history of subcutaneous fat extraction surgery contests that the father of collapsing surgery using a suction machine was Dr. George Fischer [1] of Rome, an American citizen of Hungarian extraction. He was the first to perfect specially designed instruments to extract adipose tissue to treat trochanteric lipodystrophy and to make use of a powerful suction machine to remove the fat collected by the instruments.

Fischer's instruments were the planotome, which created an intraadipose plane of dissection between 9 mm and 13 mm below the skin, and the cellusactiotome, which resected fat with a grinding motion. As the instrument descended from the top to the bottom of the working plane, it created chips of fat in a manner similar to a mining machine in a quarry.

The electromechanical cellusactiotome developed by Fischer to remove fat was, in fact, a blunt cannula with a blade at the lumen. The blade moved many times per minute, cutting the fat, which was then pushed inside the opening by slight pressure of the surgeon's hand and vacuumed out by the suction machine.

Unfortunately, although the tip of the cellusactiotome was blunt, the blade attached to the opening made it a sharp cutting instrument. The procedure of creating a wide subcutaneous plane and digging into the adipose tissue with this instrument ultimately formed a large cavity. Thus, Fischer really proceeded to do a subcutaneous block lipectomy.

Fischer's procedure caused hemorrhage and lymphorrhea of variable duration and severity, because vessels in the way of the instrument were severed. Hematomas requiring evacuation also occurred. The operation often required repeated tapping of persistent seroma. If seroma persisted, the raw cavity could undergo mesoepithelialization and, as a consequence, further ptosis of the superficial tissues could occur (see Chapter 17). Despite frequent complications, reasonable results often were obtained by Fischer, but the technique never gained lasting support.

With any new technique, there is usually considerable room for improvement. If Fischer had realized, when he analyzed his complications, that two things were *unnecessary*—the creation of a dissection plane with the planotome, and the use of a moving blade at the opening of the cannula to cut the fat—he would have discovered the right procedure in 1976.

Some years later, I invited Fischer to Paris, where Illouz and I demonstrated the concept of tunnels to him. Afterward, he returned to Rome, discarded the planotome (which was unnecessary and hazardous), and disconnected the motor that moved the cellusactiotome blade. He then had a perfectly blunt instrument with a blunt tip and blunt opening. Dr. Fischer is still using the same instrument today with the tunnel technique. For other localized adiposities, he has developed similar instruments with different calibers.

Fischer was able to make these changes because of the contributions of Dr. Illouz, the second pioneer of lipoextraction. Fischer's equipment, although commercially available, was slow in delivery and extremely expensive. So, Illouz, who became aware of Fischer's ideas in early 1977, used the equipment readily available in any hospital where abortions are performed: the common cannula and suction machine developed by Karman (an American), which for years have been employed by gynecologists.

Illouz immediately understood that this suction instrument was the most convenient tool for lipoextraction. The Karman cannula, with a blunt tip and a blunt opening, made a considerable difference in both the operation and the results. It permitted extraction from multiple tunnels, which were vastly different from the continuous plane of Fischer's technique.

The tunnel dissection method leaves connections between the deeper and superficial planes, in which vessels remain undamaged. The procedure respects, as much as a blunt dissection can, the anatomy in which we work. In addition, there is little hemorrhage, rarely hematoma, and limited lymphorrhea.

This type of cannula was chosen by serendipity to perform the specialized function of lipoextraction. Yet the technique it suggested—creating tunnels—made it possible to progress from the block lipectomy of Fischer to a "honeycomb" lipectomy. The only remaining problem was acquiring the experience necessary to perform

"blind" subcutaneous sculpturing with good aesthetic results. Eventually, all the superficial adiposities of the body, head, and neck would yield to this technique. Thanks to the pioneering work of George Fischer and the advances of Yves-Gerard Illouz, the basic technique of fat extraction surgery reached a state of advancement where other surgeons could reproduce the results.

Technical Modifications

My own contribution has been to extend and modify the original ideas of Fischer and Illouz. I also took part in the diffusion of the technique throughout the world. What is my own concept of "lipolysis," "lipoextraction," or "suction-assisted lipectomy"? First, I believe a better name is *suction lipoplasty.*

As has been said, to adopt is to adapt. In the beginning, many surgeons followed Illouz's ideas word for word. By experience and reflection over the years, we found that there was room for improvement in the application of lipoextraction, as often happens with any new surgical technique.

I believe that honeycomb lipectomy is more reliable if it is done in a criss-cross pattern. Strokes are made at right angles to each other, which permits better remodeling of the adiposity during the dressing period. The criss-cross approach is recommended with all cannulas. I prefer small-caliber lipoextractors (French #4 or #5) for all adiposities, because they allow better control of the work being done.

For the peripheral mesh undermining, which must be even and cover a large area, I use solid lipodissectors with the same caliber as the one used for the honeycomb lipectomy. The same incisions are used, or others can be made, if necessary, with the help of an awl.

The dry technique (no preceding subcutaneous injections) that is used today includes (1) criss-cross honeycomb lipectomy with limited pressure to remove fat, (2) peripheral and central mesh lipoplasty, (3) remodeling of the adipose tissue, (4) repositioning of the skin, and (5) immobilization of the treated tissues with a firm dressing, usually without drainage. I perform this procedure under decreased pressure (0.7 atmosphere), with small-caliber lipoextractors (#4 or #5 with three openings) and with multiple direct approaches through the skin openings previously made with an awl. When general anesthesia is used, the supine position is preferred, because it allows treatment of all superficial adiposities by slightly mobilizing the trunk or limbs (see Chapter 18). Ambulatory patients are treated with block or local anesthesia or with freezing.

Dissemination of the Technique

In June 1978, Illouz gave a lecture in Paris at the French National Society of Aesthetic Surgery [2] about the technique that he had been using for 1 year. I was very interested in his results, went to see him operate, and referred some of my patients to him. The results he obtained kindled my interest in his procedure, which was different from the one I already knew about used by Fischer in Rome. Little by little, I became convinced of the importance of the progress made by Illouz and in 1979 began to do the same procedure.

In May 1980, during a trip to Japan, I was invited to give a lecture on transconjunctival blepharoplasty at the Shirakabe Clinic in Osaka. I suggested that my friends, the Shirakabe brothers, should also invite Illouz (whom they did not know) to present his new procedure since he was visiting the Orient at the same time. This was Illouz's first international presentation to plastic surgeons. Among those present was Dr. Blair O. Rogers of New York City, who was also lecturing at the clinic. He was very interested in Illouz's report and offered to publish it in his journal *Aesthetic Plastic Surgery*. Illouz gave Dr. Rogers a copy of his paper, but for whatever reason it was never published. The first paper published in the United States on lipoextraction was by Drs. Teimourian and J. D. Fisher (not G. Fischer) in 1981. This publication surprised Dr. Illouz and me, since we had never before heard of anyone else's interest in this technique.

My role in popularizing the procedure began in Lake Tahoe, Nevada, in February 1982 [3]. By invitation, I regularly give a series of lectures as part of the courses on head and neck surgery organized there each year by Dr. Leslie Bernstein. During my 1982 series, I gave the first report on suction-assisted lipectomy in the United States. In my lecture entitled "A New Defatting Procedure for Head and Neck Cosmetic Surgery," I showed the results that I had achieved using the technique on double chins, nasolabial folds, jowls, and cheeks, and as an adjunctive procedure during face and neck lifts.

Another member of the faculty who was in the audience, Dr. Gregory Hetter, was one of the few who realized the full potential that the procedure had to offer. The fact that he was a specialist boarded in both otolaryngology and plastic surgery undoubtedly helped him to realize how revolutionary it truly was. Afterward, he questioned me in private to learn more details, and I showed him many of the body sculpture results, which I had on slides. The slides stimulated his curiosity so much that he decided he should go to Paris to see the operation performed.

In June 1982, Illouz, Francis Otteni, and I offered the first lipolysis course in the English language in Paris. Dr. Hetter came to Paris with two other friends, Dr. Frank Herhahn and Dr. Adrien Aiache, whom he had invited to share the experience. During the June course, the three of them decided that the procedure deserved presentation at the meeting of the world's most influential and prestigious plastic surgery organization, the American Society of Plastic and Reconstructive Surgeons.

That convention was in Honolulu in October 1982. Illouz gave his paper on the wet technique [4], and Otteni and I presented our paper on the dry procedure [5].

At Hetter's suggestion, the board of directors of the American Society of Plastic and Reconstructive Surgeons broke off their meeting to attend our lectures. As a result, Dr. Mark Gorney (ASPRS president) appointed a "Blue Ribbon Committee" to go to Europe in December 1982 to decide what stance the society should take regarding this new technique. The committee chairman was Dr. Simon Fredricks, who was already familiar with lipolysis, having seen videotapes recorded by Dr. Shirakabe at the June 1982 course in Paris and provided to Dr. Fredricks by Dr. Grazer. Dr. Fredricks expanded the committee from the original five ASPRS appointees to an eventual total of 14.

The report on surgical suction lipectomy by the society's ad hoc committee on new procedures was favorable. The report states, "The committee unanimously agrees that suction lipectomy by the Illouz blunt cannula is a surgical procedure that is safe and effective in trained and experienced hands and offers benefits which heretofore have been unavailable." This approval speeded popularization of the procedure, which had already been started by the early visitors to France— Gregory Hetter, Frank Herhahn, Frederick Grazer, and Adrien Aiache. I cannot list all of the surgeons who came, saw, and believed in the technique. There were so many.

Though it is impossible to name all of the surgeons who visited Paris in 1982 to observe the new procedure, they deserve credit. Thanks to their stimulating presence, their pertinent and accurate observations, and their enlightened criticism, great progress was made in understanding and improving the revolutionary procedure.

The American visitors to Paris included Clyde Litton from Washington, D.C., who had been interested in the technique for a long while, as well as Nicholas Georgiade, Boyd Burkhardt, Adrien Aiache, the Clarendons, Richard Mladick, and Joseph Agris. Axel Vargas came from Colombia, Simon Kirshbaum from Peru, Fossatti from Uruguay, Alejandro Vasquez Barbe from Venezuela, and Nelson de Senna, Ewaldo Bolivar de Souza Pinto, and Ricardo Baroudi from Brazil. It was Baroudi who deserves credit for the observation: "With fan-shaped dissection from the incision, you create tunnels and leave septi." We adopted his definition, which was more appropriate than the "bicycle-wheel spokes" description we previously used.

Ottermin Aguire and Mario Nosenzo came from Argentina. The latter insisted that the opening of the cannula should always be pointing down. Watanabe from Tokyo also came, as well as the Shirakabe brothers from Osaka, who faithfully recorded absolutely everything and later spread the word not only in their own country but also to plastic surgery colleagues throughout the world. Indeed, a complete television team came from Tokyo especially to record the work.

There were also visitors from Great Britain, Italy, Spain, and other countries. Once again, I apologize for not naming all the colleagues and friends of long standing who came to Paris. Preexisting professional friendships led to many visits and facilitated rapid dispersal of the technique.

In 1983, other visitors came to visit me. More important, however, were the symposiums and courses that Drs. Illouz, Otteni, and I attended in February in Norfolk, Virginia (at the Eastern Virginia Medical School), in Los Angeles, California (organized by the Lipolysis Society of North America), and in Bogota, Colombia. The round of seminars, congresses, and courses began again in April. The Educational Foundation of the American Society of Plastic and Reconstructive Surgeons and the American Society for Aesthetic Plastic Surgery sponsored a seminar in Los Angeles. Next came the VIII International Congress of the International Confederation for Plastic and Reconstructive Surgery in June in Montreal and the first International Society of Aesthetic and Plastic Surgeons (ISAPS) course with surgical demonstrations at the Royal Victoria Hospital organized by Paule Regnault. In October we went to Albuquerque, New Mexico, for the Lipolysis Society of North America's third symposium of 1983, to Dallas for their annual meeting, then to Jakarta, and finally to the Planas Clinic in Barcelona.

In addition, several courses in English were given in Paris, and trips were made by Drs. Illouz and Otteni and me, individually or in small groups, to Thailand, Japan, Italy, Germany, and Great Britain, where colleagues had invited us to teach them the technique through private instruction. It was during numerous trips to Africa and the French West Indies that Francis Otteni and I had the opportunity, because of the very special deformities seen in these areas, to develop the first circumferential lipectomies in arms and thighs, and the first combined abdominoplasty procedures, which allow successful treatment without danger to high-risk patients.

In sum, Drs. Illouz and Otteni and I watched and helped as the technique of blunt suction lipectomy spread rapidly. We did all we could to place the technique in the hands of plastic surgeons who were professionally and morally recognized as knowledgeable authorities. Grazer, Hetter (who organized symposiums during 1983), Regnault (who organized the 1983 ISAPS course in Montreal), and Gonzalez-Ulloa of Mexico (who organized the Dalinde seminar in February 1984) sponsored the technique with their moral authority, thus facilitating its popularization. A large part of the entire November 1983 issue of the *Journal of Plastic and Reconstructive Surgery* was devoted to lipoextraction. Dr. Illouz' [4] article finally was published in English, 3 years after the Tokyo meeting.

Unfortunately, this revolutionary technique is also being disseminated by physicians without special training in it—some even without training in surgery. The procedure can seem simple, but it is only so in appearance. These novice propagators make and spread the errors that we made at the beginning of our experience, putting in peril the validity of the procedure, which is safe and reliable only in well-trained hands.

Properly trained plastic surgeons have at their disposal a new instrument—the cannula or lipoextractor—that they can use as a powerful adjunct in their everyday practice. This instrument permits surgeons to obtain results that never before could be achieved in body contouring and to treat patients who previously could not benefit from treatment.

What we are doing now is certainly not the last word in lipoextraction; however, what we have done so far would not have been possible without the work of all who have taken part. As Montaigue said, "I have gathered a posie of other men's flowers, and only the thread that binds them is mine own."

References

1. Fischer, A., and Maurice, G. M. Revised technique for cellulitis fat reduction in riding breeches deformity. *Bull. Int. Acad. Cosm. Surg.* 2:40, 1977.
2. Illouz, Y. G. Communication à la Société Français de Chirurgie Esthetique, Juin 1978 et 1979.
3. Fournier, P. Facelift: New SMAS and Defatting Procedures. Presentation sponsored by the Sacramento Society of Otolaryngology and Maxillofacial Surgery. Lake Tahoe, Nevada, February 1982.
4. Illouz, Y. G. Body contouring by lipolysis: A 5-year experience with over 3000 cases. *Plast. Reconstr. Surg.* 72:591, 1983.
5. Fournier, P. F., and Otteni, F. M. Lipodissection in body sculpturing: The dry procedure. *Plast. Reconstr. Surg.* 72: 598, 1983.

Introduction of Lipolysis to the United States: A Three-Year Experience

Norman Martin

In October 1980 while vacationing in Paris, a casual inquiry to Dr. Pierre Fournier about his experience with the Fischer technique for removal of localized fat deposits led to my introduction to Dr. Yves-Gerard Illouz, also of Paris. Dr. Illouz had developed a blunt liposurgical technique—lipolysis—based on the injection of a hypotonic saline solution directly into the offending fatty mass. He had been using his technique for more than 3 years and reported dramatic results achieved via tiny incisions and with few complications. The idea sounded intriguing, and Dr. Illouz graciously consented to allow me to observe him operate.

Intrigue gave way to astonishment, followed by the realization that I was witnessing a revolutionary new surgical technique. Hours of observation, hundreds of questions, and the examination and questioning of some of his postoperative patients led me to believe that Dr. Illouz was being open and honest and that, in his hands, the procedure was valid.

I returned to the United States with a videotape of his technique and proceeded to seek peer response to my "discovery." Indifference, scorn, and ridicule were the responses of my colleagues. Nevertheless, I felt the technique was so important that it was worthy of the considerable time, effort, and risks involved in bringing it to the attention of the American public.

I was so intrigued that I returned to Paris in January 1981 to work under the direction of Dr. Illouz to learn more about lipolysis. One should never underestimate the importance of "hands on" training for this procedure.

Prior to my leaving Paris, Dr. Illouz expressed his concern regarding the dissemination of the specifics of his technique to untrained or unscrupulous individuals. He feared that they, after observing the *apparent* ease and simplicity of the lipolysis procedure, might be tempted to perform it without proper instruction (or no instruction), thereby leading to complications, poor results, and disrepute for his lipolysis procedure. I shared his concern. In addition, we were concerned with the confusion (especially in the plastic surgical community) between the various "suction" procedures. The "blunt" lipolysis technique did not share the same operative and postoperative sequelae as did the "sharp" techniques (e.g., suction curettage and lipexeresis) that were beginning to be reported in the literature. We both felt that it was vitally important to distinguish the Illouz technique (hypotonic saline injection, blunt instrumentation, high negative pressure) with a distinctive name—hence lipolysis.

After returning to California, I approached my hospital about beginning the procedure. Since lipolysis was then (and in some areas probably still may be) consid-

Table 5-1. Complications in patients of one physician resulting from lipolysis from March 1981 to February 1984

Complication	Occurrence	Number of patients	% of patients
Postoperative hemorrhage requiring transfusion	1	1	0.2
Hematoma requiring drainage	0	0	0
Hematoma not requiring drainage	11	7	1.7
Seroma	0	0	0
Wound infection	0	0	0
Skin slough	0	0	0
Persistent pain, 6 weeks or more	84	62	14.9
Persistent pain, 3 months or more	18	9	2.2
Persistent pigmentation, 3 months or more	48	48	11.6
Persistent hypesthesia, 3 months or more	22	18	4.3

Total number of patients = 415; total number of procedures = 2107.

ered experimental surgery, I obtained permission from my hospital Surgical Research Committee and developed a new surgical consent form specifically relating to it. On March 22, 1981, I performed the first lipolysis procedure in the United States using the Illouz technique. It was an overwhelming success and word spread quickly. Within weeks I was deluged with potential surgical candidates. Unfortunately, most of the candidates did not fit the stringent criteria that Illouz had recommended and had to be refused. In January 1982, Dr. Illouz was invited by the American Board of Cosmetic Surgery, Inc. to present a lecture on his technique. The talk was well received and some surgeons—on the strength of the lecture only—began performing suction procedures shortly thereafter. The initial reaction of the North American medical community ranged from disinterest to skepticism. Appearances in the media caused mild curiosity in some corners and outrage in others. Later, curiosity became intense interest, and outrage became a desire to control the technique.

Between March 1981 and February 1984, I performed more than 2000 lipolysis procedures on 415 patients. Surgical complications have been few and are summarized in Table 5-1.

Aesthetic sequelae (contour deformities) remain the largest source of physician and patient concern, despite the fact that there is an extremely high overall rate of patient satisfaction with the procedure. In my experience to date, dissatisfaction leading to malpractice suits has not occurred. Two instances of threatened malpractice suits could be traced to inadequate preoperative pyschological evaluation or intentional malicious instigation by another surgeon (perhaps the greatest cause of professional liability claims overall) or both. As with most other aesthetic procedures, careful preoperative psychological as well as motivational evaluation of the patient should be performed. Frank, open, two-way discussion of the expected results and postoperative recovery period is mandatory. In the long run, this discussion requires less physician time by allaying anxiety and apprehension in the patient.

Clinical Observations

Based on my 3-year experience using the Illouz technique in 2000 procedures on 415 patients, I believe the following observations may be of use to both the beginner and the advanced practitioner:

1. Patient selection is critical both from the standpoints of skin elasticity and patient expectations.
2. On the thighs, even minimal irregularities are of major concern to many women.
3. Most patients expect a higher degree of contour symmetry and precision with lipolysis than they do with the classical defatting procedures.
4. Certain contour irregularities are preexisting and may become more noticeable after the lipolysis procedure.
5. Upper medial thigh lipolysis should be approached cautiously and performed only in cases where a small to moderate fatty deformity exists in the presence of firm, elastic skin.
6. Lipolysis in the midmedial thigh should be avoided.
7. When presented with an asymmetry of two sides (usually hips and/or thighs), do the larger side first.
8. For fat extractions over 750 ml, bed rest for 18 to 24 hours is indicated to avoid syncopal episodes.
9. Fluid replacement should approximate fat removal plus 1000 to 1500 ml of crystalloid.
10. Using the original Illouz technique, 20 to 25% of the extracted material is blood.
11. Adding epinephrine 1:250,000 to 1:300,000 to the injection solution decreases blood loss in the extracted material to 5 to 10% of the volume.
12. Suction drains are not necessary and may increase the amount of blood loss.
13. "Third spacing" of blood has not been a problem except in patients with a preoperatively unknown bleeding problem that requires transfusion (Table 5-1).

CHAPTER 6

Human Adipose Tissue Function, Development, and Metabolism

Peter Arner

Adipose tissue was originally considered an inactive reserve of fat that insulated the body and was derived from unspecialized connective tissue cells. We know now that a certain amount of adipose tissue is fundamental to animal and human life, adipocyte fat being the main energy store of the body. It has also become evident that adipose tissue is a very active metabolic organ playing an important pathophysiological role in several common disorders such as diabetes, hyperthyroidism, and hyperlipoproteinemia. In recent years, considerable attention has been directed to the regulation of the development and metabolic functions of human adipocytes. The knowledge in this field is reviewed in this chapter, which also presents evidence that human adipose tissue is a heterogeneous organ as far as the control of metabolism and development of fatty regions is concerned.

In a newborn infant, *brown* adipose tissue is of great importance for thermogenesis, but for later life the importance of this tissue is poorly understood. This chapter presents current knowledge about the prevailing *white* adipose tissue.

Human Adipose Tissue

FUNCTION

The main function of fat cells is to release or store free fatty acids (FFA) according to the energy demands and nutritional status of the body. FFA are the most concentrated form of energy known in nature. They are stored in the adipocyte as triglyceride (TG).

Figure 6-1 illustrates schematically how FFA are liberated through hydrolysis (lipolysis) of TG and how they are stored through synthesis to TG (esterification). During lipolysis, TG are broken down to the end products glycerol and FFA, which are released to the blood stream. In the blood stream, FFA are bound to albumin and transported to peripheral tissues for oxidation or to the liver for synthesis of TG-rich lipoproteins. Regarding the storage of adipocyte FFA, three different routes are of importance in humans. First, some FFA derived from lipolysis can be reused for synthesis of new TG (re-esterification of FFA). Second, FFA can be taken up by the blood stream and directly esterified to TG. Third, circulating TG can be a source of FFA. Blood TG are broken down to FFA and glycerols through the action of the enzyme lipoprotein lipase, which is located in the endothelial wall of the adipose tissue blood vessels. FFA derived from blood TG enter the fat cell and are used for esterification to TG. In the esterification process, three molecules of FFA are coupled to one molecule of alpha-glycerol phosphate, and one molecule of TG is formed. Alpha-glycerol phosphate is formed by the glucose me-

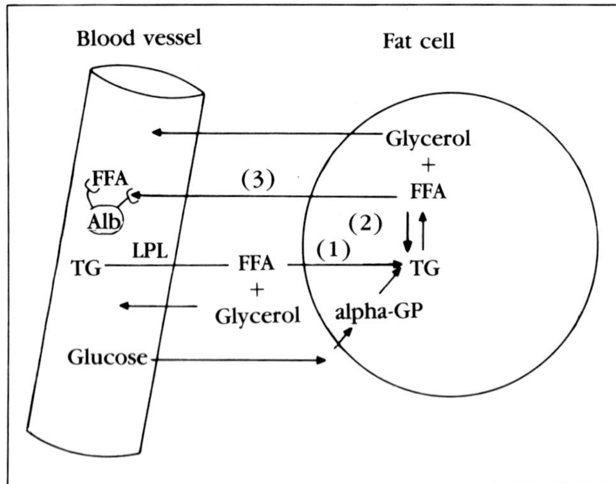

Fig. 6-1. Metabolism of human adipose tissue. TG = triglycerides; FFA = free fatty acids; Alb = albumin; alpha-GP = alpha-glycerol phosphate; LPL = lipoprotein lipase. (1) FFA formed from hydrolysis of blood TG are taken up by the fat cells and used for TG synthesis. (2) Some of FFA formed by the breakdown of TG in the fat cells are reutilized by the adipocytes to form new TG (reesterification). (3) The remaining part of FFA formed by adipocyte TG breakdown is released from the cell to the blood stream.

tabolism. Glucose enters the fat cell from the blood through a specific transport system and is then further metabolized.

The turnover of adipocyte FFA (stored through esterification and liberated through lipolysis) is 100 to 150 g/24 hr in the whole body fat of a normal weight adult subject [1]. When there is an increased demand for FFA in the periphery, such as during long-term exercise and during starvation, the turnover rate of body FFA can be doubled [1].

DEVELOPMENT

In the human fetus, white adipose tissue develops around capillary roots from arteries beneath the dermis. This development occurs in the third gestational month. Soon thereafter, the adipose tissue cells begin to enrich TG [2]. The fat cells arise from adipoblasts, which are not distinguishable from other perivascular connective tissue cells but differentiate into adipocyte precursors (preadipocytes). The preadipocytes accumulate TG to become mature fat cells [3].

The growth of adipose tissue is phasic in humans [4], as shown schematically in Figure 6-2. Adipose tissue mass expands as humans grow because of a combination of an increase in both the number and size of adipocytes. There is a replicative burst of fat cells in early childhood. The rate at which new fat cells are formed is successively reduced during puberty and adolescence.

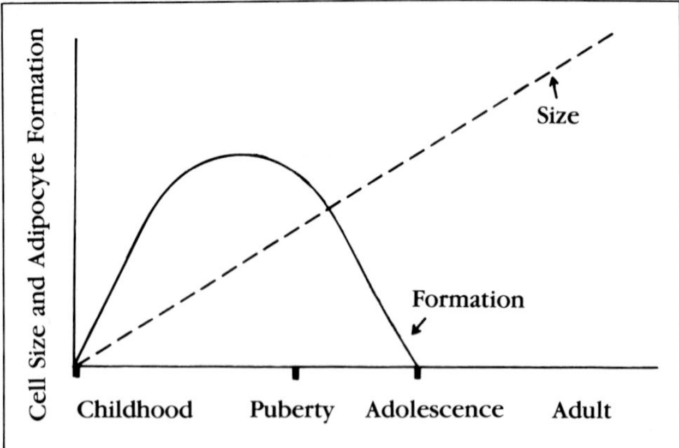

Fig. 6-2. Development of adipose tissue. There is a gradual increase in fat cell size throughout life. The increase in fat cell number is most marked in childhood. This increase is gradually reduced from puberty throughout adolescence. During adult life there is a fixed number of fat cells.

Thereafter, no new fat cells are formed and the adipocyte number is fixed throughout adult life in men and women. Although the total fat cell number may be genetically determined, it may also be modified by environmental factors such as nutritional changes during the replicative phase of adipose tissue growth. It has been shown that the most sensitive part of this period is between years 1 and 11 [5]. However, evidence is also beginning to appear that human adipose tissue growth and adipocyte replication can occur in adult life as well [6,7].

OBESITY AND DEVELOPMENT OF HUMAN ADIPOSE TISSUE

Obesity has been classified according to increasing adipocyte number or size [3]. In one less common form—*hyperplastic obesity*—there is usually an increase in fat cell number. This type of obesity usually begins in childhood. The other and much more common form starts in adult life and is generally characterized by an increase in fat cell size—*hypertrophic obesity.* The classification into these two forms of obesity is not absolute. Findings during the last decade [3,8] have led to the following conclusions: During the initial development of obesity, body fat accumulates by means of an increase in fat cell size without any change in fat cell number. There is, however, an upper limit to fat cell size at which hypertrophic growth of fat does not continue. This limit is reached when the fat cell size increases two to five times the normal size. The latter occurs in massively obese subjects (body weight exceeding 150% of the average), where almost all adipocytes are at the hypertrophic limit at this point; more fat cells are re-

Table 6-1. Various forms of human obesity

Type of obesity	Disorder	Morphology	Clinical characteristics
Adipose cellularity	Hyperplastic obesity	Increased fat cell number Normal fat cell size	Starts in childhood; poor response to conservative treatment
	Hypertrophic obesity	Normal fat cell number Increased fat cell size	Starts in adult life; may respond to conservative treatment
Fat distribution	Android obesity	Accumulation of fat in the upper body segments	Occurs most frequently among men; high risk of cardiovascular, atherosclerotic, and metabolic complications
	Gynecoid obesity	Accumulation of fat in the lower body segments	Occurs most frequently among women; low risk of secondary complications

Table 6-2. Effects of catecholamines and insulin on human fat cells

Hormone	Effect	Lipolysis	Glucose transport and metabolism	Triglyceride synthesis	Lipoprotein lipase	Phosphodiesterase
Catecholamine	Beta effect	Stimulation	Stimulation	Stimulation	Inhibition	Stimulation
Catecholamine	Alpha effect	Inhibition	?	?	?	?
Insulin	Alpha effect	Inhibition	Stimulation	?	Stimulation	Stimulation

cruited from the preadipocyte pool, and there is an increase in fat cell number (hyperplastic growth). It is of some clinical importance to distinguish between the two cellular forms of obesity, since hyperplastic obesity is more resistant to conservative therapy (diet, exercise) than hypertrophic obesity [9]. The different forms of obesity are described in Table 6-1.

We do not know which factors control the ultimate set point for body fat accumulation in a particular individual; however, the results with experimental obesity [8] in a group of otherwise healthy prison inmates indicate that such a set point does exist. The prisoners were encouraged to increase their food intake for half a year. At the end of this period all volunteers reached a 20 to 25% increase in their body weight, and they underwent metabolic studies. After the study was completed, almost all subjects returned to their prestudy body weight.

METABOLISM

All metabolic events in human adipose tissue that control adipocyte storage and mobilization of lipids (lipolysis, esterification, lipoprotein lipase activity, glucose transport, and metabolism) have spontaneous (basal) activities; that is, metabolism occurs without hormonal influence. As regards the hormonal control, humans are

unique in comparison to other species. Only catecholamines and insulin have a pronounced acute effect on metabolism in human adipocytes, whereas in animal fat cells several additional hormones play an important role [10]. The effects of insulin and catecholamines on human fat cells are summarized in Table 6-2.

Adipose metabolism is usually investigated in vitro using isolated fat cells or segments of adipose tissue that are incubated in physiologic buffers. Recently, microtechniques have been developed to specifically study lipolysis [11], glucose transport [12], and insulin [13] or catecholamine [14,15] receptor binding in human fat cells. Each of these methods requires only fractions of a gram of fat tissue for detailed investigations. Thus, it is possible to study various aspects of human fat cell metabolism in small adipose samples that can be obtained easily by a subcutaneous biopsy under local anesthesia.

Catecholamine Action

The mechanisms of catecholamine regulation of lipolysis in human fat cells are well known [16] and are illustrated in Figure 6-3. Catecholamines may stimulate or inhibit lipolysis in human fat cells. First, the hormones may bind to either of two different cell surface receptors: beta-1 and alpha-2 receptors. Both receptors are coupled to the enzyme adenylate cyclase through mech-

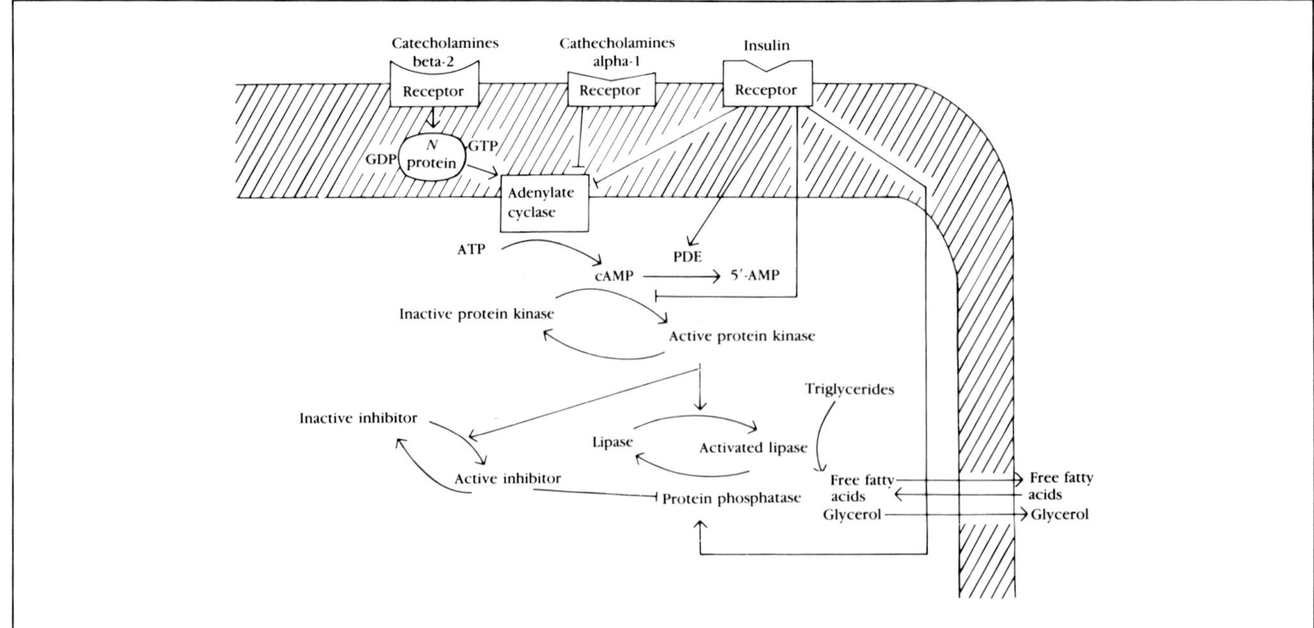

Fig. 6-3. Hormonal regulation of lipolysis in human fat cells. cAMP = cyclic AMP; PDE = phosphodiesterase; → = stimulation; ⊣ = inhibition.

anisms that involve a cell membrane–associated regulatory protein (*N*-protein). Adenylate cyclase is stimulated by beta-1 and inhibited by alpha-2 receptors. The enzyme stimulates the transformation of adenosine triphosphate (ATP) to cyclic adenosine monophosphate (cAMP), and the latter nucleotide stimulates a hormone-sensitive lipase, which regulates the breakdown of TG to FFA and glycerol. The beta-1–mediated lipolytic effect of catecholamines dominates under normal conditions. The rate of lipolysis is controlled by the level of cAMP in human adipose tissue [17]. This level is not only regulated by the production via adenylate cyclase and adrenergic receptors, but also by an intracellular enzyme, phosphodiesterase, which is important in converting cAMP to the inactive metabolite 5′ AMP. Phosphodiesterase can also be regulated by catecholamines, which stimulate the enzyme activity so that more cAMP is broken down in human fat [18].

In several common clinical conditions, the circulating level of FFA is altered presumably because of changes in adipose tissue lipolysis [10]. This alteration can be observed in obesity, diabetes, fasting, and hyperthyroidism, where there is an increase in the rate of lipolysis and an enhancement of the circulating FFA level. In hypothyroidism, the opposite phenomenon is observed. The alteration of lipolysis in these conditions can be at least partly due to changes in catecholamine function. An increased lipolytic effect of catecholamines has been described in obesity [19], fasting [20], diabetes [21], and hyperthyroidism [22], which may be explained by an enhanced beta-adrenergic effect [19,22,23] and a decreased phosphodiesterase activity [24] in these conditions. In hypothyroidism, there is a decreased lipolytic

effect of catecholamines due to enhanced alpha-adrenergic activity or enhanced phosphodiesterase activity in human adipose tissue [24,25] or both.

Catecholamines can also stimulate glucose uptake and lipid synthesis and inhibit lipoprotein lipase activity in human fat (Table 6-2). It is unclear as yet exactly how these effects are regulated under normal or pathological conditions.

Insulin Action

The first step in insulin action is binding to specific receptors on the fat cell surface [26]. Thereafter, specific intracellular bioeffects are activated. Examples of such effects are inhibition of lipolysis, stimulation of glucose transport, and stimulation of lipoprotein lipase (Table 6-2). It is not known how the signal is transformed from the insulin receptor to the intracellular metabolic process (postreceptor action of insulin). However, three potential mechanisms have currently received the most attention (Fig. 6-4). In one scheme, insulin receptor binding results in the generation of some intracellular second messenger, perhaps a small peptide of phospholipid [27]. The second model is based on the observation that the hormone-receptor complex is taken up by the cell (internalization), and the bioeffects of insulin occur after the release from the receptor of free insulin or of some biological degradation product of insulin [28]. The third model is based on the recent observation from several laboratories that insulin receptors possess

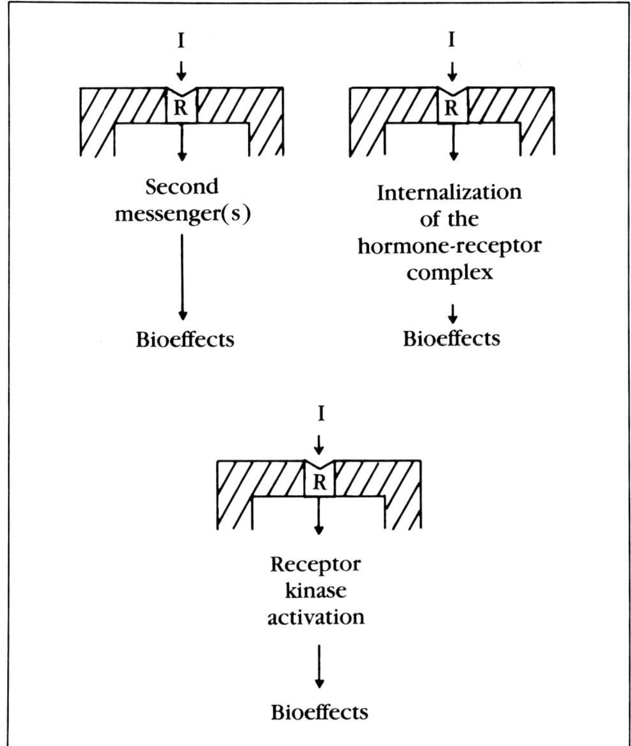

Fig. 6-4. Three current models of insulin action in fat cells. I = insulin; R = insulin receptor.

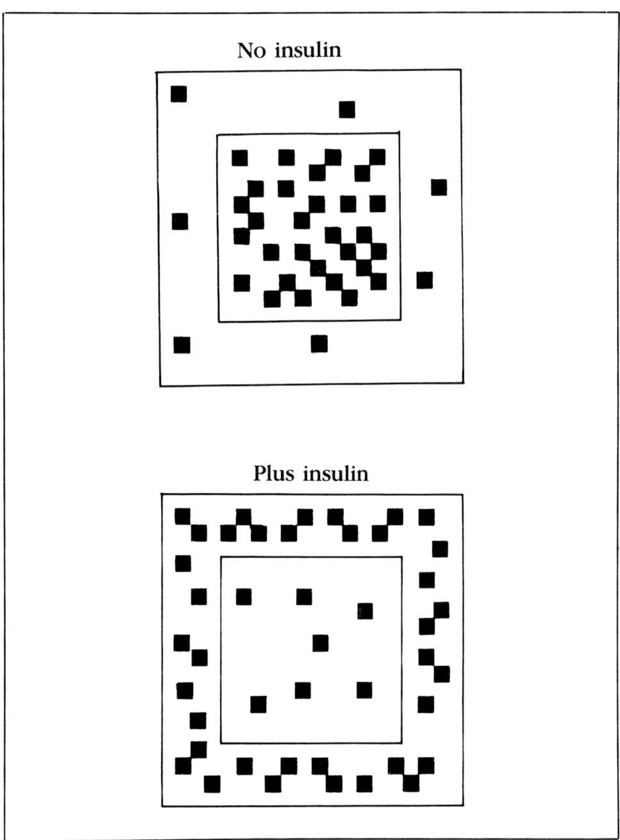

Fig. 6-5. Mechanism for insulin stimulation of glucose transport in fat cells. Glucose is transported through the cell membrane by specific carriers. These carriers are predominantly located inside the cell in the resting (basal) state. When insulin is present, there is a recruitment of glucose carriers from the intracellular pool to the cell membrane.

protein kinase activity [29]. When the receptor is occupied by insulin, this kinase is activated, causing phosphorylation of the insulin receptor. The latter turns on other phosphorylation reactions, including phosphorylation/dephosphorylation of the various enzymes that control the bioactivities of insulin.

Regarding the antilipolytic effect of insulin (see Fig. 6-3), data have been presented showing that the hormone inhibits adenylate cyclase, stimulates phosphodiesterase, and inhibits hormone-sensitive lipase [26]. These insulin effects are all associated with inhibition of lipolysis.

The model for how insulin stimulates glucose transport in fat cells is more uniform (Fig. 6-5). Glucose is actively transported by glucose carrier systems that cycle between the inside of the adipocyte and the cell membrane [30,31]. Under basal conditions, most of the transporters are localized inside the cell, and little glucose can pass through the cell membrane. When the fat cell insulin receptors are occupied by insulin, the carriers are rapidly recruited from the intracellular pool to the cell membrane, and large amounts of glucose can be transported from the outside to the inside of the cell.

It is well established that the peripheral action of insulin is impaired in several clinical conditions, the most common being obesity and maturity-onset diabetes (non-insulin-dependent diabetes, type II diabetes). The latter conditions are associated with insulin resistance; that is, the ability of the hormone to act on target tissue metabolism (fat, liver, muscle) is diminished. It is believed [32] that this resistance is due to a combination of decreased ability of insulin to bind to its receptor (receptor defect) plus diminished signals from the insulin receptor to metabolic events occurring inside the cell (postreceptor defect). The receptor defect appears first. It is associated with mild insulin resistance leading to glucose intolerance in obesity and only slightly elevated blood glucose levels in diabetes. The postreceptor defect appears later and, in combination with the already existing receptor defect, enhances insulin resistance so that glucose homeostasis is further impaired. The latter may turn obesity into overt diabetes and mild diabetes into a more severe hyperglycemic form. These conditions, however, are mainly based on studies of the hypoglycemic effect of insulin and measurements of insulin receptor binding to blood cells, which are not target cells for insulin. Recent studies have indicated that the action of insulin in human fat cells in obesity and diabetes does not fit into the current insulin resistance model. Insulin receptor binding appears to be normal in obese [33] and diabetic [34] fat cells. In both obesity and diabetes, the insulin actions on glucose transport [35,36] and glucose metabolism [34,37] are clearly blunted, whereas the antilipolytic effect of the hormone is normal or even enhanced [34,38]. These findings are best explained as follows: In obese and diabetic human adipocytes, the insulin receptor status is normal; insulin resistance is due solely to postreceptor defects, which involve only the fate of glucose, whereas the postreceptor pathways for the antilipolytic effect are normal or even stimulated. Changes of insulin action in human fat cells due to a *combination* of receptor and postreceptor defects have been recently described, however. Changes due to a combination of defects have been observed recently in conditions such as aging, fasting, and hyper- and hypothyroidism [37,39,40].

THE ROLE OF ADIPOSE TISSUE IN DISEASED STATES

According to the previous discussion of hormone action, it is obvious that lipid metabolism in adipose tissue is disturbed in several clinical conditions. In most cases, as seen in obesity and diabetes mellitus, there is an accelerated lipolysis both in the resting state and after hormone stimulation, causing chronic elevation of the circulating FFA level. A high FFA level may be harmful for the body; for example, it may be toxic for the heart [41]. Furthermore, FFA competes with glucose as energy substrate for muscle tissue. The heart may prefer uptake of the lipid instead of the carbohydrate whenever there is an excess of FFA so that glucose intolerance develops [42]. Finally, FFA is a substrate for the synthesis of TG-rich lipoproteins in the liver. An elevation of the FFA level may stimulate the production of these lipoproteins and induce hypertriglyceridemia [43]. Hypertriglyceridemia, in turn, may cause arteriosclerosis.

A direct role of adipose tissue in the development of hypertriglyceridemia has been postulated, because it has been observed that the ability of fat cells to assimilate FFA from the blood was diminished in hypertriglyceridemic patients [44]. It has recently been shown that hypertriglyceridemia may be due to a defect in the ability of fat cells to synthesize TG [45].

SITE DIFFERENCES IN SUBCUTANEOUS ADIPOSE TISSUE METABOLISM

It is well known that sex influences the distribution of body fat [46]. In women subcutaneous fat is mainly lo-

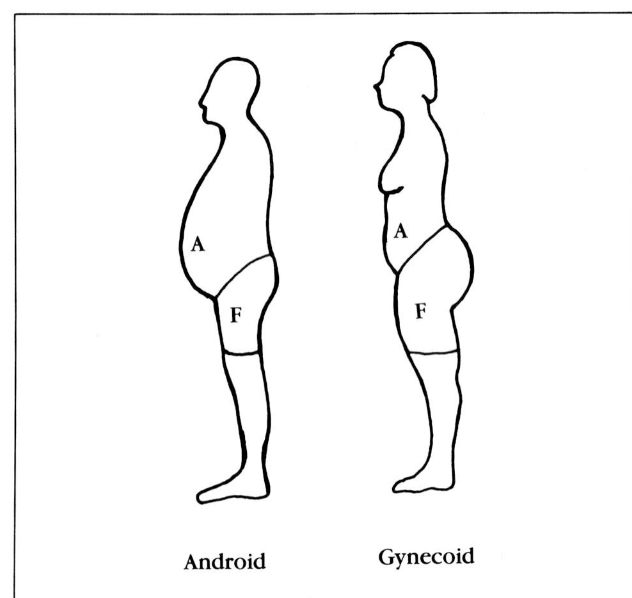

Fig. 6-6. Different distribution of subcutaneous fat in obesity. In android obesity, most frequently occurring in men, adiposity is localized in the abdominal (A) area. In gynecoid obesity, usually found among women, excess fat is confined to the hypogastric, gluteal, and upper femoral areas (F).

calized in the lower body segments (thigh, femoral, gluteal, and hypogastric regions). In males most of the subcutaneous fat is confined to the upper segment, preferentially the abdominal wall. This sex difference in body fat distribution is further pronounced in obesity. Male (android) and female (gynecoid) forms of obesity have been described (Fig. 6-6; see Table 6-1). This classification of obesity is of considerable clinical importance since the android fatness is associated with an increased incidence of arteriosclerosis, diabetes mellitus, and cardiovascular diseases. On the other hand, the gynecoid form has a lower risk of secondary complications of obesity [47]. The effect of steroid hormones on body fat distribution is well known to all physicians. In classical Cushing's patients, fat is accumulated in the trunk and lost in the extremities. Furthermore, women often complain that fat around the hip is more resistant to slimming than other adipose sites [48]. These examples indicate that there may be consistent variations in the behavior of regional subcutaneous fat.

A great deal of data has accumulated indicating that site differences in adipocyte metabolism do exist and may cause local variations in fat deposition and resistance to slimming of certain defined subcutaneous fatty regions. These regional variations in subcutaneous fat cell metabolism have been recently reviewed in detail [49]. In most studies, subcutaneous abdominal fat has been compared to femoral fat in obese women (Table 6-3). The results of these studies are summarized as follows: Fat cells are larger in the femoral than in the ab-

Table 6-3. Regional variations in subcutaneous adipose tissue metabolism of obese women

	Abdominal site (A)	Variation	Femoral site (F)
Fat cell size	A	<	F
Lipolysis	A	>	F
TG synthesis	A	<	F
Catecholamine action	A	>	F
Insulin action	A	<	F
Effect of fasting	Decrease in fat cell size Marked increase in lipolysis and marked decrease in TG synthesis		No change Less marked changes

dominal region. During 1 week of fasting, there is a decrease in fat cell size in the abdominal but not in the femoral site. In the fed state, the breakdown of TG is more pronounced in abdominal than in femoral fat, whereas the opposite phenomenon is true for synthesis of TG. During fasting there is an increased rate of TG breakdown and a diminished rate of TG synthesis in all fatty regions. These effects of fasting, however, are more pronounced in abdominal than in femoral fat. The effects of insulin (which builds up fat) and of catecholamines (which mainly break down fat) are also different in the abdominal and femoral regions. In the fed state, the action of catecholamines is marked in the abdominal site, whereas the insulin effect is most prominent in the femoral region. These site variations are further pronounced during fasting. Taken together these regional variations in metabolism go a long way toward explaining the typical distribution of body fat in gynecoid obesity and may also be a reason why many women find it almost impossible to diet away fat in the femoral (thigh) adipose region.

Summary

Adipose tissue is a metabolically active organ that plays a central role in the regulation of the energy balance of humans. The adipose tissue mass develops by an increase in the number and size of adipocytes. There is a gradual enlargement of each fat cell throughout life. The increase in cell number, however, is most prominent in early childhood and declines gradually during adolescence so that the total fat cell number usually is constant during adult life.

As far as hormonal regulation is concerned, only catecholamines and insulin have a pronounced acute effect on adipose tissue metabolism in humans. In several clinical conditions, there is an acceleration of lipid mobilization from adipose tissue that partly can be explained by changes in the action of catecholamines and insulin and may be of importance for the development of common disorders such as diabetes, cardiovascular disease, and arteriosclerosis. A direct role of adipose tissue in the development of hypertriglyceridemia has been postulated, because this disorder is associated with a decreased ability of human fat cells to store lipids.

Regional differences in fat cell metabolism are described that may cause local variations in fat deposition and resistance to slimming of some fatty regions. In obese women, it has been observed that lipid mobilization is most pronounced in the abdominal region and lipid synthesis most marked in the region around the lateral thigh. These regional differences are further pronounced if the obese women are subjected to therapeutic fasting.

Obesity can be classified according to the degree of adipose cellularity and also by fat distribution. Hyperplastic obesity (too many fat cells) responds poorly to conservative treatment with diet plus exercise. The android distribution of fat (excess abdominal fat) occurs mostly among men and carries with it a high morbidity and mortality.

References

1. Hales, C. N., Luzio, J. P., and Siddle, K. Hormonal control of adipose tissue lipolyis. *Biochem. Soc. Symp.* 43:97, 1977.
2. Wasserman, F. The development of adipose tissue. In A. E. Renold and G. F. Cahill (Eds.), Adipose Tissue. Baltimore: Williams & Wilkins, 1965. P. 87.
3. Hirsch, J., and Batchelor, B. Adipose tissue cellularity in human obesity. *Clin. Endocrinol. Metab.* 5:299, 1976.
4. Salans, L. B., Cushman, S. W., and Weismann, R. E. Studies of human adipose tissue. Adipose cell size and number in nonobese and obese patients. *J. Clin. Invest.* 52:929, 1973.
5. Knittle, J. L., Timmers, K., Ginsberg-Fellner, F., Brown, R. E., and Katz, D. P. The growth of adipose tissue in children and adolescents. Cross-sectional and longitudinal studies of adipose cell number and size. *J. Clin. Invest.* 63:239, 1979.
6. Van, R. L. R., Baytiss, C. E., and Roncarci, D. A. K. Cytological and enzymological characterization of adult human adipocyte precursors in culture. *J. Clin. Invest.* 58:699, 1976.
7. Roncarci, D. A. K., Lan, D. C. W., and Kindler, S. Exaggerated replication in culture of adipocyte precursors from massively obese persons. *Metabolism* 30:425, 1981.
8. Sims, E. A., Danforth, J. E., Horton, E. S., Bray, G. A., Glennon, J. A., and Salans, L. B. Endocrine and metabolic effects of experimental obesity in man. *Recent Prog. Horm. Res.* 29:457, 1973.

9. Krotkiewski, M., Sjöström, L., Björntorp, P., Carlgren, G., Garellick, G., and Smith, U. Adipose tissue cellularity in relation to prognosis for weight reduction. *Int. J. Obes.* 1:395, 1977.

10. Björntorp, P., and Ostman, J. Human adipose tissue. Dynamics and regulation. *Adv. Metab. Disord.* 5:277, 1971.

11. Björkhem, I., Arner, P., Thore, A., and Östman, J. Sensitive kinetic bioluminescent assay of glycerol release from human fat cells. *J. Lipid Res.* 22:1142, 1981.

12. Pedersen, O., and Gliemann, J. Hexose transport in human adipocytes: Factors influencing the response to insulin and kinetics of methylglucose and glucose transport. *Diabetologia* 20:630, 1981.

13. Pedersen, O., Hjöllund, E., Beck-Nielsen, H., Lindskov, H. O., Sonne, O., and Gliemann, J. Insulin receptor binding and receptor mediated insulin degradation in human adipocytes. *Diabetologia* 20:636, 1981.

14. Engfeldt, P., Arner, P., Wahrenberg, H., and Östman, J. An assay for beta-adrenergic receptors in isolated human fat cells. *J. Lipid Res.* 23:715, 1982.

15. Engfeldt, P., Arner, P., Kimura, H., Wahrenberg, H., and Östman, J. Determination of adrenoceptors of the alpha$_2$-subtype on isolated human fat cells. *Scand. J. Clin. Lab. Invest.* 43:208, 1983.

16. Fain, J. N., and Garcia-Sáinz, J. A. Adrenergic regulation of adipocyte metabolism. *J. Lipid Res.* 24:945, 1983.

17. Arner, P., and Östman, J. Importance of the cyclic AMP concentrations of the rate of lipolysis in human adipose tissue. *Clin. Sci. Mol. Med.* 59:199, 1980.

18. Engfeldt, P., Arner, P., and Östman, J. Studies on the regulation of phosphodiesterase in human adipose tissue in vitro. *J. Clin. Endocrinol. Metab.* 56:501, 1983.

19. Arner, P., and Östman, J. Relationship between the tissue level cyclic AMP and the fat cell size of human adipose tissue. *J. Lipid Res.* 19:613, 1978.

20. Arner, P., Engfeldt, P., and Nowak, J. In vivo observations on the lipolytic effect of noradrenaline during therapeutic fasting. *J. Clin. Endocrinol. Metab.* 53:1207, 1981.

21. Arner, P., Engfeldt, P., and Östman, J. Blood glucose control and lipolysis in diabetes mellitus. *Med. Scand.* 208:297, 1980.

22. Arner, P., Wennlund, A., and Östman, J. Regulation of lipolysis by human adipose tissue in hyperthyroidism. *J. Clin. Endocrinol. Metab.* 48:415, 1979.

23. Arner, P., Engfeldt, P., and Östman, J. Relationship between lipolysis, cyclic AMP size in human adipose tissue during fasting and in diabetes mellitus. *Metabolism* 28:198, 1979.

24. Engfeldt, P., Arner, P., Bolinder, J., Wennlund, A., and Östman, J. Phosphodiesterase activity in human adipose tissue. *J. Chronic Dis. Ther. Res.* 5:184, 1981.

25. Rosenquist, U. Adrenergic response in hypothyroidism. An in vitro study on human adipose tissue and rabbit aorta. *Acta Med. Scand.* [Suppl] 532:1, 1972.

26. Czech, M. Insulin action. *Am. J. Med.* 70:142, 1981.

27. Larner, J. Insulin mediator—fact or fancy? *J. Cyclic Nucleotide Res.* 8:289, 1982.

28. Goldfine, J. D. Does insulin need a second messenger? *Diabetes* 26:148, 1977.

29. Kahn, C. R. The insulin receptor and insulin: The lock and key to diabetes. *Clin. Res.* 31:326, 1983.

30. Cushman, S. W., and Wardzata, L. J. Potential mechanism of insulin action on glucose transport in the isolated rat adipose cell. *J. Biol. Chem.* 255:4758, 1980.

31. Suzuki, K., and Kono, T. Evidence that insulin causes translocation of glucose transport activity to the plasma membrane from an intracellular storage site. *Proc. Natl. Acad. Sci. USA* 77:2542, 1980.

32. Olefsky, J. M., and Kolterman, O. G. Mechanisms of insulin resistance in obesity and non-insulin-dependent (Type II) diabetes. *Am. J. Med.* 70:151, 1981.

33. Amatudra, J. H., Livingston, J. N., and Lockwood, D. H. Insulin receptor: Role in the resistance of human obesity to insulin. *Science* 188:264, 1975.

34. Bolinder, J., Östman, J., and Arner, P. Postreceptor defects causing insulin resistance in normoinsulinemic non-insulin-dependent diabetes mellitus. *Diabetes* 31:911, 1982.

35. Ciaraldi, T. P., Kolterman, O. G., and Olefsky, J. M. Mechanisms of the postreceptor defect in insulin action in human obesity: Decrease in glucose transport system activity. *J. Clin. Invest.* 68:875, 1981.

36. Ciaraldi, T. P., Kolterman, O. G., Scarlett, J. A., Kav, M., and Olefsky, J. M. Role of glucose transport in the postreceptor defect of non-insulin-dependent diabetes mellitus. *Diabetes* 31:1016, 1982.

37. Pedersen, O., Höllund, E., and Schwartz Sörensen, N. Insulin receptor binding and insulin action in human fat cells: Effects of obesity and fasting. *Metabolism* 31:884, 1982.

38. Arner, P., Bolinder, J., Engfeldt, P., and Östman, J. The antilipolytic effect of insulin in human adipose tissue in obesity, diabetes mellitus, hyperinsulinemia, and starvation. *Metabolism* 30:753, 1981.

39. Bolinder, J., Östman, J., and Arner, P. Influence of aging on insulin receptor binding and metabolic effects of insulin and human adipose tissue. *Metabolism* 32:959, 1983.

40. Arner, P., Bolinder, J., Wennlund, A., and Östman, J. Influence of thyroid hormone level on insulin action in human adipose tissue. *Diabetes* In press, 1984.

41. Oliver, M. F. The vulnerable myocardium. *Lancet* 2:560, 1973.

42. Randle, P. J., Garland, P. B., Hales, C. N., and Newsholme, E. A. The glucose—fatty acid cycle, its role in insulin sensitivity and the metabolic disturbances of diabetes mellitus. *Lancet* 1:785, 1963.

43. Havel, R. J. Conversion of plasma free fatty acids into triglyceride of plasma lipoprotein fractions in man. *Metabolism* 10:1031, 1961.

44. Walldins, G. Fatty acid incorporation into human adipose tissue (FIAT) in hypertriglyceridemia. *Acta Med. Scand.* [Suppl] 591:1, 1976.

45. Arner, P., Engfeldt, P., and Östman, J. Changes in the metabolism of fatty acids in obese patients with primary hypertriacylglycerolemia. *J. Lipid Res.* 23:422, 1982.

46. Vague, J., Boyer, J., Jubelin, J., Nickolino, C., and Pinto, C. Adipo-muscular ratio in human subjects. In J. Vague and R. Denton (Eds.), Physiopathology of Adipose Tissue. Amsterdam: Excerpta Medica, 1969. P. 460.

47. Krotkiewski, M., Björntorp, P., Sjöström, L., and Smith, U. Impact of obesity on metabolism in men and women. Importance of regional adipose tissue distribution. *J. Clin. Invest.* 72:1150, 1983.

48. Garn, S. M. Fat patterning and fat intercorrelation in the female. *Hum. Biol.* 29:19, 1956.

49. Arner, P. Site differences in human subcutaneous adipose tissue metabolism in obesity. *Aesth. Plast. Surg.* In press, 1984.

CHAPTER 7

Body Image Disturbance and Eating Disorders

James M. Ferguson

Background

Many women feel uncomfortable about the size and shape of their body. Recently a popular magazine [1] surveyed 33,000 women and asked them a variety of questions about their self-esteem and their degree of satisfaction with the size of their body and its proportion. A startling picture emerged of body dissatisfaction. Seventy-five percent of the sample felt too fat despite weight measurements indicating that only 25% were by any measure overweight. Actual body weight correlated poorly with self-image. Those who were too thin had the same feelings as those who were demonstrably overweight. Forty-five percent of the underweight women felt they were too fat and dieted regularly. Only 6% of the 33,000 women were happy with their bodies.

The surveyors asked the sample of women about areas of their body that embarrassed them or with which they were dissatisfied. Twenty-nine percent were dissatisfied with their breasts, 64% with their stomach, 61% with their hips, and 72% with their thighs.

When asked how they feel when they see their nude bodies in a mirror, 32% felt anxious, 12% felt depressed, and 5% felt repulsed, while only 12% were proud and 27% content. Twelve percent were "neutral." This obsession with weight and body size is often socially disrupting in both single and married women. Nineteen percent said weight affected their desire for or enjoyment of sexual activities, and 46% felt self-conscious and inhibited if they felt overweight. Eighty percent felt they had to be slim to be attractive to men, and 67% felt that other women would judge their appearance unfavorably according to weight.

During the past recession in a similar survey, a magazine asked women readers what their most pressing problem was on a day-to-day basis. The answer was not finances or women's rights, *but rather diet and body size and shape.*

These concerns are not confined to the readers of *Glamour Magazine* or to upwardly mobile independent young women. Johnson et al. [2] surveyed 1286 adolescent females between the ages of 13 and 19 in Chicago public schools. Forty-eight percent of the girls surveyed felt they were either overweight or very overweight; however, only 14% of these girls were seen as overweight by friends. Fifty-two percent had begun to diet seriously before the age of 14, and 37% had been urged to diet by their parents despite the lack of demonstrable obesity in most of the sample. Among these girls, 16% self-induced vomiting after eating too much as a way of controlling their weight.

This dissatisfaction with body size is not new. In 1966 Huenemann et al. [3] reported that 63 to 70% of teenage subjects were dissatisfied with their bodies and wanted to lose weight. Theander [4] reported that up to 70% of Swedish teenage girls were dissatisfied with their body weight and shape in a survey done more than 20 years ago. Although these earlier surveys indicate widespread dissatisfaction with body size, they fail to show the high incidence of resulting psychopathology in the teenage and postadolescent population we see today.

Some of the societal factors that mirror the result of these surveys were reported by Garner et al. [5]. They made a study of the winners of the Miss America Pageant Contest and found that, over time, the average weight of the contestants declined at a rate of 0.13 kg per year, with the winner's weight declining at an average yearly rate of 0.17 kg despite an increase in height year after year. The winner was always thinner than the average contestant. The most recent contest winner in this publication was approximately 20% under ideal body weight for her height. In his study, Garner also showed that measurements of *Playboy* centerfold playmates have changed significantly during the past 20 years: bust measurements are significantly smaller, waists are larger, hips are smaller, and there has been an overall increase in height. Total body weight, despite the increase in height, has remained constant or decreased slightly.

With this widespread societal preoccupation with body size and shape, and the large number of individuals caught up in this intense preoccupation, it is not unexpected that, for some individuals, body weight regulation will become pathological. The body image disturbance is most frequently seen in the two eating disorders—anorexia nervosa and bulimia.

The concept of body image disturbance was developed in the 1930s to explain or understand individuals who have a difficult time perceiving their body as it physically exists [6]. Initial examples of this type of disorder included neurological illnesses that affected a part of the peripheral or central nervous system, disorders that were the result of metabolic or toxic disturbances, disorders occurring after an acute dismemberment (the phantom limb syndrome), and those cases in which the individual, for psychological reasons, could not perceive himself as he really was [7].

Most adolescents go through a period of confusion about their body size, shape, and function at the time of puberty. For an adolescent girl to not believe others who tell her she is normal, or that breast development and wider hips are a sign of sexual maturation, is not unusual. It is common to develop fears of this development, to be unduly shy, and to want to turn back the clock and be a little girl again. Some girls, however, do not grow out of this stage, and they retain a very poorly defined concept of their body, usually accompanied by anxiety and a fear of sexuality, growing up, and being independent. Society today reinforces this adolescent confusion about body size, shape, and function in many young women with these concerns by strongly suggesting that "thin is in," that if one is thin enough, one will be happier, more successful, sexier, and in general have an easier lot in life. Many, if not the majority of young women, make drastic attempts to reshape their body by dieting during this period in their life. Dieting is undertaken regardless of whether any amount of dietary restriction could possibly give them the size and proportions they desire. In past eras, this has perhaps been accomplished more by dress than by body reshaping. Today, it is not uncommon for a young woman to check out the size of her body undressed in front of a mirror several times a day, accompanied by elaborate measurements.

Most young women grow out of this intense preoccupation with shape, size, and weight and go on to live a normal life. Others remain intensely preoccupied and futilely pursue diet and exercise as ways of undoing what often is *genetically predestined.* These women often become anorexic or bulimic [8].

The purpose of this chapter is to make the reader aware of these disorders and to point out the high probability that individuals with them will seek out surgeons in the vain hope that there is some cure. The cure for which they are searching is to not grow up, to not be responsible, and to not age. Two brief clinical vignettes point out the type of individual:

Case 1. The patient is a 19-year-old single white female from an upper-class family. Her father is a prominent attorney. She has had a lifelong dissatisfaction with her body, and remembers at age 3 ripping her clothes off and screaming that she could not stand the feeling of constriction on her body. This history is verified by both parents independently. By age 10 the patient had experimented with drugs; by age 13 she was promiscuous and was a polydrug abuser. By age 15 she had undergone several months of inpatient treatment for drug and alcohol addiction. Despite the "cure" of her addictions and a cessation of her promiscuity, she usually ate and threw up ten times a day. She had a constant preoccupation with body size and shape. She made multiple suicide attempts and was quite depressed. Her family was distraught. The patient felt that if only she could become thin enough, all of her problems would cease. When asked what she would like to change about her body, she indicated she would like her breasts reduced in size, along with the sides of her chest. She wanted smaller hips and thighs and some off her abdomen. If somehow this could be done, she was certain that she would have no problems. At the time of complaining that she needed body reshaping, the patient weighed 90 pounds with a height of 5'2". Her real wish, of course, was to be totally asexual and have the body shape and size of a small child. This would help her to not be grown up in any way, and not to have to face issues of sexuality, education, and leaving home, or the consequences of her previous behavior. The patient's diagnoses were bulimia, depression, and a borderline personality disturbance.

Case 2. The patient is a 17-year-old woman of divorced parents. She had been a national roller-skating champion and thought that she was overweight and ill-proportioned, even though public acclaim and feedback from friends and critics told her she was neither. Particularly, she felt her legs were too large, despite the knowledge that their size was primarily the result of her extensive physical conditioning and the exercises she did daily as part of her skating routine. The patient began starving in an effort to change these proportions. She presented to the emergency room at 62 pounds after a suicide attempt. When asked about her body image, she stated she was fat and we should not allow her to eat so that she could become thinner. As she regained weight during an inpatient hospitalization, she was desperately unhappy, not particularly about body shape or the resumption of a feminine figure, but because this feminine figure made her look more mature. With an age-appropriate body, parents and friends expected her to become independent, to go to college, and to grow up.

Anorexia Nervosa

Two disorders of body image—anorexia nervosa and bulimia—have been well defined. Anorexia nervosa has been described since 1694, when Richard Morton described his first case as looking like a skeleton clad only in skin [9]. Anorexia nervosa is characterized by:

1. An intense fear of becoming obese that does not diminish as weight loss progresses
2. A disturbance of body image; for example, claiming to "feel fat" even when emaciated
3. Weight loss of 25%
4. A refusal to maintain body weight over minimal normal weight for age and height
5. No known physical illness that would cause weight loss

Approximately 1 of every 100 high school girls meets these diagnostic criteria today. Many more meet some of these criteria, but they may not progress beyond a "forme fruste" of the disease. These incidence figures make it apparent that anorexia nervosa is the most common life-threatening disorder of adolescence. There are four ages of onset of the disease:

1. The young anorexic, age 11 to 15, who is usually involved in family disturbances
2. The teenage anorexic, age 15 to 20, who has difficulty with separation from home, growing up, and sexuality
3. The newly married anorexic who develops the disorder after the birth of her first child, almost as though

to compete with the baby for the attention of her husband and parents
4. The woman who develops anorexia nervosa in middle age

The middle-aged anorexic patient often has a profound body image disturbance and desperately tries anything she can think of to hold off the ravages of age, to look adolescent, and to perfect her body. Usually this struggle begins when her husband is in mid-career and very emotionally and physically involved elsewhere, and when her children are in their late teenage years or leaving home. This group of patients is frequently hospitalized for the evaluation of their thinness, without the physician thinking of the teenage disorder, anorexia nervosa, in the differential diagnosis.

Most patients with anorexia nervosa suffer from a severe psychobiological illness. They try to reduce their size in order to become nothing. Often this begins in the pursuit of beauty, but soon it turns into a nightmare, called by Hilda Bruch "the cult of thin and beautiful" [10].

A few patients, however, may become anorexic because of the desperate attempt to become more proportional rather than thin per se. An example of this is a young woman with small breasts and relatively large thighs who reduces her weight in order to reduce the size of her thighs in a futile attempt to become proportionate. Since there is a relative sparing of the tissue in the thigh compared with the breasts during starvation, the disproportion persists into severe emaciation. This type of patient has a better prognosis and might, when at normal weight and psychologically stable, be a candidate for a cosmetic reshaping of her body to put an end to her need for self-starvation.

Bulimia

Bulimia is a common disorder of adolescence and early adulthood. Up to 30% of high school and college-age girls use vomiting as a significant way to control their weight [11]. Up to 10% cannot stop vomiting, even when urged by their physicians, parents, or boyfriends. Every time they eat something high in calories, they have an intense fear of becoming overweight. After a few months of self-induced vomiting after each "excessive" eating episode, the patients begin to binge eat and lose control of their eating. These binges can include enormous quantities of food, up to 40,000 calories a day. The desperate attempts at getting rid of the food include self-induced vomiting with repeated "cleansing" ritual, starvation, laxative (up to 200 a day) or enema abuse, the inappropriate use of diuretics, amphetamines, and over-the-counter diet preparations, and the use of syrup of Ipecac for weight control.

Bulimia is diagnosed in an individual who has the following symptoms:

1. Recurrent episodes of binge eating (defined as a rapid consumption of a large amount of food in a discrete period of time)
2. An awareness that the eating pattern is abnormal and a fear of not being able to stop eating voluntarily
3. A depressed mood with self-deprecating thoughts following eating binges
4. Binges not due to anorexia nervosa or any known physical disorder
5. At least three of the following characteristics are present:
   a. Consumption of high-caloric, easily ingested food during a binge
   b. Inconspicuous eating during a binge
   c. Termination of binge eating by abdominal pains, sleep, social interruption, or self-induced vomiting
   d. Repeated attempts to lose weight by severely restrictive diets, self-induced vomiting, the use of cathartics or diuretics
   e. Frequent weight fluctuations greater than 10 pounds due to alternating binge-eating and fasts

These patients are often attractive young women at or near normal weight. Despite this, they try to control their weight excessively because of a feeling of being fat and bloated or a morbid fear of becoming fat. They usually begin to crave carbohydrates after having been bulimic for some time; at the same time, they fear foods that contain carbohydrates. These patients put off eating until they finally give in to their urge to eat; then, having eaten something, they decide to go ahead and binge, knowing they will subsequently purge themselves of all the food. This cycle may be repeated 20 times a day. They usually do not want to be sexless like the majority of anorexics, but want to be more attractive partly as a way of combating their negative feelings about themselves. Within this group, most have extremely poor self-esteem and tend to project this negative opinion of themselves. Although the majority start the bulimic pattern as a way of weight control, within a few months the binging takes on new characteristics. Bulimics find that it is an antidote to feelings of loneliness, boredom, frustration, anger, and even happiness. With the habit, they can gorge on all types of fattening foods, knowing full well they will not have to suffer the consequences.

Within the group of bulimics there are several other diagnoses that are significant, particularly in a clinical situation. At least one-third of these patients are polydrug abusers or alcoholics, one-third compulsively steal, and one-third are episodically promiscuous. When one looks at the personality structure of the bulimic, approximately 50% have a borderline personality disturbance. This personality disturbance is diagnosed in patients who have at least five of the following traits:

1. Impulsivity in at least two areas that are potentially self-damaging; for example, spending, sex, gambling, substance abuse, shoplifting, overeating, or physical self-damaging acts
2. A pattern of unstable and intense interpersonal relationships
3. Inappropriate or intense anger and lack of control of anger with frequent displays of temper or constant anger
4. An identity disturbance manifested by uncertainty about self-image, gender, long-term goals, career choice, values and loyalties, affective instability with marked shifts of mood from normal to depression to irritability to anxiety within a few hours
5. Intolerance of being alone
6. Physically self-damaging acts
7. A chronic feeling of emptiness or boredom

Individuals with this constellation of psychological traits expect the physician or any authority figure to make everything perfect. When their expectations are not realized, they tend to focus an intense anger and blame on the other person rather than look at their own unrealistic expectations. In the case of cosmetic surgery, these individuals often believe that a change in body size or shape will change their entire life. These patients expect miracles and become extremely angry when they are not forthcoming.

Lipolysis offers individuals a rapid, radical way to reshape their body size and proportions. Never in history has there been such a satisfactory technique for giving people the power to transform their bodies from a genetically determined shape to a cosmetically determined shape. As with many types of plastic surgery, most patients will undoubtedly be benefited by, and pleased with, the outcome. However, the question must be asked: Are there some foreseeable psychological consequences to this type of intervention with one's body size and shape? There are no psychological outcome studies in the area of suction lipectomy, although there have been detailed studies of patients who had surgical intervention for morbid obesity.

It was initially feared that this radical intervention with a subsequent weight loss of 150 to 200 pounds would lead to severe depression or some other serious psychological consequence. This fear was based on the observation that total fasting often leads to depression in the obese population, and the then popular theory that somehow fat was a "character armour" that protected people from their impulses and aggressiveness. What was found was exactly the opposite. Patients successfully undergoing weight loss after gastrointestinal bypass surgery did extremely well; their image of themselves improved; their assertiveness improved; the quality of their interpersonal life improved; the quality of their sexual relations improved; and many felt like they had a new lease on life [12,13]. In the area of facial and breast surgery, the majority of patients do extremely well, given the proper informed consent and given realistic expectations about the outcome of the procedure.

There are broad predictors of successful psychological outcome, both from the plastic surgery literature and from the intestinal and gastric bypass surgery literature, many of which confirm what is standard practice. These predictors of successful outcome include a realistic discussion with the patient before surgery about the outcome and the exclusion of patients who have magical expectations of lifestyle change and believe there is no need for them to be involved in this change. Patients who are psychotic, extremely argumentative, or those with multiple psychosomatic complaints do poorly. Likewise, patients who are ambivalent about surgery or come in wanting their mind to be made up for them should probably be told to go home and think about it. Those patients with a marked body image disturbance should be excluded, at least until they undergo a period of counseling to help set some limits on their expectations. These are the patients who feel fat at a low body weight and those who complain bitterly about the size of various parts of their body beyond what could be reasonably expected given the actual measurements. Finally, those patients who have the characteristics of a borderline personality disturbance with poor impulse control, exaggerated anger, polydrug abuse, and poor

relationships should be included only with great caution.

When patients are properly screened, lipolysis should both enhance the quality of life for these patients and fulfill realistic expectations for success.

References

1. *Glamour Magazine.* Feb., 1984. P. 198.
2. Johnson, C. L., et al. A Descriptive Survey of Dieting and Bulimic Behavior in a Female High School Population. In *Understanding Anorexia Nervosa and Bulimia.* Columbus, Ohio: Ross Laboratories, 1983. P. 14.
3. Huenemann, et al. A longitudinal study of gross body composition and body conformation and their association with food and activity in a teenage population. *Am. J. Clin. Nutr.* 18:325, 1966.
4. Theander, S. Anorexia nervosa: A psychiatric investigation of 94 female patients. *Acta Psychiatr. Scand.* [Suppl.] 214:1, 1970.
5. Garner, D., et al. Cultural expectation of thinness in women. *Psychol. Rep.* 47:483, 1980.
6. Schilder, P. *The Image and Appearance of the Human Body: Studies in the Constructive Energies of the Psyche.* London: Kegan-Paul, 1935.
7. Kolb, L. D. Disturbances of the Body Image. In M. Reiser (Ed.), *The American Handbook of Psychiatry* (vol. 4) (2nd ed.). New York: Basic Books, 1975.
8. Crisp, A. Anorexia Nervosa: Let Me Be! In *Extensive Aspects of Maturation.* London: Academic Press, 1980.
9. Morton, R. *Phthisiologica—or a Treatise of Consumption.* London: Smith and Walford, 1694.
10. Bruch, H. *Eating Disorders.* New York: Basic Books, 1973.
11. Halmi, K., Falk, J. R., and Schwartz, E. Binge-eating and vomiting: A survey of a college population. *Psychol. Med.* 2:697, 1981.
12. Solow, C., Silverfaub, P. M., and Swift, K. Psychosocial effects of intestinal bypass surgery for severe obesity. *N. Engl. J. Med.* 290:300, 1974.
13. Halmi, K., Stunkard, A. J., and Mason, E. E. Emotional responses to weight reduction by three methods: Gastric bypass, jejunoileal bypass, and diet. *Am. J. Clin. Nutr.* 33:446, 1980.

CHAPTER 8

Harmony and Proportion in the Female Form

Hale Tolleth

Humans, from the earliest times, have drawn, painted, or carved images of the human figure, as illustrated by the stick-like figures of the Hawaiian petroglyphs (Fig. 8-1) and the repeated geometric volumes of the Ice Age Venus (Fig. 8-2). They have decorated and shaped their bodies, even to the present, with tattoos, knives, and assorted devices to conform to some cultural logic [1]. The anthropologists may be able to explain such fashions, but only supposition exists to explain why such distortions appear attractive. Clearly, standards of form and beauty vary both in time and place; the bound foot of the Chinese does not appear attractive to the African, where steatopygia or the stretched neck is the mode. Within a culture, however, studies have shown a remarkable similarity in choices of beauty, suggesting that there are common bases for aesthetic judgment [2].

Standards of Shape and Proportion

Standards of shape and proportion have been sought in Western culture for at least 2500 years by artists, philosophers, and mathematicians [3,4]. Polycletus, a great sculptor of the fourth century BC, produced sculpture that has been described as "of exquisite beauty with a perfection of symmetry and balance and compensation which is the essence of classic art." He said that "a well-made work is the result of numerous measurements made to within a hair's breadth" (Fig. 8-3). His system and its rules, however, have been lost, although assuredly his system was complicated, arithmetic, and geometric. All that remains is a simplistic formula redrawn in art manuals to the present [5] (Fig. 8-4). Vitruvius, architect of the first century, knew of this system, wrote of it, and ultimately produced a rather homely figure drawn within a circle and a square. It illustrated well the burden of rigid formula preceded by imperfect analysis. It required the talent of Da Vinci to increase the size of the head and diminish the feet, producing the familiar "Vitruvian" diagram of human proportion (Fig. 8-5).

Koestler, in typical penetrating fashion, noted that "the philosophers of classicism saw beauty wherever mortal flesh testified to the immortal axioms of Euclidean geometry" [6]. The sculptor of the classic period in Greece attempted to illustrate the ethos of the culture—strength, purity, harmony, beauty, and knowledge of perfect form—which must be adduced from philosophic principles. The Pythagorean doctrine [7] that everything is arranged according to number and the theme of Plato that the cosmos has been harmoniously arranged had the appeal of great truth, however difficult to prove. Plato asserted that "the qualities of measure and proportion invariably constitute beauty and excel-

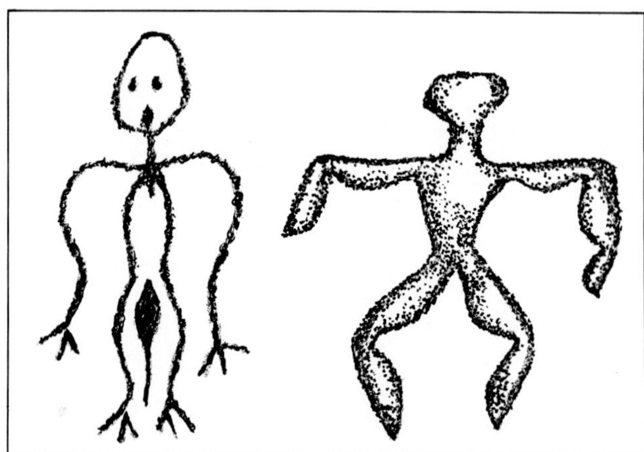

Fig. 8-1. Petroglyphs of rock designs from Hawaii.

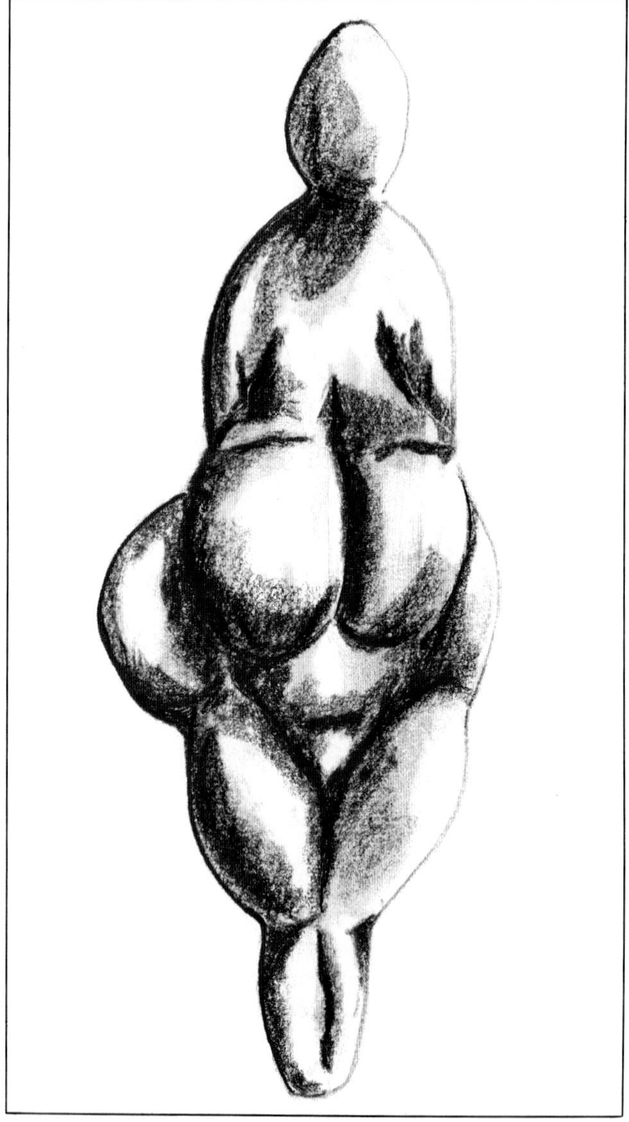

Fig. 8-2. One of a number of "Venuses" from prehistoric time. Detail is lacking. Relationship between volumes and the abstraction of the figure is striking.

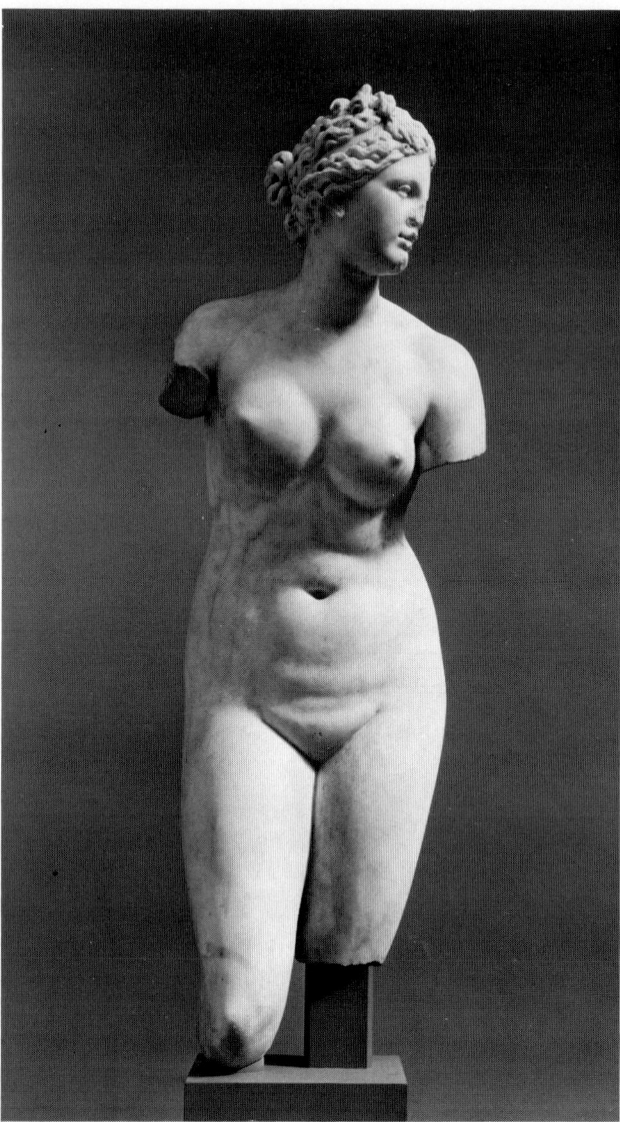

Fig. 8-3. Aphrodite, probably a Hellenistic copy of a fourth century BC original, shows exquisite attention to proportion. (Courtesy of the Metropolitan Museum of Art, Fletcher Fund.)

lence" [7]. The secrets of the pentagram and the magic of the divine proportion are still studied in certain societies and lodges to explain the mysteries of the universe.

The glorification or even the acknowledgment of the human body disappeared in Western art for more than one thousand years because the artist's vision was clouded for religious reasons. The flat and lifeless figure, neither anatomic nor proportioned to our eye, served until the Middle Ages when it gave way to the Renaissance. Around 1500 AD, Alberti devised a system called "Excupeda" where the body was divided into sixths called "pedes," the pedes into ten "inches," and the inches into ten "minuta"; any part of the body could

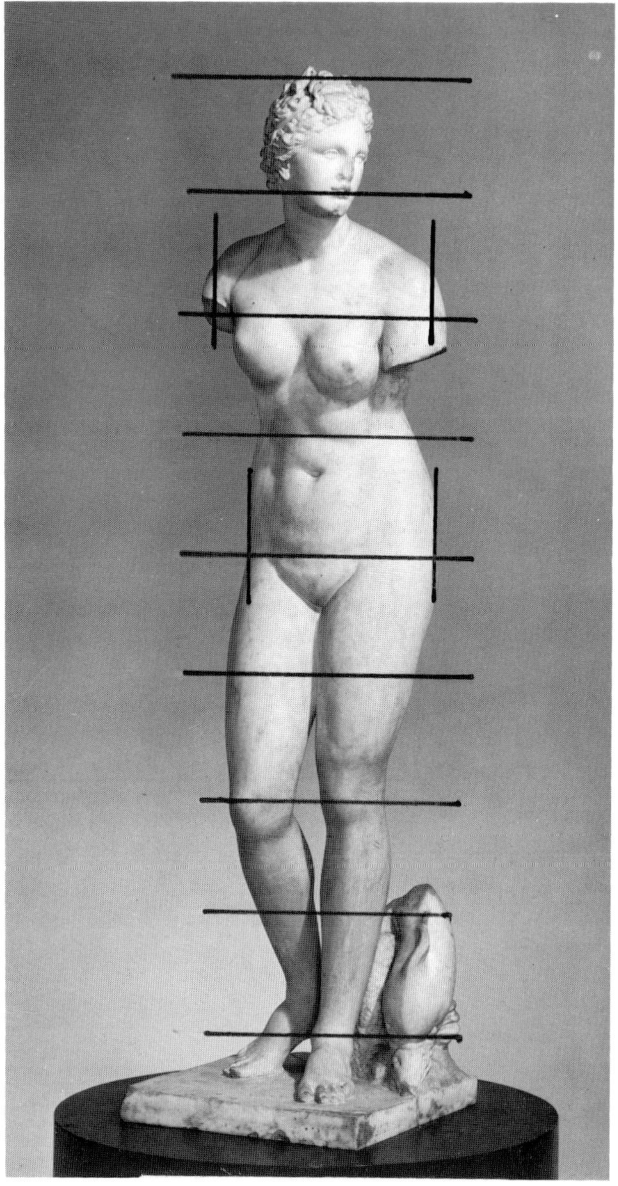

Fig. 8-4. The classic proportion: The figure is 7½ to 8 heads high, the hips 1½ heads wide, and the shoulders 1½ to 2 heads wide. (Courtesy of the Metropolitan Museum of Art, Fletcher Fund.)

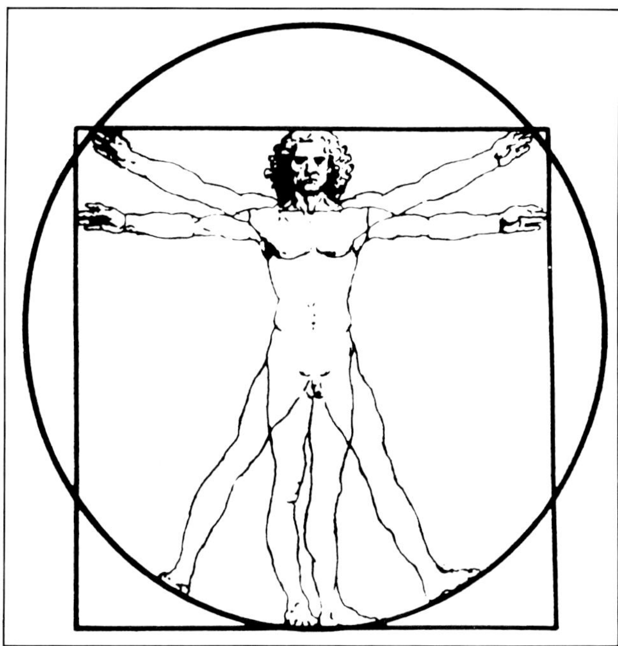

Fig. 8-5. Vitruvian Man as redrawn by Leonardo Da Vinci. A number of similar designs are extant.

then be described as a three-figured number. Da Vinci established "analogies" using head length as a primary unit; other parts of the body were compared to this unit. "From the chin to the starting part of the hair is the tenth part of the figure, from the pit of the stomach to the top of the chest is the sixth part, the foot is a sixth part and the forearm to the elbow a fourth part" [8].

Albrecht Dürer, also of great talent and mathematical bent, examined and discarded arithmetic, geometric, and aliquot part systems (Figs. 8-6 to 8-9). He had measured classical Greek sculpture and several hundred living persons, recognizing finally that the average is not necessarily beautiful and that proper numbers observed do not always result in beauty. He said, "good and better, in respect to beauty, are not easy to discern for it would be quite possible to make two different figures, neither conforming with the other, one stout and one thinner, and yet we might scarce be able to judge which of the two excelled in beauty" [9].

MATHEMATICAL STANDARDS

Several hundred years before Dürer, Leonardo of Pisa (also called Filius Bonacci or son of Bonacci), having been educated in Algeria by the Hindu-Moslems, published a book on mathematics that, among other things, promoted the Arabic numeral system with its decimal and zero. As part of the solution of a trivial mathematical riddle, he developed a sequence of numbers later called the Fibonacci series by Lucas, a nineteenth-century numbers theorist [10]. Beginning with two positive integers, 1 and 2, subsequent numbers in the series are obtained by adding the two previous numbers (e.g., 1-2-3-5-8-13-21---). These numbers have been analyzed with great interest since they demonstrate many curious mathematical properties. For example, the ratio between any two adjacent numbers (beginning with 3) is always 1 to 1.61803. It has been found that the sequence has application in computer programming, data sorting, data retrieval, and in random number generation.

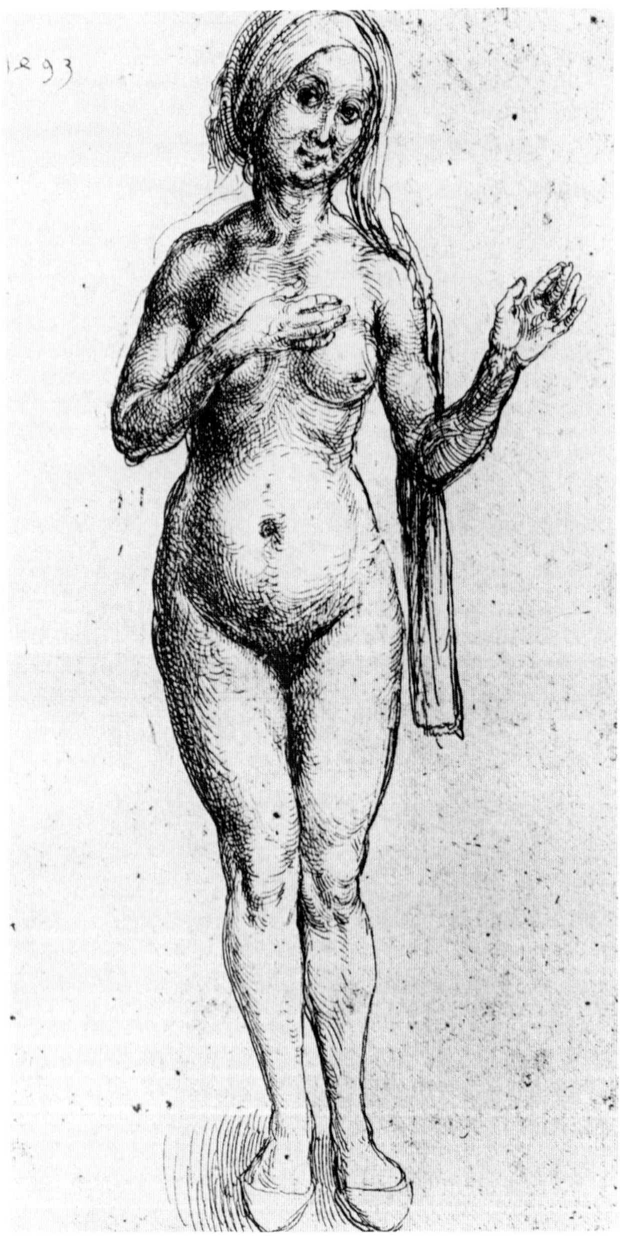

Fig. 8-6. Drawing of a young woman by Albrecht Dürer. Note roundness of forms and the sense of correctness imparted by attention to proportion. Compare volume of upper torso with hip and belly area.

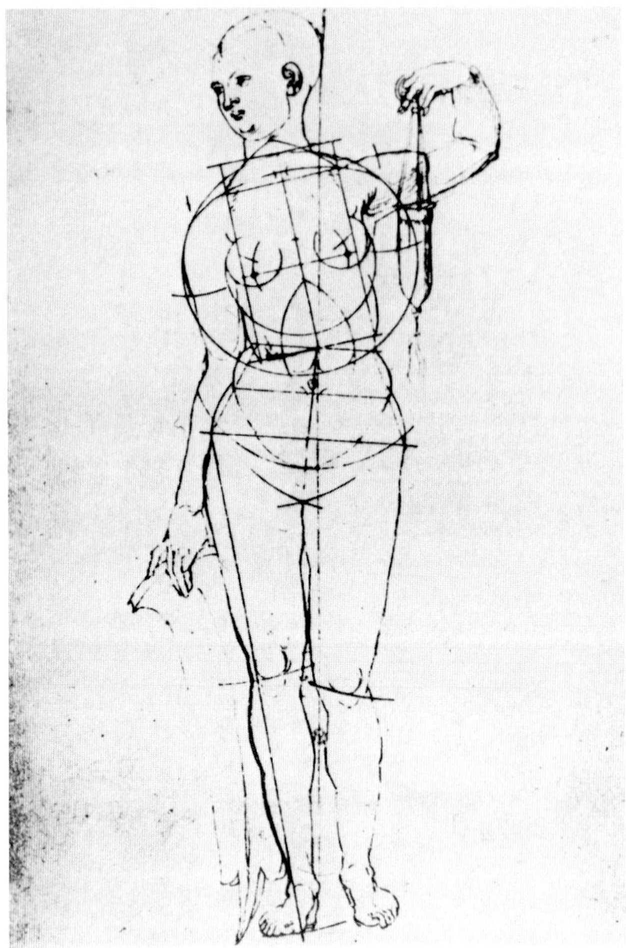

Fig. 8-7. One of many analytic approaches to the female figure used by Dürer.

Curiously, this irrational number, also called phi, φ, or the "Golden Proportion" by Pacioli, can be developed in another way. If a line is divided into two parts so that the ratio between the smaller of the lines and the longer is the same as the ratio between the longer and the whole, the proportion will always be 1.61803 to 1. A rectangle with sides of this dimension is called "golden," and a triangle with two sides in the same ratio is also called a "golden" triangle (Fig. 8-10). For the past several hundred years, the rediscovered ratio, which the Greeks knew, has been a basis for analysis of architecture, art, poetry, biologic structure, growth sequence, and the human body [11]. In recent years, use of the Fibonacci series has been used in facial analysis by dental specialists. "Traditionally and psychologically the proportion 1.618 has been considered particularly satisfying because of its combination of unity and dynamic variety. Whole and parts are nicely adjusted in strength so that

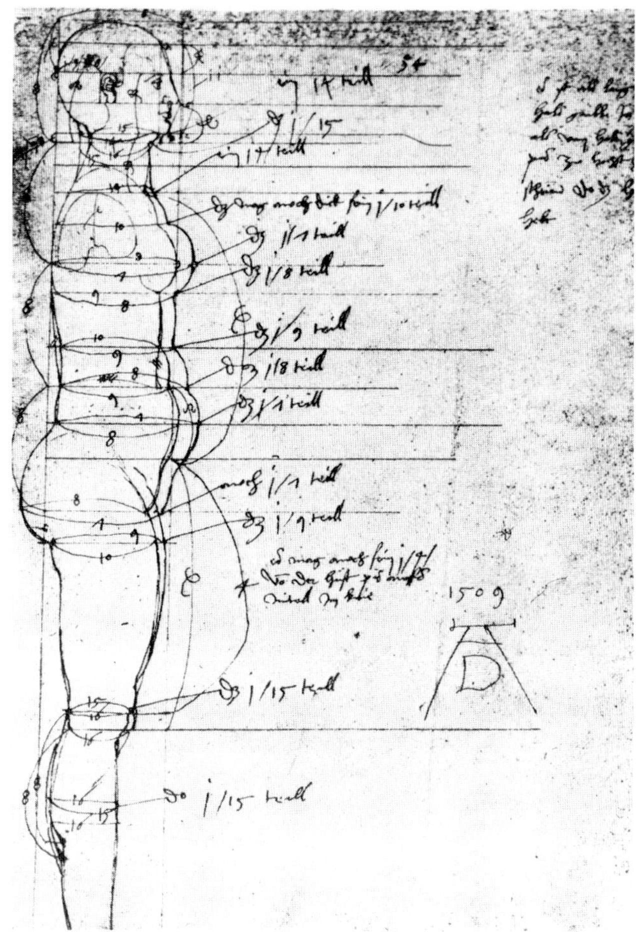

Fig. 8-8. Arithmetic and geometric analyses combined in a drawing done by Dürer.

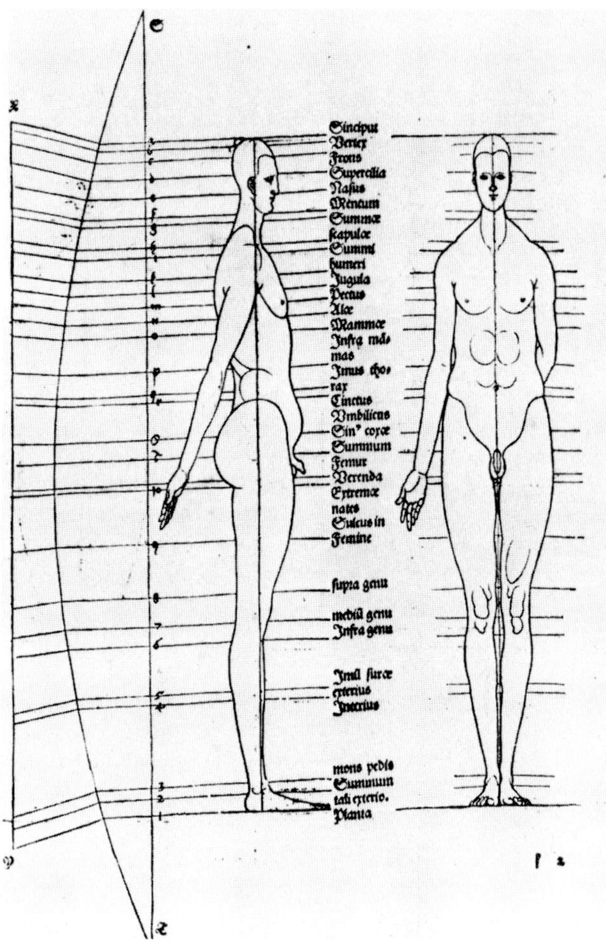

Fig. 8-9. An extraordinary, idealized design done by Dürer. On the left, the orthogonal lines can be extended into logarithmic curves allowing the possibility of proportional distortion.

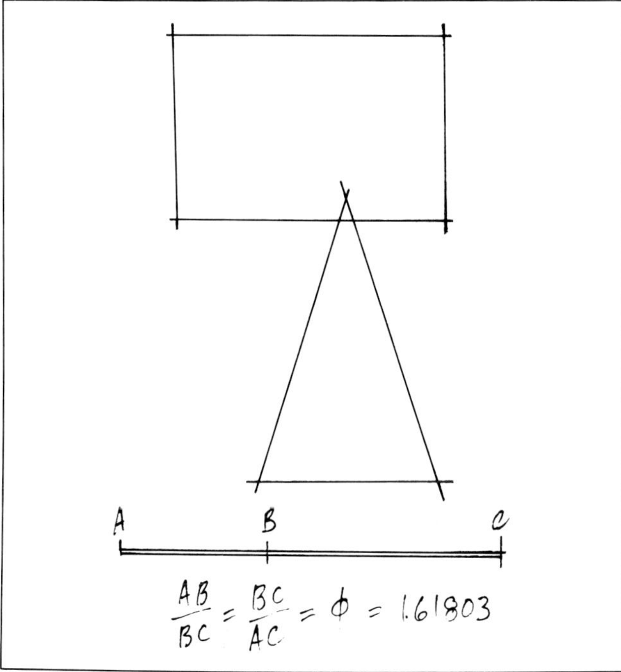

Fig. 8-10. The "golden" rectangle, triangle, and the primary proportion or phi. It has been widely used for analysis in art, architecture, and biology.

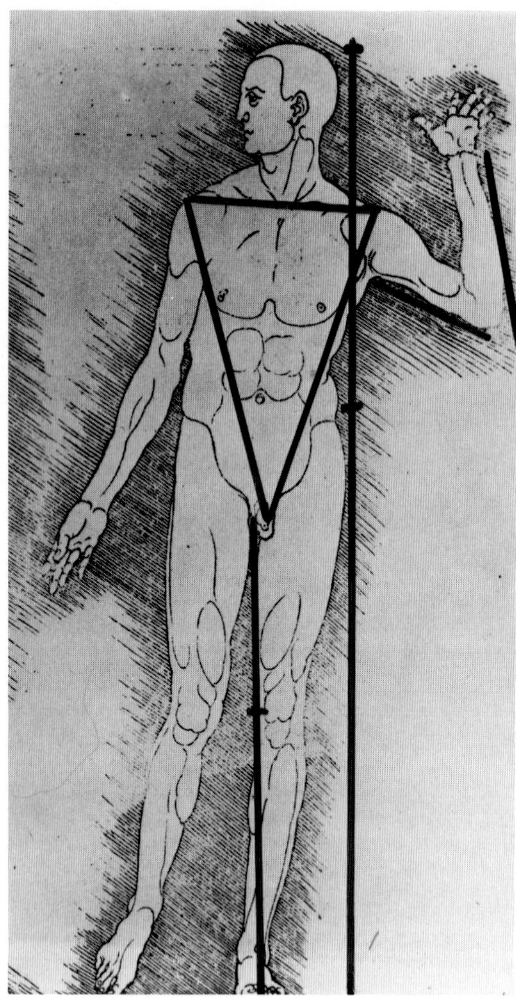

Fig. 8-11. The golden proportions superimposed on a Dürer drawing. A large number of φ relationships have been found in the human, especially in skeletal analysis.

the whole prevails without a split but at the same time the parts retain self-sufficiency" (Fig. 8-11) [7,12,13,14].

Perceptions of Form and Proportion

The preceding analyses are essentially linear; however, a well-ordered face or body in silhouette may be less attractive than in full view. The plastic surgeon, the sculptor, and the ordinary person see a rounded figure with size, shape, planes, shadows, and color. They may consciously know nothing of the numbers yet are quite able to determine what they perceive to be beautiful or not. Arnheim [12] points out, ". . . Just as a living organism cannot be described by an account of its anatomy, so the nature of a visual experience cannot be described in terms of inches of size, distinct degrees of angle, or wavelengths of hue."

The perception of what exists is not merely the pattern of light waves stimulating some of the 130 million rods and cones but is inevitably a product of age, culture, personality, training, and other factors, including the object itself and what is known about it. A picture of a dancer who has been stopped in mid-action looks different from a single frame taken from a filmstrip of the same dance. There are sufficient clues that the eye, in concert with some part of the brain, can often tell the difference between the photograph of a real tiger and that of a stuffed one. With that degree of subtlety demonstrated, it is no wonder that the brain can perceive proportions with little difficulty.

Until relatively recently, concern about human form was academic in the sense that derived rules, formulas, systems, and analyses were to be applied in understanding or producing objects of utility or beauty. Modification of the living human was limited by physiologic possibility and steered by some peculiar cultural force. Examples include the shaped skull of the Aztec or the stretched lip and ear of the Western African. The milliner's art allowed nonanatomic alterations that could be reversed or modified as fashion dictated (which was fortunately true in the case of the bustle). For the last 100 years or more, substantial anatomic alteration of the human form has become increasingly possible and popular to the point that restorations toward "normal" have given way to creating some "ideal." Fashion no longer dictates only to the designer of clothes and hair but to the surgeon as well, who, like the art student, must now learn the somewhat esoteric language of harmony and proportion. Mere science and technique will no longer suffice in aesthetic surgery; consideration of size, form, shape, symmetry, dynamic symmetry, balance, proportion, and harmony must become a part of the surgeon's considerations before surgical intervention [15].

Symmetry is the identical or orderly disposition of units on either side of a plane or about an axis. Vitruvius indicated that "symmetry resides in the correlation of measurements between various elements of the plane and between each of these elements and the whole" and "symmetry is harmoniously ordered or rhythmically repeated analogies" [7]. In the human figure, the relationships between the geometric form of the head and torso, between the upper torso and hips, and between the body above and below the waist should be studied. They are in "dynamic" symmetry if the repeated volume ratios appear consistent; some would say that these ratios and proportions should be golden [16]. Women recognize the necessity of balance between the volume and shape of the upper torso and bust *and* the hips and buttocks. Similarly, the slimness of arms or thickness of thighs should be in a satisfactory and symmetrical relationship to each other and to the torso.

Volume and mass are but a part; the shape and contours of the head, breast, or buttock are evaluated by their outline and by the shadows and highlights that define them [17,18], using the exquisite capacities of the right brain. Even in extreme postures, distortion, protrusion, interruptions, angularity, or abrupt changes should not be seen. Abnormal folds, creases, textural, or color changes are tolerable to the eye only to a point. Any peculiarity of joint position or abnormality of muscle prominence during activity will be immediately seen as "wrong" or unaesthetic and will be described as clumsy, awkward, or graceless. Unbalance or disturbance of the equilibrium relative to gravity, such as leaning forward or to one side, suggests an incomplete transition or an arrest of a normal movement and may be sensed as unpleasant, humorous, or pathologic.

Modifications of the Body

If one accepts the broadest view that any alteration of appearance is a modification of the body, then it appears to be an almost universal human trait. The plucking of eyebrows, removal of facial hair, haircutting, weight loss or gain, and muscle building are so common as to be dismissed as trivial, although they are not. Apparent changes in body form can be made by adjusting the length, fullness, or pattern of clothing and by wearing high heels, which increase height and definition of the calf muscles. Breasts are modified, shaped, uplifted, compressed, or separated by the brassiere; the derriere can be padded, compressed, or controlled. The fullness of a blouse or skirt, the judicious and cunning arrangement of pleats, the use of belts, sashes, and other accessories emphasize or camouflage according to a problem or fashion's dictates. Although fashion persists, it always changes and the surgeon must beware lest some anatomy be distorted, requiring a revision at a later time. The too-small, turned-up nose or excessively augmented breasts have been observed.

BODY WEIGHT AND MEASUREMENT

The first and most commonly modified parameter is body weight, since exercise and adjustment of diet often can be easily done. The briefest research shows that more than 30 million Americans carry 20% or more than their ideal weight and as many as 70 million are dieting. Atkin's book on dieting has sold more than 6½ million copies. It has been said that if the excess pounds were averaged, everyone over 18 years of age would have 14.3 excess pounds.

Obviously, there should be an ideal height-weight proportion, and there are many schemes and tables, including body mass nomograms, skin fold thickness measurements, and water displacement tests. Many women use the scale, measuring tape, and "rule of thumb," which indicates adding five points to a base 100 pounds for every inch of height over 5 feet to give an ideal weight. The airlines supposedly use this same method, adding only 3 or 4 pounds for every inch over 5 feet. Another standard of overweight is bust measurement exceeding the waist by 9 inches, the hips exceeding the bust by 3 inches, the thigh exceeding the calf by 8 inches, or the calf exceeding the ankle by 6 inches. Using the weight tables available from the Air Force, Blue Cross, Metropolitan Life Insurance Company, or Pinters Underwriters, a 5'5" female of medium frame could weigh between 124 and 141 pounds. Balanchine, the choreographer, on the other hand, would have been distressed at this weight since he believed the ideal dancer to be 5'7" and weigh but 95 pounds. Excess fat can also be determined by skin fold thickness, commonly checked on the back of the arm; 1 inch is critical, although ½ inch is better.

The localized accumulation of fat on an otherwise proportioned figure has been called cellulite, a term coined by the beauty expert Nicole Ronsard in 1973. Although the word has yet to make the dictionary, women's magazines suggest it to be an epidemic problem requiring special diets, massage, and exercise for its reduction. Cellulite is described as abnormal fat due to accumulation of metabolites and is distinguished by a ripply appearance when grasped between the thumb and forefinger. It is located on the arms, back, belly, buttocks, thighs, and knees. There is no acceptable evidence that cellulite differs in any regard from the normal human fat, which again places science and beauty on opposite sides of the fence.

Women assess the adequacy of their own figures using clothes size and fit and relationship between bust, waist, and hips. It is notable that expensive garments run a little larger. The centerfold subjects of *Playboy* magazines were reviewed and the figures given analyzed [19]. Average height was 5'6" and weight was 117.7 pounds. The bust varied from 34 to 36 inches, the average being 35.5 inches. The waist average was 23 inches, varying from 20 to 26 inches. The waist never exceeded 70% of the hip size. The bust and hip averages were the same; only in a few instances did the hip size exceed the bust measurement.

In a major anthropometry reference [20], measurements were recorded for WAC and WAF recruits, female pilots, and nurses. These measurements were compared with those of the *Playboy* centerfolds. The approximate averages were noted to be as follows: height, 5'4"; bust, 35 inches; waist, 26½ inches; and hip, 37½ inches. Relatively small differences were noted between these figures and those in *Playboy* magazine, although it is notable that the women in *Playboy,* on the average, were 2 inches taller and their hips were somewhat

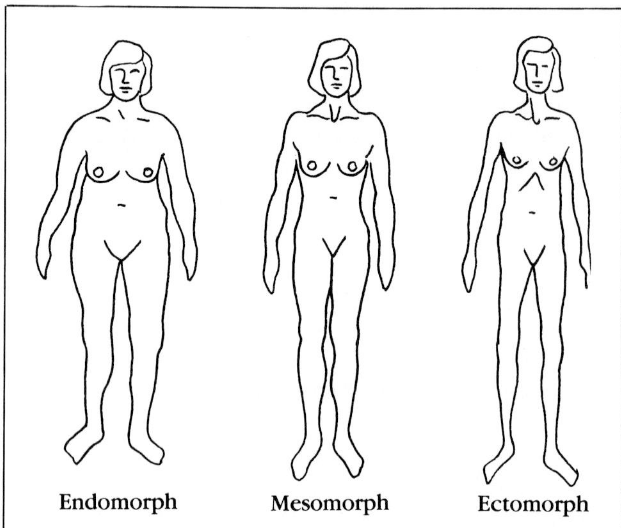

Fig. 8-12. The endo-, meso-, and ectomorph configurations as described by Sheldon. In his somatotyping, a figure is described by a three-digit code indicating the degree of presence of the characteristics.

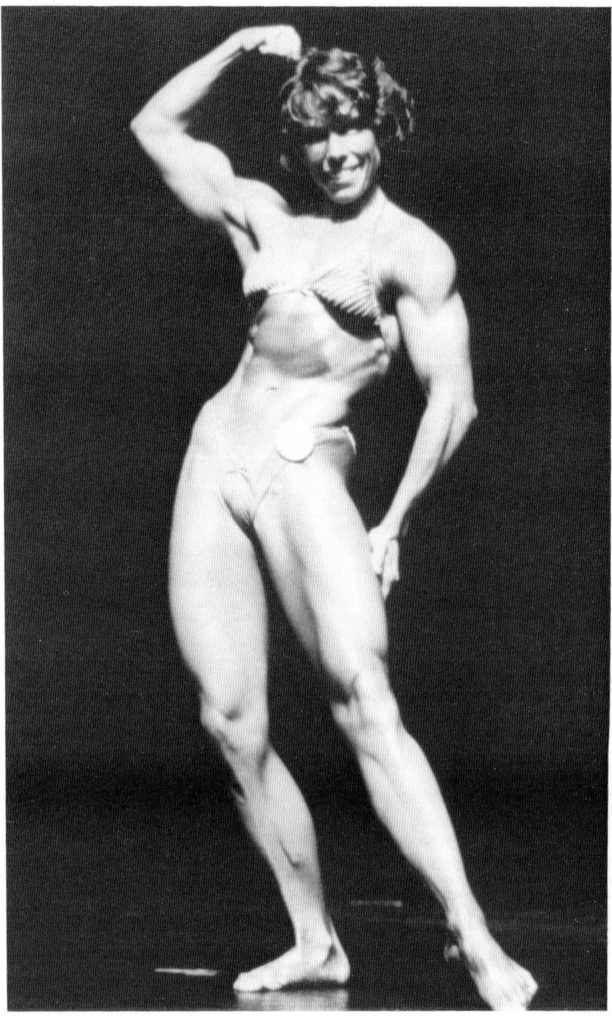

Fig. 8-13. A classic example of alteration of body form by muscle development and decrease in total body fat. The pose intentionally accentuates definition. (Photo courtesy of Michael Neveux and The Joe Weider Photo Library.)

smaller. The other measurements that were of interest included the circumference of the arm at the axilla, 11 inches; midforearm, 7½ inches; the thigh just below the buttock crease, 22 inches; the calf, 13½ inches; and the ankle, 8½ inches.

But measurement, as Dürer proved to himself, is inadequate to define the parameters of form. Great efforts have been made, notably by Kretschmer, the psychiatrist, and later by Sheldon, to not only categorize body shape and form but also to correlate these measurements with psychological characteristics, longevity, and pathology. The acceptability of the psychological judgments is probably considerably less important than the order that Sheldon created in somatotyping his subjects as endo-, ecto-, or mesomorphs [21] (Fig. 8-12). Briefly, the ectomorph is a body dominated by the ectoderm, with a fragile linear shape, flat chest, slender extremities, and the greatest surface area; the ectomorph is called cerebrotonic. The mesomorph is of essentially athletic build with a firm, upright physique, thick skin, and a dominance of mesodermal structures; the mesomorph has a high specific gravity. The endomorph has a predominance of endodermal, or visceral structures, with softness, sphericity, weakness, and obesity. The majority of Sheldon's work was done on men with the standardized, three-view photographs, although several thousand young women were also analyzed. Findings indicated that most of the women were far more endomorphic than men and heavier in proportion to stature. There was essentially a bell curve with endomorphism as the peak and ecto- and mesomorphy at the extremes; women clustered about the center of the curve, unlike men who showed considerably more scattering.

If parameters of beauty are at least partially cultural and the culture is sufficiently large, subcultures could be anticipated with distortions or modifications found. Worth considering are those cultural influences sufficiently large or important to affect either the surgeon or the patient such as news media, print, magazines, television, and movies. In these forms of media, the female form is illustrated, glorified, and possibly exploited, but in any case these media have a large and potentially receptive audience of women who might desire to imitate and therefore deserve our attention.

The woman's figure of fashion magazines is seen to be linear with long, smooth limbs, slim torso, limited breast protrusion, and little muscle definition. All appear to be at least eight heads tall, recalling the proportion of sev-

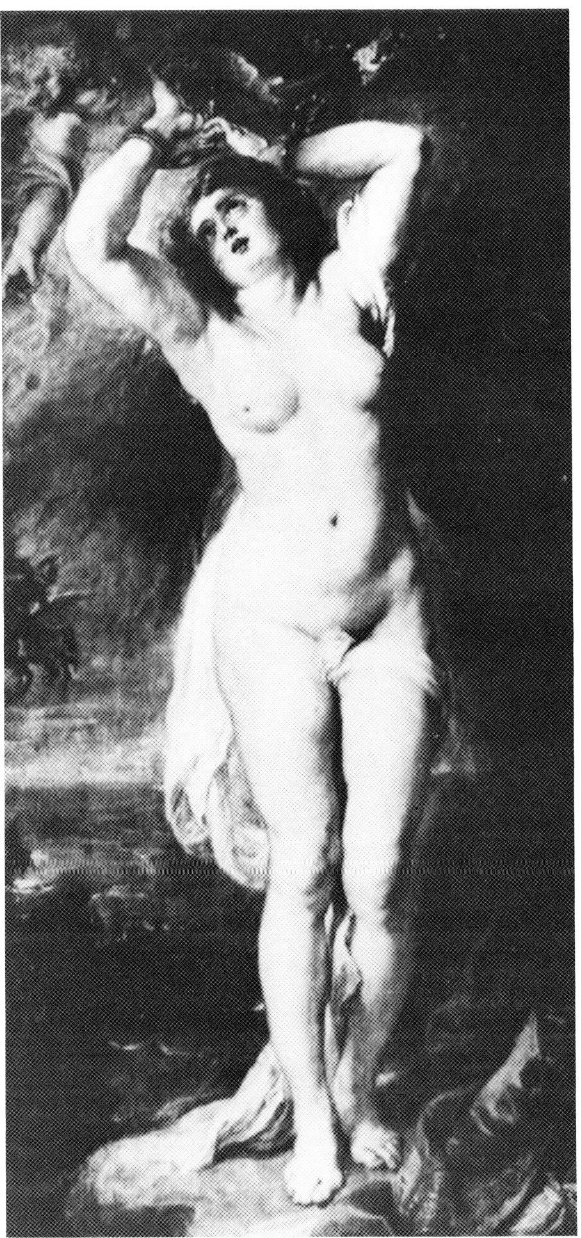

Fig. 8-14. A Rubens' nude, possibly less ample than some, but preserving classic proportion and form.

eral thousand years ago, and sometimes appear taller when exotic photographic angles are used. They might be described as smooth ectomorphs or very slim endomorphs. In contrast, in the muscle development publications, the women show well-developed musculature with significant muscle definition, but not necessarily resembling the male (Fig. 8-13). Body fat appears to be much less than the 25% normally given for a female. Bellies are not perfectly flat but are tucked in, and rectus definition is much less than in males. Breasts and buttocks are small. In the fitness books, form seems to follow low fitness [22]. Hips and thighs are smooth, breasts are not protrusive but seemingly compressed by garments, and obesity or cellulite is not seen. All have feminine figures appearing to be slim endomorphs with little muscle definition. Comparison with the current fashion photographs and Greek sculptures suggests that again the measurements will be very close and that the eye perceives the significant differences.

Summary

Analysis of beautiful form in a human female (Fig. 8-14) by diagrams or photographs has its limitations, as do the numbers. However, the terms of the artist and critic—shape, form, harmony, balance, symmetry, proportion, tension, movement, stress, color, and mass—must be considered and studied. Analysis by lines, axes, planes, curves, and spirals have worked well enough for the world of art, but those endeavors were significantly broadened and improved as physiology and psychology of vision and perception were studied. The methods of the mathematician continue to be utilized; numbers, lines, and angles are used by orthodontists, who rely on the radiographic profile of the mandible and the maxilla to plan their course [23].

Until the present, aesthetic considerations of form have not been easily quantifiable. Possibly with new tools, the hologram, computerized tomography, and the computer combined with older methods of arithmetic, geometric, and logarithmic/orthogonal projections, better judgments will be made in the future. Although it appears that in this "modern" age we modify the body for the sake of fad, fashion, or beauty (to a greater degree than before), we are merely doing the same thing that other societies have done for the same deep and uncertain cultural reasons. Modification of body image continues in a multiplicity of ways, including make-up, hairstyling, dress, weight change, and muscle building, aside from surgical methods. The perception of the ideal, or at least better, shape is undoubtedly influenced by our efficient communication system; however, the final arbiter of harmony, beauty, and proportion remains the human eye.

References

1. Brain, R. *The Decorated Body.* New York: Harper & Row, 1979.
2. Iliffe, A. H. A study of preferences in feminine beauty. *Brit. J. Psychol.* 51:267, 1960.
3. Adler, M. J. *Six Great Ideas.* New York: Macmillan, 1981.
4. Clark, K. *The Nude: A Study in Ideal Form.* Princeton, N.J.: Princeton University Press, 1956.

5. Sheppard, J. *Drawing the Female Figure*. New York: Watson Guptill, 1975.

6. Koestler, A. *The Act of Creation*. New York: Macmillan, 1964.

7. Ghyka, M. *The Geometry of Art and Life*. New York: Dover, 1977.

8. MacCurdy, E. *The Notebooks of Leonardo Da Vinci*. New York: George Braziller, 1958.

9. Panofsky, E. *The Life and Art of Albrecht Dürer*. Princeton, N.J.: Princeton University Press, 1955.

10. Gardner, M. Mathematical games. *Scientific American* 236:134, 1977.

11. Thompson, D. *On Growth and Form*. Cambridge, Eng.: Cambridge University Press, 1961.

12. Arnheim, R. *Art and Visual Perception*. Berkeley, Calif.: University of California Press, 1974.

13. Huntley, H. E. *The Divine Proportion*. New York: Dover, 1970.

14. Pacioli, L. Divina Proportione. Weingraser: Winterberg, 1896.

15. Grazer, F. M., and Klingbeil, J. R. *Body Image: A Surgical Perspective*. St. Louis: Mosby, 1980.

16. Hambidge, J. *The Elements of Dynamic Symmetry*. New York: Dover, 1967.

17. Hogarth, B. *Dynamic Figure Drawing*. New York: Watson Guptill, 1970.

18. Kramer, J. *Human Anatomy and Figure Drawing*. New York: Van Nostrand Reinhold, 1972.

19. *Playboy Magazine*. Chicago, Ill. Issues June 1980–January 1984.

20. Garrett, J. W. *A Collation of Anthropometry* (vols. 1 and 2). Wright-Patterson Air Force Base, Ohio: Aerospace Medical Research Lab., 1971.

21. Sheldon, W. *Atlas of Men*. Darien, Conn.: Hafner, 1970.

22. Fonda, J. *Jane Fonda's Workout Book*. New York: Simon and Schuster, 1981.

23. Lombardi, R. Principles of visual perception and their clinical application to denture esthetics. *J. Prosthet. Dent.* 29:358, 1973.

CHAPTER 9

Nomenclature

Gregory P. Hetter
Carson M. Lewis
Peter Arner

To increase the accuracy of our communication relative to lipolysis, it has become imperative that we establish a standard nomenclature for the areas on which we are working. The French have used interesting descriptive terms that often have been transliterated to English, such as *culotte de cheval* (riding breeches) and *déformation en violin* (violin deformity) (Figs. 9-1 and 9-2). The American "square bottom" is another descriptive term (Fig. 9-3).

Fat researchers [1] have given us other descriptive terms such as android and gynecoid fat distributions (Figs. 9-4 and 9-5). Interestingly, the android habitus carries with it associated disease states and an implication about shortened longevity, but the gynecoid form does not. Thus, the presence of excessive fat in certain locations or perhaps the presence of certain kinds of fat may indicate a difference of appearance as well as of metabolism or disease.

Difficulties arise because even common English words such as *hip* may be used by some to refer to the trochanteric area, while others refer to the iliac crest. Colloquialisms, such as *love handles*, are often used, in this case to describe male flank fatty accumulations.

The need for accuracy of description and for the common use of less colloquial words prompted the Lipolysis Society of North America to work on appropriate nomenclature for English usage. Dr. Carson Lewis of La Jolla, California, and Dr. Peter Arner of Stockholm joined me in examining the terms most used and abused at this time and in suggesting a glossary of terms.

Wherever possible, modern English words, or common medical terms of Latin or Greek derivation that have passed into Middle English via French, have been used. We have particularly rejected terms of improper or imprecise usage (e.g., trochanteric lipodystrophy, since no dystrophic process has ever been demonstrated) for simpler and hopefully more accurate and less ambiguous terms. Occasionally, clearly descriptive anatomical terms are used where they serve most concisely.

Since we are usually dealing with localized fatty deposits in excess of generalized deposits, there are areas where these fatty deposits have been observed to be far more common than others. The male and female distribution of fat is usually different; however, the gynecoid distribution of fatty excess (usually seen in females) can be seen in males, and the android form (usually seen in males) can be seen in females. The most common localized lower body deposits have been treated in France since the late 1970s. In the female these deposits are shown in Figures 9-6 and 9-7 and in the male in Figures 9-8 and 9-9. The lower body will be described first.

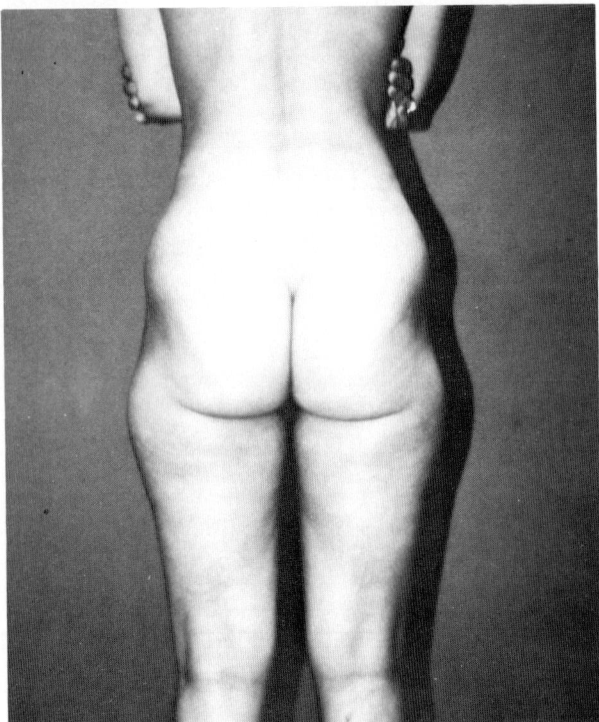

Fig. 9-1. Typical single patient in her twenties seeking consultation for hereditary localized fatty deposits known in French as culotte de cheval and in English as riding breeches or saddlebags.

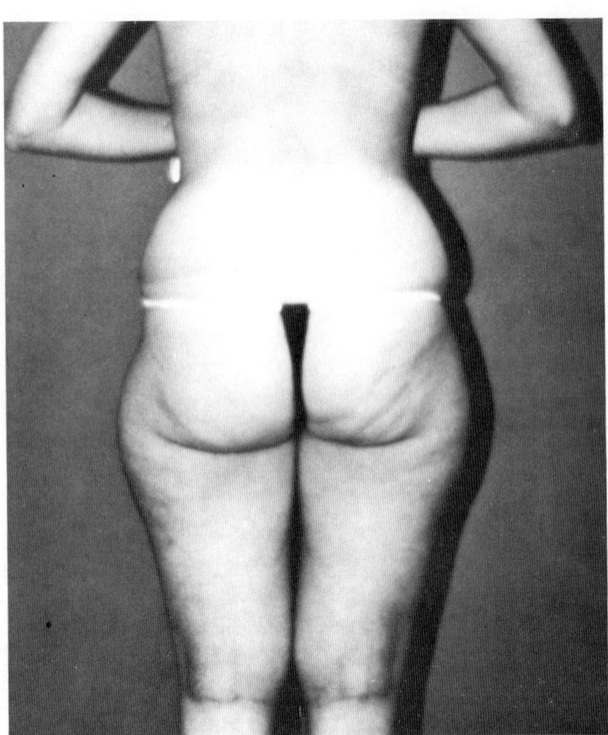

Fig. 9-2. Typical married patient in her thirties with children seeking consultation for diet-resistant fatty deposits overlying iliac crest and lateral thigh described in French as déformation en violin and in English as violin deformity.

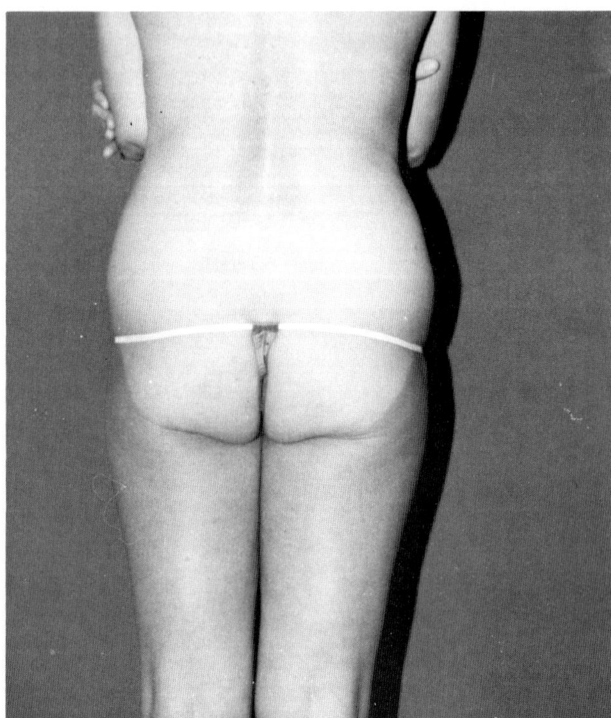

Fig. 9-3. Buttock anatomy given the descriptive term of "square bottom" because of the horizontal infragluteal crease running perpendicularly into the vertical buttock cleft.

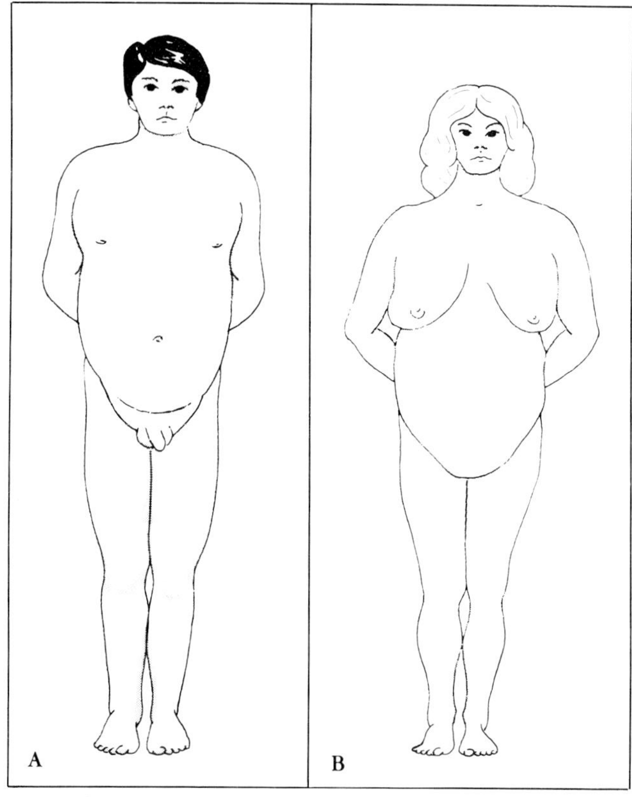

Fig. 9-4

A. Male with an android fat distribution.

B. Female with an android fat distribution, often indicating pathology.

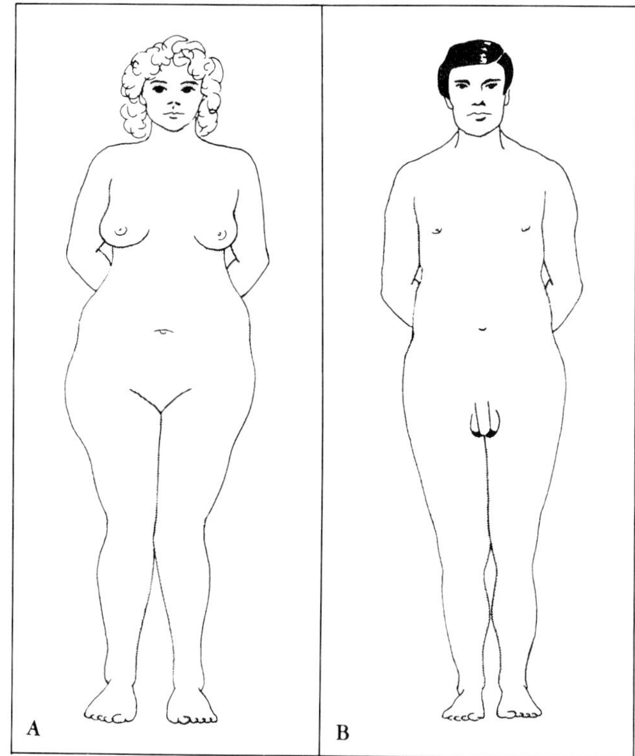

Fig. 9-5

A. Female with a typical gynecoid fat distribution. This carries no increase in morbidity.

B. Male with a gynecoid fat distribution seen occasionally in young men.

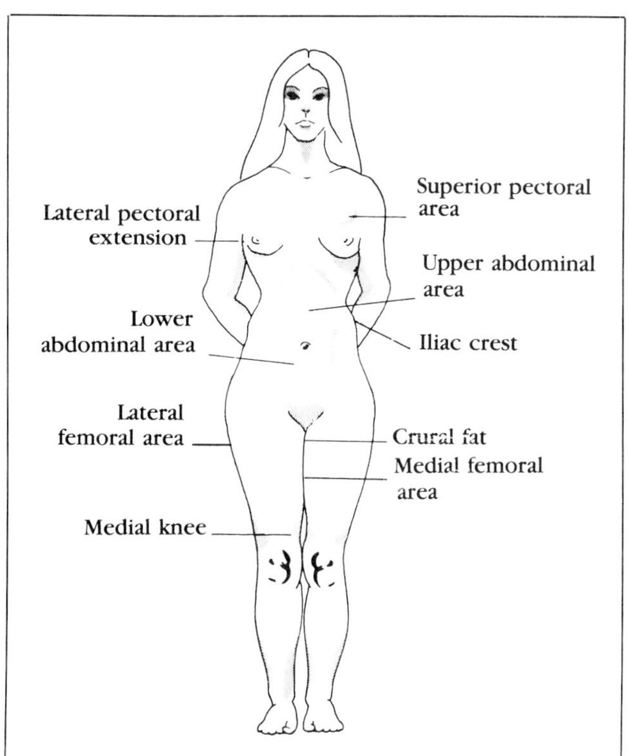

Fig. 9-6. Female, anterior view.

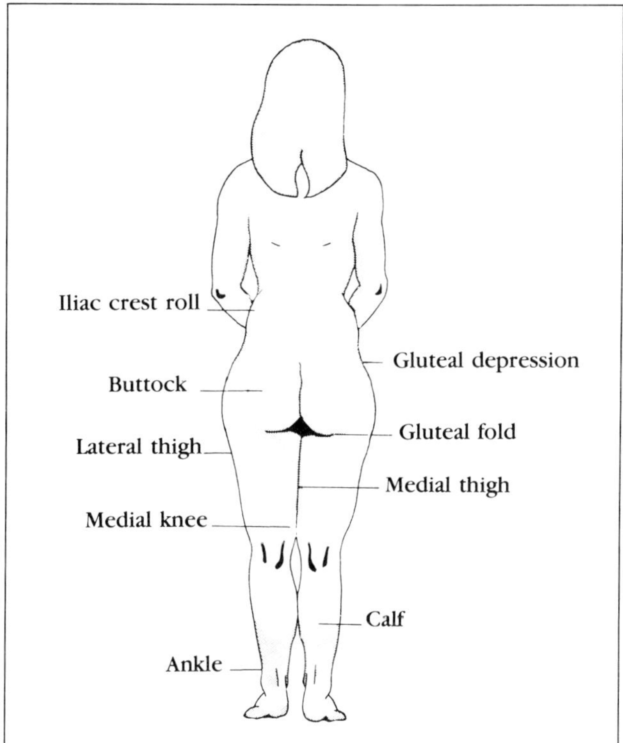

Fig. 9-7. Female, posterior view.

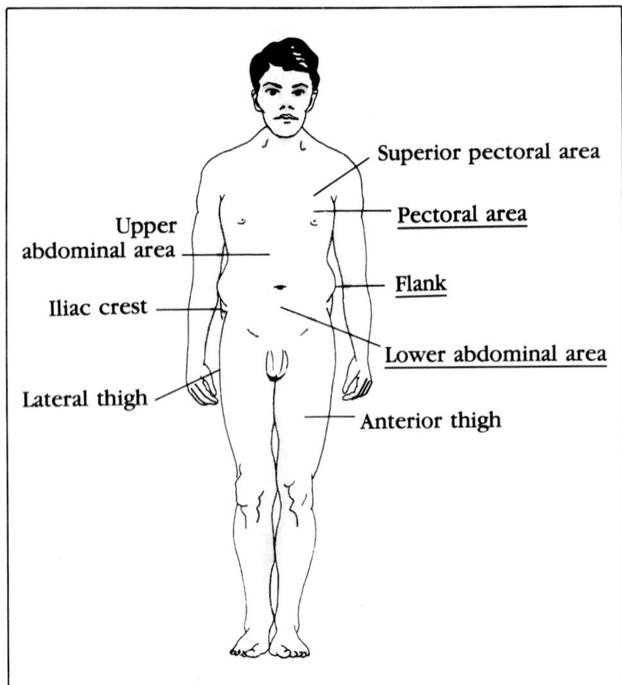

Fig. 9-8. Male, anterior view. Underlined areas are typical male problem areas.

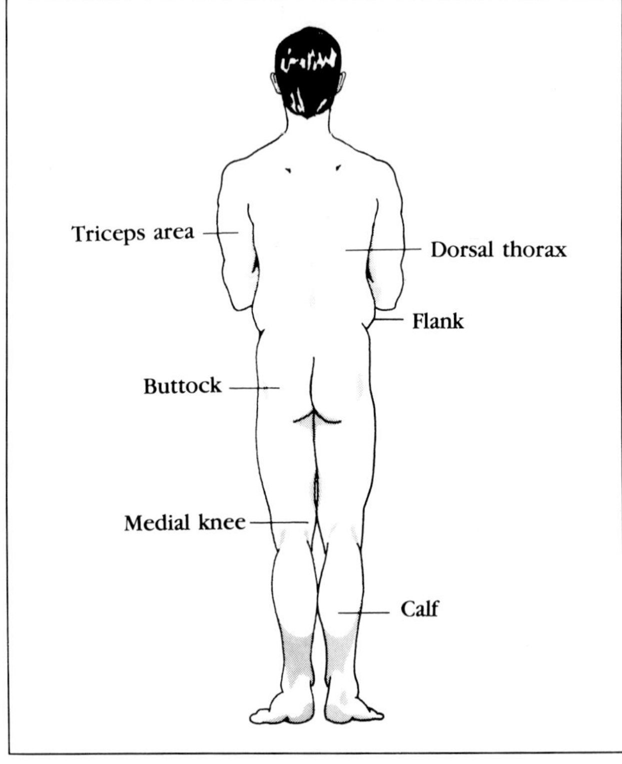

Fig. 9-9. Male, posterior view.

LOWER BODY

Upper abdominal   Epigastrium (Greek). The area below the xiphoid and above the umbilicus overlying the rectus abdominus muscles.

Lower abdominal   Hypogastrium (Greek). The area below the umbilicus, above the mons pubis, extending laterally as far as the anterior superior iliac spine.

Flank   Flanc (Old English via Old French from Germanic root). Here defined *only* as that area between the ribs and the iliac crest on the side of the torso. The flank fat in males commonly has an extension onto the lumbar area, and it is commonly confluent with the lower abdominal fat. The colloquial term "love handles" is often used to describe excess in this area.

Iliac crest roll   Ilium (Latin). The area overlying the junction of the ilium with the sacrum and extending forward laterally along and just below the iliac crest. (Hip roll was rejected because of the imprecise usage of the word *hip* referring to both the ilium and the trochanteric area of the femur.)

Violin deformity   Déformation en violin (Modern French). When an iliac crest roll combines with a lateral femoral deposit, a violin deformity results (Fig. 9-10).

When an iliac crest roll combines with a lower abdominal fatty deposit, a pear-shaped deformity occurs, giving a typical cowish appearance (Fig. 9-11).

Buttock   Buttok (Middle English). The area overlying the pelvic bones posteriorly and posterolaterally, bounded inferiorly by the gluteal or buttock fold, laterally and superiorly by the gluteal depression (see Fig. 9-7).

Gluteal fold or buttock fold   Gluteus (Latin), buttok (Middle English). The usually well-defined crease delineating the buttock from the posterior thigh (see Fig. 9-7).

Double fold   (English). A second lesser fold below the gluteal fold is described as a double fold (Figs. 9-12 and 9-13). The French authors describe the intervening tissue as a "banana" because of its shape.

Gluteal depression   Gluteus (Latin). This area overlies the gluteus musculature and often fat is lacking. This lack, combined with excess on the iliac crest and lateral femoral area, gives the violin silhouette (Fig. 9-14A,B).

Crural fat   Crura (Latin). The area of soft fat covered by thin, fine skin where the thighs kiss just beneath the labia in the female. The removal of this fat results in a slot-like appearance between the legs (Fig. 9-15). This area is prone in middle age to become irregular and wavy as the thin skin loses its elasticity. In old age, the fat atrophies and gives the characteristic slot-like appearance.

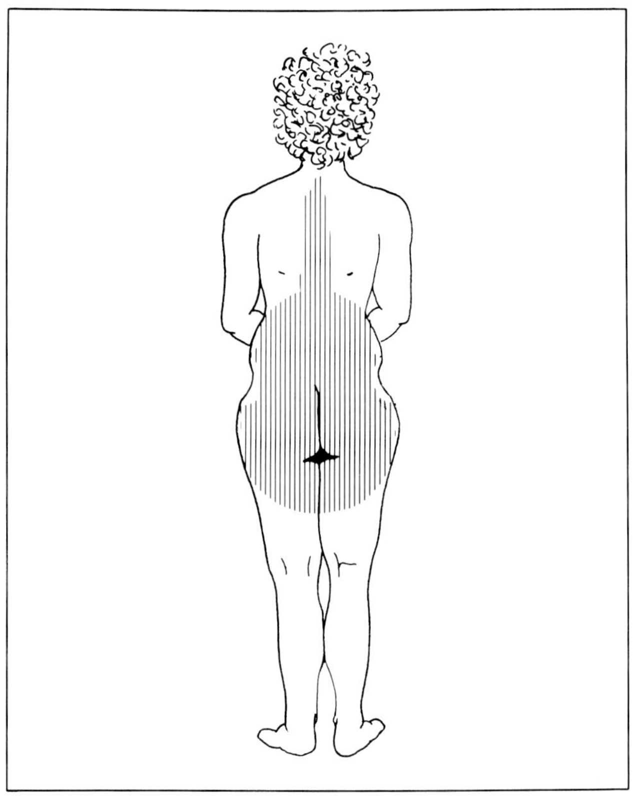

Fig. 9-10. Violin deformity.

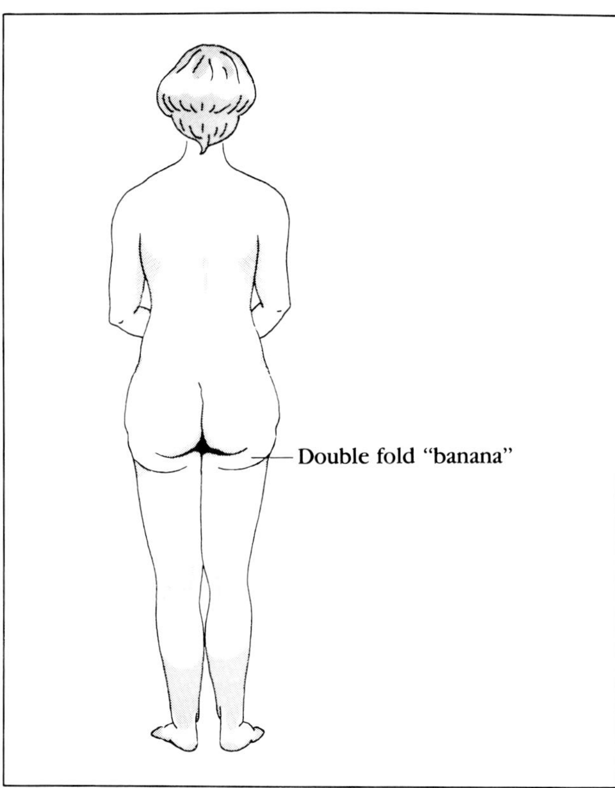

Fig. 9-12. The double fold is a common complaint in otherwise thin females.

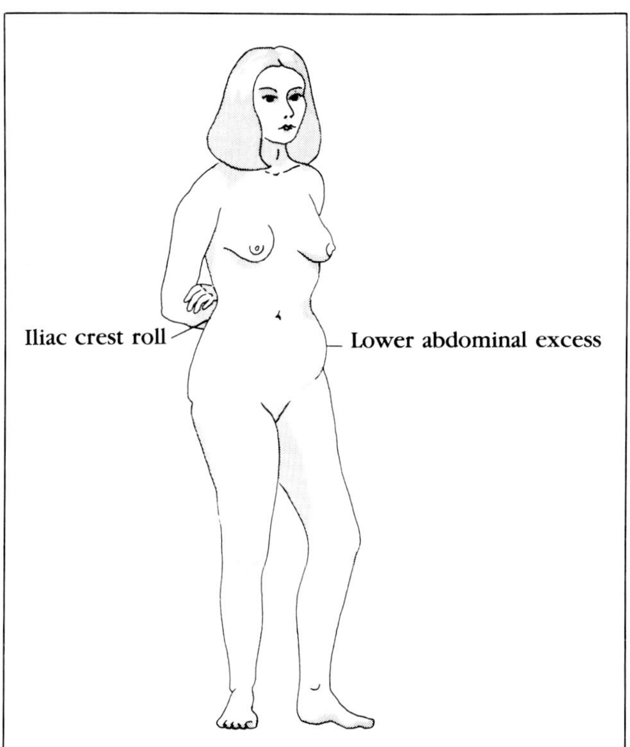

Fig. 9-11. Pear-shaped appearance caused by iliac crest and lower abdominal fat creating a lower torso ring of fat.

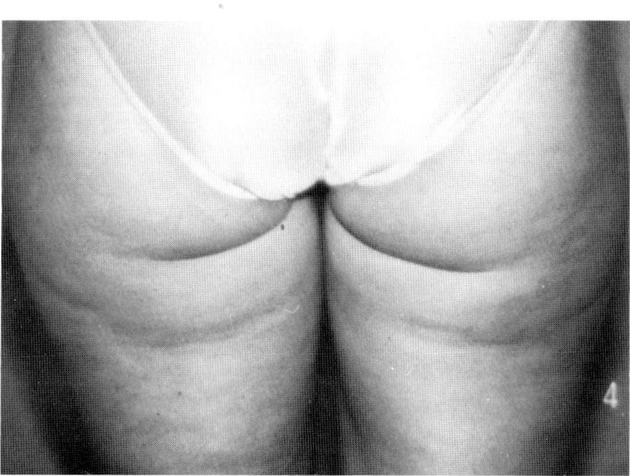

Fig. 9-13. Female showing double fold. This patient had dieted and exercised until she had only ½″ of lower abdominal integument, which could be pinched up between the fingers.

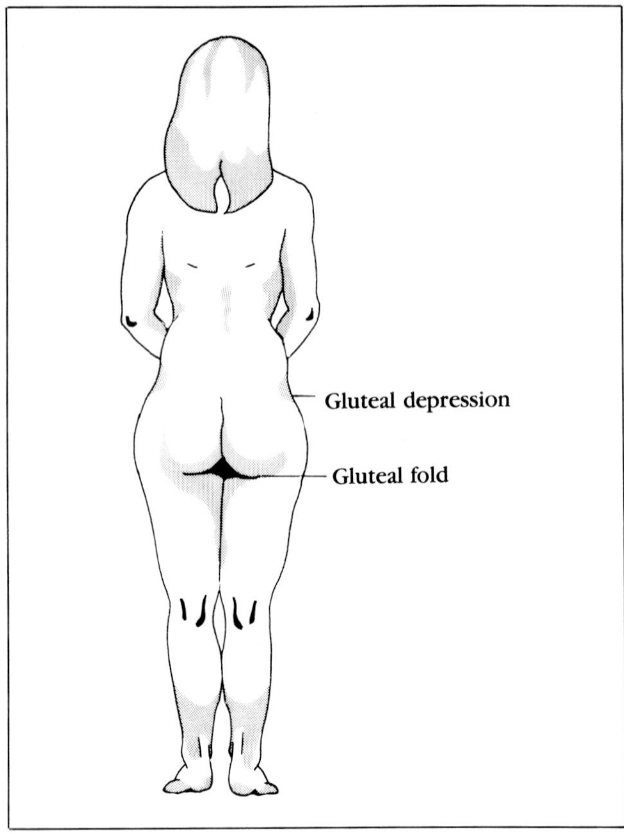

A

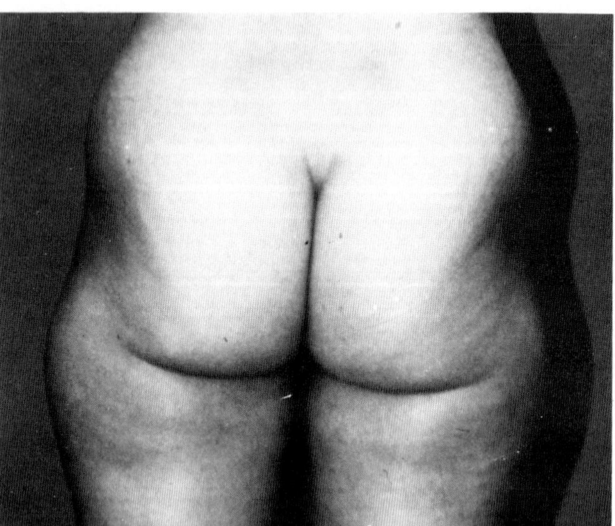

B

Fig. 9-14.
A. Drawing illustrating that the gluteal depression often
   lacks the thickness of the iliac crest fat above and the lateral thigh fat below.
B. Photograph showing a marked gluteal depression.

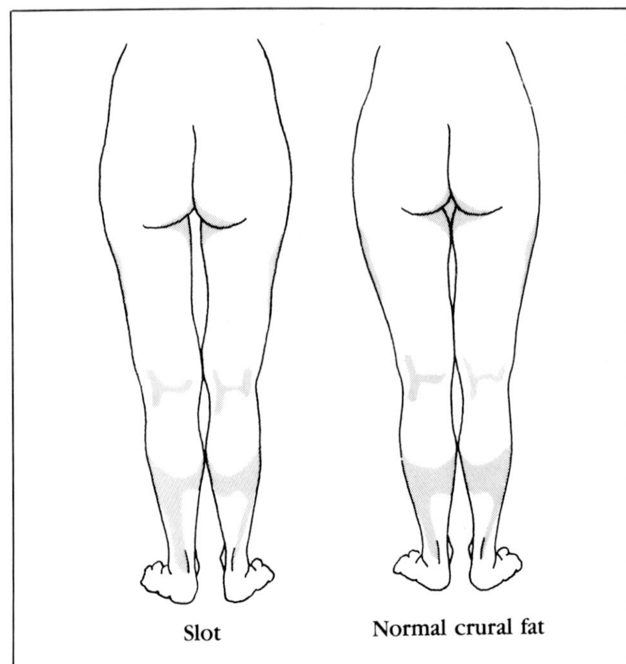

Fig. 9-15. Normal-shaped crural area and slot-like appearance when the crural bulge is deficient or has been overly
operated or has atrophied with age.

Medial femoral fat   Femoris (Latin) or *medial thigh
   fat:* theogh (Old English), thjo (Icelandic). The area
   below the crural fat to the medial knee fat.
Anterior femoral fat   Femoris (Latin) or *anterior thigh
   fat:* theogh (Old English), thjo (Icelandic). The area
   from below the inguinal crease to the suprapatellar
   area.
Lateral femoral fat   Femoris (Latin) or *lateral thigh
   fat:* theogh (Old English), thjo (Icelandic). The most
   common area for localized fatty deposits. Words in
   common usage to describe this fat are trochanteric
   lipodystrophy (a misnomer since there is no dystrophic process), peritrochanteric fat (a misnomer since
   the iliotibial fascia separates the trochanter from the
   subcutaneous fat of the saddlebags, riding breeches,
   and culotte de cheveau). This fat has been proven to
   be metabolically and morphologically different from
   abdominal fat (see Fig. 9-14B) (see Chap. 6.).
Medial knee fat   Knee (Middle English). An area of
   common complaint colloquially called "chubb." A
   well-shaped knee is seen in Figure 9-16; a typical excess of fat is seen in Figure 9-17.
Suprapatellar fat   Patella (Latin). Some patients have
   an accumulation of fat just above the patella, giving
   the appearance of the anterior thigh ptosing over the
   patella (Fig. 9-18).
Posterior calf fat   Calf (Middle English). The accumulations in the inferior posterior area give the calf a
   sausage-like appearance ending in a "pursestring" just

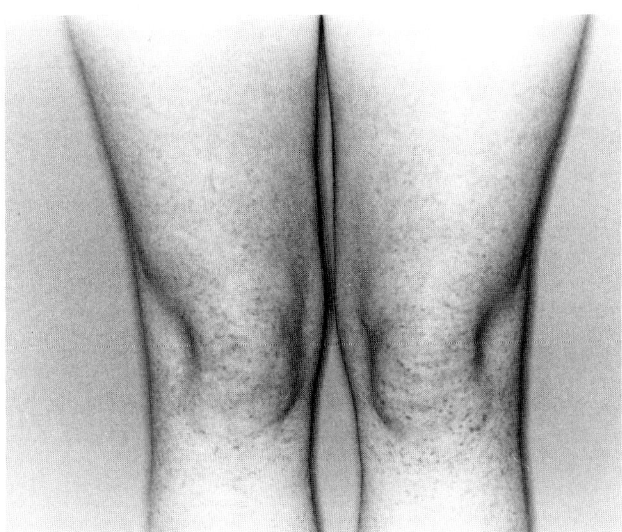

Fig. 9-16. Shapely knee with prominence of condyle.

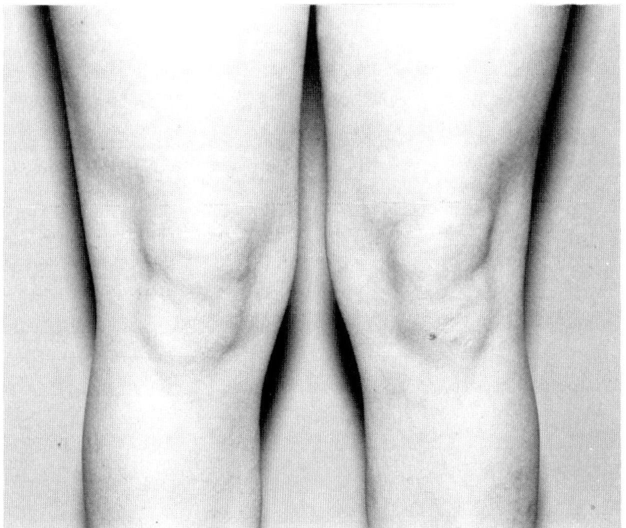

Fig. 9-17. Excessive medial superior knee fat.

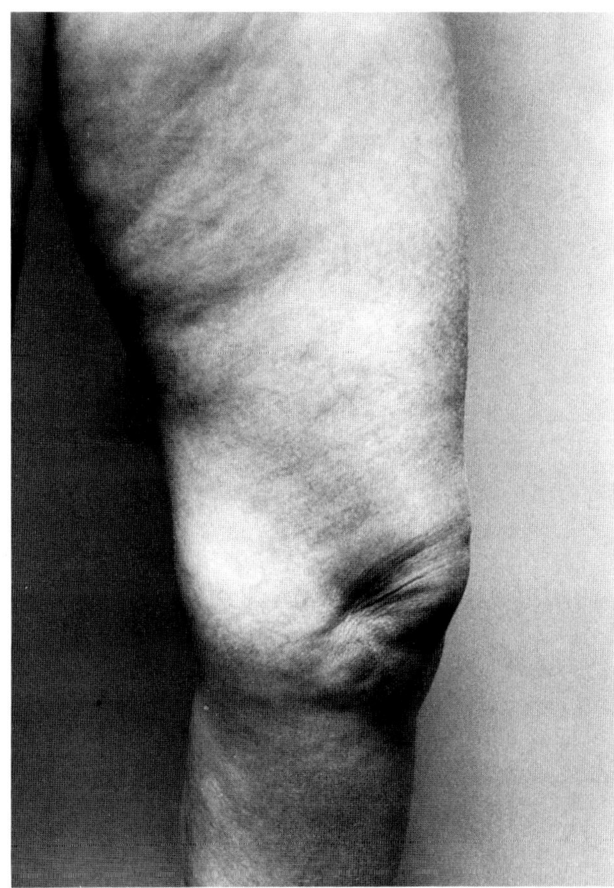

Fig. 9-18. Suprapatellar fat ptosing over the patella.

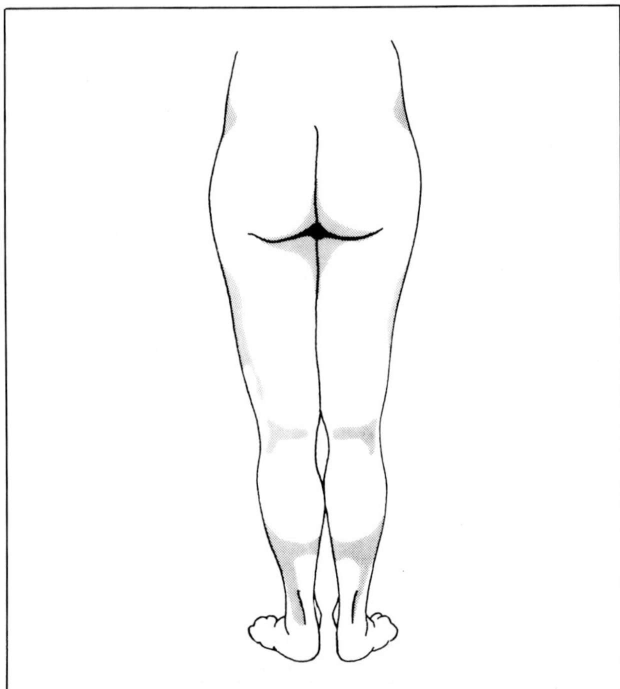

Fig. 9-19. Shapely calf and ankle. Note gastroc shadow.

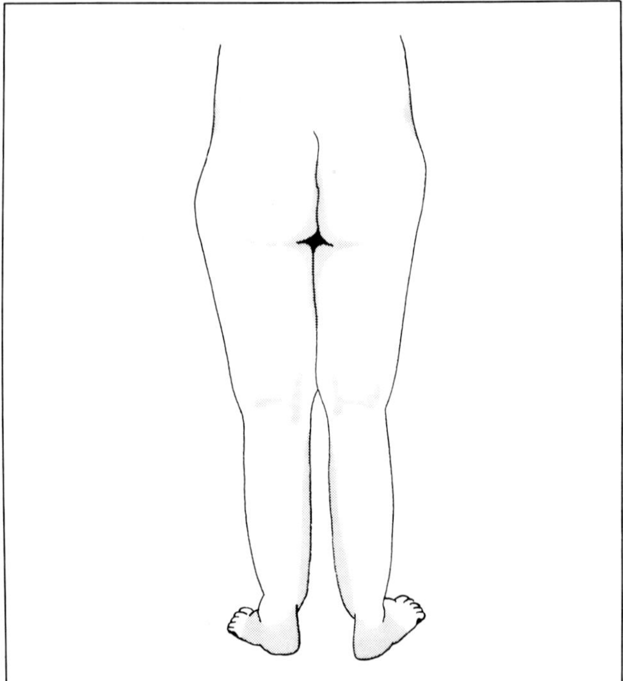

Fig. 9-20. Heavy lower calf fatty accumulation obliterating normal gastroc shadow and ending in a "pursestring" appearance just above the malleoli.

above the malleoli. A normal calf with well-defined gastrocnemius shadow and pleasant curves is seen in Figure 9-19, and the typical hereditary deformity is seen in Figure 9-20.

Ankle Ankle (Middle English). Ankle refers to the area of the malleoli and attachment of the Achilles tendon just above the calcaneus. This area has little fat and is rarely a problem.

FACE, NECK, AND UPPER BODY

Lipolysis has been applied to the face, neck, and upper body only since its worldwide popularization late in 1981 and 1982. The terminology will certainly grow as new areas are added to those presently being treated. This glossary makes no claim to be inclusive or exclusive but can contribute to the accuracy of our communication.

Malar area Mala (Latin). The area just below and lateral to the infraorbital rim where a bulge may persist following blepharoplasty or may be present as a discrete bulge (Fig. 9-21).

Preantral area Antron (Greek via Latin). The area in front of the maxilla bordered inferiorly by the nasolabial fold. A heavy fatty accumulation here may give an apparent deep fold because of the shadow thrown by its prominence (Fig. 9-21).

Cheek Cheke (Middle English). The area between the upper and lower jaw overlying the masseter muscle and parotid gland. Excessive fat accumulations above the parotid fascia may be the object of suction removal (Fig. 9-22).

Anterior carotid triangle area Karotides (Greek via Latin). The area bounded superiorly by the submandibular triangle, posteriorly by the sternocleidomastoid muscle, anteriorly by the strap muscles. Superficial to the platysma, significant fat may be found obliterating the definition of these contours. This fat may be confluent with the precricoid fat (Fig. 9-22).

Submandibular triangle area Mandibula (Latin). This area is bordered superiorly by the body of the mandible but extends forward to the submental area anteriorly and extends inferiorly into the superior carotid triangle. The typical jowl fat that appears in middle age is seen here and must be differentiated from a prominent or ptotic submaxillary gland. The jowl fat is usually confluent with the submental fat (Fig. 9-22).

Submental area Mentum (Latin). This area extends from the midline of the mandible to the hyoid bone and is confluent laterally with the submandibular triangle area. The fat is superficial to the platysma except between the medial platysma bands where it is

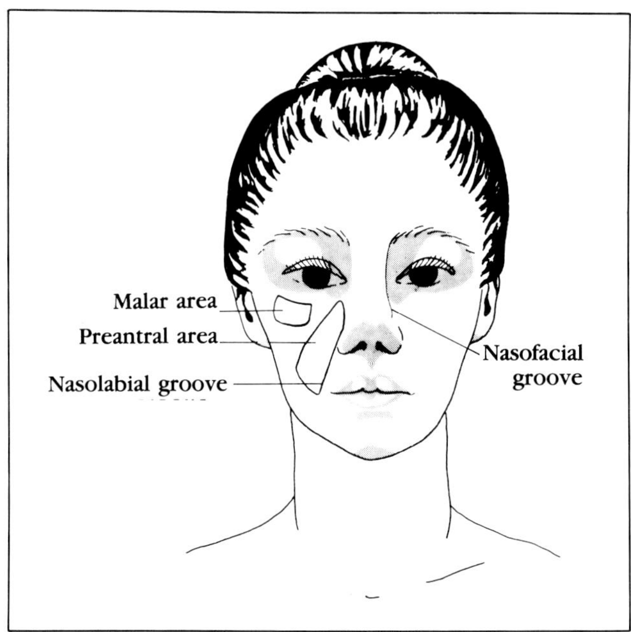

Fig. 9-21. Anterior view of head and neck.

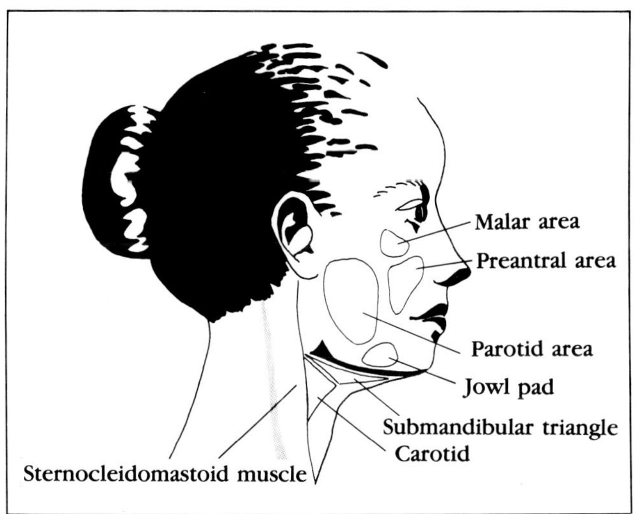

Fig. 9-22. Lateral view of head and neck.

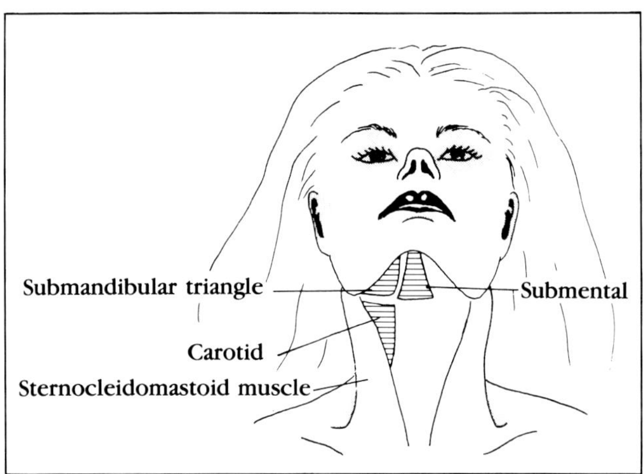

Fig. 9-23. Anterior view of neck with head extended on neck.

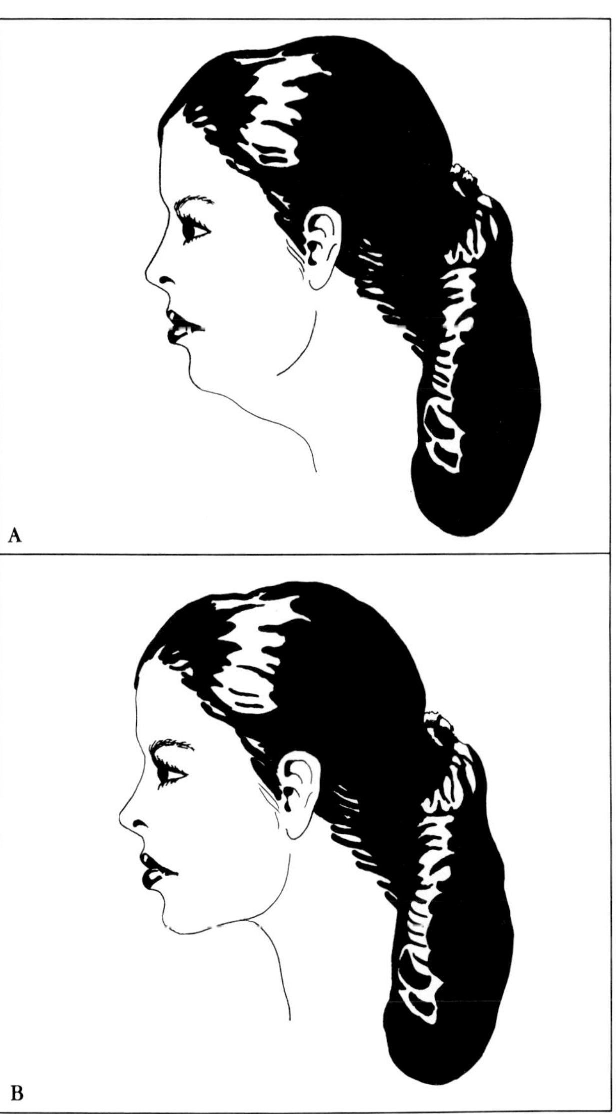

Fig. 9-24
A. Cervicomental angle filled with fat.
B. Normal cervicomental angle.

easy to enter into deeper fat between the bellies of the digastric since the fascia is usually deficient here (Fig. 9-23).

Cervicomental angle   Cervix (Latin), mentum (Latin); (accepted aesthetic descriptive term). This area overlies the hyoid bone (which is usually the deepest point of the angle), the cricoid cartilage, and the laryngeal cartilage. Fat obliterating these landmarks may be removed with astonishing improvement in appearance (Fig. 9-24A and B).

Posterior humeral area   Umerus (Latin). The area over the back of the upper arm overlying the triceps muscle, extending from axilla to olecranon (part of the elbow) (Fig. 9-25).

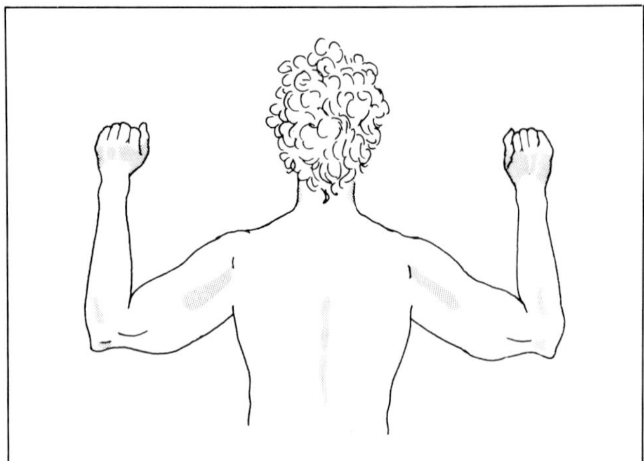

Fig. 9-25. Posterior view of arms demonstrating localized fatty accumulations in the posterior humeral area.

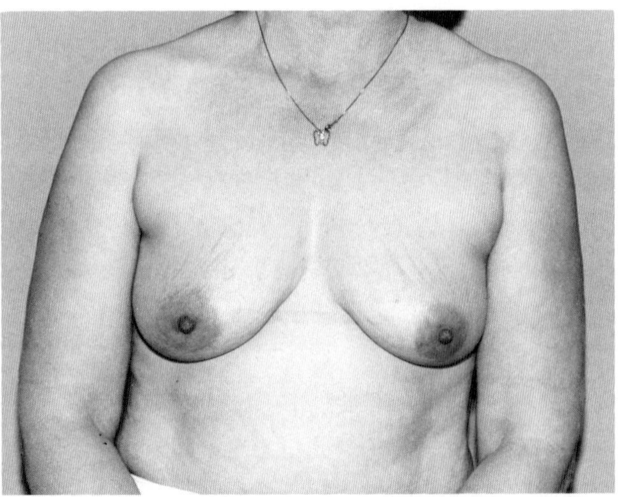

Fig. 9-27. Superior pectoral fat bulge where subcutaneous fat may be extensive, leaving a valley before the breast fat begins.

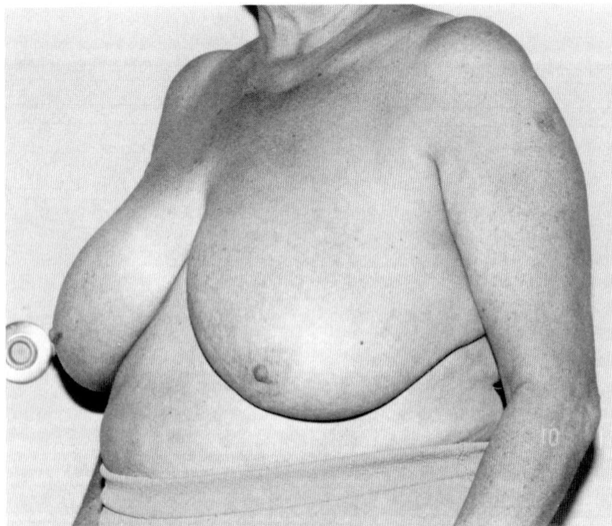

Fig. 9-26. Oblique view showing extension of breast fat laterally along the thoracic ribs beneath the arm.

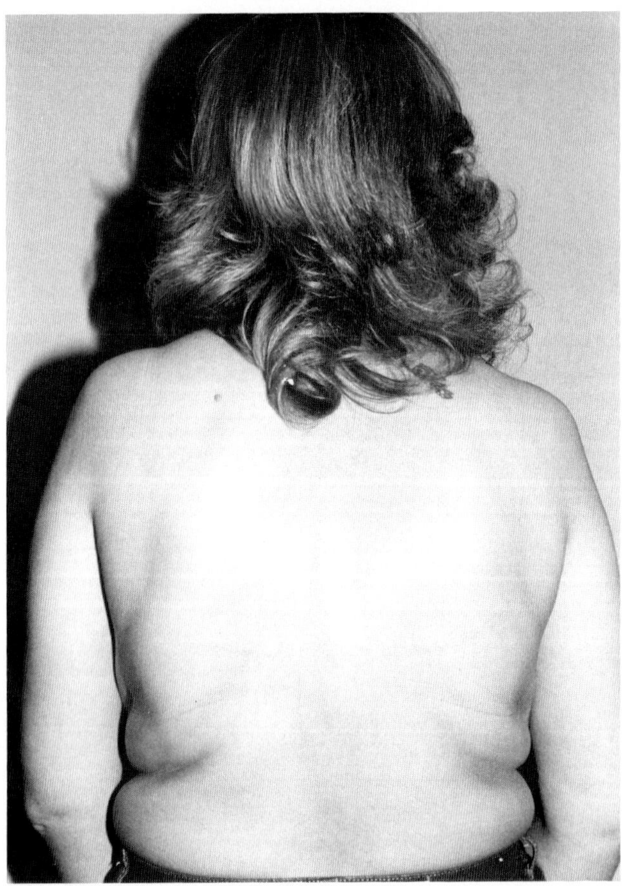

Fig. 9-28. Redundant folds of skin and fat on the dorsal thorax.

Pectoral area   Pectoralis (Latin via Middle English). The area surrounding the breast. The two most important subareas are the *lateral extension* seen in macromastia (Fig. 9-26) and the *superior pectoral area* (Fig. 9-27) seen often in nonobese subjects.

Dorsal thoracic folds   Thorako (Greek via Latin and Middle English). These folds are seen in persons with truncal obesity and are often confluent with lateral extensions of pectoral fat (Fig. 9-28).

GENERAL TERMS

A number of terms have been used since Dr. Illouz [2] first called his procedure lipolysis and are examined in the following section.

Lipolysis

Lipolysis   Lipo (Greek "lipos") meaning fat; lysis (Greek) meaning dissolution, loosening, setting free, releasing.

Lipolysis literally means dissolution or setting free of fat and is linguistically sound as formed by the two Greek words. Its meaning is clear. Lipolysis is also used to mean the enzymatic breakdown of fat, and therefore some do not wish to use the term in a mechanical as well as a biochemical meaning. Any resistance to the word's usage obviously cannot rest on linguistic or entymological reasons.

Concerns of personal notoriety by those seeking to associate their name with another new term appear to account for most of the flurry of terms that were rapidly rushed into print to try to replace the choice of the originator of the procedure, Dr. Illouz.

Suction-Assisted Lipectomy (SAL)

Lipectomy   Lipo (Greek "lipos") meaning fat; ectome (Greek) meaning excision.

This clearly descriptive term was copyrighted by Dr. Frederick Grazer [3] in late 1982. It was used by Mr. Guenter Grams, a manufacturing associate of Dr. Grazer, to market the Grazer-Grams vacuum pump in 1983. Its use was subsequently prohibited by the Food and Drug Administration in connection with the labeling of pumps or cannula.

The term *lipectomy* is clear. It is generic in the sense that any procedure in which suction is used to remove adipose tissue is covered. Thus, all procedures from Schrudde onward are covered by this term.

Blunt Suction Lipectomy

I (Hetter) used this term in late 1982 [4] to describe more specifically the Illouz technique and to differentiate the blunt technique from all the previous sharp techniques. The term highlights the specific feature of the technique, which has the most important implications for the complication rate. Blunt suction lipectomy refers only to the Illouz technique and not to the Schrudde technique [5] or to the unmodified techniques as originally reported by Fischer [6], Kesselring [7], and Teimourian [8]. The term is particularly useful because there are many de novo practitioners of suction lipectomy who are currently repeating many previous errors. These practitioners are designing cannulas that are very sharp or that have lumens at the tip causing all the problems of the sharp techniques, which are being or have been abandoned by more serious practitioners. The term therefore has validity not only for descriptive reasons but also for its clinical implications.

Liposuction

Liposuction   Lipo (Greek "lipos") meaning fat; suction (Latin "sugere") meaning to suck.

This term is a combination of a Greek root and a Latin root. The proper term is *adiposuction*, combining the Latin root *adipo*, meaning lard or fat, to the Latin *sugere*, meaning to suck.

The term *liposuction* has been used by a variety of practitioners, especially by those otolaryngologists (ear, nose, and throat surgeons) and dermatologists who are going far outside of their disciplines by attempting body contour procedures. Since both lipolysis and suction-assisted lipectomy were copyrighted terms in California, another term, *liposuction*, was coined.

Suction Extraction of Fat

Suction extraction of fat   Suction (Latin "sugere") meaning to suck; extraction (Latin "ex" and "trahere") meaning to draw out.

This term is accurate and highly descriptive. It is useful in describing what we are doing in clear modern English. For those reasons it has much to recommend it.

Lipoplasty

Lipoplasty   Lipo (Greek "lipo") meaning fat; plasty (Greek "plassein") meaning to form, mold, or shape.

A number of leading international plastic surgeons have suggested the term *lipoplasty* be used as the generic term for this surgery for change in fatty contours. This generic term covers all procedures used toward that end, including (1) lipolysis alone, (2) lipolysis with minor dermatolipectomy, (3) lipolysis with glandular removal (e.g., gynecomastia), and (4) dermatolipectomy with minor lipolysis.

Lipoplasty defines these procedures as plastic surgical procedures to mold and change the shape of fatty areas with a view toward improvement of form. *Lipo-*

plasty, although performed for years by a variety of procedures, is now a most important area of concern for plastic surgeons because the technique of *lipolysis* (blunt suction lipectomy) offers safety, reliability, and reproducible results in its application.

Summary

As with any new area, a search for terminology develops as the fervor of expansion occurs. Most contribute to this vocabulary as knowledge advances. For a few, the motivations for new terms, as for new journals, is to attempt to self-servingly carve out new "turf" for themselves [9].

In view of this, it is suggested that *lipoplasty* be the generic term for all remodeling of fatty tissues. *Blunt suction lipectomy* is suggested as the generic term for the *Illouz technique of lipoplasty.*

The use of the terms described and depicted in this chapter will help us to be more accurate in our verbal presentations and written articles. More terms will be added as the field expands and changes. We have tried to have clarity and entymologic accuracy as our guides in presenting this nomenclature for lipoplastic procedures.

References

1. Vague, J. (Ed.) Diabetes and Obesity. Clinical Features of Diabetogenic Obesity. Amsterdam: Excerpta Medica, 1979. Chap. 127.
2. Illouz, Y. G. Reflexions apres 4 ans et demi d'experience et 800 cas de ma technique de lipolyse. *Rev. Chir. Esthet. Lang. Franç* 6:27, 1981.
3. Grazer, F. Discussion: Suction-assisted lipectomy, suction lipectomy, lipolysis, and lipexeresis. *Plast. Reconstr. Surg.* 72(5):620, 1983.
4. Hetter, G. P., and Herhahn, F. Experience with "lipolysis": the Illouz technique of blunt suction lipectomy in North America. *Aesth. Plast. Surg.* 7:69, 1983.
5. Schrudde, J. Lipexeresis in the correction of local adiposity. In *First Congress of the International Society of Aesthetic Plastic Surgery,* Rio de Janeiro, 1972.
6. Fischer, A., and Fischer, G. M. Revised technique for cellulitis fat reduction in riding breeches deformity. *Bull. Int. Acad. Cosm. Surg.* 2:40, 1977.
7. Kesselring, U. K., and Meyer, R. Suction curette for removal of excessive local deposits of subcutaneous fat. *Plast. Reconstr. Surg.* 62:305, 1978.
8. Teimourian, B., and Fisher, J. B. Suction curettage to remove excess fat for body contouring. *Plast. Reconstr. Surg.* 68:50, 1981.
9. Newman, J. Lipo-suction surgery: Past, present, future. *Am. J. Cosm. Surg.* 1:19, 1984.

Chapter 10

Photographic Documentation

Gregory P. Hetter

Plastic surgeons sculpt in living flesh in which the only certainty is change and not always for the better. For our own sense of achievement, if for no other reason, we need accurate photographs to depict the changes wrought by our work. Our review of these photos is often the beginning of dissatisfaction, which leads to new concepts, techniques, and variations. At other times, the photographs are a source of great ego gratification as we see the documented results of artistry combined with skill.

Patients need accurate photography, too. They soon forget the unsightly bulge or blemish that brought them to the plastic surgeon. The ability to bring the blemish or bulge back via photography, with accurate comparison photographs of the result, aids the memory and perhaps alleviates the discontent.

Sometimes, unfortunately, the photographs serve as a witness for or against the surgeon in civil judicial procedures. More often than not, the photographs protect the surgeon and are of the utmost value to counter emotional allegations.

Photography for the Plastic Surgeon

GOOD PHOTOGRAPHY DEFINED

By good photography we mean photography that is *consistent* in:

1. Type of film
2. Background
3. Lighting
4. Focal length of lens
5. Distance
6. Focus
7. Patient position and attire
8. Film processing

IDEAL PHOTOGRAPHY DEFINED

By ideal photography we mean the unattainable for a plastic surgery practice, where a knowledgeable professional photographer would set up cameras, lighting, and background with no regard to expense, time, or personnel to obtain the photographs.

AVERAGE PHOTOGRAPHY

The 35-mm through-the-lens reflex camera is the standard in most plastic surgery offices. Slide film (diapositive) is most commonly used because it is inexpensive and can be projected at medical meetings without further expense. Often a 50- or 55-mm lens is used—even for the face—which produces a distortion of the parts.

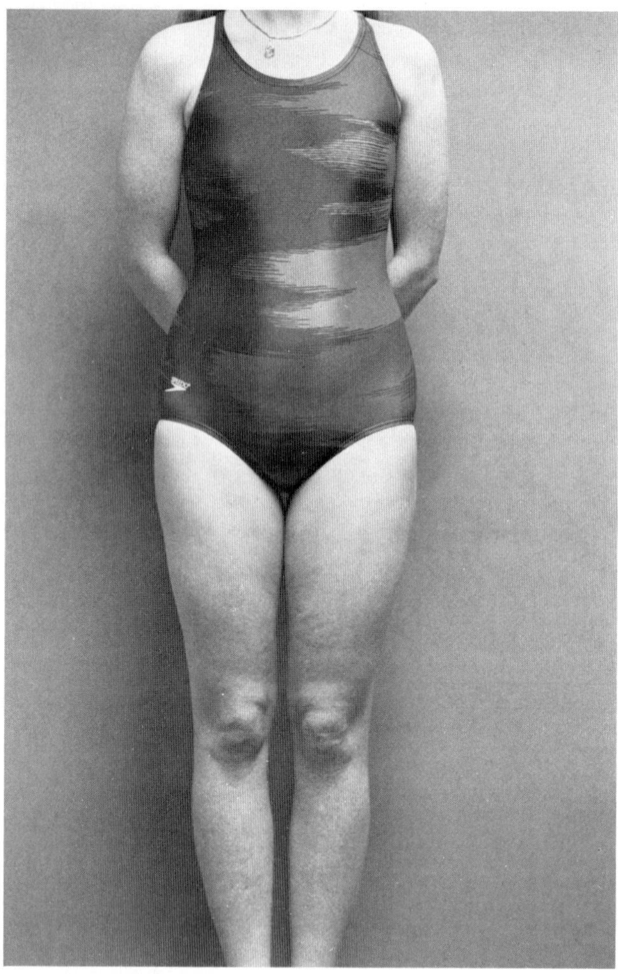

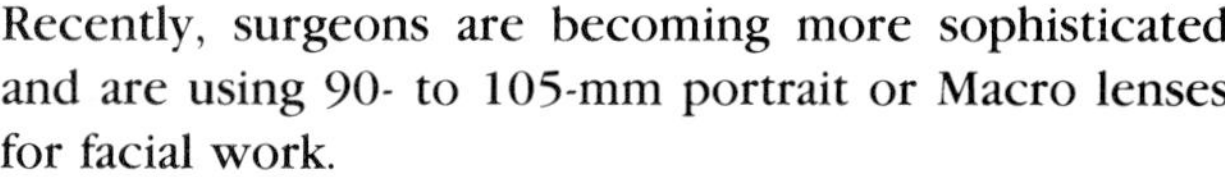

Fig. 10-1. Black and white print showing medium-blue background and white skin as nearly equal gray shades. Taken with ambient overhead light.

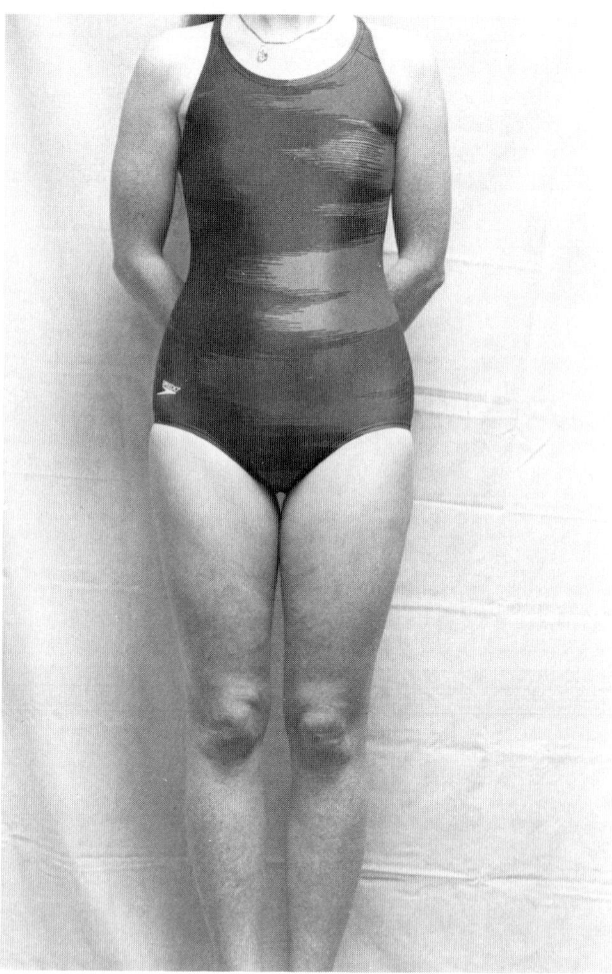

Fig. 10-2. Same model as in Figure 10-1 photographed with Kodak Tri-X against light background with ambient overhead light.

Recently, surgeons are becoming more sophisticated and are using 90- to 105-mm portrait or Macro lenses for facial work.

The light source is almost always an electronic flash, usually body mounted to the camera, or a ring light around the lens, which allows very close-up photography with Macro lenses. (Macro lenses allow pictures up to 1:1 ratio between the object and the image on the film.)

FILM

The choice of film is important. If slide film is chosen, background color almost automatically becomes a medium blue. This color is good for white or black skin, blonde or black hair, and is excellent for projection at national meetings. A matte paint on rough wall board and felt material are the most common backgrounds because they are nonreflective.

BLACK AND WHITE PRINTS FROM SLIDES

Problems arise when a black and white print is desired because the medium-blue background has the same gray density as the average "white" skin tone, and the contrast between the blue background and the skin is poor (Fig. 10-1). This is the reason for the minimal contrast seen in black and white reproductions of slides in most surgical publications, including many of the photographs in this textbook.

BACKGROUND

If a good black and white print is desired, the background color should be an off-white (Fig. 10-2) or black (Fig. 10-3). This background can be provided by a cloth shade of either color available to roll down in front of the medium-blue background whenever desired. A very dark blue or black cloth is good for body photography if one is willing to sacrifice the loss of black hair into the

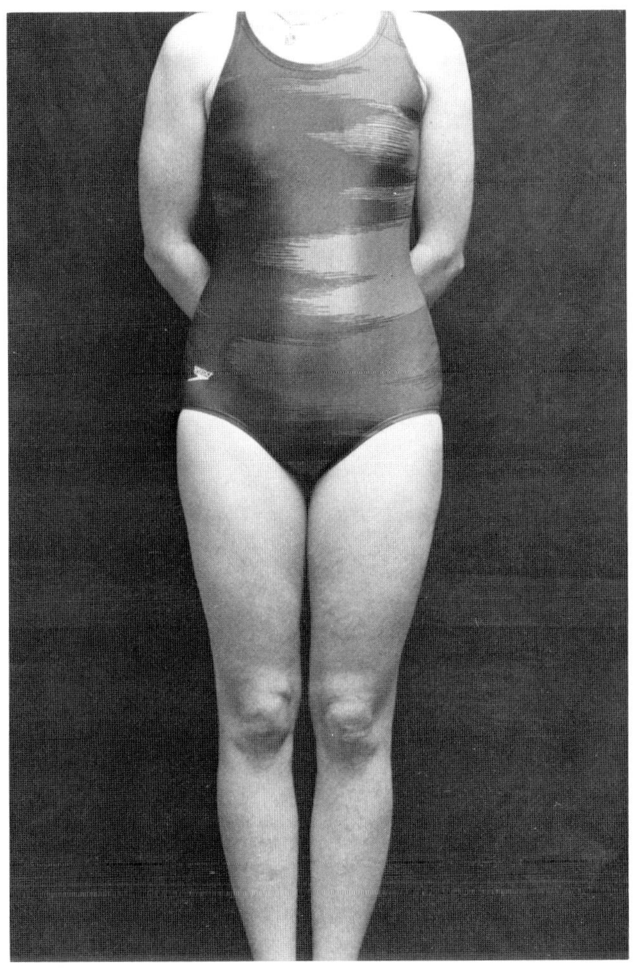

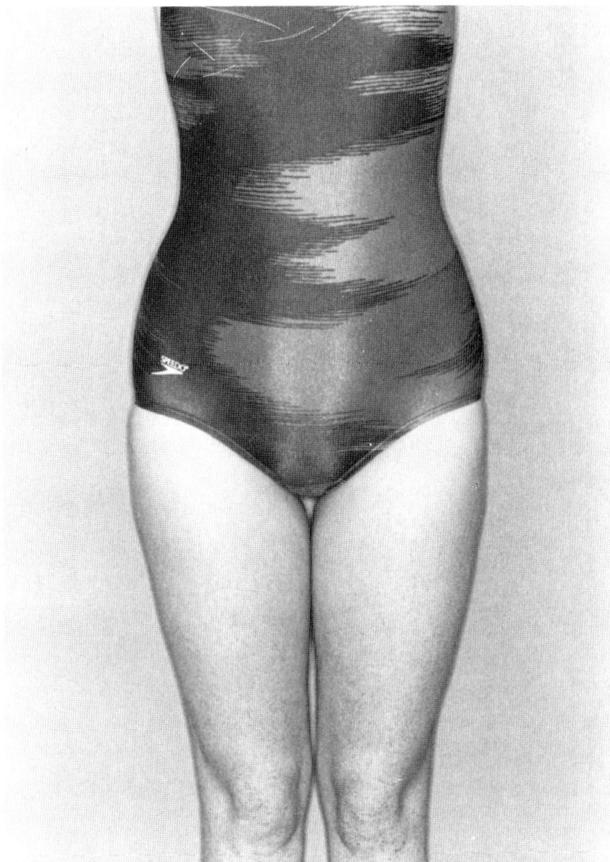

Fig. 10-4. Body photo showing small, equal shadows and loss of skin detail (flattening) caused by ring light. Notice fuzzy appearance of edge contours. Compare to Figure 10-6.

Fig. 10-3. Same model as in Figure 10-2 photographed with same film against black background with ambient overhead light.

background color. There is no perfect solution short of going to two background colors and shooting two sets of slides, or shooting one set of slides and one set of black and white negatives. With the problems most of us face with our office personnel, two sets of slides and two backgrounds would present us with almost unsolvable problems and create patient annoyance.

LIGHTING

Most plastic surgeons know that a photographic facelift is caused by using light from above for the preoperative picture and a ring light for the postoperative picture. The patient's wrinkles, bags, and sags are exaggerated by the shadows thrown by the overhead light while the ring light produces few shadows except laterally. The reader is referred to one of Dr. B. Teimourian's [1] articles in which the lighting as well as the backgrounds and contrasts are so different between the preoperative and

postoperative photographs that absolutely no conclusion about the surgery could possibly be drawn from them, either by the editor or the reader. Yet such photographs are accepted by some journal editors.

In body photography, the ring light throws small equal shadows on either side of the patient (Fig. 10-4) and flattens any contour irregularity. Light from above reveals the irregularity of the skin; note the knees and thighs in Figure 10-5. The ring light is not recommended for accurate skin detail because it washes out the waves and irregularities of which the patient and the physician need to be aware.

A single electronic flash used in the side-mounted mode throws a dense black shadow to one side (Fig. 10-6). This parallax between the light source and the lens, however, also causes the texture of the skin to show better and thus is exactly what we are interested in. A second flash unit fired by an electronic "slave" shaded to hit only the background area where the shadow appears can ameliorate this problem (Fig. 10-7). This set-up is a recommended arrangement. There are many flash units that operate on 110 volts and are triggered by the on-

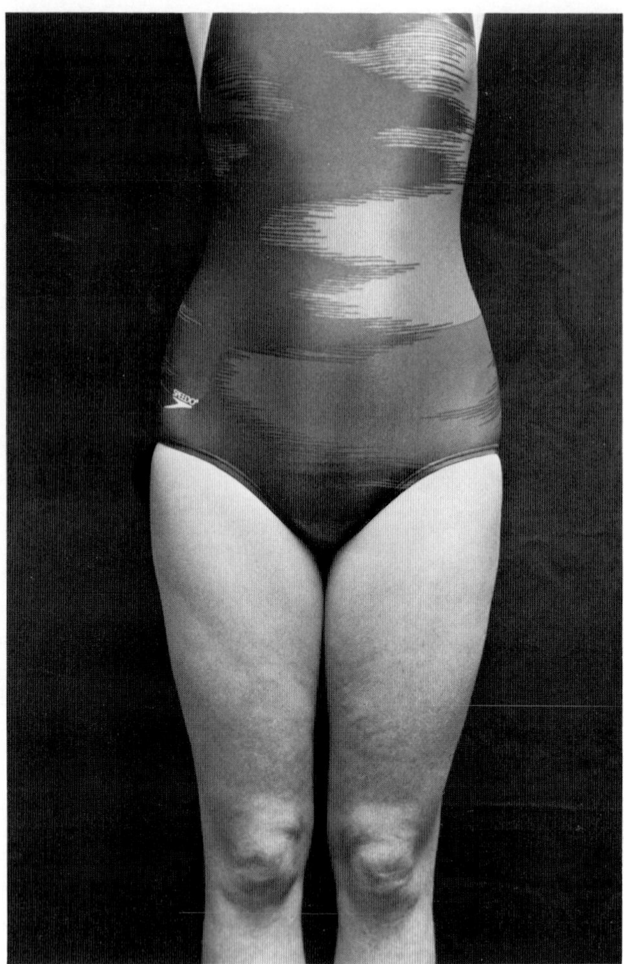

Fig. 10-5. Body photo showing skin detail revealed by ambient light from above.

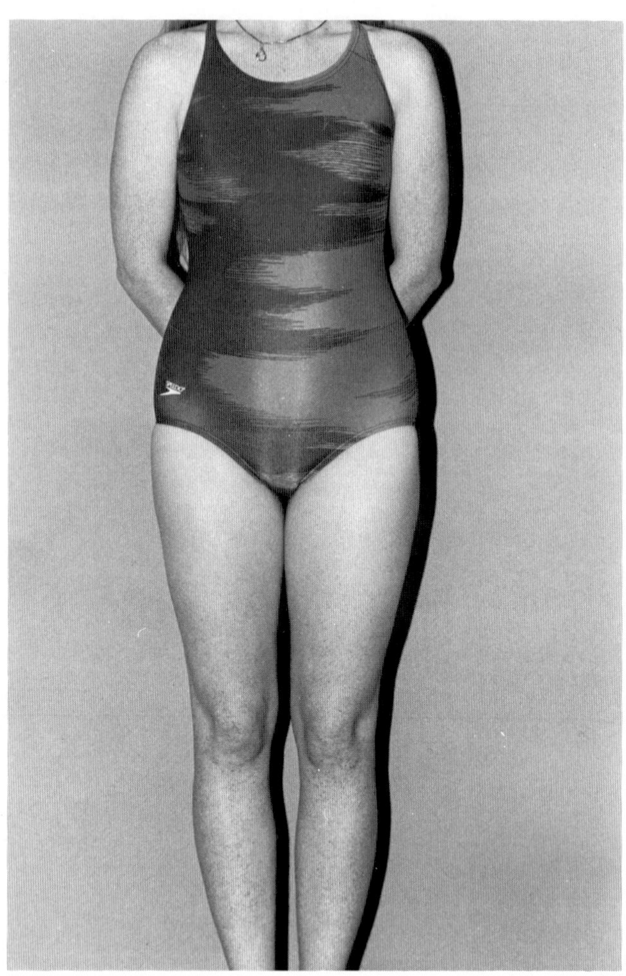

Fig. 10-6. Average office photograph with side mounted flash. Note sharp detail. Compare to Figures 10-4 and 10-5.

camera flash unit. The light output is limited by black "barn doors" to hit only the background where the shadow would fall.

A double set of flash units provides even better color and black and white pictures by eliminating shadows and by giving a bright, light background that is good for publication. This is a good alternative for those desiring very high quality pictures (Fig. 10-8). Special effect lighting for the face is mentioned in Chapter 24.

FOCAL LENGTH OF LENS

For *facial pictures* a 90- to 105-mm portrait or Macro lens is best. The distance from the patient is 4 to 6 feet, which produces a normal relationship between ears and nose. Figures 10-9, 10-10, and 10-11 show the distortion that short focal length causes when working at short distances of less than 4 feet.

For *torso pictures* a 50-mm lens is adequate. To fill the frame, a camera-to-subject distance of 5 to 6 feet is necessary and produces no distortion. A 90-mm lens

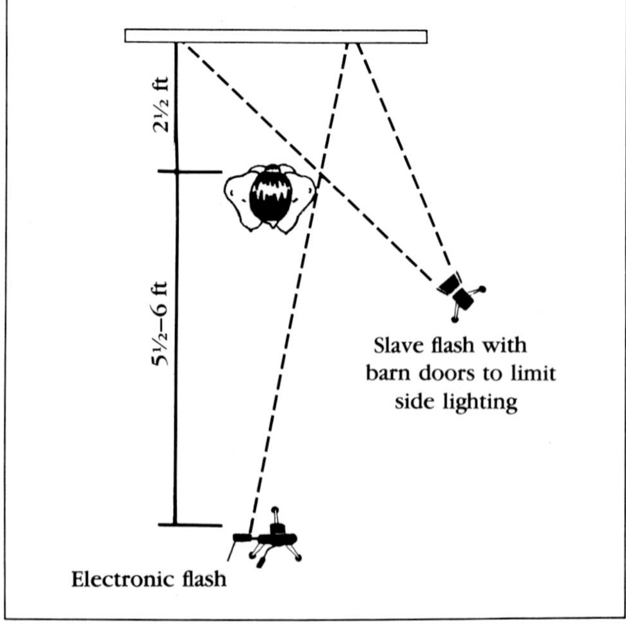

Fig. 10-7. Drawing to show method of illuminating background to eliminate shadow from camera mounted flash.

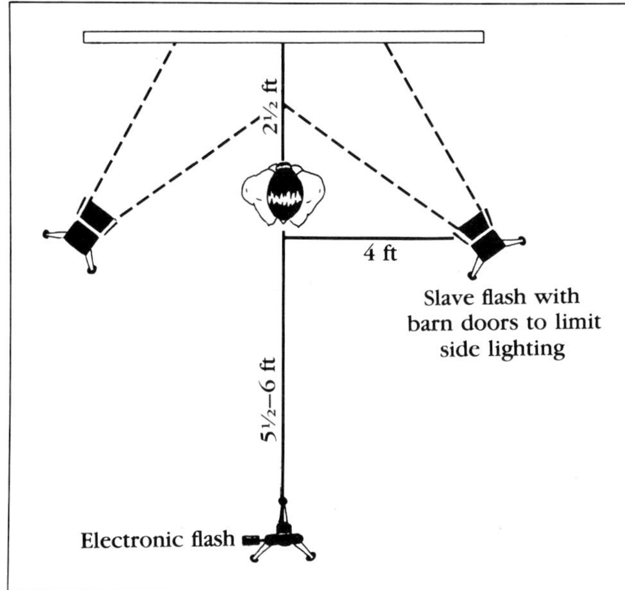

Fig. 10-8. Drawing to show best method of taking photographs for publication.

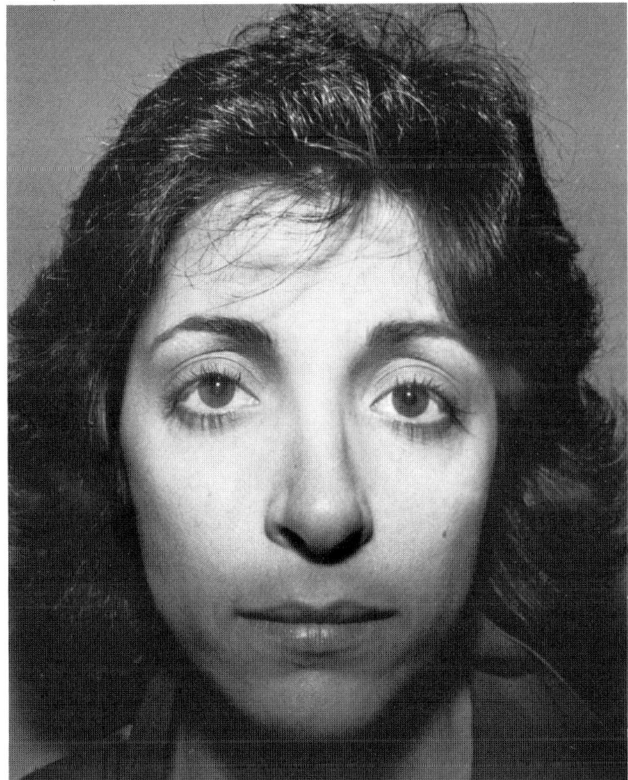

Fig. 10-9. 28-mm lens at 14 inches. Obvious distortion of nose size to rest of face.

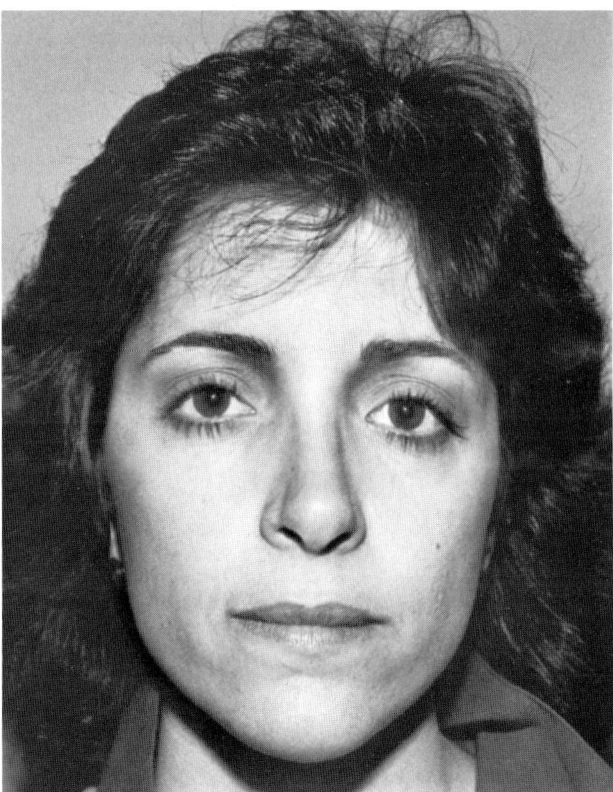

Fig. 10-10. 50-mm lens at 2 feet. Slight enlargement of nasal tip and wider cheek bones.

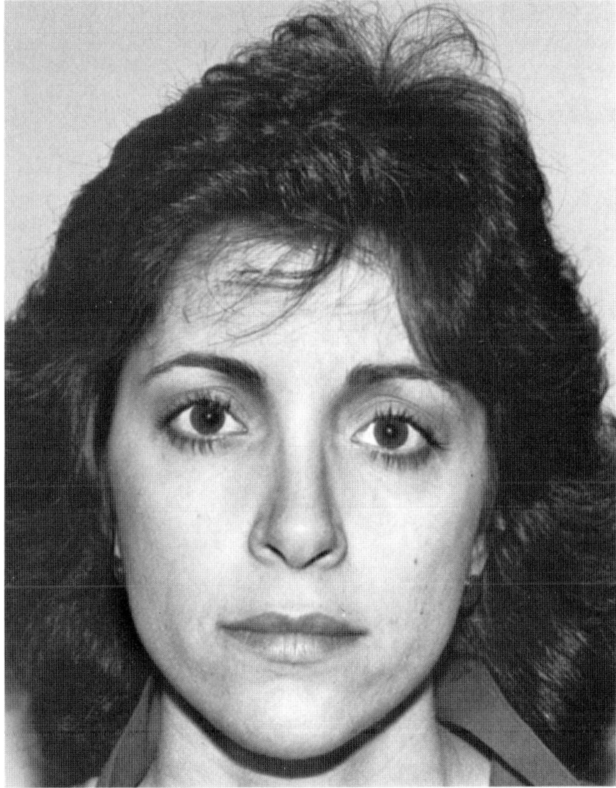

Fig. 10-11. 90-mm lens at 4 feet. Normal proportions.

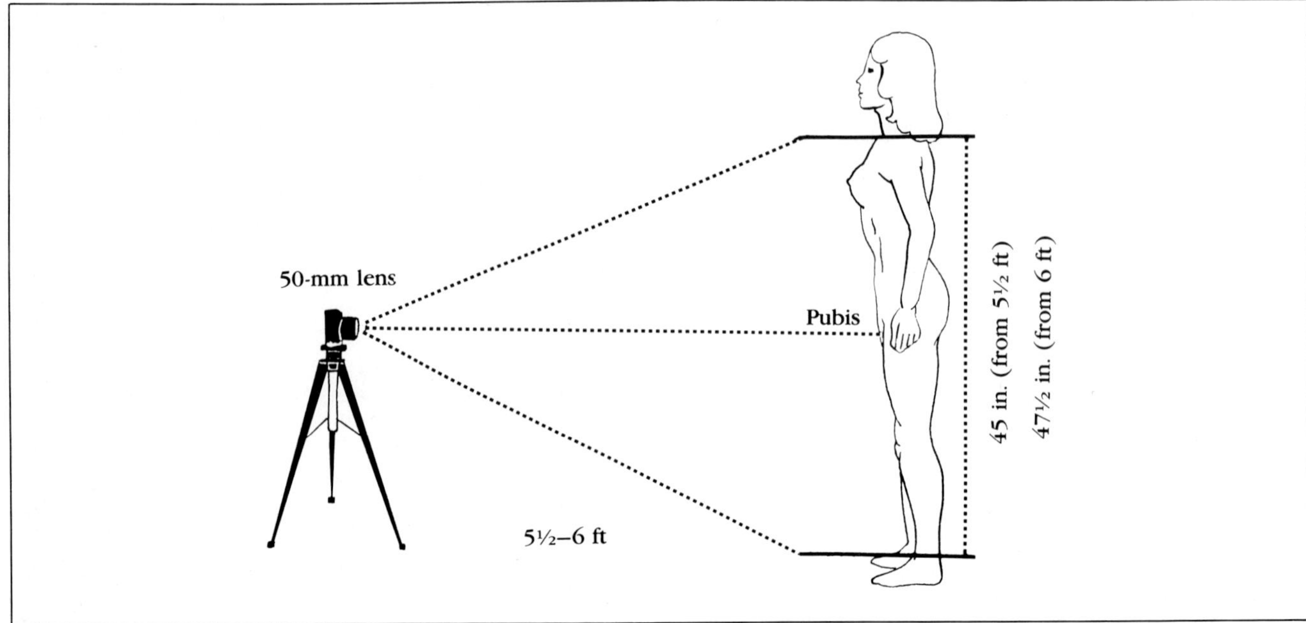

Fig. 10-12. Camera set up for lipolysis pictures to exclude head and feet from picture and to provide consistent distance for pre- and postpictures.

would give as good a picture as the 50-mm, but it would require 9 feet camera-to-subject distance, which is impractical if tripods and background are to be used in an office setting.

DISTANCE

The 50-mm lens allows a torso, less the head and the feet, to fill the frame, as shown in Figure 10-12 at 5 to 6 feet. Whatever distance is chosen should be permanently marked on the floor, with tape indicating where the patient stands and where the tripod will stand. If no tripod is used, the person taking the pictures will weave back and forth sufficiently to alter the size of the image, thereby making inconsistent pre- and postoperative pictures as well as causing possible depth of focus problems.

FOCUS, f-STOP, AND FILM SPEED

The distance from heel mark to lens should be measured and the camera focus control adjusted accurately to that distance. Focus on either side will be clear to an extent dependent on the f-stop. I recommend a minimum of f5.6. Films are now available that allow the use of f5.6 or f8, even with modestly priced electronic flash units set on automatic or "dedicated" mode. Whereas a few years ago ASA 25 was the Kodachrome standard, ASA 100 films are now comparable in quality. Soon ASA 200 and ASA 400 will be the norm, which will allow higher f-stops with even better depth of field. Seek competent advice at a good photo store on the choice of electronic

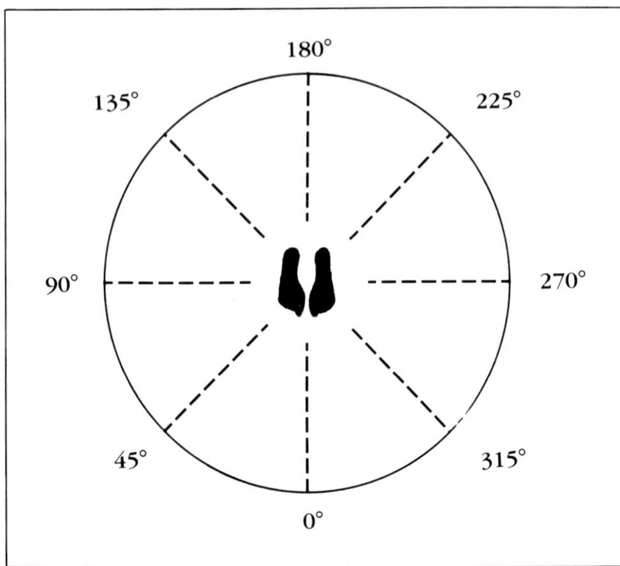

Fig. 10-13. Drawing showing floor markings for the eight positions taken of a body sculpture patient.

flash units to provide an f-stop of at least 5.6, or preferably higher, if you are not knowledgeable in these areas.

PATIENT POSITION AND ATTIRE

We have all seen slide presentations where various articles of clothing are shown in the picture in a state of partial removal. The postoperative photo is equally messy but totally different. This type of picture is simply

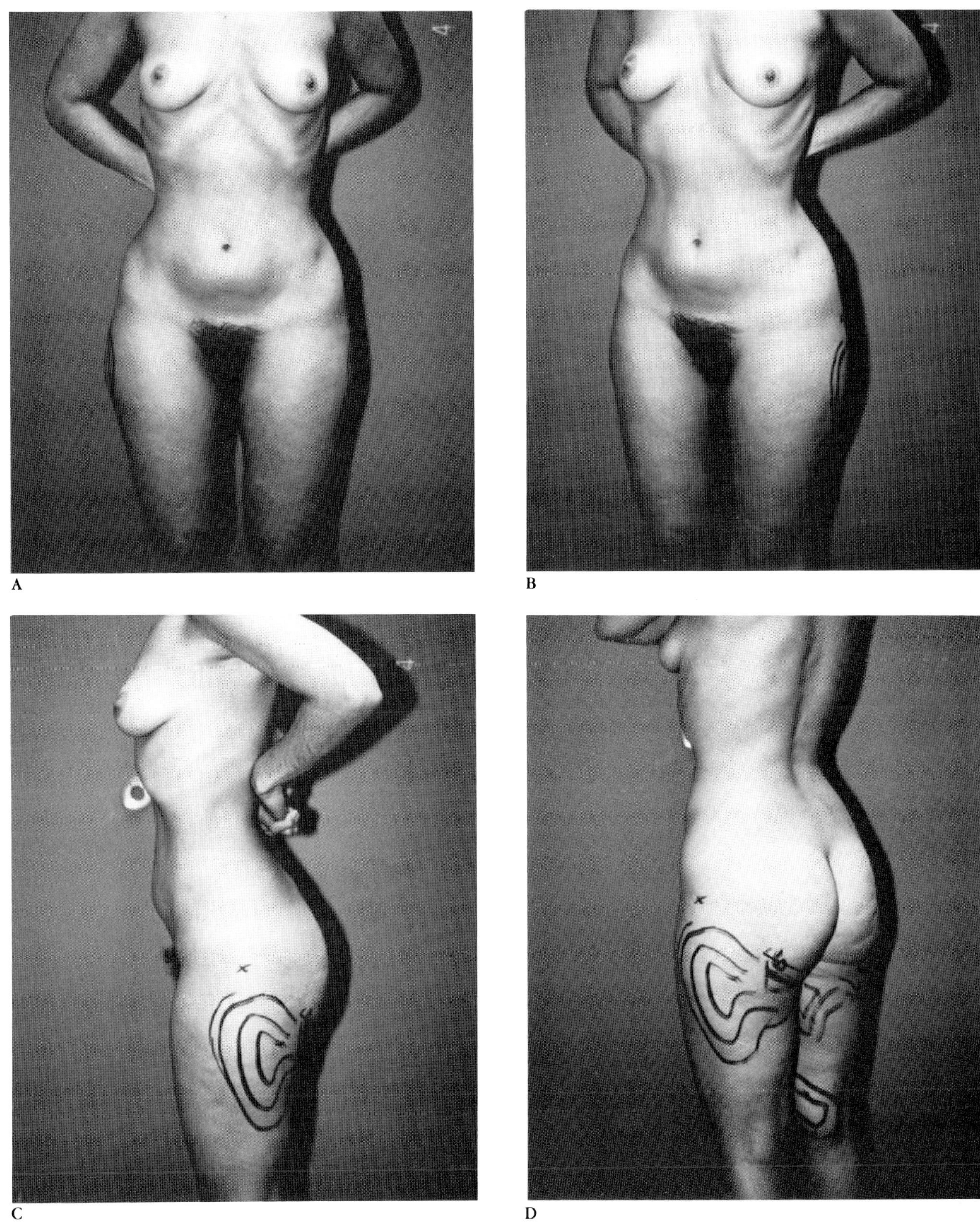

Fig. 10-14. Eight positions for complete photographic evaluation.
A. Frontal view.
B. Right anterior oblique view.
C. Right profile view.
D. Right posterior oblique view.

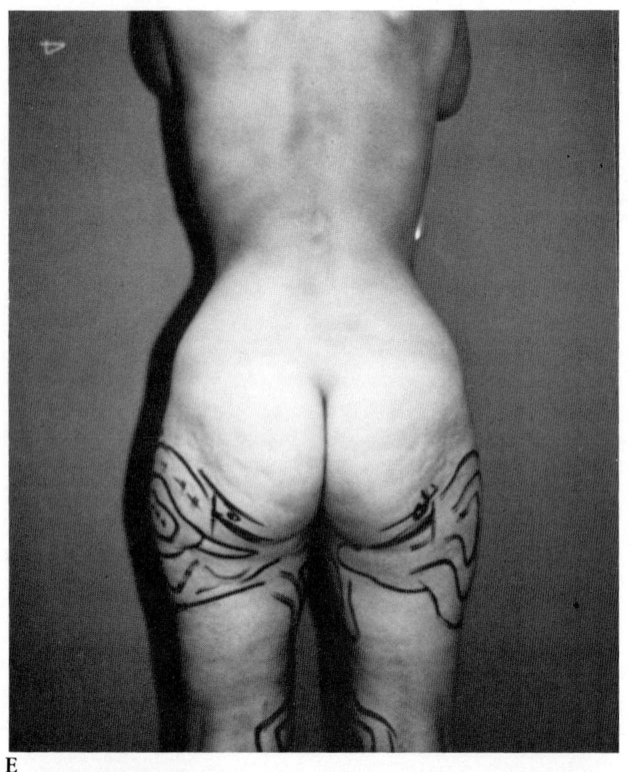

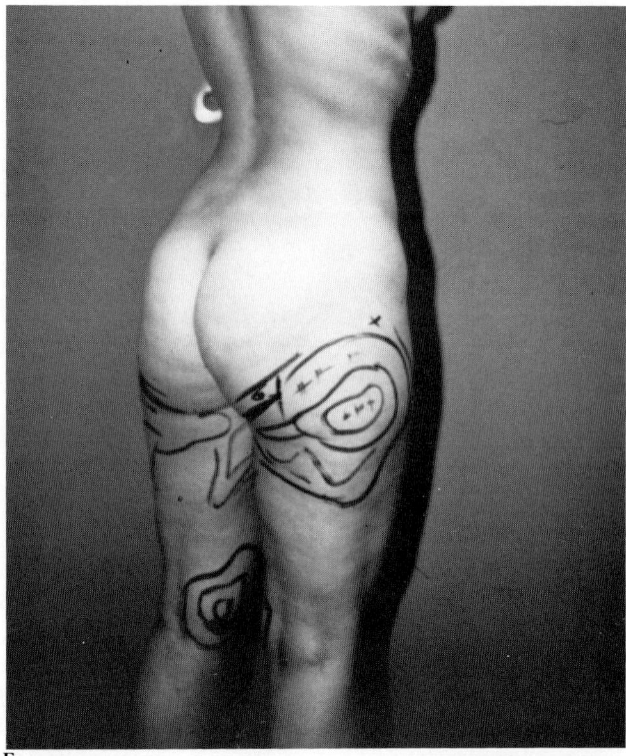

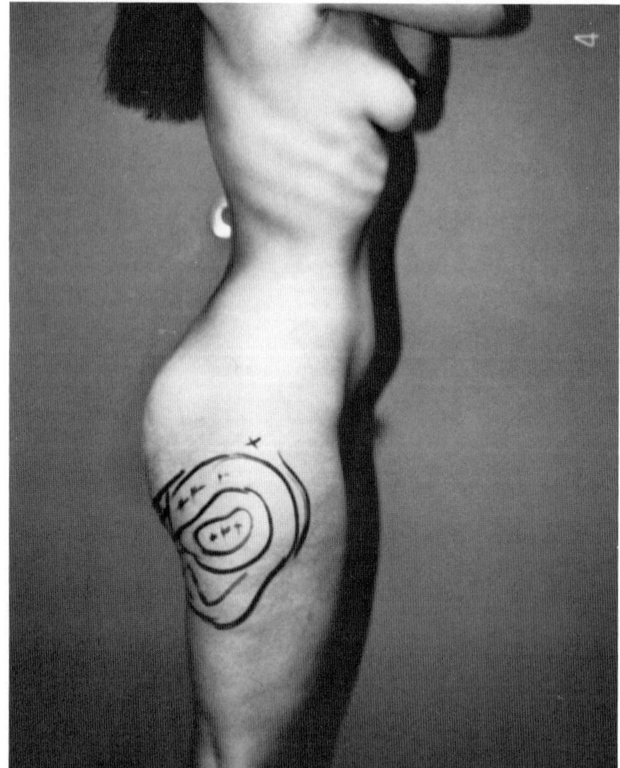

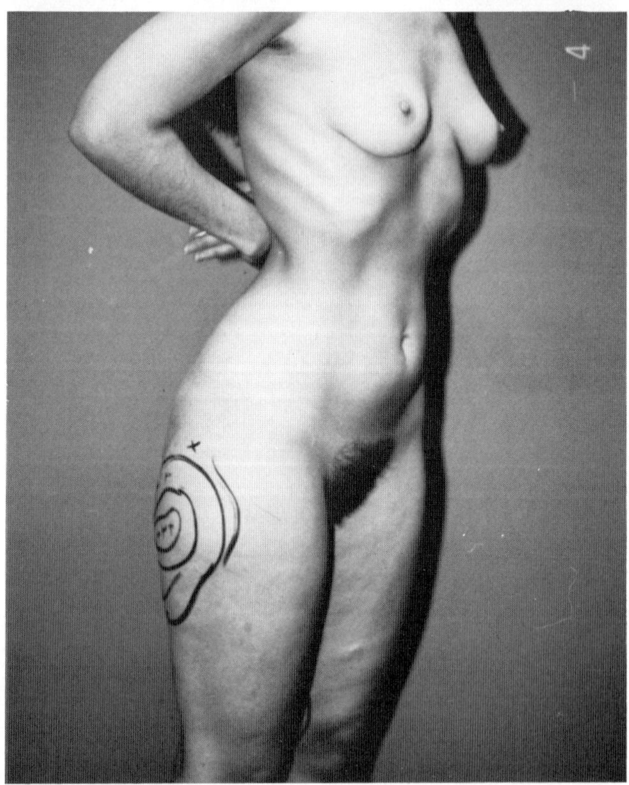

Fig. 10-14 (continued)
E. Posterior view.
F. Left posterior view.
G. Left profile.
H. Left anterior oblique.

not adequate, and we all must strive for better photographs.

The plastic surgeon should determine whether the patient should be totally nude (ideal) or wear a small G-string; either way, neither clothing nor heavy jewelry should be worn. As shown in Figure 10-13, the eight positions necessary for complete evaluation should be marked on the floor: front and rear, right and left quarter oblique, right and left profile, and right and left three-quarter oblique (Fig. 10-14A-H). The heel position should remain marked on the floor as this is the axis of rotation and the toes should rotate around this point.

The camera is adjusted in height on the tripod to the level of the patient's pubic bone (Fig. 10-12), which provides the approximate midpoint of the body. The camera is then adjusted to exclude the face, obviating the necessity of requesting permission from the patient to show the photographs subsequently.

Photographs of the upper torso alone, or pelvis and thighs alone, taken in the hand-held mode are obviously inconsistent and should be avoided. In lipolysis patients, it is the relation of the part to the whole that is awry, and we need to view the whole body from neck to ankles to appreciate these relationships.

FILM PROCESSING

Kodak laboratories have the most consistent processing of Kodachrome slide film and, despite occasional loss of film in the mail, it is recommended. If the preoperative slides have not been returned by the day of surgery, either another set should be taken or Polaroid pictures should be taken to fulfill medicolegal concerns. Local laboratories can handle Ektachrome reasonably well but have greater inconsistency than Kodak laboratories.

Internegatives for black and white prints and color montage slides are a custom service. It is hard to find good work outside of university audiovisual departments, large urban area commercial laboratories, or a dedicated amateur photography buff, although advances in films and processing may well solve some of the dilemmas presented in this chapter. The new Polaroid instant slide system in which you develop the slides immediately is a safe back-up system made to order for plastic surgery offices. However, the slides will be no better than the lighting, background, position, and lens system that you employ. Take the time to set it up well and enjoy seeing good results consistently well presented.

References

1. Teimourian, B. Face and neck suction-assisted lipectomy associated with rhytidectomy. *Plast. Reconstr. Surg.* 72(5):627, 1983.
2. Dickason, W. L., and Hanna, D. C. Pitfalls of comparative photography in plastic and reconstructive surgery. *Plast. Reconstr. Surg.* 58(2):166, 1976.

Suggested Reading

The Time-Life Revised Library of Photography, New York: Time-Life Books, 1970. The following volumes are especially valuable: *The Camera, Photography as a Tool, Light and Film*, and *Color.*
Kodak Workshop Series: Electronic Flash. Rochester, NY: Kodak Publication KW-12, 1981.

CHAPTER 11

Risk Management for Blunt Suction Lipectomy

George Greenberg

This chapter is limited to consideration of injury prevention and actions to be taken at the time of injury. These recommendations result from experience gained over the past years on the committee of the Doctors' Company, the second largest physicians' own medical malpractice carrier in California.

Photographs

Cosmetic surgery is indefensible without preoperative photographs. These photographs constitute the best rebuttal to a patient who contends no improvement has occurred, and they should be present in the chart before surgery. If not in the chart, a Polaroid picture should be used to ensure documentation of the preoperative status. Standard photographs at a set distance and rotation should be taken on all patients (see Chapter 10). Photographs must show normal as well as involved areas, pinpointing the amplitude of the defect.

Photograph collections showing results to patients should be discouraged. If photographs are shown, they must demonstrate the full range of potential results, including good, fair, and unsatisfactory results. By showing this spectrum, patients will not recognize any implied warranty in the procedure.

Appropriate Patient Selection

Patients who have unrealistic expectations are poor candidates for any aesthetic surgery. They will present a very uncomfortable postoperative course as they have not realized their desired result. Patients suffering a minor deformity to be corrected through a large surgical procedure have unrealistically high expectations. Patients seeking aesthetic surgery to satisfy the demands of other individuals, such as spouse or companion, are poor operative risks. Surgeons who "sell" a procedure without adequate informed consent or who foster an unrealistic expectation are setting the groundwork for litigation.

Informed Consent

An adequate informed consent is mandatory and must be presented verbally to the patient by the physician. A detailed preoperative discussion with the patient, including the informed consent and reasonable postoperative expectations, is mandatory. Presentation of complications should not be minimized in an effort to avoid scaring patients away from lipolysis. An accurate discussion of the problems, as well as the expenses involved, should be discussed. A consent listing all complications should be obtained in the physician's office and witnessed. The patient then should be allowed to question any statements and sign a release to that effect. Chart documentation should contain a specific description of the discussion of the procedure with the patient. The simple notation "complications explained" is not satisfactory, particularly in this procedure at this time.

With an adequate informed consent and an outline of the lipolysis discussion, including the extremes of problems, the physician will place himself or herself in a defensible position. The current state of mind of some staff members of the Food and Drug Administration, with regard to the equipment used for lipolysis, does create a question of merit in the plaintiff bar. Plastic surgeons are therefore advised to give close attention to their records.

Patients from another geographical area should understand the time frame for complete resolution of the effects of the surgical procedure. They should be encouraged to remain within the treating physician's geographical area to receive maximal attention during the early healing process. These patients should be encouraged, in addition, to return for follow-up visits in the future. Postoperative photographs are important.

Unrealistic Expectations

It should be emphasized that, as yet, lipolysis is not considered a treatment for generalized obesity but is an accepted treatment for localized fat deformities not responsive to the usual dietary and exercise regimens. The possibility that the patient may not recognize significant improvement should be pointed out, and volume limitations of removed tissue strictly emphasized. The anatomical appearance of the treated area must be discussed with the patient preoperatively. In areas such as the legs, the anatomical landmarks (including the trochanteric and tibial prominences) should be specifically pointed out as natural occurrences. Avoidance of the straight-line appearance on an extremity should be discussed with the patient so he or she understands the normal contours.

Patients over the age of 40 or with poor skin tone need to be told that they have a decreased contractility of the skin. In preoperative evaluation, the presence of skin laxity should alert the physician to the possibility of skin excision in addition to, or in combination with, lipolysis.

The calf area is the area of most delayed results and hence least patient satisfaction. Preoperative discussion should be approached with this in mind. Again, the physician should remember that patients with minimal deformities often have maximal expectations.

Preoperative Evaluation

Careful screening preoperatively is necessary. A history including previous surgeries, medical history, medications, allergies, and bleeding history are necessary. Routine bleeding time, PTT, and blood count prior to lipolysis are recommended. Any patient with a history of bleeding should have a complete coagulation panel before any surgery.

Medications should be evaluated with attention to salicylates, diuretics, steroids, and anticoagulants. Simple blood pressure evaluation may pick up patients with labile hypertension who may present a postoperative bleeding problem.

In cases of any temperature elevation, abnormalities in blood count or other newly discovered medical problem, surgery should be cancelled. Lipolysis is an elective procedure and nonperformance of surgery when a possible medical problem is discovered can save hours of postoperative anguish.

Postoperative Medications and Instructions

The use of pain medication containing any salicylates should be avoided in the postoperative period. The use of salicylates is indefensible in cases of postoperative bleeding. Excessive demands for medication should be carefully evaluated to rule out the possibility of creating a drug dependency.

An instruction sheet should be given at the time of the patient's discharge, including a phone number for any emergency as well as the time of the patient's next appointment. Postoperative surgical instructions must be simple and specific. The patient should be advised to contact the physician's office should anything occur that has not been discussed or is unexpected.

Billing Disputes

All charges for physician, anesthesiologist, and hospital services must be discussed with the patient in advance. Responsibility for any costs incurred in the treatment of complications should be delineated preoperatively. As a rule, preoperative collection of the physician's fee will weed out many patients who, in an attempt to mitigate the doctor's bill, become unhappy postoperatively with the results.

Touchup and redo procedures should be discussed with the patient preoperatively and a policy established as to the fee charged the patient for the procedure. In many practices, touchups and redos are usually done for the cost of supplies and, if necessary, hospital and anesthesiologist. The number of lawsuits filed because of billing disputes of noncollected money is significant. Postoperative dissatisfaction with a request for return of fees should be carefully evaluated to ascertain any real basis for dissatisfaction. In cases where there is no basis for dissatisfaction, the money should not be returned. The writing off of a bill, however, is not an admission of guilt. It may be helpful in cases in which the results are less than desirable, and allow the physician to avoid becoming entangled in a legal process to resolve the problem.

Office Personnel

Patients undergoing lipolysis will need positive reinforcement from the office personnel. The office personnel should provide a positive atmosphere postoperatively and treat the patient in a fashion to assure them that their appearance is not an aberration of the normal postoperative course. The postoperative appearance after bandage removal should be carefully dealt with by office personnel who will comfort the patient that this is an accepted appearance. They will reassure the patient that the bruising, edema, waviness, and any other changes will resolve.

The patient is encouraged to call the physician's office for any question regarding postoperative problems. Office personnel should be instructed that postoperative patients complaining of problems should be evaluated within a short period of time and should not be allowed to wait several days before being seen. The tendency for office personnel to protect a physician must not be allowed to prevent possible complications from being seen in the office promptly.

Lipolysis Privileges

Because of the potential surgical problems involved in the technique of lipolysis, in the care and handling of the skin, it would be wise to have each physician performing this procedure obtain surgical credentials from the hospital to fall within the realm of the Plastic Surgery Department. Other specialties wishing to do this procedure should be limited to areas in which they have surgical privileges. All suction equipment should be approved by the appropriate Biomechanical Department in the hospital and approved for use.

Repeat Procedures

Repeat procedures are best treated by the original physician under his or her original agreement with the patient. The use of a 4- or 6-mm cannula in the office, under a local anesthetic, can usually correct small areas of unevenness. By maintaining the cost of a repeat procedure within the original surgery, patients will not seek other physicians, and this will avoid the very common problems of "Who did that?"

Record Keeping

After lipolysis, operative records should be kept as in any surgical procedure. These records should never be altered. Any change should be noted as an addendum to the chart. During the operative procedure, any problems should be mentioned and appropriate actions or consultations documented without delay to show that early recognition and treatment was performed. It should be strictly emphasized that the patient, as well as any attorney, has a right to obtain a copy, not the original, of these records, and that they may be subjected to very careful scrutiny and semantic interpretations.

The Next Physician

"Who did that?" is the most common source of litigation arising from aesthetic surgery. The magnification of a possible unsatisfactory result by another plastic surgeon, in his or her attempt to obtain ultimate perfection, provides the plaintiff's bar with an excellent case for litgation. Subsequent treating physicians should show concern for the patient's problem rather than attempting to place blame on the initial surgeon. Inflammatory statements referring to the original physician and the operative procedure may present a major problem to insurance companies insuring plastic surgeons.

It should be emphasized that the "new" physician did not see the patient before the first surgery. Variations in patient's healing, as well as the fact that time may provide further resolution of the problem, should be discussed. Effort should be made to have the patient contact the original physician to rectify the problem, which often concerns billing or an area of scarring. It is imperative that all plastic surgeons realize that they face similar scrutiny and comments from their peers. Statements such as "only I can obtain perfection" and similar feelings passed onto the patient should be avoided. A concerted effort to show patient concern and the recognition that we are all human would help avoid many lawsuits.

CHAPTER 12

Patient Selection: Psychological Aspects

Carson M. Lewis

What is the ideal end point of an aesthetic surgical procedure? The end point may vary, depending on the level of experience: For the plastic surgery resident in training, it may simply mean getting from point A to point G in a complicated cleft lip repair; for the teacher it may mean seeing his or her resident progress safely through an operative procedure; for the young surgeon it may mean an operative procedure without complications. For the experienced aesthetic surgeon, however, the satisfactory end point lies in patient satisfaction. When the patient, at the completion of the convalescent period, expresses happiness with having had the procedure, this is the successful surgical experience.

Successful Patient Selection

The path to a satisfied postoperative patient is treacherous and filled with many dangers. The first step begins with the initial patient interview. We plastic surgeons should realize that in our specialty, as in no other, patients come to us wanting the operation. They see an aesthetic operation as a solution to their problems. With other surgical specialties, patients reluctantly see their consultants, hoping there are other ways to treat their problems, dreading the moment the surgeon will recommend an operation. Our specialty is unique in that they seek us out, wanting an operative procedure to change their appearance; therefore, it is not difficult to find patients on whom to operate. Ross Musgrave [1] states, "In our residency, we learn how to operate. Probably more time should be spent on learning on whom to operate and, more appropriately, on whom not to operate." Our responsibility is to be selective so that most patients will be satisfied at the completion of the operative procedure. Nothing builds a practice faster than satisfied patients singing your praises. On the other hand, a disgruntled patient, whether justified or not, will keep other potential patients from your door.

In the initial interview, important decisions are made. The surgeon decides if the patient is a satisfactory candidate. The evaluation includes both physiological and psychological components. Physiological criteria are tangible and more readily assessed. Ideal patients for lipolysis are those under 40 years of age and with localized areas of fat. Criteria are easily noted. Pathological contraindications such as hypertension, bleeding, and clotting abnormalities are readily identified.

EVALUATION OF PSYCHOLOGICAL ASPECTS

Evaluating the psychological aspects of a patient is difficult. The plastic surgeon, without benefit of specialized training in psychology, must decide whether a patient should be chosen or rejected for an operative procedure. Most frequently, this decision is based on an intuitive feeling. With experience, the surgeon is better able to avoid the undesirable patient, having been "burned" in the past. However, even the most experienced surgeons, on occasion, regret their selection of certain patients.

Plastic surgeons walk a fine line in patient selection. On the one hand, they must reject patients who they believe will be dissatisfied. Dissatisfaction is an important factor in the etiology of medical malpractice suits. It is estimated that some plastic surgeons reject up to 30% of patients interviewed for aesthetic procedures. If surgeons are too rejecting, however, their practice suffers. If they are too accepting, the plethora of unreasonable and dissatisfied patients makes each day a burden and increases the risk of a lawsuit.

What qualities are helpful in the analysis of patient selection? Several investigators have performed studies of patients undergoing cosmetic surgery; both facial cosmetic and torso procedures have been evaluated [2,3,4]. There appears to be no discernible difference in approaching patient selection between facial cosmetic surgery and cosmetic surgery of the body. The criteria evaluated for potential aesthetic patients are the same. There appears to be no apparent difference between those seeking lipolysis and other types of aesthetic surgery.

Several general rules of thumb have stood the test of time and experience. These rules suggest questions that can be easily answered by the plastic surgeon to help determine the patient's chance of a satisfactory result from a psychological standpoint.

1. Self-motivation. Is there motivation from within the patient? Studies indicate that the patient should have the operation for him- or herself, not because of the motivation of others. The patient who is in the plastic surgeon's office because her husband wants her to have larger breasts or her mother wants her to have a different nose has a greater risk of dissatisfaction. If the patient does not desire the surgery but goes through it to please others, the inconveniences of surgery are exaggerated and the pain enhanced. These patients become irritated with those who have insisted or encouraged them to be operated on. The surgeon becomes a party to this process and a more convenient target for vengeance than those on whom the patient may be emotionally or sexually dependent. Ask yourself if the patient is motivated from within or without.

2. Duration of complaint. The concern that brings the patient to the doctor should be present for several months. The prolonged duration indicates a chronic

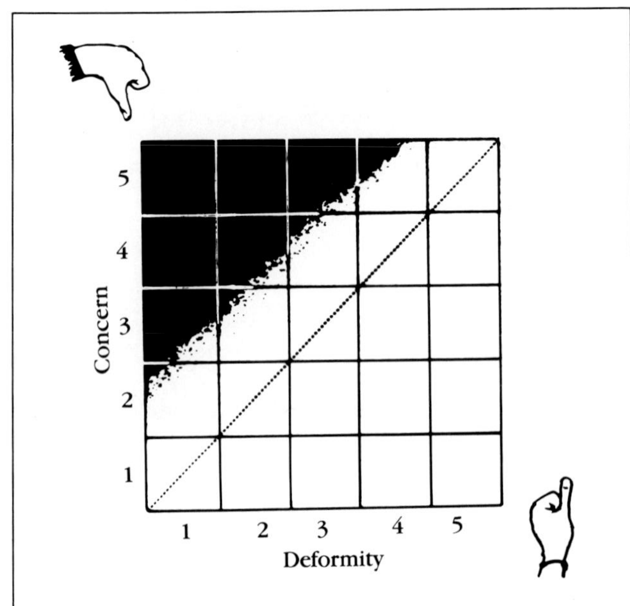

Fig. 12-1. Graph plotting the degree of concern of the patient against the degree of anxiety. This graph is helpful in patient selection. (Developed by Dr. Mark Gorney; reproduced with permission.)

source of concern. If the patient, on the other hand, is seen soon after having heard of the procedure, the patient may not have been concerned long about his or her problem.

3. Anxiety compared to deformity. Dr. Mark Gorney [5] developed a graph that plots degree of anxiety or concern of the patient against the degree of deformity. If there is a great deformity and low anxiety, there is a high chance of success. If the patient exhibits minimal deformity and a high degree of anxiety, the patient becomes more difficult to please. The graph is placed on the patient's chart (Fig. 12-1).

4. Wanting to be made over. Some patients with multiple areas of concern essentially want to be made over. They want their face, their breasts, and their torso operated on. We see reports from South America that multiple surgeons perform multiple procedures on such patients. In my experience, these patients are difficult to satisfy. What they are saying is that they are dissatisfied with everything about themselves. They frequently have associated turmoil in their lives such as divorce, separation, vocational problems, or other unresolved emotional conflicts. This patient is really saying, "I'm not satisfied with anything about my body or my entire existence." I have found that they are a group of patients difficult to satisfy and are best avoided.

5. Severely depressed patients. The severely depressed

patient represents an unsatisfactory candidate because of lack of emotional reserve. Operative procedures require mental as well as physical energy. These patients have little or none to give. The stress concomitant with any operative procedure may bring on a profound depression and psychomotor immobilization.

6. Psychotic patients. This group lives in a world out of contact with reality. Psychotic patients are not always easily identified or labeled. Many are ambulatory schizophrenics functioning more or less well in our society, and some are bound to enter your office.

These patients are difficult to communicate with, and they may have a distorted impression of the result. This type of patient may kill his surgeon.

Dr. Sharie Lavell, who is working on her Ph.D. thesis in my office, and I evaluated aesthetic facial surgery patients in a postoperative patient satisfaction study. Certain areas of patient personality appeared important to determine patient satisfaction. We coined the acronym "SAFE," and we asked the question, "Is the patient SAFE for surgery? SAFE refers to four areas investigated:

S: Self-esteem
A: Anxiety
F: Fear or paranoia
E: Expectations

These areas provide the surgeon with other criteria to assist in the patient selection process. The surgeon should ask questions that begin with words such as who, what, when, how, and why. Open-ended questions of this type require an explanation and cannot be answered with a simple yes or no. The evaluation of SAFE by the surgeon is based on patients' answers to questions and on observing the patient during the answering process.

"S" refers to self-esteem. Patients who have a high esteem of themselves are better operative candidates. One question to help determine the self-esteem is, "How would you rate yourself in attractiveness from 1 to 10?" Candidates with good self-esteem rate themselves a 6 or above. Also, the patient who is concerned and interested about what others think about their appearance is a better candidate for surgery.

"A" refers to anxiety. Anxiety is the state of being ill at ease. Anxious patients appear as though they expect to be scolded. They have body gestures such as wringing their hands, wet hands on handshake, or other evidence of apprehension. Patients with anxiety have a higher risk of dissatisfaction.

"F" refers to fear, more aptly classified as paranoia. These patients have difficulty relinquishing control to others. They spend an inordinate amount of time asking and reasking questions. They go into meticulous detail. Paranoid patients see more than two plastic surgeons. These characteristics are manifestations of an inability to relinquish control and fear. In our survey, patients who had seen more than two plastic surgeons or who had an inability to relinquish control to the professionals were poor operative candidates.

"E" refers to expectations. Are the patient's expectations realistic? What do they expect to happen in their lives as a result of the surgery? If they expect to retain a spouse who is unfaithful and wandering, or to have a job promotion by having surgery, these are unrealistic expectations. These factors can be evaluated by the surgeon.

The surgeon can ask himself or herself, "Did the patient exhibit evidence of not being SAFE, that is, lacked self-esteem, showed evidence of anxiety and/or fear and paranoia, or had unrealistic expectations of the procedure?" If present, the patient is less likely to be satisfied.

EDUCATION OF PATIENTS

In addition to plastic surgeons fulfilling their responsibilities in selecting patients for operative procedures, they have the responsibility to educate patients about the procedure, providing realistic information so patients may better decide for themselves if they wish to undergo the procedure. This information should include, not necessarily in any order, possible complications and morbidity, and alternative treatments. As surgeons we must personally inform the patient of the surgical risks to legally fulfill our obligation of informed consent. In my office, this is done with a film clip about the procedure, followed by my consultation in which I personally discuss the risks of the operative procedure with the patient.

Morbidity should also be discussed with the patient. How long will the patient have pain, be unable to walk, how long should they take off from work, and when can they resume full athletic activities? These questions should be answered in a realistic way. It is easy to be cavalier and underestimate time off from work and the time necessary to resume normal activities, and thus give the patient an unwarranted sense of simplicity regarding the procedure. If you err, it is far better to overestimate the time necessary to resume normal activities. If the patient is able to return to work earlier, both you and the patient are pleased because he or she is a "good healer." Disappointment and certain dissatisfaction occurs when the convalescent period is prolonged beyond what is anticipated. The informed patient is a better patient. The surgeon has the responsibility to provide this information. If the information is omitted or misleading, this will be a source of dissatisfaction and possibly litigation.

Summary

Patients seeking lipolysis (blunt suction lipectomy) need to be evaluated by the surgeon on the same basis as any patient seeking an aesthetic operation. Physical findings and psychologic make-up of the patient should be analyzed at the initial interview. Time-tested rules of patient suitability for aesthetic procedures should be applied. The acronym SAFE can help the surgeon to analyze the patient's psychology in a systematic manner. This analysis helps identify those who have a good chance of being satisfied postoperatively. The surgeon also has the responsibility to properly inform patients about the operative procedure. Educating the patient increases the chances for a high patient satisfaction rate.

References

1. Musgrave, R. The Difficult Patient. Presented at the American Society of Aesthetic and Plastic Surgeons Annual Meeting, 1982.
2. Lavell, S. The Female Patient's Experience of Aesthetic Regenerative Facial Surgery. Doctoral dissertation, United States International University, 1980.
3. Linn, L., and Goldman, I. B. Psychiatric observations concerning rhinoplasty. *Psychosom. Med.* 11(5), 1949.
4. Webb, W. L., Jr. Mechanisms of psychosocial adjustment in patients seeking "face-lift" operations. *Psychosom. Med.* 27(2):183, 1965.
5. Gorney, M. Personal communication, 1982.
6. Lavell, S. Patient psychological reactions to surgery. How the office-based setting makes them different. Presented at the Third Annual Meeting for the Society for Office-Based Surgery, 1981.

CHAPTER 13

Physical Evaluation and Informed Consent

Frank T. Herhahn

The clue to success in lipolysis, as in all other surgical procedures, is patient selection. Selection does not focus mainly on the exclusion of a particular patient, but rather on the selection of the proper procedure, or combination of procedures, that may apply to a particular patient. If no procedure is applicable, the patient necessarily is excluded.

Early in a surgeon's experience, patient selection should be limited to those who will obtain the best overall result with minimal aesthetic complications. As experience is gained with the lipolysis technique, extended applications and the inclusion of the not-so-ideal patient become more manageable. As plastic surgeons gain experience with this procedure, it is conceivable that an increase in medical indications for the surgical removal of the localized adiposities will appear.

The Ideal Candidate

As Dr. Illouz has pointed out, the ideal candidate for lipolysis is the young, relatively thin, motivated woman (or man) with a localized contour deformity consisting of fat with smooth, taut overlying skin. Ethnic background, skin color, and a history of hypertrophic scarring are minor considerations in selecting the ideal patient.

To bridge the gap from an ideal candidate to a happy patient, one must educate that person on the expectations, limitations, and consequences of lipolysis. This education requires detailed counseling by the surgeon and his or her staff. The surgeon must be well educated about the technique and must establish rapport with and instill confidence in the patient. His or her staff must also be knowledgeable and reinforce that image. Adequate data should support the surgeon's convictions. If possible, postoperative patients should be available to allay new patient fears and to demonstrate the efficacy of the procedure.

The ideal patient is usually less than 35 years old and falls within the ideal limits of weight for his or her height and body type. The best characteristics are good skin turgor without "cellulite," a distinct firmness of adiposity, and little or no tendency toward skin sagging. The skin should be free of striae. This patient usually has excess fat less than 250 ml in the abdomen; less than 300 ml in each lateral thigh; less than 200 ml per side in the iliac crest rolls; and a negligible amount in the inner thigh or knee region. Ideal candidates for lipolysis are presented in Figures 13-1 to 13-3.

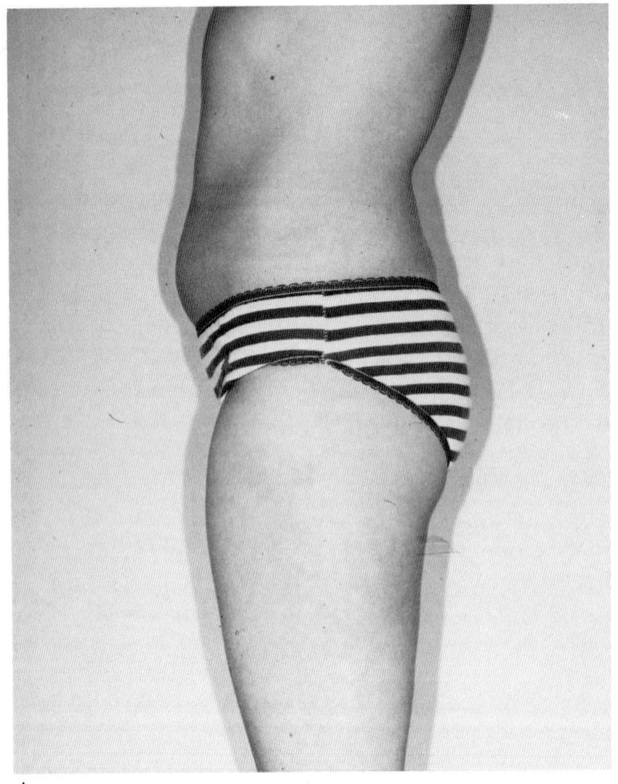

A

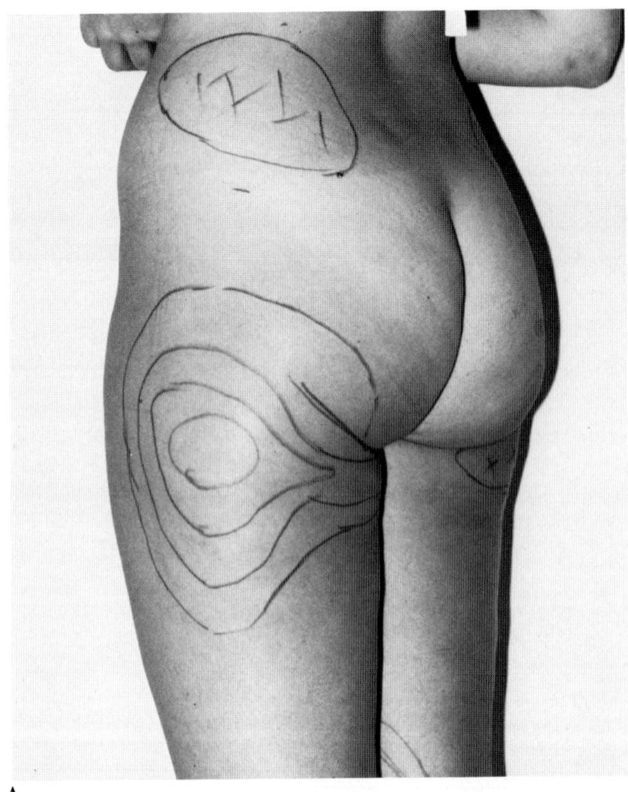

A

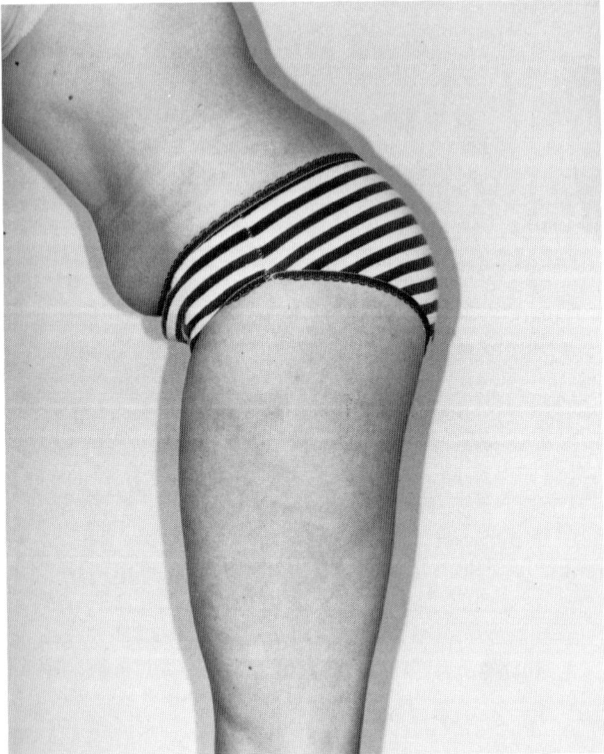

B

Fig. 13-1. A. and B. A 35-year-old jazzercise instructor with one child. Patient is 5′5″ tall and 114 pounds with primary complaint of a "pot belly" resistant to diet and exercise. Preoperative view.

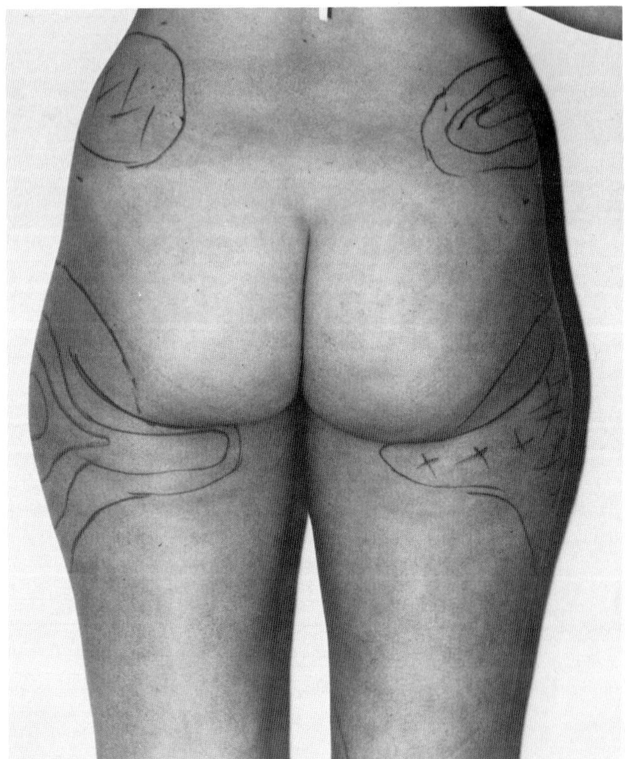

B

Fig. 13-2. A 24-year-old model and dance choreographer with diet-resistant adiposities of hips, lateral femoral area, and inner knee region, present since age 14. Patient is 5′6″ and weighs 130 pounds.
A. Posterior oblique preoperative view.
B. Posterior preoperative view.

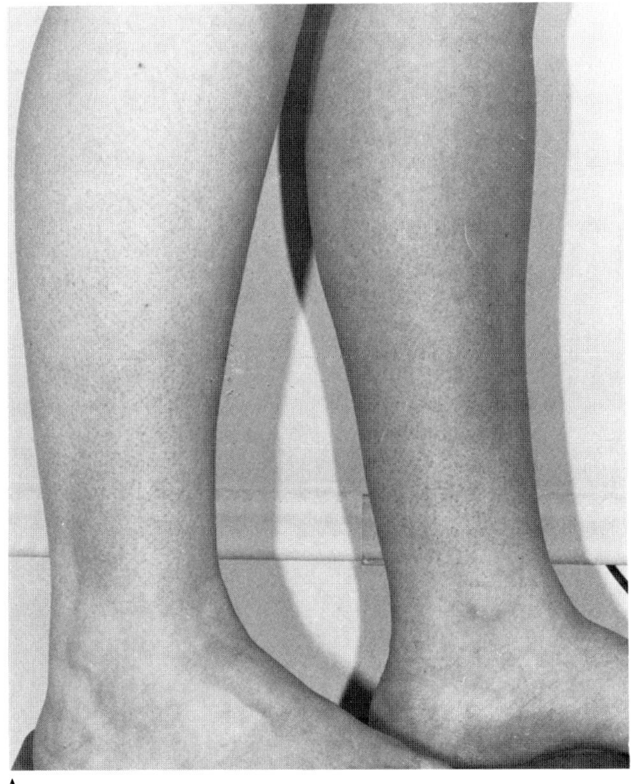

A

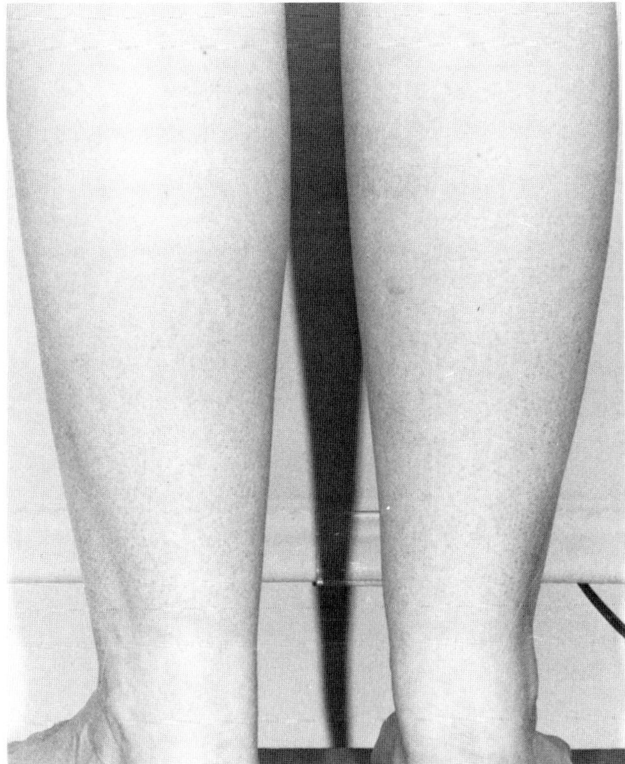

B

Fig. 13-3. A 27-year-old female nurse with inherited lower calf adiposity, present since age 15. Note tight skin.
A. Lateral preoperative view.
B. Posterior preoperative view.

The Average Patient

The average patient varies from practice to practice but is between 30 and 45 years old. This patient is usually 5 to 10 pounds above the ideal weight for his or her height and body build. Many have striae over the abdomen or hips (caused by pregnancy), and there may be very early sagging with loss of the "smile" in the gluteal fold. Lipolysis combined with limited dermolipectomy of the abdomen is a fairly common procedure in this group.

The average patient typically has excess fat in one or more areas. The total fat removal in these patients is usually in the 1000 to 2000 ml range: 200 to 500 ml in the abdomen, 200 to 300 ml in each iliac crest roll, 400 to 800 ml in each lateral thigh, 150 ml from each inner thigh, and 100 ml from each knee. Examples of average patients are presented in Figs. 13-4 and 13-5. See Chapters 26 and 33 for information on the arms and calves.

Most patients are satisfied with the procedure, and the surgeon need not hesitate to recommend lipolysis to this group. Cellulite, striae, and loose skin may compromise the results to a degree, and thus the surgeon or the patient may be critical of the result. In middle-aged women, lateral thigh deformities exceeding 800 ml per side may be removed at 6-month intervals; this allows better skin contraction. The average patient is often more satisfied than the surgeon.

The Less-Than-Ideal Patient

The less-than-ideal patient is usually over 35 years of age and 10 to 20 pounds overweight, but may have been significantly overweight at one time. This patient frequently has striae, cellulite, and loose overlying skin. The beginning of an apron may be seen in the abdomen, and the buttocks frequently are flat or sag and have a downturning crease. It is difficult to view one's buttock and posterior thigh anatomy. These patients are aware that they have a problem but rarely can they appreciate the exact appearance of this area. They are quite critical of their body result postoperatively. The surgeon's ally in these instances is careful and extensive, accurate measurements and preoperative records and good photographs.

Combined lipolysis and abdominal dermolipectomy is the usual treatment for this group. Fat removal usually includes 500 to 1500 ml from the abdomen, 600 to 800 ml from the iliac crest rolls, 800 to 1000 ml from the lateral thighs, 200 to 250 ml from the inner thighs, and 200 or more ml from the knees (Figs. 13-6 to 13-9.) The less-than-ideal patient is generally not enthusiastic about his or her results and frequently inquires about

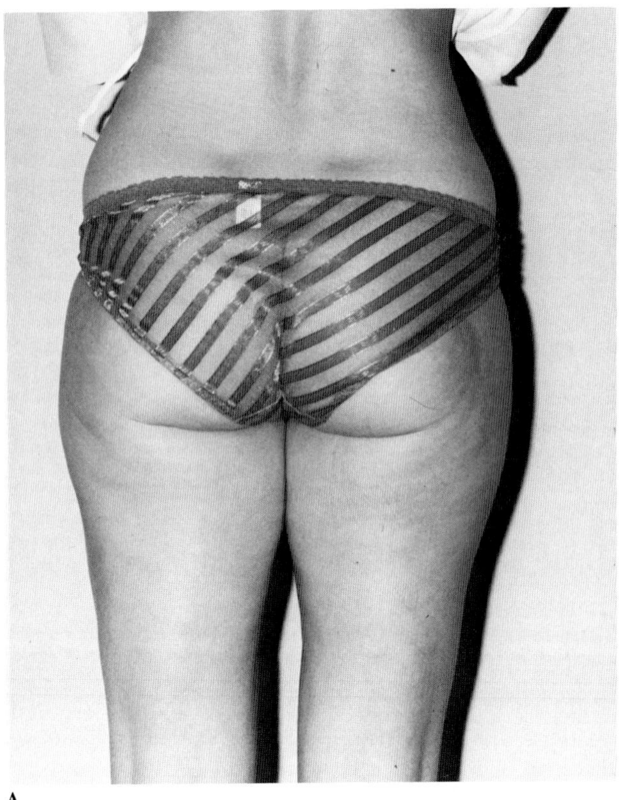

A

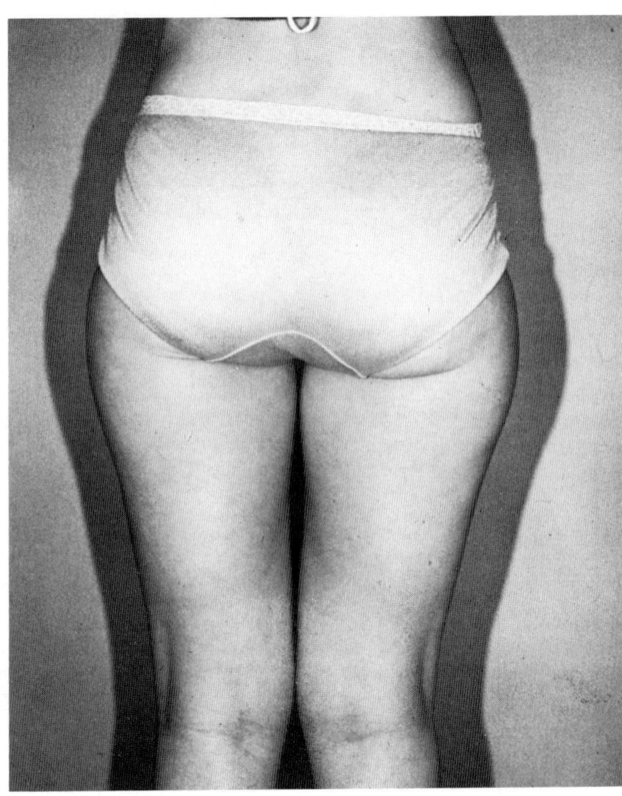

A

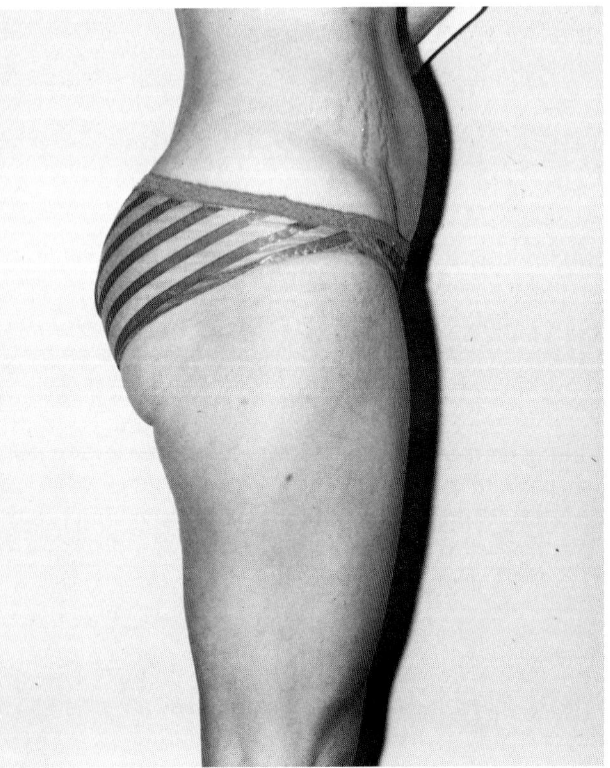

B

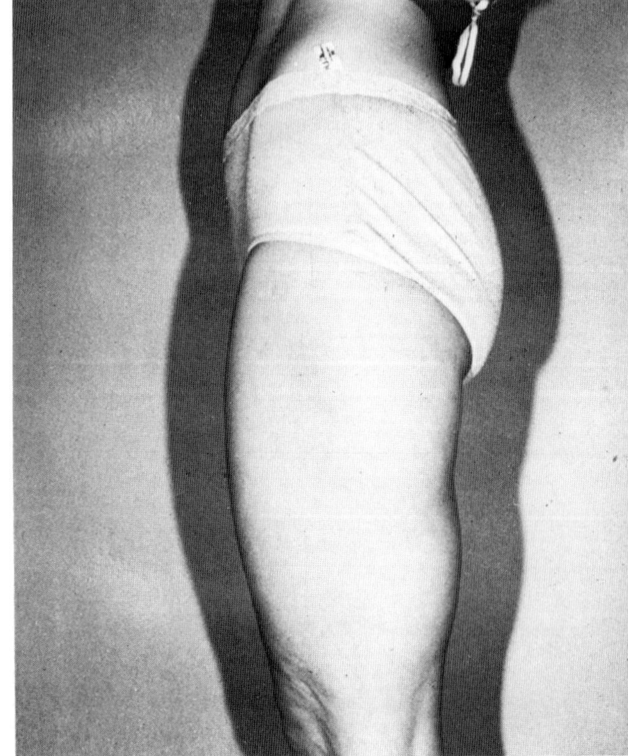

B

Fig. 13-4. A 32-year-old dancer with two children with adiposities of the hip, buttocks, and medial femoral areas. The patient is 5′7″ tall and weighs 140 pounds.
A. Posterior preoperative view.
B. Lateral preoperative view.

Fig. 13-5. A 36-year-old woman with adiposities of the hips, lateral and medial femoral area, and the knees with early ptosis of the buttocks. The patient is 5′6″ tall and weighs 124 pounds.
A. Posterior preoperative view.
B. Lateral preoperative view.

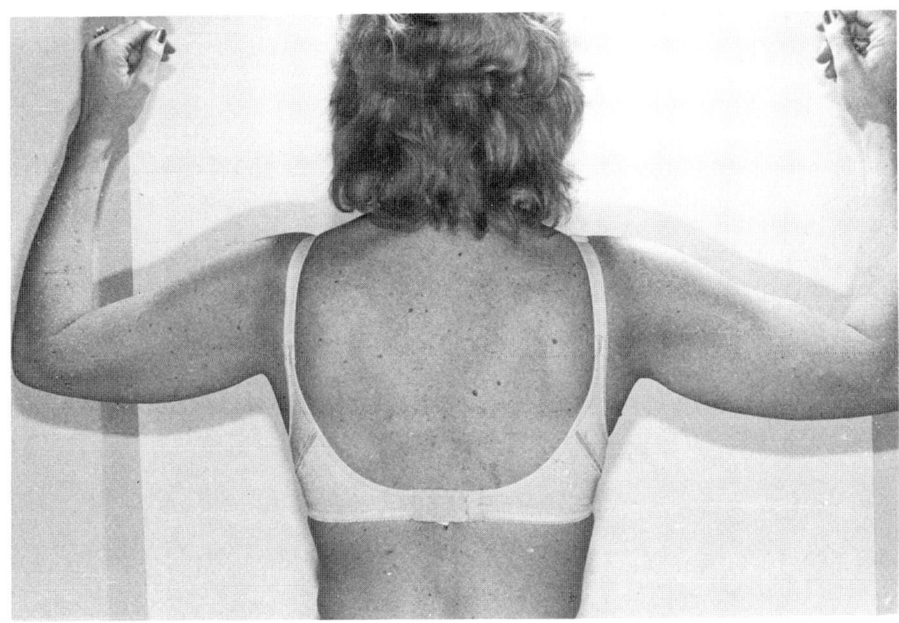

A

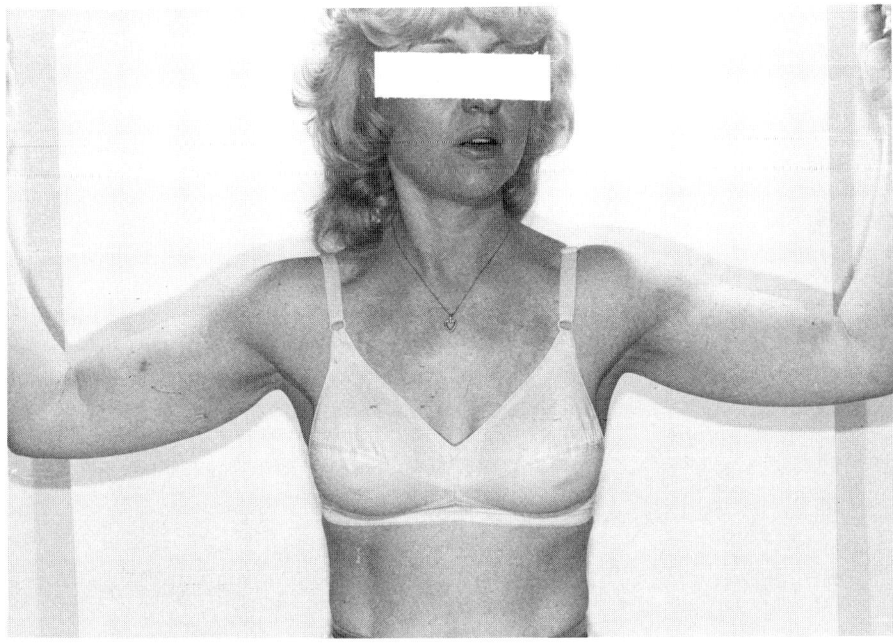

B

Fig. 13-6. A 32-year-old woman with brachial adiposities after a 100-pound weight loss. Skin excess beyond fatty excess. The patient is 5'7" tall and now weighs 140 pounds.
A. Posterior preoperative view.
B. Anterior preoperative view.

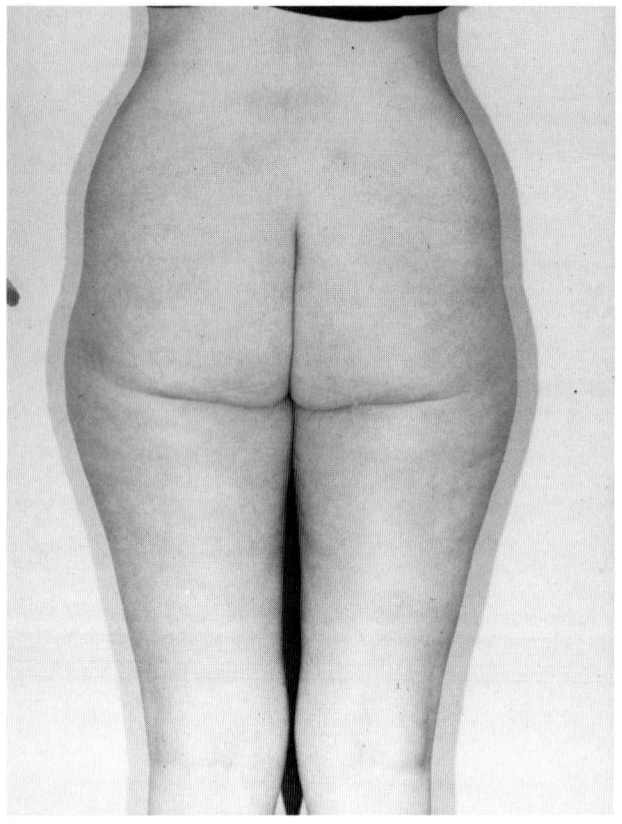

A

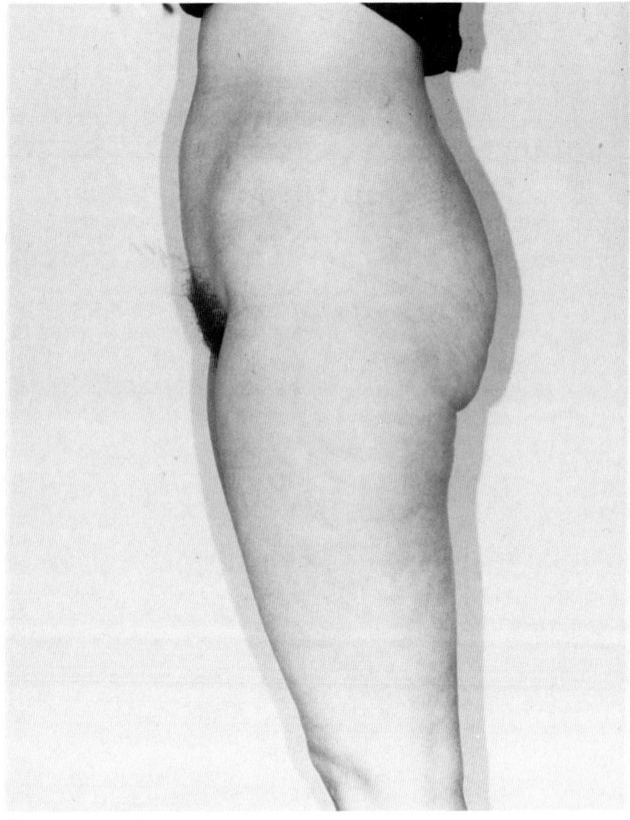

B

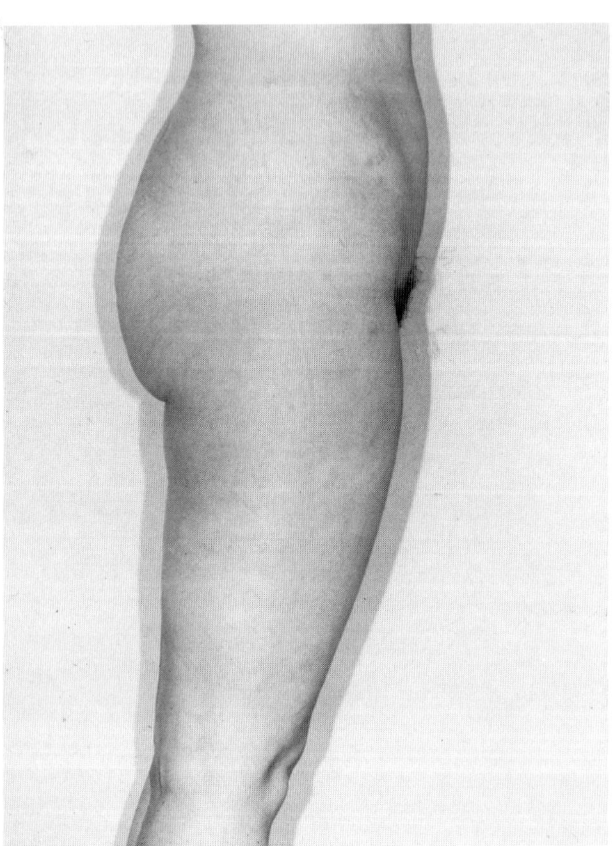

C

Fig. 13-7. A 26-year-old woman with early poor skin tone and lack of subgluteal support. Note early buttock ptosis and straight buttock fold. The patient is 5′4″ tall and weighs 123 pounds.
A. Posterior preoperative view.
B. Left lateral preoperative view.
C. Right lateral preoperative view.

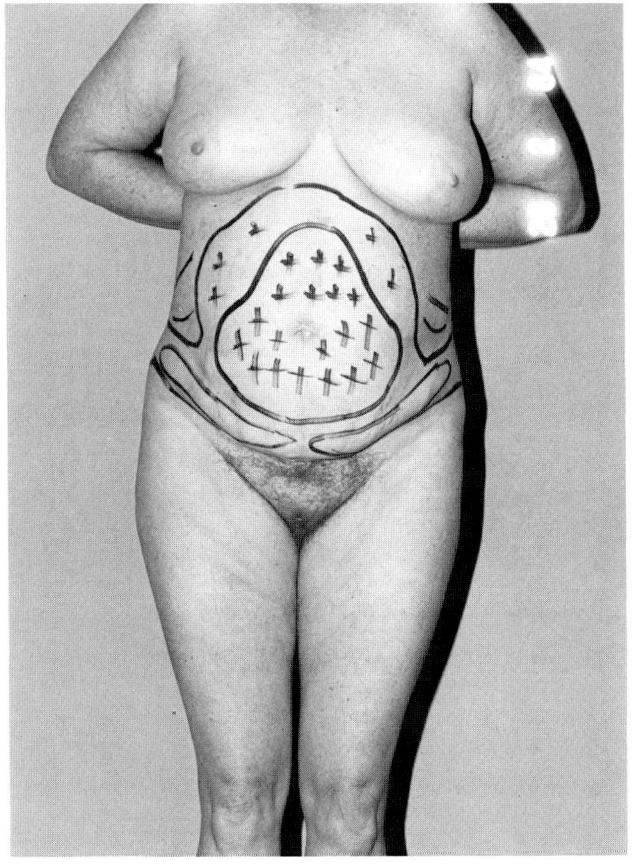

A

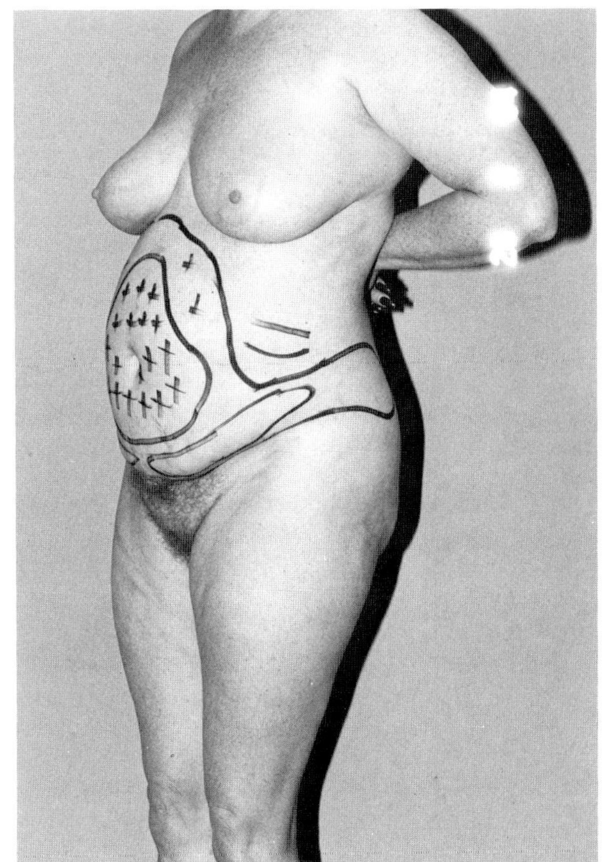

C

Fig. 13-8. A 54-year-old woman with excess adiposities of epigastrium, hypogastrium with flank extensions. Note beginning apron. The patient is 5′9″ and weighs 190 pounds.
A. Anterior view.
B. Lateral view. Note apron.
C. Oblique view.

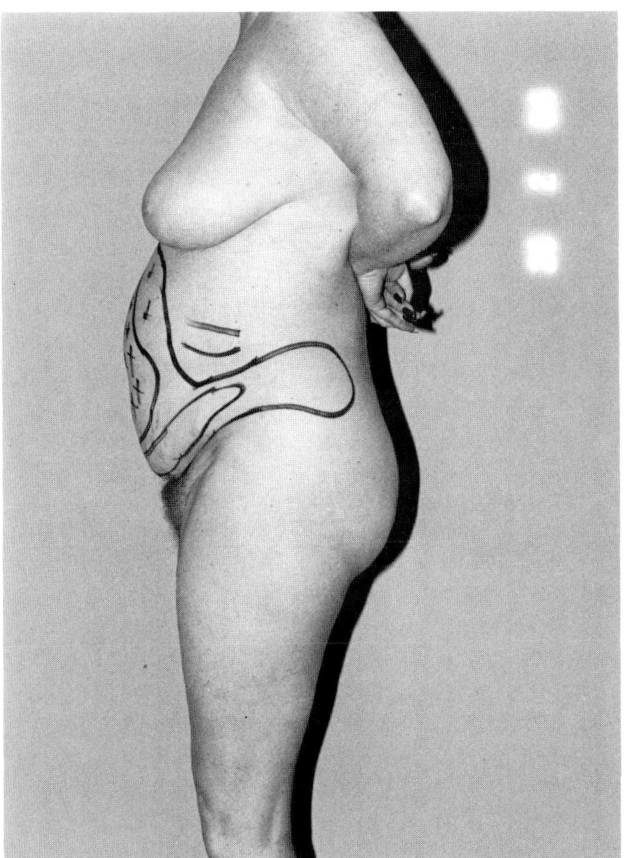

B

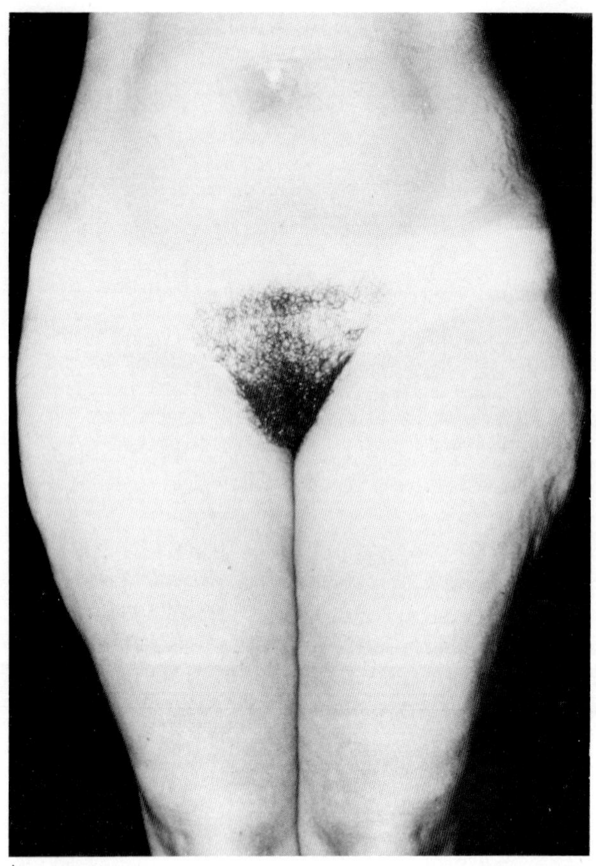

A

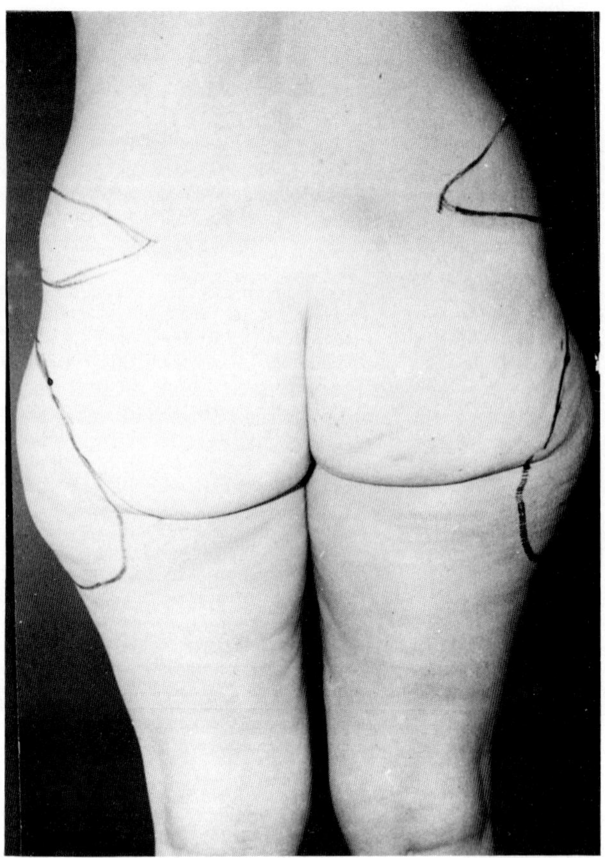

B

Fig. 13-9. A 39-year-old woman with unfirm skin and marked flabbiness by manual exam. Suction amount will be limited by flabbiness.
A. Anterior view.
B. Posterior view.

"touchups." *Before* the first surgical procedure is performed, the surgeon should adequately warn this patient of the need for secondary procedures. A clear understanding about finances, timing, and who makes the final decision between the surgeon and prospective patient will save the surgeon embarrassing moments 4 to 6 months later.

Limiting Factors

In any age group, the surgeon will encounter anatomical findings that limit the result of lipolysis no matter how perfectly the technique is executed. These findings can be separated into skin, soft-tissue, and bony conditions.

Skin conditions include loss of turgor, cellulite, striae, and loss of subcutaneous support. Soft-tissue conditions include asymmetries and differences in fat consistency. Bony anatomical deformities such as are occasionally found in the greater trochanter of the femur, knee joint, lower leg, and ankle may contribute to a less than satisfactory result or lead the untrained surgeon into overresection with resultant depressions. Careful preoperative evaluation, patient counseling, and meticulous technique assist the surgeon in obtaining satisfactory results with the Illouz technique.

The Interview and Examination

Communication is the most valuable tool for the surgeon since it creates patient confidence, empathy in both parties, mutual agreement, and a clear financial understanding.

After preparatory education through the use of written material and audiovisual aids, the surgeon should clearly explain the procedure and its limitations. This period allows a "sizing up" on the part of both the patient and the surgeon. During this time, a good relationship must begin; after the more formal discussion, the surgeon proceeds to the examination.

The patient should be clothed with an adequate, but brief, bikini-type suit and robe because the examination is so vitally important, and relieving embarrassment facilitates an accurate examination. During the examination, just as during the procedure, evaluation of fat, skin, and bone by touch and pinch is important. The exam confirms and extends the diagnosis and often gains the patient's confidence.

Marking the proposed surgical removal on one side with a skin marker and including this in the preoperative photographs is helpful to the surgeon in reviewing his or her operative plan before surgery. It also aids the patient in discussing the examination with his or her spouse.

After the examination, the patient should be allowed to redress in private while the physical findings are recorded. From here, the informed consent may be formulated so as to explain the procedure, the expected results, the need for possible combined procedures, plus the alternatives, limitations, and risks.

Informed Consent

If we were always successful in fulfilling patient expectations, there would be no need for this section. Unfortunately, there are times when the patient misunderstands the procedure or the surgeon's presentation.* In these instances, documentation of the interview is of paramount importance.

A consent form should be given to the potential patient, providing sufficient time for the patient to appreciate its seriousness. The consent form should be returned to the physician for proper signature and witnessing. Sufficient copies for all interested parties should be made available. All consent forms, as well as other printed information from the surgeon's office, should have revision dates in the lower right hand corner and should be reviewed at regular intervals to maintain current perspectives.

The importance of an informed consent to cover a new procedure with relatively limited long-term experience cannot be overemphasized. The informed consent form should be drawn up by the surgeon, the staff, and legal counsel.†

First of all, the consent form should be well labeled with proper heading information: name, address, age, and date of signing. The heading should be followed by the authorizing statement and a brief historical note.

I hereby authorize _______________ and such assistants as may be selected and supervised by him or her to perform lipolysis on my _______________. I fully understand that this procedure has had limited application, consisting of more than 3000 cases, in France since 1977. No guarantee or assurance has been given to me by anyone as to the results that may be obtained.

A paragraph to cover the nature and purpose of the procedure should follow.

Dr. _______________ has discussed in detail with me the information that is briefly summarized below:

A. Nature and Purpose of Lipolysis

Lipolysis is a relatively new body contouring technique. It is a means of reducing localized fat deposits that are difficult or impossible to remove with diet or exercise. It is not a proper technique for treating obesity.

In lipolysis, a hypotonic saline and enzyme solution may be injected under the skin to break down the fatty tissue before it is removed. Afterward, the skin is taped or a girdle is worn for support. Patients usually return to work after 4 to 7 days. Hydrotherapy, physical therapy, and massage may be necessary for several months.

Of course, the inherent risks, both surgical and aesthetic, should be listed as comprehensively as reasonable. As medical articles appear, such listed items as fat emboli, pulmonary emboli, and skin slough should be amended. Currently, it is not clear whether these reported complications are related to blunt suction lipectomy, lipectomy, or to other techniques described by Schrudde, Fischer, Kesselring, or others. To date, I have not encountered any of these problems.

B. Risks

I understand that among the known risks are bruising, lumpiness, dimpling, sagging of the skin, scarring, numbness, minor depressions, and periodic swelling of the lower legs. If skin sagging occurs, a second operation incorporating skin excision with additional scarring may be needed.

An effective way to soften the reality of such complications is to follow with a paragraph about alternatives to lipolysis. Standard body contouring procedures with pictures as shown in *Body Image: A Surgical Perspective* [1] will immediately give support to lipolysis.

C. Alternatives to Lipolysis

Alternative methods of body contouring do exist. Some of them have caused serious complications; however, these techniques have been used longer and are more widely accepted than lipolysis.

I include a paragraph listing a partial list of other complications that may occur with any surgical procedure. This list is a general statement alluding to some of the many things that can but rarely do occur.

I am aware that, in addition to the risks specifically described in section B (Risks), there are other risks, such as severe loss of blood, infection, and cardiac arrest, that may accompany any surgical procedure.

Because general or regional anesthesia is frequently required with this procedure, a paragraph specifically addressed to anesthesia has been included.

---

*Editor's comment: It has been shown that patients retain about 30% of what the surgeon tells them.
†Ellen Thorne, Albuquerque, NM, assisted in preparation of this informed consent form.

I am aware that, in addition to the risks specifically described in section B and in the preceding section, risks are involved with the administration of anesthesia. I understand that general anesthesia is normally required when lipolysis is performed and that general anesthesia is riskier than local anesthesia. I consent to the administration of anesthesia by or under the administration of ___________________.

The next paragraph is perhaps one of the most important. It acknowledges that the patient has had sufficient opportunity to ask questions and get satisfactory answers. It also makes a statement indicating that the patient has obtained sufficient knowledge on which to base an informed consent.

I have had sufficient opportunity to discuss my condition with _______________ and all of my questions have been answered to my satisfaction. I believe that I have adequate knowledge on which to base an informed consent to the proposed treatment.

One of the last areas covered relates to the problem of third party coverage and also to the fact that the treatment of complications may also not be covered by insurance.

Because lipolysis is a new procedure in the United States, third party payment (insurance) does not cover any costs related to lipolysis. This may include further medical or surgical care incurred as a result of a complication to this procedure.

Closing statements are fairly standard and relate to imposed limitations and cooperation in aftercare.

I impose no specific limitations or prohibitions regarding treatment other than the following: (if none, state so)

____

____

I agree to keep _______________ informed of any change in my permanent address so he or she can inform me of any important new findings about lipolysis. I agree to cooperate with my physician in my aftercare.

Not only is a signature required at the completion of the consent form, but also initialing each page read is recommended.

Summary

In summary, the most important key to success in lipolysis, as with most aesthetic surgical procedures, is patient selection. Adequate time should be spent with patients to gain their confidence. Accurate office and photographic records are absolutely necessary with this new procedure. Many patients rapidly forget their original deformity, and preoperative photographs will reveal the extent of their improvement.

References

1. Grazer, F., and Klingbeil, J. *Body Image: A Surgical Perspective.* St. Louis: Mosby, 1982.
2. Goldwyn, R. *The Unfavorable Result in Plastic Surgery.* Boston: Little, Brown, 1972.
3. Illouz, Y. G. Reflexions apres quatre ans et demi d'experience et 800 cas de ma technique de lipolyse. *Rev. Chir. Esthet. Lang. Fr.* 6:27, 1982.
4. Illouz, Y. G. Personal communication. June and October, 1982.
5. Schrudde, J. Suction curettage for body contouring. *Plast. Reconstr. Surg.* 69:903, 1982.
6. Fischer, A., and Maurice, G. M. Revised technique for cellulitis fat reduction in riding breeches deformity. *Bull. Int. Acad. Cosm. Surg.* 2:40, 1977.
7. Fournier, P. F. Personal communication. June and October 1982; September 1983.

CHAPTER 14

Anesthesia

Michael C. Braunstein

The administration of anesthesia for lipolysis involves no new techniques, skills, or drugs. There is an infinite combination of drugs that can be used to achieve satisfactory general anesthesia. As an alternative, a regional anesthetic technique may be used. Physiologic alterations caused by lipolysis should be considered in trying to achieve optimal anesthesia. Techniques are discussed in this chapter that can help promote early ambulation during the recovery stage.

Preoperative Visit

The preoperative visit is necessary to both evaluate and counsel the patient. The physical examination concentrates on the heart, lungs, and airway. The history may be facilitated by having the patient complete a medical questionnaire. Careful evaluation must be made of all medication that the patient is taking. Most drugs should be continued, but any that are likely to cause problems in the perianesthetic period must be noted. Of particular interest are tricyclic antidepressants, lithium carbonate, phenothiazines, isoniazid, levodopa, narcotics, anticonvulsants, ethanol, beta blockers, antihypertensives, diuretics, anticholinesterases (Prostigmin, Mestinon, Mytelase), organophosphates, antibiotics, anticoagulants, antiinflammatory drugs (aspirin), and monoamine oxidase inhibitors. *The monoamine oxidase inhibitors, phenelzine (Nardil), isocarbozid (Marplan), and pargyline (Eutonyl), should be discontinued at least 2 weeks before surgery.* While it is not mandatory that birth control pills be discontinued preoperatively, it should be mentioned that they do cause an increased risk of postoperative venous thrombosis.

Proper counseling of the patient has long been known to be more effective than pentobarbital premedication. This is true even when the pentobarbital is given in a dose sufficient to cause drowsiness; *drowiness does not ensure that a patient is calm.* The patient should be informed of the estimated duration and the scheduled time of surgery. If any premedication is given, the type (I.M. or P.O.) and time of its administration should be discussed as well as the type of anesthesia to be used. The patient must be told of the importance of not eating or drinking for at least 8 hours before surgery. Many surgery centers distribute a booklet to patients explaining anesthesia in some detail.

Premedication

Premedication is largely a matter of personal preference. Administering heavy sedation just to achieve a smooth induction is not necessary with the use of ultrafast-acting barbiturates (Pentothal, Surital, Brevital) specifically for induction. Some patients may be sufficiently prepared psychologically by the preoperative visit alone and will not require premedication. Narcotics, sedatives, and tranquilizers are used alone or in combination to decrease apprehension. If early recovery from anesthesia is desired, however, premedication should be kept to a minimum or simply eliminated altogether.

Diazepam (Valium) is a specific antianxiety drug that is extremely safe when given orally. It does not cause nausea and, in usual doses, does not cause significant respiratory depression or cardiovascular changes. *Diazepam should not be used intramuscularly* since the injection is painful and its absorption is slow and unpredictable. Diazepam blood levels peak in less than 1 hour after oral administration. Rapid redistribution gives it a short duration of action. Because of its long biological half-life (54 hours) and active metabolites, however, drowsiness may persist for 24 hours or longer. Oral diazepam given with 50 ml of water does not increase volume or acidity of gastric fluid and therefore does not increase the risk of aspiration. Newer benzodiazepines that are rapidly redistributed and have faster ultimate elimination may prove superior to diazepam.

Lorazepam (Ativan) is a benzodiazepine that is three to four times longer acting than diazepam and is more likely to produce amnesia. Patients receiving lorazepam, 2.0 mg P.O., will probably be significantly sedated 6 hours later. Therefore, it has little indication in outpatients unless it is given long before surgery.

Droperidol (Inapsine) is a butyrophenone tranquilizer. It is a powerful antiemetic that may prove to be useful in patients who also receive a narcotic. It should not be used alone since it may cause an unpleasant dissociative reaction, even in a patient who is extremely drowsy. Narcotics are not potentiated by droperidol, but their duration of action may be prolonged.

Anticholinergics were once used routinely to decrease oral and tracheobronchial secretions. This treatment helped prevent bronchospasm and laryngospasm caused by irritating gases such as diethyl ether. Occasionally a patient will salivate excessively; for this reason anticholinergics are still very popular. An anticholinergic should be administered preoperatively if ketamine is used since ketamine causes excessive salivation.

Atropine and scopolamine can cause sedation and delirium (central cholinergic syndrome); these side effects are less likely to occur with atropine. Glycopyrrolate (Robinul) is an excellent drying agent and does not have any central nervous system effects since it does not cross the blood-brain barrier. Ideally, it is given just before surgery so the patient does not suffer from a dry mouth for a lengthy period of time. None of the anti-

cholinergics prevent reflex vagal bradycardia when given intramuscularly in the customary dosages.

Aspiration of stomach contents is a potentially lethal complication. In a patient who has had no oral intake, aspiration of gastric acid can still occur, resulting in pneumonitis, pulmonary edema, and/or bronchospasm. The risk of a serious complication is increased if the gastric pH is less than 2.5 and the gastric volume exceeds 25 ml (0.4 ml/kg). Antacids were once popular to neutralize gastric acid but have since fallen into considerable disfavor because they increase stomach volume and their particulate matter may cause complications if aspirated. Sodium citrate is a clear antacid that does not contain particulate matter. Reports of its efficiency are conflicting.

Cimetidine (Tagamet), an H_2-(histamine) receptor antagonist, is a potent inhibitor of gastric acid secretion. In addition, it may decrease gastric volume significantly. *Cimetidine, 300 mg P.O., 1 to 3 hours before surgery reduces but does not eliminate the risk of complications from aspiration.* No complications have been reported with the preoperative use of oral cimetidine, but intravenous cimetidine can cause life-threatening arrhythmias and cardiac arrest. Ranitidine (Zantac) is a new H_2-receptor antagonist that is longer acting (8–12 hours) than cimetidine. It has not been as well studied as cimetidine, but would seem preferable if extubation is anticipated more than 4 hours after premedication. The usual dose is 150 mg.

Preoperative Screening Tests

Preoperative screening tests for healthy individuals are ordered to detect unrecognized disease states. Such unrecognized disease may or may not have a bearing on the type of anesthesia to be used or whether surgery should be performed. Other reasons for doing preoperative screening tests would be to initiate early treatment of previously undetected diseases, for medicolegal reasons, and to detect diseases that may present a hazard to medical personnel.

The question of which tests should be given is a controversial issue because of the complexity of risk-benefit-cost analysis. From an anesthesia standpoint, hemoglobin or hematocrit is requisite in operations involving significant blood loss. Serum glutamic pyruvic transaminase (SGPT), serum creatinine, and blood glucose are used to detect liver disease, renal disease, and diabetes, respectively. A urinalysis is of little additional value if the above tests are done. While a chest x-ray is performed almost uniformly as a screening test, it is now coming under attack when done on patients under the age of 40. It is unlikely that it would change the type of anesthesia to be administered, but it may detect an unrecognized disease at an early stage of development. EKGs are strongly recommended for males over 40 years of age and for females over 60. Further tests may be needed as a result of specific findings on the history and physical. The Phoenix Surgicenter limits routine screening tests to hemoglobin, urinalysis, and clotting time. To date there is no consensus as to which screening tests should be ordered.

Induction of Anesthesia

General anesthesia is the usual anesthetic technique for lipolysis. In addition to drugs given by the anesthesiologist, the surgeon may be injecting a local anesthetic with epinephrine. Induction utilizing an ultrashort-acting barbiturate such as thiopental (Pentothal), thiamylal (Surital), and methohexital (Brevital) is standard for routine anesthesia. Unless there is a contraindication, there is little reason to use any other agent in healthy patients. Contraindications against using a barbiturate include porphyria and allergy to barbiturates. Other induction agents could include ketamine, etomidate (Amidate), diazepam (Valium), and/or narcotics. Induction can also be achieved with inhalation agents.

Etomidate provides a fast and smooth induction with rapid recovery. Common adverse reactions are pain on injection (20%), myoclonia (32%), and apnea. Other reported reactions are snoring, hiccup, hyperventilation, hypertension, hypoventilation, tachycardia, bradycardia, and postoperative nausea and vomiting. Etomidate is thought to produce better cardiovascular stability than thiopental (Pentothal); however, it should be used with caution in patients with porphyria. The myoclonia and pain on injection are likely to limit its use.

To attenuate the adverse circulatory and psychic effects of ketamine, diazepam can be administered before the ketamine. Hallucinations can still occur after diazepam-ketamine, and intellectual function may be impaired for at least 3 months [1]. The patient should be premedicated with an anticholinergic drug (glycopyrrolate or atropine) to prevent excessive salivation. Ketamine used alone is a cardiovascular stimulant and therefore has some popularity for patients who are in shock. It has no value as an induction agent for healthy adults having lipolysis surgery.

Induction with narcotics is usually reserved for very ill cardiac patients. Such an induction results in prolonged drowsiness and apnea. The possibility of recall also exists. New, short-acting narcotics such as sufentanil may hasten recovery. Induction with diazepam results in prolonged drowsiness and is usually reserved for patients with severe cardiovascular disease. *Intravenous diazepam is painful and can cause thrombophlebitis.*

Slow injection of a dilute solution into a large vein is recommended to prevent thrombophlebitis. An injection of 2.0 ml of 1% lidocaine given immediately before the diazepam will prevent burning pain.

Airway Maintenance

In all general anesthesia techniques except, possibly, ketamine, the patient requires assisted or controlled ventilation after the induction. If the patient remains supine, the anesthesiologist must decide whether or not intubation is necessary. This decision is made on the basis of personal preference, length of the surgery, and ability to maintain a good airway by mask. Other positions generally require intubation. Advantages in using a mask, rather than intubation, include (1) not having to give a neuromuscular blocking drug, (2) less chance of trauma to the larynx and pharynx (fewer sore throats), (3) the ability, in some cases, to maintain a lighter state of anesthesia, and (4) avoidance of the cardiovascular stress associated with intubation and extubation. Disadvantages to using a mask, which are potentially more serious, include (1) the increased likelihood of aspiration, (2) the anesthesiologist not having both hands free in a crisis, and (3) the increased skill and attention that mask anesthesia demands. Patients tolerate hypoventilation much better with a direct oxygen line to their trachea than with oxygen flowing over their faces.

To facilitate intubation, the patient is usually paralyzed with succinylcholine. This step may or may not be preceded by a defasciculating dose of a nondepolarizing muscle relaxant, such as curare, given 3 to 5 minutes before the succinylcholine. This pretreatment may reduce the likelihood of muscle pain postoperatively as a result of the fasciculations and is also popular for patients with full stomachs to prevent a rise in intragastric pressure.

Other adverse effects of succinylcholine are hyperkalemia, malignant hyperthermia, myotonic response, prolonged apnea, and increased intraocular pressure. In healthy individuals only the triggering of malignant hyperthermia and prolonged apnea are of any importance.

Prolonged paralysis can occur following succinylcholine and is clinically significant in 1 per 1800 anesthetics. This problem does not represent a crisis since ventilation can be supported until recovery. Pseudocholinesterase is formed in the liver and is responsible for the rapid breakdown of succinylcholine. Pseudocholinesterase may be insufficient in quantity or may be atypical and have reduced activity. Reduced pseudocholinesterase activity is an inherited disorder. Reduced quantities of pseudocholinesterase are of little clinical significance. Pseudocholinesterase levels and activity can be quantitated, but this is not a routine practice. Pseudocholinesterase activity can be measured by determination of dibucaine, fluoride, scoline, chloride, and urea numbers. In clinical practice, only the dibucaine number is routinely available; even if all tests were done, a significant number of patients with atypical pseudocholinesterase would be missed [2]. Thus, *prolonged apnea can occur after succinylcholine even if all screening tests were normal.*

Succinylcholine can be avoided either by not intubating or by using a nondepolarizing neuromuscular blocking drug (atracurium, metocurine, pancuronium, tubocurarine, gallamine). To achieve adequate muscle relaxation for intubation, a large dose of a nondepolarizing drug is needed; it takes up to 3 minutes to achieve satisfactory conditions. More important, with the exception of atracurium (Tracrium), this large initial dose will keep patients paralyzed for 1 hour or longer.

Atracurium is the newest drug of its type and has a duration of action three times shorter than other nondepolarizing neuromuscular blocking drugs. It can be easily reversed even if anesthesia lasts less than a half hour; when anesthesia lasts longer, reversal is usually not necessary. Atracurium is not cumulative, has no risk of "recurarization," is not metabolized by the liver or excreted by the kidneys, and in usual doses does not have cardiovascular side effects [3].

The major disadvantage with this technique is encountered in very short procedures. Another disadvantage is that respiration has to be controlled for about a half hour, thus eliminating one of the clues to depth of anesthesia. However, *the high incidence of succinylcholine-induced pain in women and in ambulatory patients should make atracurium a popular drug.* Reversal of nondepolarizing neuromuscular blocking drugs is achieved by giving an anticholinesterase agent. These agents include neostigmine (Prostigmin), pyridostigmine (Mestinon, Regonol), and edrophonium (Tensilon). Anticholinesterase-induced bradycardia can be prevented or treated by giving atropine or glycopyrrolate. *Glycopyrrolate results in fewer cardiac disturbances than atropine.*

The circulatory response to intubation and extubation includes tachycardia, hypertension, and arrythmia. A variety of drugs can be given to blunt this response and have included laryngeal lidocaine, intravenous lidocaine, nitroprusside, narcotics, and deep inhalation anesthesia. Hypertensive patients should be treated medically up until the time of surgery.

Malignant Hyperthermia

Malignant hyperthermia refers to a hypermetabolic crisis precipitated by a variety of agents or stress in patients with an underlying muscle disease that is inherited. Symptoms include tachycardia, tachypnea, arrhythmias, elevation of temperature, rigidity (sometimes absent), skin mottling, profuse sweating, and unstable blood pressure. Rigidity induced by succinylcholine may be the first sign. Testing reveals hypoxemia, hypercarbia, low pH (respiratory and metabolic acidosis), hyperkalemia, hypocalcemia, myoglobinemia, and hypermagnesemia. Fatality rates of up to 70% were reported before the use of dantrolene sodium (Dantrium). The incidence of malignant hyperthermia is about 1 in 50,000 anesthetics.

Preoperatively the diagnosis is extremely difficult to make. Some of the associated features are localized muscle weakness, generalized muscle bulk, muscle cramps, club foot, joint hypermobility (especially of the knee), deformities of the spine, joint dislocations, hernias, difficulty in controlling temperature, strabismus, and ptosis. In most cases, the patient seems normal. Serum creatinine phosphokinase (CPK) is elevated in 70% of these patients but is nonspecific. The only definitive diagnostic test for susceptibility to malignant hyperthermia is a muscle contracture test, which involves obtaining a muscle biopsy. This test can be carried out reliably in only a few medical centers.

Potent volatile anesthetic agents and succinylcholine are precipitating agents of malignant hyperthermia; isoflurane and enflurane are less likely than halothane to trigger the syndrome. Local amide anesthetics (lidocaine, bupivacaine, mepivacaine, and etidocaine) should not be used. *Malignant hyperthermia has occurred in patients given "safe" anesthetics and may have been precipitated by stress.* A protocol treatment for malignant hyperthermia, as well as the necessary drugs, should be available near the operating room.

Maintenance of Anesthesia

Anesthesia is maintained with narcotics, ketamine, or volatile anesthetic agents in all but the shortest operative cases. As a general rule, nitrous oxide is added to any technique since it allows a linear decrease in the amount of other agents needed, has comparatively little adverse physiological effects, and is rapidly eliminated. Nitrous oxide may produce undesirable cardiovascular effects in patients who are cardiac cripples.

Fentanyl (Sublimaze) is currently the most popular narcotic used for high-dose narcotic techniques. It produces greater cardiovascular stability than morphine. In low doses fentanyl is short-acting because of its rapid redistribution. When it is used as a sole anesthetic agent, the dose required (≥ 50 µg/kg) converts it into a drug comparable to morphine in its length of action. Actually its biological half-life, about 4 hours, is longer than that of morphine. In patients over 60 years of age, its half-life is nearly 16 hours. Because this technique results in prolonged drowsiness and respiratory depression, it is generally reserved for patients with severe cardiac disease. In high doses, fentanyl has no place among the choices of anesthetic techniques if the goal of early ambulation is desired.

Fentanyl is a very useful drug for ambulatory surgery when it is used in conjunction with other anesthetic agents. It is frequently used in small doses to provide both a smoother induction and emergence. A continuous infusion of fentanyl with nitrous oxide is an acceptable outpatient technique, but will cause an increased incidence of nausea and vomiting.

Maintenance of anesthesia with ketamine is possible but results in prolonged drowsiness. This type of anesthesia is usually reserved for pediatrics or situations where access to the patient's airway could cause trauma, such as in the case of facial burns. As a maintenance agent, it has no other notable advantages in skilled hands. Even in patients pretreated with diazepam, 0.4 mg/kg, there is likely to be significant tachycardia and hypertension. In unskilled hands, it leads to a false sense of security when it is assumed that there will be no airway problems. Ketamine can lead to hypoventilation, apnea, laryngospasm, and vomiting with aspiration [4]. At that point, an airway will have to be secured in the patient whose heart is already stressed by the tachycardia and hypertension. There is also the possibility of psychomimetic effects, even in patients given diazepam before the ketamine.

Ketamine alone, without preoperative medication or diazepam, is considered a general anesthetic when administered in an intravenous dose of 1 mg/kg. This dosage is recommended for cesarean section and works very well [5]. When used in combination with other drugs, ketamine is considered a general anesthetic at an even lower dosage. As such it should usually be administered by a competently trained professional versed in general anesthesia. Furthermore, it is imperative one individual not be placed in the role of both an operator and an administrator of general anesthesia.

Inhalation anesthetics include methoxyflurane (Penthrane), halothane (Fluothane), enflurane (Ethrane), and isoflurane (Forane). Methoxyflurane is seldom used today because induction and recovery are slow, and it causes a dose-related nephrotoxicity. The popularity of halothane began to decline when it was linked, in rare instances, to postoperative hepatitis. It also sensitizes the myocardial conduction system to epinephrine; therefore, *great caution must be exercised if epinephrine is given during the course of a halothane anesthetic.*

The chief advantage of halothane is that it provides a smooth induction with little respiratory irritation. Since lipolysis surgery involves the injection of epinephrine for hemostasis, halothane should probably not be used.

Enflurane (Ethrane) hepatotoxicity has not been firmly established. If it does exist, it is extremely rare. At this time, it does not pose the medicolegal threat that halothane hepatitis does. Renal dysfunction has occurred but no case of renal failure has been documented. Recovery is theoretically faster than with halothane, but is probably not clinically significant. Induction may be slowed due to its irritating effects on the respiratory system. Epinephrine is better tolerated with enflurane than with halothane. The published safe limit dose of epinephrine used in conjunction with enflurane is 2.0 µg/kg injected subcutaneously over a period of 10 minutes and is not to exceed 6.0 µg/kg per hour. Thus, up to 40 ml of a 1:400,000 (10 µg/ml) solution can be used on a 50-kg patient if it is injected over a period of 10 minutes. It should be emphasized that this guideline dosage limitation assumes delivery by subcutaneous injection and not accidental intravenous or intraarterial injection. Also, *there is great individual variability in response to epinephrine with enflurane* [6]. *An occasional patient may exhibit toxicity with what is considered to be a safe dose of epinephrine.* Enflurane given to a patient with marked hypocapnia can produce seizure activity.

Isoflurane (Forane) is the newest general inhalation agent. It is the intention of Ohio Medical Products to eventually replace enflurane with isoflurane. Isoflurane undergoes minimal metabolism; therefore, nephrotoxicity, due to the release of fluoride ions, is not a concern. Hepatitis from isoflurane is unlikely to occur since there should be few, if any, active metabolites produced. Induction and recovery are slightly more rapid than with enflurane, if the induction is not slowed by coughing, breath holding, bronchospasm, or laryngospasm. Isoflurane is more irritating to the respiratory system than enflurane, so these side effects are more likely to occur. Clinically, induction and recovery rates are not significantly different between the two agents. Isoflurane may produce less myocardial depression than halothane or enflurane; this is not well established and may not even be desirable. Hypotension can occur secondary to a decrease in peripheral vascular resistance or cardiac output or both. Isoflurane does not cause seizure activity. Like halothane and enflurane, it can trigger malignant hyperthermia.

Epinephrine is better tolerated with isoflurane than with enflurane. The safe limit is given as 6.7 µg/kg if it is injected submucosally [6]. In a 50-kg patient, the safe limit would be 134 ml of a 1:400,000 solution. The addition of lidocaine probably increases this limit. Furthermore, this study was done by injecting into a vascular submucosal area. Blood levels of lidocaine given subcutaneously are considerably less than those obtained after an intercostal injection. Injection into adipose tissue results in even less absorption, lower blood levels, and a higher toxic dose limit. While no data is available on the toxic dose limit of epinephrine injected into adipose tissue, it is presumably very high. Dr. Hetter has had no complications using 325 ml of lidocaine 0.23% with epinephrine 1:435,000. If premature ventricular contractions (PVCs) occur, injection should be stopped. The PVCs can be treated with lidocaine or propranolol.

Intravenous Fluids

Great variety exists in the routine administration of fluids intraoperatively. This is testimony to the ability of healthy humans to adapt. Maintenance fluids are used to replace insensible fluid losses. In healthy adults, this loss is about 2 ml/kg per hour. Replacement is accomplished by giving hypotonic fluids that range from sodium-free fluid (D5W) to one-half normal saline solutions. In a 50-kg patient who has been without oral intake for 10 hours, fluid replacement would be 1000 ml. Many anesthesiologists routinely give only replacement-type fluids without apparent ill-effect [7].

Replacement fluids are nearly isotonic with saline and are used to correct loss of blood or nearly isotonic body fluids such as edema fluid. Lipolysis involves moderate to extreme trauma to tissue, which causes fluid loss due to the formation of acute sequestered interstitial edema. The amount of edema fluid that is functionally lost relates to the degree of surgical trauma and not to blood loss. Replacement of this edema fluid loss requires 6 to 8 ml/kg per hour. Adding the nonsurgical loss of 2 ml/kg per hour puts replacement fluids at 8 to 10 ml/kg per hour. D5LR and normal saline are commonly used replacement fluids. Also, additional fluids are given because of blood loss.

The crystalloid versus colloid controversy in the resuscitation of shock continues. Crystalloids are used to replace lost extracellular fluid. Smaller volumes of colloids restore plasma volume. Lipolysis patients, with recommended volume removals (<2000 ml), are not in shock. There is little doubt that crystalloid fluid therapy will be sufficient in patients without acute bleeding or renal or cardiovascular dysfunction. If it is desirable to minimize interstitial edema formation, colloids may be used. Hetastarch (Hespan) is a synthetic colloid that stays in the circulation longer than albumin, does not increase lung water, and is less expensive than albumin.

Blood is given to increase oxygen-carrying capacity. Healthy adults who have their plasma volume maintained probably do not lose significant oxygen-carrying capacity until the hematocrit falls below 30. This is because of an increase in cardiac output brought about by a decrease in blood viscosity. Assuming a starting hematocrit of 45 in a 50-kg woman, a blood loss of about 1500 ml is needed to reach a hematocrit of 30 [8]. Should major blood loss be anticipated, up to 4 units of

blood can be removed preoperatively through a series of phlebotomies. Autologous blood avoids many of the complications of blood transfusions. The hematocrit drop at 2 days reported by Dr. Hetter [13] indicates that transfusion of blood is seldom needed. Only one patient had a postoperative hematocrit below 30 and that patient had a starting hematocrit of only 38.6.

Fat embolism may be observed 12 hours to 10 days after injury or surgery. An intravenous drip of ethanol has been advocated to thwart the possibility of pulmonary complications after lipolysis. There is little rationale for such treatment and there are even several possible disadvantages. First, the ethanol will cause increased postoperative sedation. Second, ethanol inhibits the production of serum lipase. This is not desirable soon after the trauma of surgery, since efficient lipase activity is necessary to clear fat from the blood. Elevation of serum lipase activity is associated with a good prognosis [9].

Pulmonary lipase converts innocuous triglycerides to irritating fatty acids that can cause chemical pneumonitis. Ethyl alcohol inhibits the rate of hydrolysis of fat and has therefore been advocated to prevent and treat fatty embolism. It has not been proven effective clinically, however, and is no longer a recommended treatment. Furthermore, fat embolism has not been observed clinically after lipolysis surgery.

Some of the symptoms of fat embolism may be confused with manifestations of malignant hyperthermia. These symptoms include tachycardia, elevated temperature, tachypnea, and hypoxemia. Associated with fat embolism are the appearance of petechiae, hypotension, changes in sensorium, and a decrease in the platelet count. Treatment consists of supplemental oxygen, respiratory support, and massive doses of steroids.

Local Anesthetics

Local anesthetics act on nerves by blocking their sodium channels, thereby preventing depolarization and nerve conduction. When local anesthetics inactivate nerve membranes, the desired response is achieved. When they block the electrophysiological activity of other membranes, the untoward response is called *toxicity*. Local anesthetics block membranes in the brain, heart, and arteriolar smooth muscle, and they do so in much lower concentrations than it takes to block nerve conduction. Cocaine is an exception in that it does not cause arteriolar dilation when given in the usual doses. It is therefore essential to inject local anesthetics properly to keep blood levels at a minimum. Injecting the proper dose slowly is of prime importance since this will allow early detection of toxicity symptoms before a catastrophic event occurs.

Manifestation of toxicity usually first appears clinically as central nervous system excitation. Symptoms of central nervous system excitation include lightheadedness, dizziness, auditory and visual disturbances, and convulsions. These symptoms are caused by initial inactivation of the inhibitory synapses in the brain before facilitory neurons are inactivated. *Central nervous system excitation should be taken as a sign of impending danger* since higher blood levels depress the brain, impair impulse conduction in the heart, decrease myocardial contractility, and dilate arteriolar smooth muscle. Toxicity reactions can also occur suddenly and without warning if local anesthetic blood levels are rising rapidly. Pretreatment with diazepam may raise the seizure threshold for local anesthetics; however, diazepam can also mask central nervous system excitation, thus eliminating an early sign of local anesthetic toxicity.

Some surgeons advocate infiltration of the operative site with a local anesthetic containing epinephrine. The epinephrine aids in hemostasis, prolongs the duration of action of local anesthetic agents and decreases potential toxicity. The length of duration for lidocaine 0.5% with epinephrine 1:200,000 is approximately 228 minutes. Duration of bupivacaine 0.25% (Marcaine) with epinephrine 1:200,000 given percutaneously for infiltration averages 429 minutes. The duration of effect of the bupivacaine on the heart will be in proportion to its duration of effect on nerves; therefore, *cardiac arrest after the injection of bupivacaine may necessitate prolonged resuscitation.* In some cases the cardiac arrest is not preceded by convulsions.

Bupivacaine appears to be more cardiotoxic than lidocaine; however, the possibility of toxicity is extremely remote if injection is extravascular. Local anesthetic injection for lipolysis is given into an area with poor vasculature. If the needle is continually moving during injection, it is very unlikely that toxicity to bupivacaine will occur.

Local anesthetic infiltration for lipolysis surgery is into deeper planes of fatty tissue than is done by percutaneous injection. Because injection is made into an area where blood flow is relatively slow, absorption into the circulation will be slow, resulting in a prolonged effect from the local anesthetic and a decreased chance of toxicity. Bupivacaine with epinephrine is safe to adminster in a dose of up to 400 mg when it is given for an intercostal block. Lidocaine without epinephrine is safe in a dose of up to 400 mg [10]. Adding epinephrine and injecting into fat will allow a much larger dose to be administered. Epinephrine is the drug of choice should cardiovascular collapse occur secondary to bupivacaine.

Anaphylaxis has been reported with local anesthetics as well as with most drugs. Fortunately, allergy to ester-type local anesthetics is rare, and allergy to amide locals is extremely rare. In some reported cases the offending agent may have been a preservative and not the local per se. The mainstays of anaphylaxis treatment are epinephrine and ventilatory support.

Central Neural Block

Epidural (lumbar or caudal) or subarachnoid anesthesia represents a useful anesthetic technique for lipolysis surgery. Thus, the patient who objects to being put to sleep has an alternative.

Advantages of regional anesthesia include a lower incidence of aspiration, possibly a decreased risk of deep venous thrombosis, and greater respiratory and cardiovascular stability if the block is kept below the level of T10. Abdominal lipolysis requires a block to T6 or higher. The major disadvantage of any of these nerve blocks is the possibility of a serious neurological complication. Urinary retention is a frequent problem if the block is prolonged. Since this problem necessitates catheterization, blocks lasting more than 2 hours should be avoided in outpatients.

Hypotension can occur secondary to sympathetic block and vasodilation. If significant sympathetic block occurs, prolonged postural hypotension is a risk that would prohibit early ambulation of the patient. It should also be mentioned that intravascular injection can cause local anesthetic toxicity.

Subarachnoid anesthesia has the advantage of using such a small amount of local anesthetic that there will be no systemic effect from the drug itself. Even accidental intravascular injection is unlikely to lead to any adverse consequences other than failure of the block to work. It is also very unlikely to produce a total spinal block when a subarachnoid block is done, since an incredible error in the dosage or volume would have to be made. The disadvantage of subarachnoid block is the possibility of postoperative spinal headache. This side effect is more likely to occur in young, ambulatory patients. The incidence can be reduced by using a 26-gauge needle. If conservative treatment fails, the patient may require an epidural block patch to treat a spinal headache. A prophylactic blood patch is not recommended.

Epidural anesthesia commonly results in a backache. More important, the amount of local anesthetic used is enough to cause systemic toxicity, if given by intravascular injection. Both the lumbar and caudal blocks can lead to accidental dural puncture, although this is rare with a caudal block. Since large needles are used for these blocks, dural puncture frequently causes a spinal headache. If dural puncture is not noticed, the injection of the large volume and dose of the local anesthetic agent used for epidural anesthesia will result in a total spinal block.

In summary, epidural or subarachnoid anesthesia is a viable alternative to general anesthesia. In healthy patients there is no clear superiority of regional versus general anesthesia. If early ambulation is desired, however, general anesthesia is usually preferable.

Problems Seen in the Recovery Room

Respiratory complications are probably the most common serious postanesthetic complication. Certainly they are by far the leading cause of mortality and morbidity [11]. Airway obstruction is very common postoperatively, with the tongue being the most frequent culprit. This obstruction most commonly occurs when patients have high levels of circulating anesthetic remaining in their system and are in the supine position with the head flexed.

The problem of airway obstruction is diagnosed by observation of snoring, flaring of the nostrils, retraction of the suprasternal notch, intercostal space narrowing, or little excursion of the anterior chest wall coupled with vigorous abdominal contractions. Late signs include cyanosis, hypertension, hypotension, tachycardia, bradycardia, and arrhythmias. Treatment can include hyperextension of the head, cephalad displacement of the mandible, head-up tilt, lateral positioning, or insertion of a nasal or oral airway.

Hypoventilation can also occur secondary to residual anesthesia. Surgical manipulations and endotracheal tubes are powerful respiratory stimuli to patients. When surgery is over and the patient is extubated, respirations may slow because these stimuli are gone. Hypoventilation should immediately be treated by assisting or controlling ventilation. If there is significant residual paralysis from a nondepolarizing neuromuscular-blocking drug, reversal should be undertaken. Narcotics can be reversed with naloxone (Narcan). Naloxone is a pure narcotic antagonist, so there is no reason to use any other narcotic reversal agent. Reversal of narcotics can cause a patient to have sudden, severe pain. Such pain can cause tachycardia and hypertension, and thus stress the myocardium. Naloxone can cause pulmonary edema or cardiac arrest in healthy patients. *Reversal with naloxone should not be undertaken lightly.* The half-life of naloxone is short so that renarcotization is a real possibility. Patients reversed with naloxone must be watched very closely. Intramuscular injection is less likely to result in renarcotization.

Delayed emergence is usually due to an anesthetic overdose, but can be secondary to hypothermia and depressant drugs reaching their peak at the end of surgery (e.g., diphenylhydantoin (Dilantin) therapy or late narcotic premedication). Doxapram (Dopram) is a centrally acting respiratory stimulant with many potential adverse reactions and a brief duration of action. *It is therefore of little value.*

Patients exhibiting postoperative delirium is a common cause for anxiety among recovery room nurses. Hypoxia, hypercarbia, and hypotension must be ruled out first, as possible etiologies. Pain can cause delirium, and low-dose narcotics can reverse delirium occurring from many causes. Postoperative pain after lipolysis surgery does not appear to be a major problem. Some patients report minimal or no postoperative pain, while others may have mild to moderate pain. *Patients should be forewarned about the possibility of pain postoperatively, so their anxiety about the pain, should it occur, is reduced.* Narcotics given in the recovery room should be administered intravenously so that the dose can be titrated to the patient's individual need. Furthermore, the drug reaches its peak effect in only a few minutes, when recovery room personnel are more likely to be attentive. Fentanyl (Sublimaze) is presently the narcotic of choice for outpatient anesthesia because of its short duration of action (30–60 minutes).

Treatment of pain with injection of spinal (intrathecal or epidural) narcotics is a popular topic in the anesthesia literature. Injection of spinal narcotics allows these drugs to act directly on pain receptors in the substantia gelatinosa of the spinal cord. The hope is that this method will achieve prolonged pain relief with few systemic effects. This has not been the case, however, since respiratory arrest may occur up to 24 hours after the injection. The respiratory arrest can occur without warning; *close observation of patients for 24 hours after the last dose of spinal narcotics is mandatory. Injection of spinal narcotics is still experimental* but the proper narcotic, route of administration, and technique may be found in the near future.

Other sources of postoperative restlessness may stem from the side effects of ketamine, scopolamine, or atropine or from drug withdrawal, alcohol withdrawal, and a full bladder. The antiacetylcholinesterase drug physostigmine (Antilirium) readily reverses scopolamine and atropine reactions and possibly other drugs that cause sedation as well. Physostigmine can cause hypertension, nausea, and bradycardia, so it should be given slowly. The bradycardia can be reversed with glycopyrrolate, if necessary. Sedation may return some hours after physostigmine reversal.

Nausea is common postoperatively with many possible etiologies. Hypotension and hypertension can cause nausea; therefore, *blood pressure should be checked immediately in any patient who develops nausea.* Narcotics are especially likely to cause nausea. Fentanyl seems to have less emetic effect than other narcotics. Attempts at prevention of nausea have been made with a variety of antiemetics. *Droperidol (Inapsine) is a potent antiemetic that is effective in a dose (1.25 mg) that causes little sedation* [12]. Given prophylactically, patients need less recovery room time.

Cardiovascular problems include hypotension, hypertension, bradycardia, tachycardia, and arrhythmias. There are many etiologies for postoperative hypotension, but underreplacement of fluids is the most likely culprit. Removal of the stimulus of surgery, in conjunction with persistent anesthesia, is also a common cause. Other possible causes of hypotension that may need to be eliminated include pain, hypothermia, hypoxemia, myocardial depression, myocardial infarction, electrolyte disturbances, hypoglycemia, blood transfusion reaction, adrenal failure, gastric distention, tamponade, anaphylaxis, and aspiration. Initial treatment of hypotension should be immediate elevation of the patient's lower extremities until a diagnosis is made.

Hypertension is most commonly seen in patients who were hypertensive preoperatively. They may be known hypertensives or simply nervous patients who are otherwise normotensive. Other causes of hypertension include such conditions as hypercarbia, shivering, pain, bladder distention, circulatory overload, and drugs like doxapram, ketamine, and vasopressors. Both hypertension and tachycardia increase myocardial oxygen demand, so that moderate hypotension, in conjunction with a fast heart rate, may need to be treated. Treatment should be directed at the etiology if it can be determined.

Bradycardia can be caused by pain, vagal stimulation, nausea, heart block, sick sinus syndrome, hypoxia, residual anesthesia, and anticholinergic drugs. Bradycardia needs to be treated if it results in hypotension or arrythmia. Marked bradycardia can be a normal phenomenon in well-conditioned individuals. Treatment using an anticholinergic drug has the potential of causing life-threatening tachycardia, but this is less likely to occur with the use of glycopyrrolate (Robinul) rather than atropine. *Failure of either atropine or glycopyrrolate to increase the heart rate should make one suspicious of the existence of hypoxia* or, in rare instances, heart block or sick sinus syndrome.

Tachyarrhythmia is a common problem and is usually a case of sinus tachycardia. Tachycardia can be seen as a response to volume depletion, pain, pyrexia, myocardial infarction, delirium, malignant hyperthermia, heart failure, pulmonary embolism, hypercarbia, hypoxia, and from such drugs as gallamine, pancuronium, and anticholinergics. The treatment should be specific when the etiology of the tachyarrhythmia is known. In many instances, the etiology cannot be found and, in such cases, the treatment can be nonspecific with the use of propranolol (Inderal), calcium channel blockers such as verapamil, edrophonium (Tensilon), or by vagal stimulation.

Shivering is a common postoperative problem and can be secondary to a decrease in body temperature or to residual anesthesia. Shivering is not only very distressing to the patient but also greatly increases oxygen consumption. Shivering is often due to hypothermia but, in some instances, it seems to be secondary to residual anesthesia. Efforts to maintain the patient's temperature will help prevent shivering. Means of maintaining the patient's temperature can include warm humidified gases for inhalation, warm irrigating fluids, warm intravenous fluids, a warming blanket, covering of areas of the patient not in the operative field, and *a reasonable room temperature without a draft.* Prevention and treatment of shivering can usually be achieved with a small dose of a narcotic, such as fentanyl 25 µg.

Supplemental oxygen should be routinely given in the recovery room. Anesthesia and the supine position both decrease functional residual capacity (FRC), which can result in shunting and a decrease in blood oxygenation. Shivering, tachycardia, and hypertension are common causes of increased oxygen demand. Anemia, hypoventilation, and a decrease in cardiac output can all decrease oxygen delivery to the tissues.

Many other potential complications can occur in the recovery room. It is mandatory that postoperative patients be taken to a recovery room where they will be placed with trained personnel and where there is equipment for monitoring and resuscitation.

References

1. Klausen, N. O., Wiberg-Jørgensen, F., and Chraemmer-Jørgensen, B. Psychomimetic reactions after low-dose ketamine infusion. Comparison with neuroleptanaesthesia. *Br. J. Anaesth.* 55:297, 1983.
2. Viby-Mogensen, J., and Hanel, H. K. Prolonged apnoea after suxamethonium: An analysis of the first 225 cases reported to the Danish Cholinesterase Research Unit. *Acta Anaesthesiol. Scand.* 22:371, 1978.
3. Hunter, J. M., Jones, R. S., and Utting, J. E. Use of atracurium during general surgery monitored by the train-of-four stimuli. *Br. J. Anaesth.* 22:371, 1978.
4. Coppel, D. I., and Dundee, J. W. Ketamine anaesthesia for cardiac catheterization. *Anaesthesia* 27:25, 1972.
5. Hodgkinson, R., Bhatt, M., Kim, S. S., et al. Neonatal neurobehavioral tests following cesarean section under general and spinal anesthesia. *Am. J. Obstet. Gynecol.* 132:670, 1978.
6. Johnston, R. R., Eger, E. I., and Wilson, C. A comparative interaction of epinephrine with enflurane, isoflurane, and halothane in man. *Anesth. Analg.* (Cleve.) 55:709, 1976.
7. Giesecke, A. H. Perioperative Fluid Therapy-Crystalloids. In R. Miller (Ed.), *Anesthesia* (vol. 2). New York: Churchill Livingstone, 1981. Pp. 865–883.
8. Furman, E. B., Roman, G., Lemmer, I. A. S., et al. Specific therapy in water, electrolyte and blood-volume replacement during pediatric surgery. *Anesthesiology* 42:182, 1975.
9. Peltier, I. F. The diagnosis and treatment of fat embolism. *J. Trauma* 11:661, 1971.

10. Moore, D. C., Bridenbaugh, L. D., Thompson, G. B., et al. Factors determining dosages of amide-type local anesthetic drugs. *Anesthesiology* 47:263, 1977.
11. Stoddart, J. C. Postoperative respiratory failure: An anaesthetic hazard? *Br. J. Anaesth.* 50:695, 1978.
12. Korttila, K., Kauste, A., and Auvinen, J. Comparison of domperidone, droperidol, and metoclopramide in the prevention and treatment of nausea and vomiting after balanced general anesthesia. *Anesth. Analg.* (Paris) 58:396, 1979.
13. Hetter, G. P. The effect of low dose epinephrine on the hematocrit drop following lipolysis. *Aesthetic Plast. Surg.* 8:19, 1984.

CHAPTER 15

The Use of Low-Concentration Epinephrine

Gregory P. Hetter

Patients undergoing suction lipectomies have often been hospitalized by many surgeons for several days [1,2]. Although hematoma and seroma formation are reported in 30% of the curette cases [2], this complication is minimal in the cannula cases [1,3]. Nevertheless, major shifts of intravascular fluids causing orthostatic hypotension have caused Dr. Illouz to keep most patients as inpatients for 1 to 3 days. He frequently administers albumin in removals of more than 1000 ml, which may be accounted for by the French tendency to give considerably less crystalloid than is common in North America.

I have shown that large drops in hematocrit frequently follow blunt suction lipectomy [3]. In my preoperative protocol, patients who have a demonstrable bleeding tendency by laboratory tests, including bleeding time, are eliminated as candidates for lipolysis. I suggested that the removal of each 100 to 150 ml removed results in a hematocrit drop of at least 1% by the second postoperative day.

To quantify the hematocrit drop, I followed the hematocrit in 10 patients who underwent lipolysis. Before the removal of tissue, the usual Illouz formula was injected subcutaneously: 100 ml saline, 20 ml distilled water, and 1 unit per milliliter of Wydase. Approximately 5 ml was injected every 5 cm. The maximal injection was 300 ml. The preoperative hematocrit was compared to the hematocrit on the second postoperative day. The amount of tissue removed was compared to the hematocrit drop, and the ratio of milliliters removed per percentage point hematocrit drop was calculated. Table 15-1 illustrates the hematocrit drop from lipolysis in a series of 10 patients.

The following observations were made from the series:

1. The average removal was 772 ml.
2. The range was 475 ml to 1100 ml.
3. The average hematocrit drop was 8.7%.
4. The range was 3.5% to 15.4%.
5. For each 89 ml removed, a hematocrit drop of 1% occurred on average.
6. The number of milliliters removed divided by the hematocrit drop varied from a worst case of 52 ml to a best case of 200 ml removed per 1% hematocrit drop.
7. The worst case was an abdominal lipolysis and the best case a lateral femoral area ("saddlebag") lipolysis.
8. Of the 10 patients, 6 were hospitalized postoperatively in this series at a total cost of $7220 for 19 hospital days.

Table 15-1. Hematocrit drop from lipolysis in a series of ten patients

Patient	Amount removed (ml)	Albumin	Hospital	Hct fall (%)	Ml removed ÷ Hct fall = ml/%
1	550	No	Yes	38.0 − 30.6 = 7.4	550 ÷ 7.4 = 74.3
2	475	No	No	44.4 − 38.5 = 5.9	475 ÷ 5.9 = 80.5
3	750	No	Yes	41.3 − 34.6 = 6.7	750 ÷ 6.7 = 111.9
4	1000	No	Yes	40.7 − 32.7 = 8.0	1000 ÷ 8.0 = 125.0
5	700	No	No	41.5 − 38.0 = 3.5	700 ÷ 3.5 = 200.0
6	550	No	No	42.5 − 37.2 = 5.3	550 ÷ 5.3 = 103.0
7	800	Yes	Yes	48.7 − 40.0 = 8.7	800 ÷ 8.7 = 92.0
8	800	Yes	Yes	38.6 − 23.2 = 15.4	800 ÷ 15.4 = 52.0
9	1100	Yes	Yes	40.2 − 33.3 = 6.9	1100 ÷ 6.9 = 159.0
10	1000	Yes	Yes	40.9 − 30.4 = 10.5	1200 ÷ 10.5 = 114.0
Average 772				**Average 8.7**	**Range 52–200** **Average 88.7**

Table 15-2. Hematocrit drop in a series of ten patients administered low-concentration epinephrine (1:435,000)

Patient	Amount removed (ml)	Albumin	Hospital	Hct fall (%)	Ml removed ÷ Hct fall = ml/%
1	1350	No	No	45.8 − 38.7 = 7.1	1350 ÷ 7.1 = 190.1
2	1200	No	No	38.8 − 31.5 = 7.3	1200 ÷ 7.3 = 164.4
3	650	No	No	50.1 − 40.5 = 9.6	650 ÷ 9.6 = 67.7
4	1500	Yes	Yes	42.6 − 29.4 = 13.2	1500 ÷ 13.2 = 113.6
5	500	No	No	43.6 − 36.0 = 7.6	500 ÷ 7.6 = 65.8
6	550	No	No	37.4 − 34.3 = 3.1	550 ÷ 3.1 = 177.4
7	250	No	No	41.7 − 40.7 = 1.0	250 ÷ 1.0 = 250.0
8	1500	No	Yes	40.7 − 33.7 = 7.0	1500 ÷ 7.0 = 214.3
9	520	No	No	42.2 − 36.5 = 5.7	520 ÷ 5.7 = 91.2
10	900	No	Yes	45.0 − 41.0 = 4.0	900 ÷ 4.0 = 225.0
Average 892				**Average 6.56**	**Range 66–250** **Average 136**

To investigate the effect that low-concentration epinephrine might have on the hematocrit drop, a similar series of 10 patients underwent lipolysis using a solution to which Xylocaine and epinephrine were added. The formula was

250 ml saline
75 ml Xylocaine 1% with epinephrine 1:100,000
300 units of Wydase

This mixture provides Xylocaine 0.23% and epinephrine 1:435,000. Wydase, 0.92 units per ml, is present. It differed from the previous solution in that it was isotonic. The technique and amounts of injected solution were similar to the first series of patients as was the actual performance of the surgery. Anesthesia agents were similar and performed by the same anesthetists. Isoflurane (Forane) was used. It allows a higher concentration of epinephrine before extrasystoles occur than do other agents [4] (see Chapter 14). Injection of multi ple areas was carried out incrementally. No more than 300 ml was used on any case. Fluid replacement with Ringer's lactate was the same except that less albumin was given, since the removed tissue was obviously far less sanguinous than in the previous series. Table 15-2 illustrates the results.

The following observations were made from the second series:

1. The average removal was 892 ml.
2. The range was 250 ml to 1500 ml.
3. The average hematocrit drop was 6.6%.
4. The range was 1.0% to 13.2%.
5. For each 136 ml removed, a hematocrit drop of 1% occurred on average.
6. The number of milliliters removed divided by the hematocrit drop varied from a worst case of 66 ml to a best case of 250 ml.
7. The worst cases were abdominal lipolysis. The best case was a *very small* abdominal lipolysis of only 250

Table 15-3. A comparison of observations from Tables 15-1 and 15-2

	Series I	Series II
Average removal	772	892
Range of removal	475–1100	250–1500
Average Hct drop	8.7%	6.6%
Range of drop	3.5%–15.4%	1.0%–13.2%
Average amount of removal per 1% of Hct drop	89 ml/%	136 ml/%
Average Hct drop per 100 ml removed	1.12%	0.74%

ml. The next best was a large lateral femoral area ("saddlebag") lipolysis. This pattern is the same as the first series (see Table 15-1).

8. Of 10 patients, 3 were hospitalized postoperatively in the second series at a total cost of $1900 for 5 hospital days. This amount was $5320 less than the first series.

A comparison of the observations between the two series is shown in Table 15-3.

Clinical Observations

Certain clinical observations were made at the time of surgery and are pertinent and worthy of mention. It was immediately evident when beginning the series in which epinephrine-containing injections were used that the tissue removed consisted of more fat and less blood. Larger removals were performed more often in the second series, which may reflect the increased confidence generated by less blood seen in the removed tissues. The second side was more often bloodier than the first on bilateral procedures. This occurrence was interpreted as the epinephrine effect "wearing off" during lengthy removals. There appeared to be less postoperative pain; this was attributed to the Xylocaine.

Conclusions

1. Lipolysis may be performed with or without a preceding injection of an epinephrine- or Xylocaine-containing solution.

2. The use of a solution containing a weak concentration of epinephrine (1:435,000) showed a demonstrable effect on the hematocrit drawn on the second postoperative day as compared to not using epineph-

rine. Approximately 50% more fatty tissue could be removed for the same drop in hematocrit; that is, 136 ml with epinephrine versus 89 ml without epinephrine caused an average 1% drop in hematocrit.

3. The size of removal considered safe for ambulatory discharge using epinephrine is larger. Removals in the general area of 1000 ml are usually treated as outpatients. Clinical judgment, of course, prevails. Less postoperative pain required less postoperative analgesics, which aids early ambulatory discharge.

4. Hospitalization days were reduced by 70% (5 versus 19) by the use of epinephrine, with a savings of $5320 ($7220 − $1900) in a series of 10 patients.

Summary

The hematocrit drop on the second postoperative day after lipolysis is dependent on the size of the removal but has a wide variation. The preparation of the localized area by the subcutaneous injection of a solution containing a weak concentration of epinephrine lessens the magnitude of this drop by about one-third. Expressed another way, for the same hematocrit drop, 50% more tissue may be removed when using subcutaneous epinephrine than without. Ambulatory discharge is more often possible when using epinephrine- and Xylocaine-containing solutions; as a result, there is a significant reduction in hospital days.

The use of low-dose epinephrine is recommended for lipolysis to increase safety, lower morbidity, reduce economic outlay, and reduce hospitalization. Since the original presentation of this work at the first annual meeting of the Lipolysis Society of North America in 1983, and its subsequent publication in the *Aesthetic Journal* [5], the benefit of low-concentration epinephrine has been adopted by most practitioners.

References

1. Illouz, Y. G. Une nouvelle technique pour les lipodistrophies localisées. *Rev. Chir. Esthet. de Lang. Fr.* 4(19): Avril, 1980.
2. Teimourian, B., and Fisher, J. B. Suction curettage to remove excess fat for body contouring. *Plast. Reconstr. Surg.* 68:50, 1981.
3. Hetter, G. P. Experience with "lipolysis": The Illouz technique of blunt suction lipectomy in North America. *Aesth. Plast. Surg.* 7:69, 1983.
4. Eger, E. *Isoflurane (Forane).* Madison, WI: Ohio Medical Products, 1981.
5. Hetter, G. P. The effect of low dose epinephrine on the hematocrit drop following lipolysis. *Aesth. Plast. Surg.* 8(1):19, 1984.

CHAPTER 16

Physics and Equipment

Gregory P. Hetter

This chapter is divided into three parts. Each part overlaps in some respects, as does the following chapter on technique. Repetition may be annoying to some while others will be appreciative. The physics of pressure have been forgotten without regret by most surgeons, who remember only the units but not their meaning or interrelationships. This chapter attempts to explain why the Illouz technique depends on certain physical properties and why and how alterations in the equipment may affect the technique.

Physics

AIR PRESSURE

The column of air above us out into space has weight. In 1643 Evangelista Torricelli filled a glass tube closed at one end with mercury and everted it with the open end in a cup of mercury. The mercury fell in the closed top tube until it was 76 cm (760 mm), or 29.9 inches, in height (Fig. 16-1). Torricelli drew the conclusion that the column of air pressure on the surface of the mercury in the cup was equal to the pressure of the column of mercury pressing out against the column of air. This device persists to this day in the form of mercury barometers and is still the most accurate.

Most mechanical gauges on pumps work by connecting a metal chamber to the suction line. The chamber is made of pliable metal; as the inside pressure changes, the chamber wall moves in or out (much like a balloon) because of the outside air pressure. By connecting this movement to a dial and a scale, the change in pressure can be read. The outside atmospheric pressure becomes the *reference pressure* or *zero point*. Since atmospheric pressure changes both in relation to altitude and weather, the zero point is always changing.

UNITS OF MEASUREMENT FOR PRESSURE

Pressure is expressed in many units. The metric system expresses it in the height of a mercury column. Absolute vacuum supports 0 mm of mercury (Hg). At sea level a full atmosphere supports approximately 760 mm of mercury, as Torricelli's experiments proved. One could use a column of water as has also been done, but this is impractical since the water evaporates and the column is an unwieldy 34 feet high. When expressed in English units, 760 mm becomes 29.9 inches of mercury.

Pressure also is expressed as weight per surface area. In the metric system, this is calculated as follows: A column of mercury 76 cm high (760 mm) has a density of 13.6 grams per cubic cm. Thus:

$$\frac{76\ cm \times 13.6\ g}{cm^3} = \frac{1033.6\ g}{cm^2}$$

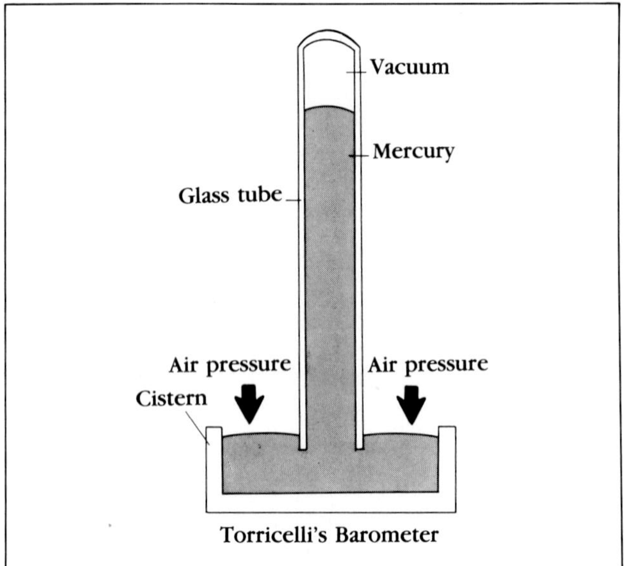

Fig. 16-1. Illustration of Torricelli's original experiment with the atmospheric pressure equaling the pressure of the column of mercury.

Table 16-1. Air pressure values in relation to increasing altitude

	Hg (mm)	Hg (in)	g/cm^2	lb/in^2
Sea level	760	29.9	1034	14.7
1000 ft	734	28.9	999	14.2
2000 ft	706	27.8	961	13.7
3000 ft	680	26.8	926	13.2
4000 ft	655	25.8	892	12.7
5000 ft	632	24.9	861	12.2
6000 ft	607	23.9	826	11.7
7000 ft	584	23.0	795	11.3
8000 ft	564	22.2	768	10.9
9000 ft	541	21.3	737	10.5
10,000 ft	521	20.5	709	10.1

The figure of 1034 g/cm^2 is shown on the gauges of French suction machines as the value of 1 atmosphere. The English system equivalent is measured in pounds per square inch and is equal to 14.7 pounds per square inch.

Another measurement that may be confusing and ought not to be used in discussions of pumps and pressures is the millibar. The U.S. Weather Service defined a *bar* in 1939 as the pressure equivalent to 75.01 cm of mercury (29.53 inches Hg). A millibar equals $\frac{1}{1000}$ of a bar. Thus, 76 cm of mercury (760 mm Hg), or 1 atmosphere, is approximately 1020 millibar. This scale is seen on weather barometers. Because the value of this unit (1020) is so similar to the metric expressions of grams per square centimeter (1034 g/cm^2), many uninformed persons confuse the two scales. Once understood, confusion between the two scales is prevented. On European pumps, g/cm^2 is the usual mode of expression. Many small American manufacturers use inexpensive gauges marked in inches of mercury ($\pm$10% accuracy). Ideally, millimeters of mercury should be used.

THE EFFECT OF ALTITUDE ON PRESSURE

At sea level the air column above us will support 76 cm of mercury as discussed. As we climb from sea level the pressure falls, until at 10,000 feet the pressure is 52.1 cm (521 mm) of mercury. This fall is not exactly arithmetical, but for all practical purposes the values in Table 16-1 are more than adequate for those in high mountain areas to use for calculation purposes.

THE TORR: THE PROPER UNIT OF MEASUREMENT FOR VACUUM

One torr is the pressure necessary to support a column of mercury 1 mm high at 0°C and standard gravity. This unit is easily confused with the way we normally speak of pressure in millimeters of mercury. This measurement is unrelated to the surrounding air pressure and is an absolute value. This absolute molecular pressure is different from what we may read on the gauge of a suction pump, as explained below.

When the manufacturer states that a surgical suction pump provides a "suction pressure" of 730 mm Hg, *what is meant is that the pump will remove all but 30 mm of pressure from within the system* (760 mm − 730 mm = 30 mm). If we would place the cup of mercury at the base of the mercury barometer on the inside of the suction system and turn the pump on, as the air molecules were extracted, the mercury column would fall from 760 mm to 30 mm of mercury. The 30 mm is the absolute pressure within the system, and the 730 mm is the difference between atmospheric pressure and the absolute pressure within the system. Since the pump is not capable of extracting more molecules, the remaining molecules are exerting a pressure sufficient to hold up a column of mercury 30 mm high. This is 30 torr* whether the machine is on top of a mountain, at sea level, or deep in a mine shaft.

The gauges on all machines measure the difference between the pressure remaining in the system and the outside air pressure but not the pressure in the system directly. In that sense, significant elevation above sea

---

*The correction to 0°C for the mercury is a negligible value and is neglected for the purpose of this discussion.

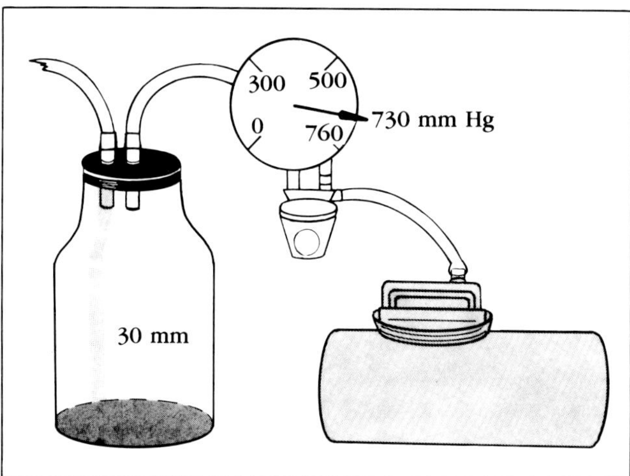

Fig. 16-2. Vacuum pump capable of producing 30 torr used at sea level. Gauge pressure shows 730 mm Hg. Atmospheric pressure is 760 mm Hg.

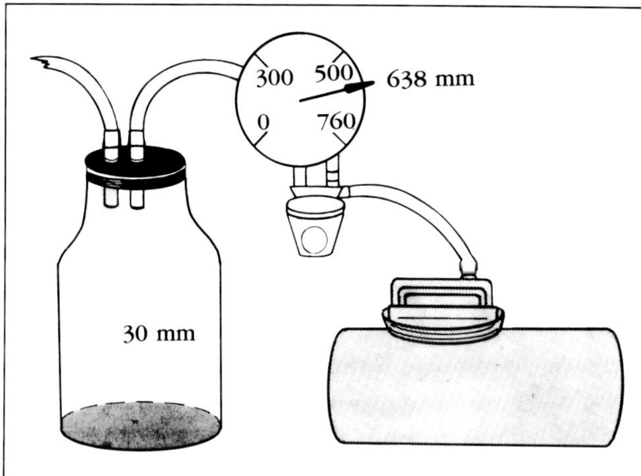

Fig. 16-3. Same vacuum pump producing same degree of vacuum of 30 torr but used at 4000 feet above sea level, where the atmospheric pressure is only 668 mm Hg. Gauge reads only 638 mm giving a falsely low impression.

level gives a falsely low impression of the true vacuum in the system.

Example: One surgeon is at sea level. The atmospheric pressure is 760 mm Hg. His pump shows a gauge reading of 730 mm Hg at sea level (30 mm Hg pressure remains in the system). This is 30 torr (Fig. 16-2).

Another surgeon is at 4000 feet. The atmospheric pressure is 668 mm Hg. The gauge on the same pump will read the difference between 668 mm and the pressure remaining in the system of 30 mm Hg and show a gauge reading of 638 mm. Yet the true pressure within the system remains at 30 mm or 30 torr, just as it was at sea level. The apparent pressure on the gauge, however, will read only 638 mm (Fig. 16-3).

Table 16-2. Vaporization pressure of water at various temperatures

Temperature	Vaporization pressure
15°C	13 mm Hg
20°C	17½ "
25°C	24 "
30°C	32 "
35°C	42 "
37°C Body temp.	47 "
40°C	55 "

The surgeon at higher elevations should use Table 16-1 to correct for his altitude. He may calculate the capability in torr of his pump by subtracting his gauge reading from the average air pressure at his altitude as found in Table 16-1.

THE VAPOR PRESSURE OF WATER

Water will vaporize under one atmosphere of pressure at sea level (760 mm Hg) at 100°C (212°F). As the pressure against the surface of the water decreases, for example, in the mountains, the water will vaporize at progressively lower temperatures. It takes longer to boil an egg in Denver or Aspen than it does at sea level because the lower temperature at which the water boils requires a longer exposure at this lower temperature to achieve the same degree of heat coagulation inside the egg. Table 16-2 shows the vaporization pressure of water at various relevant temperatures.

If the air in a suction bottle containing water at 37°C is exhausted by a powerful vacuum pump, the pressure will fall until it reaches 47 mm Hg (47 torr). At that point the water will begin to vaporize. If this vaporization is rapid, the water will boil vigorously. The pressure will not fall below 47 mm no matter how powerful the pump, as long as water remains at that temperature. The vaporization of water, however, requires a heat exchange of 80 cal per gram, so the temperature of the water, if not kept constant, will rapidly fall. If the temperature is kept constant, the pressure will not fall below 47 mm as long as water remains to vaporize.

The molecules of vaporized water rush toward the pump just as the air molecules did before they were exhausted from the system. Exactly the same phenomenon of vaporization occurs during lipolysis with tissue fluids such as interstitial fluid, serum, or blood. With powerful vacuum pumps, this vaporization can be observed in the tubing and collection jar as a bubbling action (boiling).

WHAT PRESSURE IS ADEQUATE?

Controversy exists as to the suction pressures necessary to perform "suction lipectomy." On the one side, Dr. Illouz of Paris, after performing 5000 procedures, states that pressures close to 1 atmosphere (30 in or 76 cm Hg) are necessary to perform his procedure properly. Characteristic of his procedure are blunt cannulas with blunt openings, individual tunnels in the fat, and the closed technique (no air leak). He describes this procedure in his articles in French [1,2,3,4]. My article [5] describes the technique in English. The Educational Foundation (EF-ASPRS) basic videotape on lipolysis demonstrates the technique and shows the vaporization of water by a powerful suction pump.

Dr. Kesselring [6], after performing fewer than 100 procedures, stated that 0.5 atmosphere (15 in or 38 cm Hg) is enough suction pressure for his curette technique. Characteristic for his technique (as seen at the Educational Foundation Symposium in Los Angeles in April 1983) is air leak to the operated space, confluency of the spaces, and sharp curettes to carve away the fat.

Dr. Courtiss [7], after performing fewer than 100 procedures, stated at the same symposium that the suction pressure is unimportant. As viewed on his videotape presented in April 1983, his technique appeared to have air leak to the operated space and curettes were used.

Dr. Teimourian [8], after performing 200 procedures, stated that a very high vacuum pressure is necessary for adequate performance. Dr. Teimourian's 1983 technique appears to be a closed technique.

Dr. Chajcher [9], after treating 150 patients, stated that 450 mm (0.59 atmosphere) is enough for his curette technique (his instruments appear to be copies of Kesselring's).

The Illouz technique is performed with the blunt cannulas described in the next section. When such a cannula is driven into the deep subcutaneous fat without suction attached (Fig. 16-4) and withdrawn (Fig. 16-5), chunks of fat will be found in the barrel. This is especially true of the "shark mouth" #10, which is Dr. Illouz's favorite for large fat extractions (Fig. 16-6). The mechanical nature of the fat extraction is clear.

When suction is applied, fat globules are drawn into the lumen. The greater the suction, the more securely the fat glob is held as the cannula edge is moved across its base. If the attachments are stronger than the suction, the glob pulls away from the lumen as the cannula is moved. If the suction is strong enough to hold the glob, the edge of the lumen opening will avulse the glob from its attachment (Fig. 16-7A). The stronger the suction, the more fat that is avulsed. With sharp-edged curettes [6,9], the amount of suction need not be very great (0.5 atmosphere or less), because cutting rather than avulsion occurs. This must be clearly comprehended. Suc-

tion pressures higher than 0.5 atmosphere are necessary for reasonably efficient avulsion to occur. This pressure is probably not critical, however.

Once the fat is in the barrel of the cannula or curette, the movement of that fat may occur by way of one of two separate physical processes. This aspect has been poorly understood by many surgeons who did not have the great advantage of being in Dr. Illouz's operating room watching him perform the procedure with the equipment designed for him.

MOVEMENT BY VAPORIZATION

With high-pressure machines producing a residual pressure of 15 to 20 torr or less (740–745 mm Hg gauge pressure or more *at sea level*), tissue fluids including serum, blood, and interstitial and intracellular fluids are vaporized by the pressure [10]. As previously outlined, the machine cannot lower the pressure to less than the vaporization pressure of a liquid present in the system. The molecules of vapor traveling in the cannula collide with the fat globs in the cannula and the tubing and push these globs toward the pump. The globs are therefore slowly "bumped" along down the tube by these molecular collisions (Fig. 16-7B). Fluid in the tube will be seen to "boil" indicating vaporization (Fig. 16-7C).

The Illouz technique is essentially a closed technique; that is, the cannula is buried in fatty tissue during the whole procedure and does not depend on air leak to clear the cannula. The cannula is rarely withdrawn from the tissues. Dr. Illouz states that a complete lateral femoral defatting or abdominal defatting can be accomplished without withdrawing the cannula; this has been adequately verified.

MOVEMENT BY AIR LEAK

Without a high-pressure machine capable of vaporization, the fat can be propelled out of the cannula and down the tubing only by withdrawing the cannular lumen to or near the site of entry, allowing atmospheric air at 760 mm Hg to leak into the cannular lumen. The fragments of fat and liquid are propelled by this dense air into the collection bottle with a splash. The disadvantages of this technique are several. First, returning to the site of entry repeatedly runs the risk of unwanted excessive defatting in that general area. Second, the extracted tissue is not clearly observed for content of blood or type and amount of fat removed from each tunnel because it is so quickly propelled to the collection bottle where it disperses with a splash. Third, the procedure is unnecessarily prolonged by repeated withdrawals and reinsertions. Fourth, the accuracy of the removal is impaired by the necessity to relocate the interface between extracted and unextracted areas. The chance of

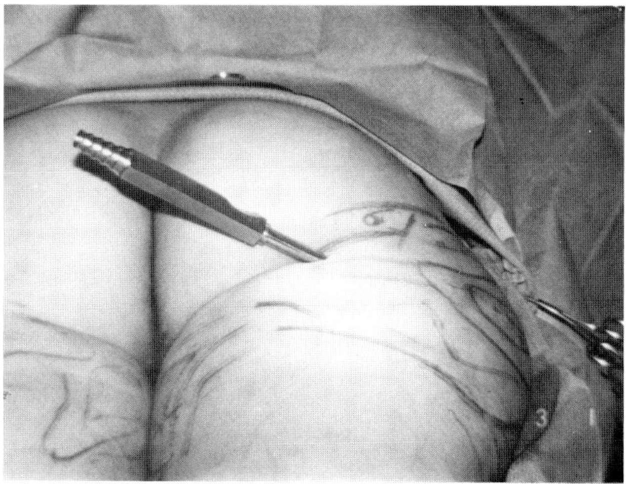

Fig. 16-4. #10 Illouz cannula driven into subcutaneous fat with no suction attached.

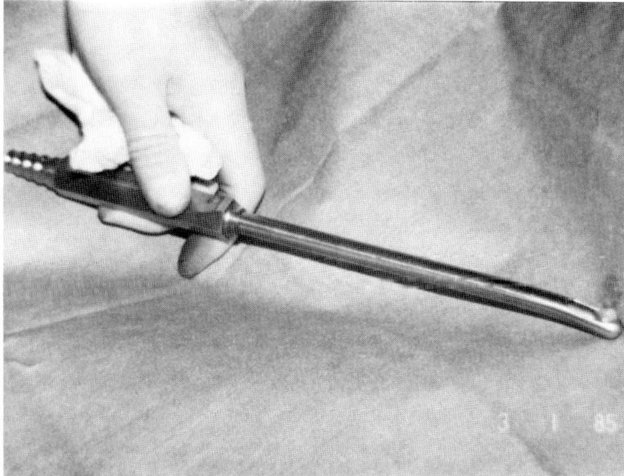

Fig. 16-5. Same cannula withdrawn showing evulsed fat in lumen *without* suction.

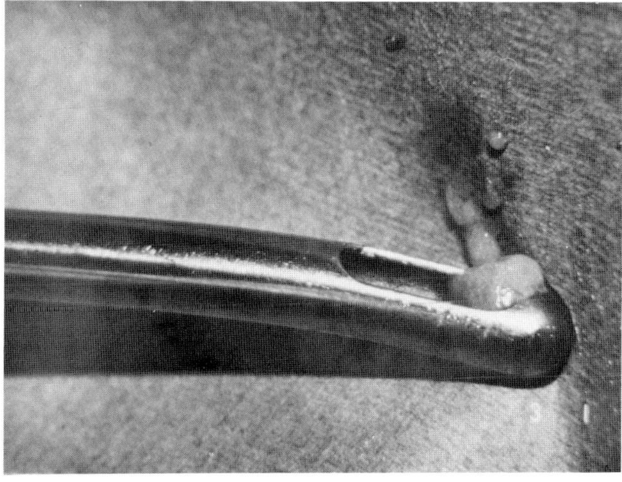

Fig. 16-6. Close-up of lumen of cannula.

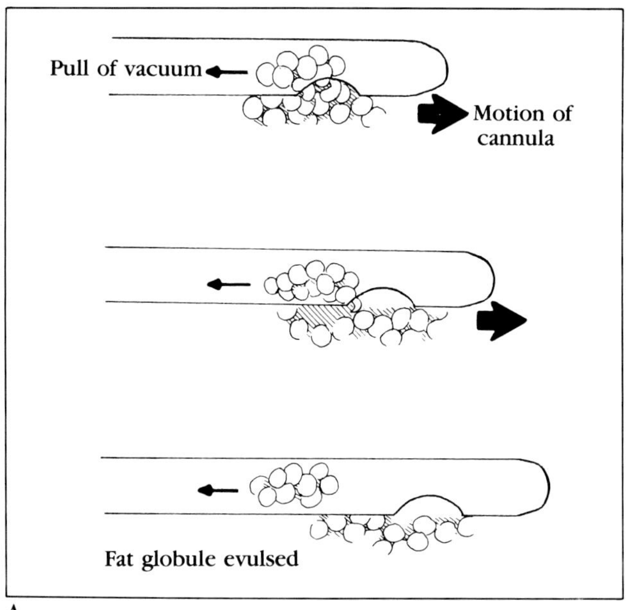

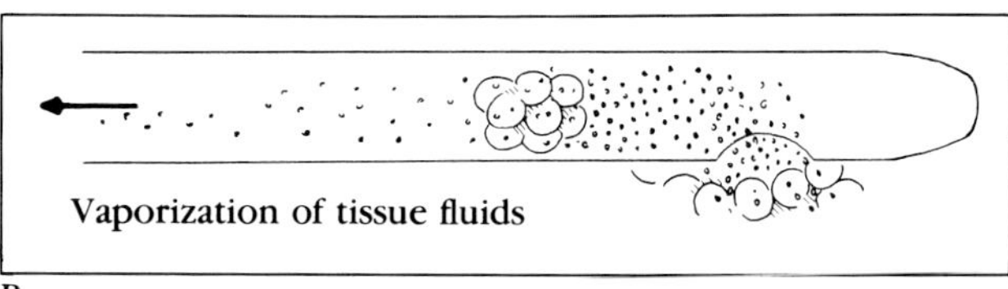

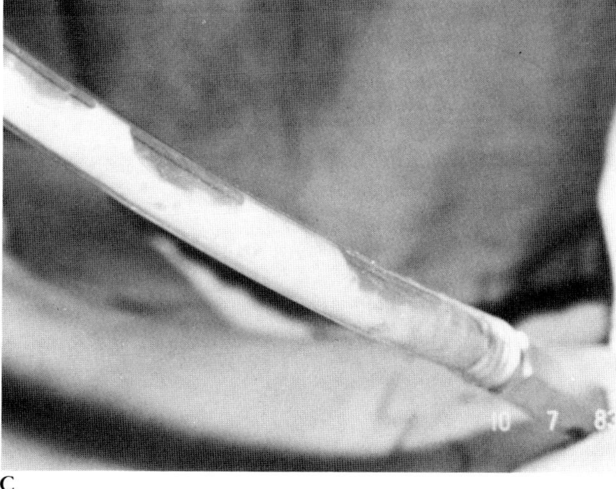

C

Fig. 16-7.
A. Fat globules held in the lumen of the cannula by suction are evulsed by the movement of the cannula by the surgeon.
B. Molecules of vaporized tissue fluids collide with fat chunks and propel them out of cannula.
C. Fatty fluids vaporize ("boil") in tubing producing bubbles.

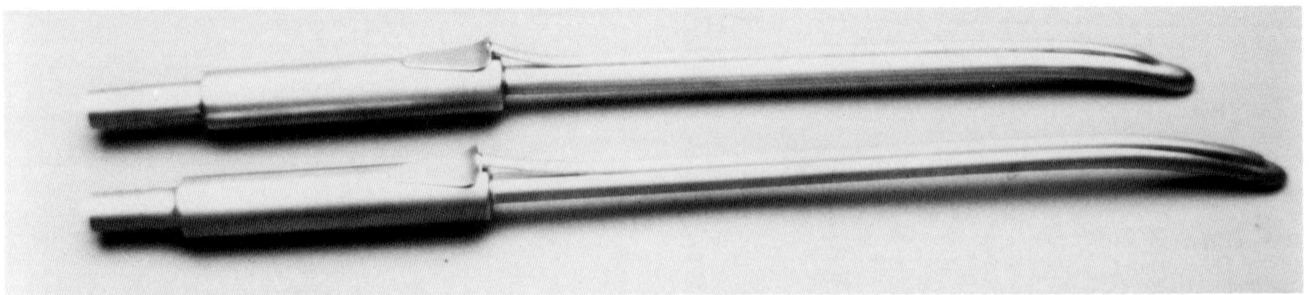

creating an island or peninsula of fat or irregularity is greater.

If surgeons are forced by circumstances to use this manner of performing the fat extraction, they should understand that they are performing the procedure in a less efficient manner than is possible and unnecessarily adding to the uncertainties of a blind procedure.

In South America both cannulas and curettes have been machined to eliminate the need to withdraw the instrument to obtain an air leak when using a low-pressure machine (Fig. 16-8A). An air leak or "sump" line has been incorporated into the cannula, controlled by the thumb, which runs to the tip in front of the lumen (Fig. 16-8B). In this way, air may be leaked to the lumen at will and with some degree of control to clear the cannular contents or to release a vacuum. This is a good mechanical solution for the problems caused by the use of lower-pressure machines.

Equipment

CANNULAS

The first cannulas used for fat extraction were existing curettes or cannulas. Surgeons have advanced their own techniques by modifying these instruments. Cannulas that have been used or are now being used for extraction of fat include

Abortion curette: plastic uterine curette (Fig. 16-9)
Teimourian curette: modified fascia lata stripper (Fig. 16-10)
Kesselring curette: Fig. 16-11A,B with inset
Illouz cannula: Fig. 16-12 with inset
Grazer-Grams modification: Fig. 16-13 with inset
Hetter-Padgett modification: Fig. 16-14 with inset

The original Kesselring technique [11] used a curette with a sharp back-cutting blade introduced through a substantial incision into a plane developed with scissors. It was introduced close to the muscle fascia with the opening toward the surface. The blade shaved fat as

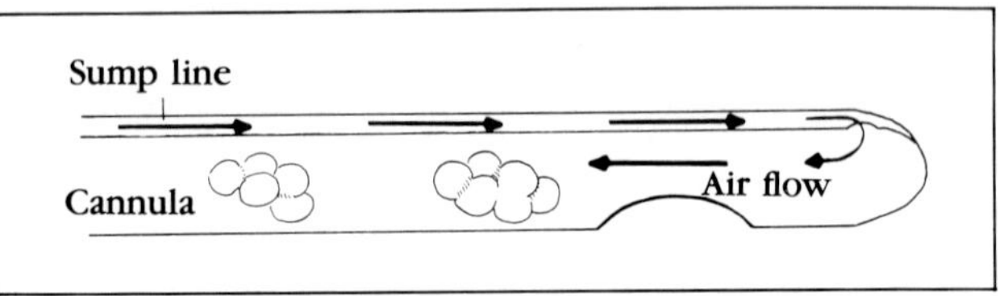

B

Fig. 16-8.
A. Picture of Brazilian cannulas with "air leak" channel.
   (Courtesy of R. Baroudi, M.D., Sao Paulo, Brazil.)
B. Drawing showing the way the cannula functions.

the curette was drawn back, and the suction pressure evacuated the fat, which was thus carved away. At the annual American Society of Plastic and Reconstructive Surgery (ASPRS) meeting in October 1982, in Hawaii, Dr. Kesselring said that his technique was used only on "saddlebags" and small deformities and fewer than 50 patients had been treated to that date over several years; the exact date was not then and has never been made clear [6]. Seroma was acknowledged as a frequent problem.

Dr. Teimourian [12] reported on 4 years' experience comprising 54 patients in 1981. He started with the uterine curette, modified a fascia lata stripper, and then used the Kesselring instrument. Sharp instruments similar to the Kesselring instrument were modified over the years. Dr. Teimourian, however, extracted fat from a variety of areas. The reported seroma rate was high, indicating lymphorrhea or hematoma or both.

Dr. Illouz [1,2,3,4] states that he began his technique in 1977. He reported on his first 300 cases in 1980. The reported seroma rate was 0. That seroma is negligible has been confirmed by those practicing his technique. His cannula has a blunt tip and rounded edges at the opening, as shown in Figure 16-12.

Derivatives of the Illouz cannulas are the Fournier, Grazer-Grams, Hetter-Padgett, Robbins, and others.

Note the difference between the tips of the Illouz and the Grazer-Grams cannulas as seen in Figures 16-13 and 16-14 insets. The sharp edges of the latter can tear muscle fascia or vessels more easily than the blunt opening of the original Illouz cannulas.

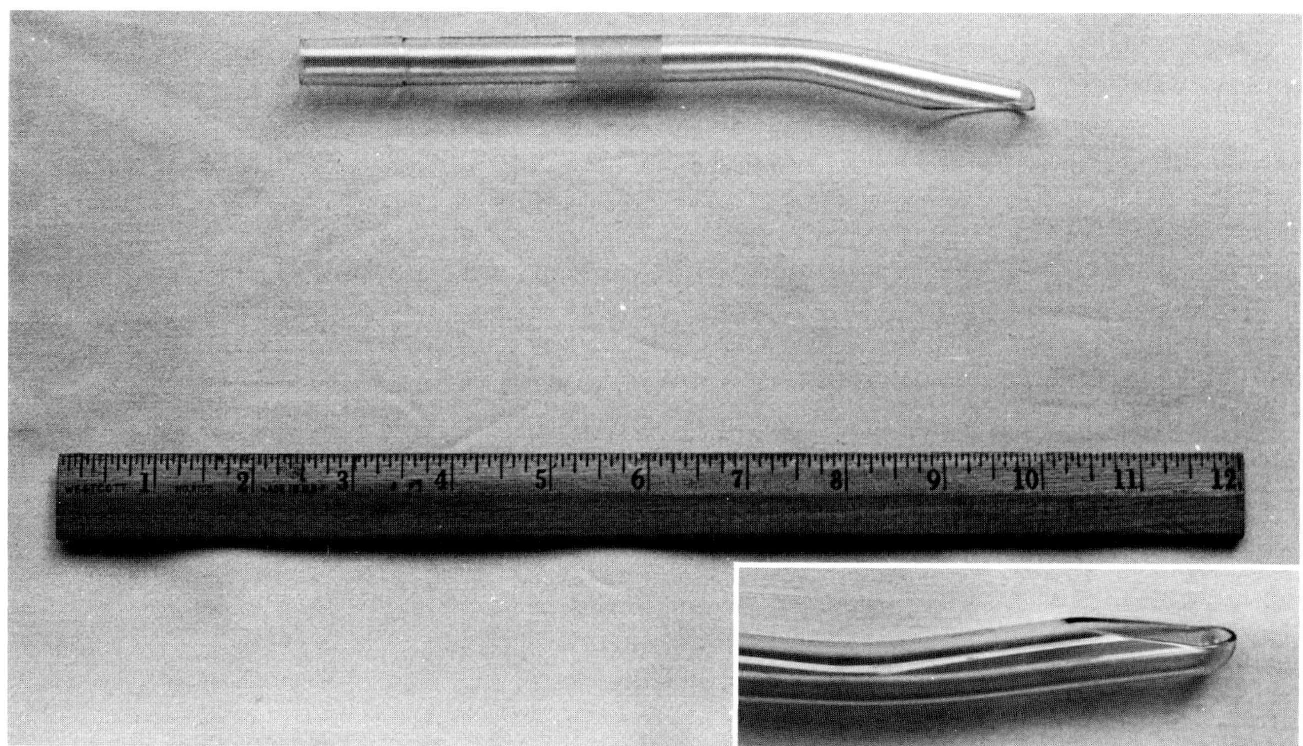

Fig. 16-9. Plastic uterine curette supplied by Cabot Medical Corporation. Inset shows sharp edges.

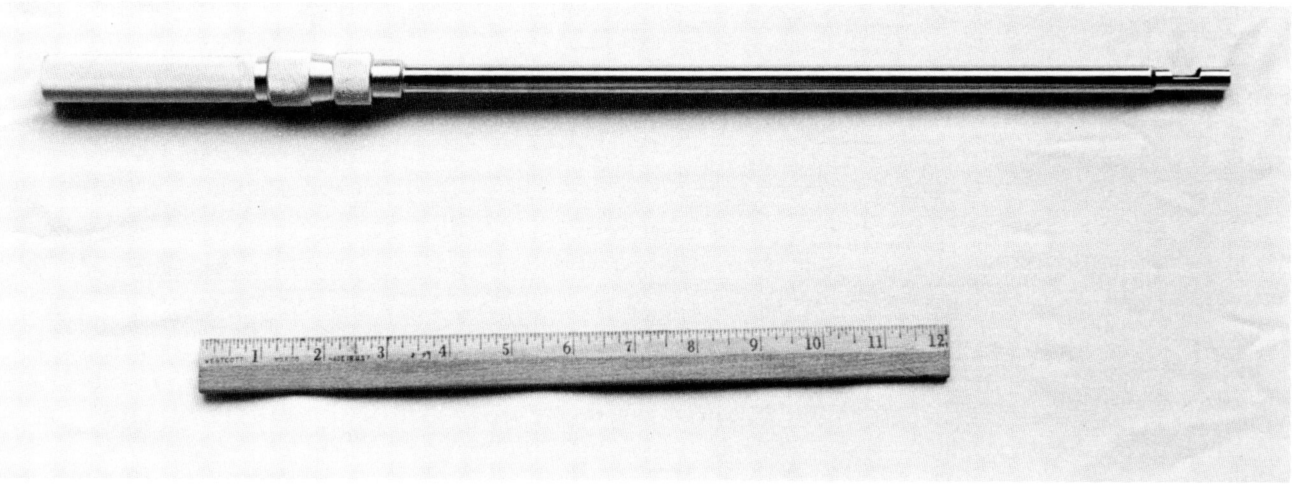

Fig. 16-10. Fascia lata stripper modified by Teimourian as reported in 1981.

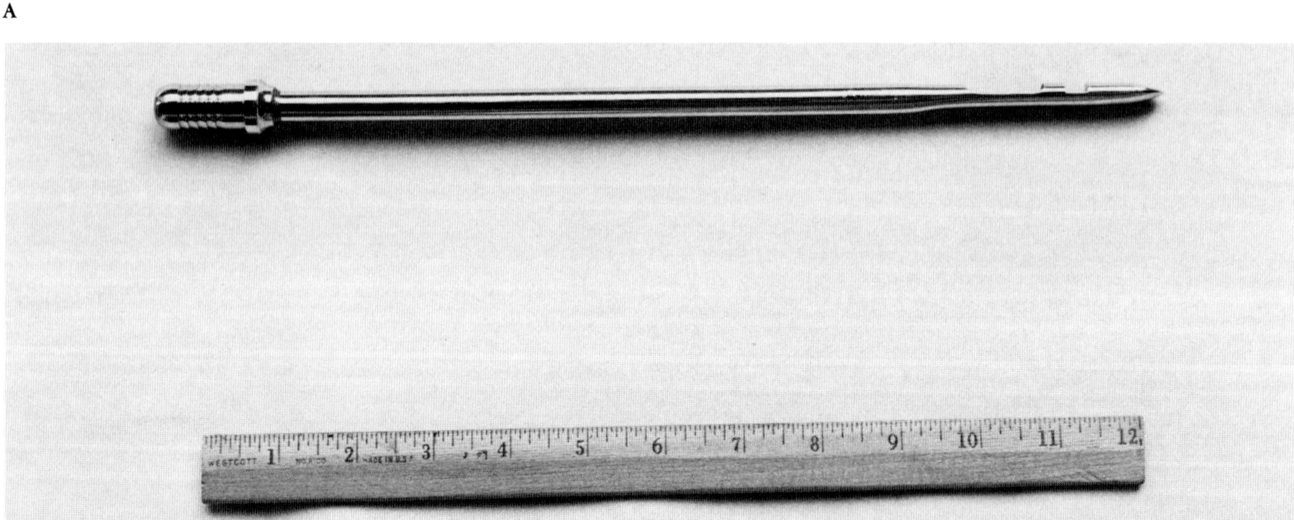

A

B

Fig. 16-11.
A. Kesselring sharp curette reported in 1978. Inset shows
   close-up of blade. Top view.
B. Kesselring curette. Side view.

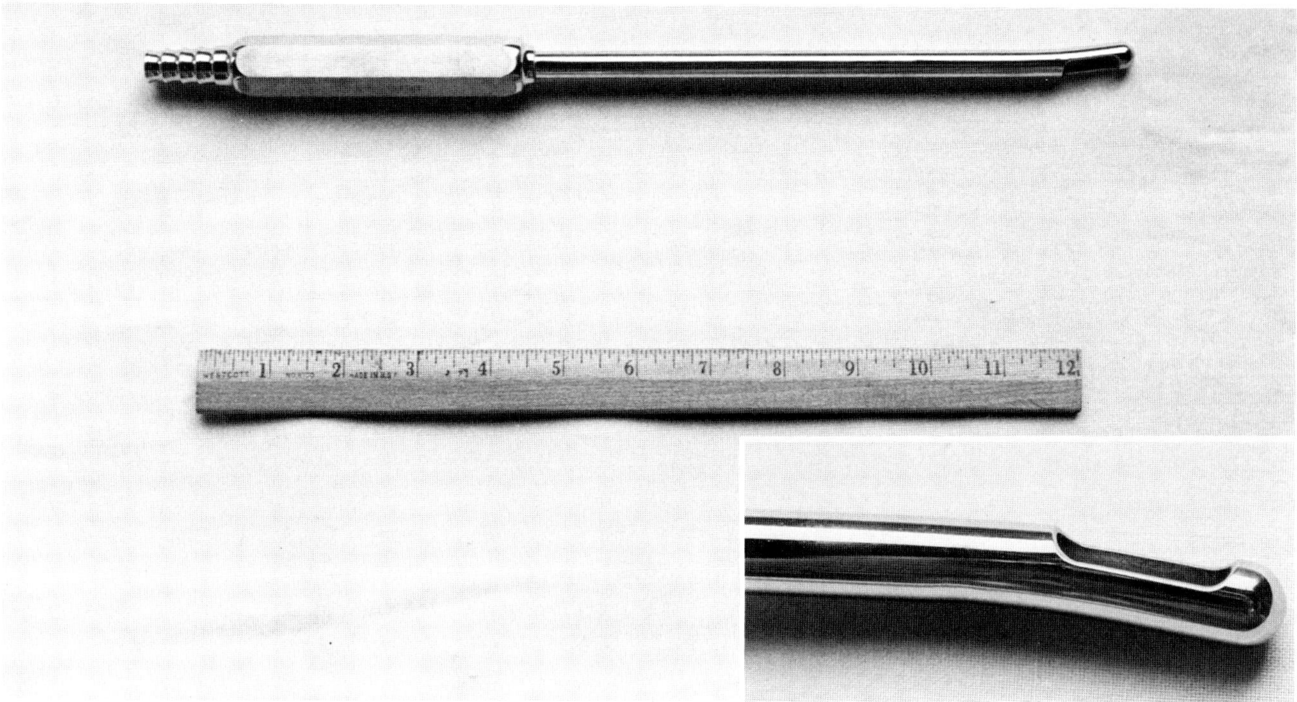

Fig. 16-12. Illouz blunt cannula. Groove on handle is same side as lumen. Inset shows blunt rounded lumen.

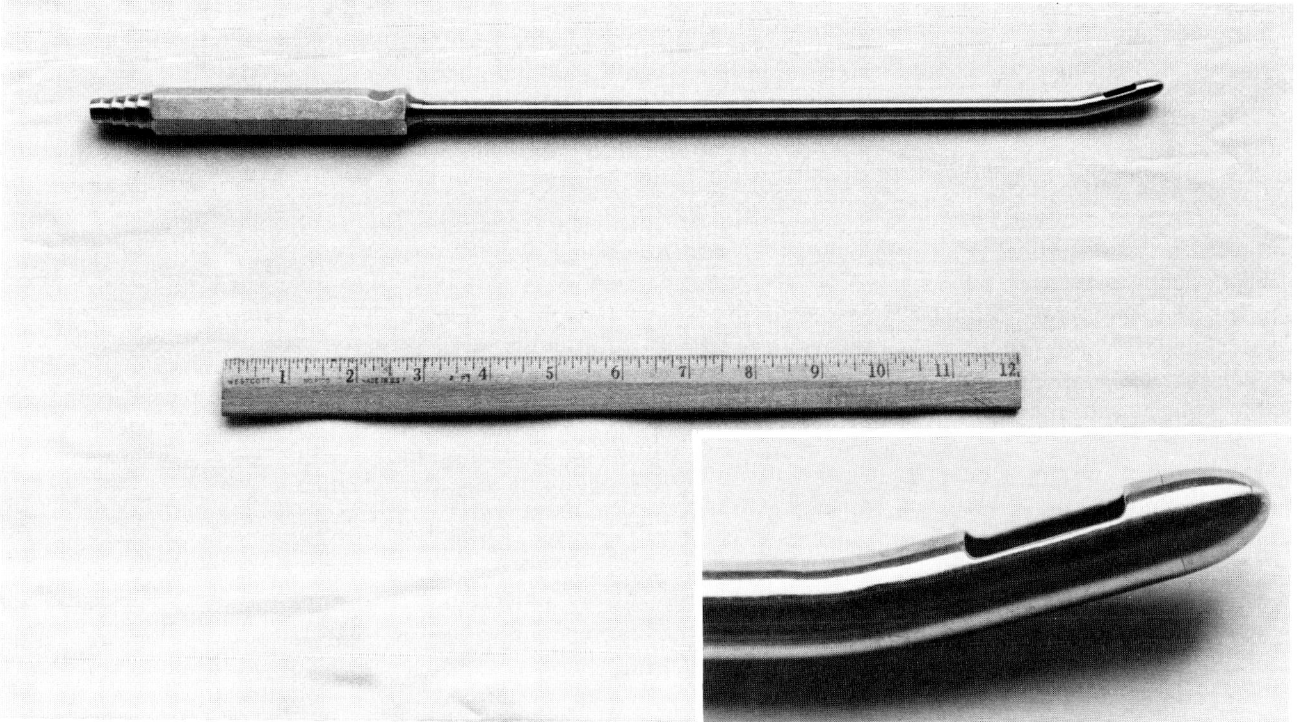

Fig. 16-13. Grazer-Grams version of Illouz cannula. Inset shows straight, fairly sharp edge instead of rounded opening.

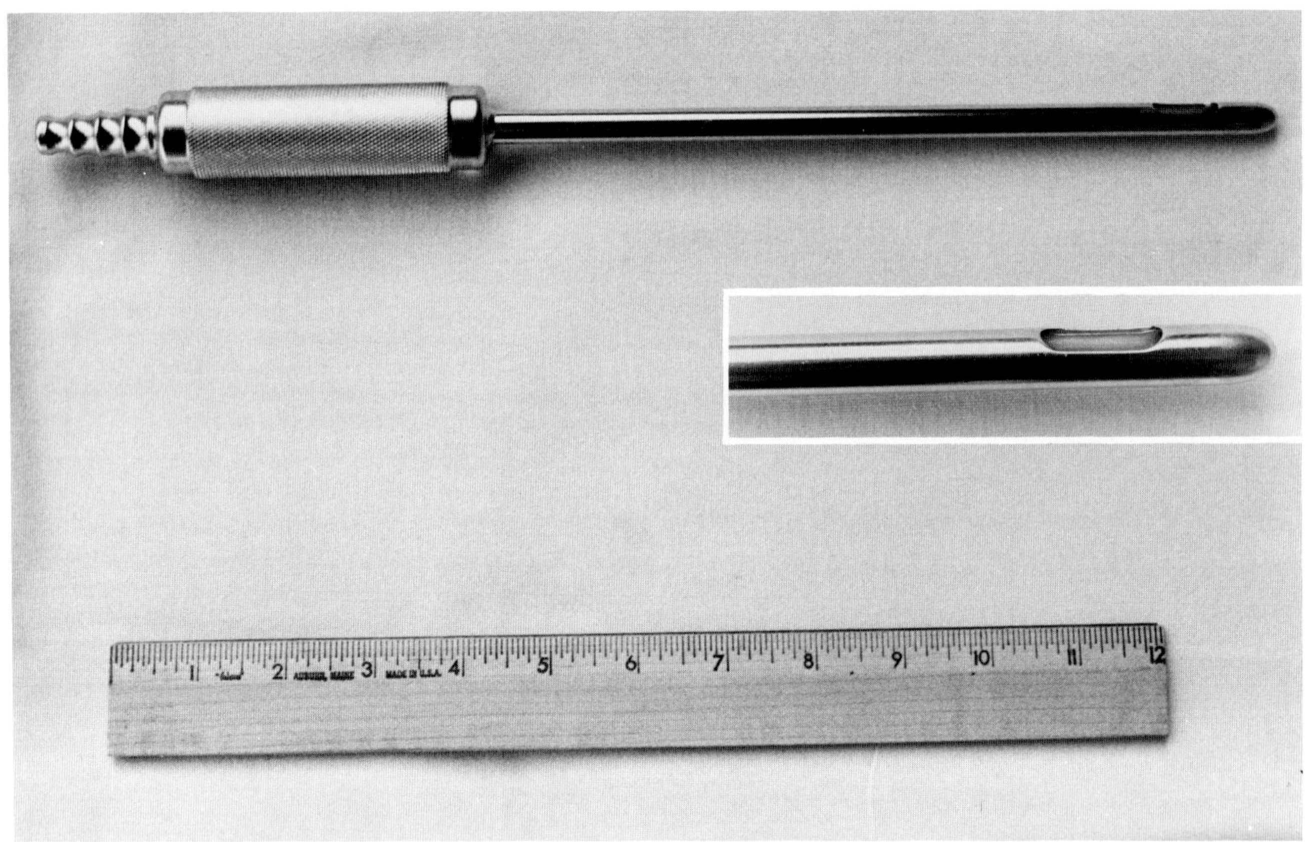

Fig. 16-14. Hetter-Padgett version of Illouz cannula with thumb stop opposite to opening. Inset shows rounded lumen at least 2.5 cm back from tip.

General Considerations

On the basis of experience, I believe the following observations are worth mentioning. The blunt tip tends not to enter the somewhat firmer subdermal fat unless forced. The more pointed the instrument, the more chance of tearing a furrow in the subdermal fat, piercing the skin and piercing the muscle fascia or abdomen.

The opening should be several centimeters behind the tip so that it does not suck away subdermal fat when pushed out against the skin on a curved surface, for example, the thigh (refer to Fig. 16-26).

The rounded opening lessens the chance of tearing the fascia and lessens the tearing of veins, arteries, nerves, and fibrous strands stretching from muscle fascia to skin.

Any surgeon who has used the instrument with the opening up has had the experience of having a chunk of subdermal fat sucked away, leaving a sudden dent or saucerized area. By using the instrument opening down, as suggested by Illouz, there is little chance of suctioning away a chunk of subdermal fat, causing an untreatable dent.

The smaller the diameter of the cannula that can reasonably be used, the more even the surface. As one progresses in the technique, one generally moves toward smaller diameter cannulas.

The shorter the shaft of the cannula, the better the surgeon's control of the instrument. Therefore, it is much better to make a second small incision to treat a far away area than to lose control of the tip of a very long cannula, especially in a nonforgiving area such as the abdomen.

Resistance

The resistance of any round tube or hose to flow is determined by the formula

$$R = r^4 (1) K$$

In this formula, "R" is the resistance, "r" is the radius of the tube, "l" is the length, and "K" is a factor. It is then obvious that the overriding function is the radius. The increasing resistance of the cannula as the diameter diminishes is readily seen in Table 16-3 (using outside dimension for simplicity sake).

These relationships help to understand the surgeon's relative time necessary to remove the same amount of fat with the different sized cannulas.

Although the relationship is certainly not exact, it

Table 16-3. Theoretical relationship between
the resistance of the cannula and its diameter

Cannula	Diameter	r^4	Resistance compared to #10 cannula
#10	1.0 cm	0.0625	1.00
# 8	0.8 cm	0.0256	2.44
# 6	0.6 cm	0.0081	7.71
# 4	0.4 cm	0.0016	39.10

probably takes about 2 or 3 times as long to remove the same amount of fat with a #8 cannula as with a #10 during the actual active part of the procedure. Since there are frequent rest periods and since less physical effort is required using smaller cannulas, the total elapsed time may not be greatly increased.

Cannulas for Specific Areas

THE CHIN, JOWL, AND CHEEK

A small #4 lightweight cannula used with a soft, flexible Silastic hose makes extraction of the submental, jowl, and preantral fat much easier than the usual #6 cannula (Fig. 16-15A and B).

THE ABDOMEN

A short #6, #8, and #10 are useful here (Fig. 16-16A and B). Control is better with short cannulas. The reach of the cannula through a periumbilical incision is excellent (Fig. 16-17). The #6 can be used through a small suprapubic incision to clear the periumbilical fat and the fat between the paramedian vessels (and less chance of vessel injury) (see Fig. 16-16A).

The #6 and #8 pass into the more fibrous epigastric fat with greater ease than the #10, which is ideal for the softer hypogastric fat (Fig. 16-17).

THE FLANK

The long curved #10 is useful to reach the flank excess in the male or female if it is confluent with the hypogastric fat (Fig. 16-18).

THE ILIAC CREST

The short #8 and short #10 passed through a direct posterior or gluteal region incisions allow excellent control and rapid defatting (Figs. 16-19 and 16-20).

THE THIGH

Here the #8 or #10 regular is the workhorse (Fig. 16-21), but to reach and feather the edges, especially in the big patient, the long #8 downcurve is useful (Fig. 16-22). This feathering and loosening of the edges allows for a smoother transition between the untouched and heavily defatted areas.

Fournier uses a rod to "mesh undermine" the edges

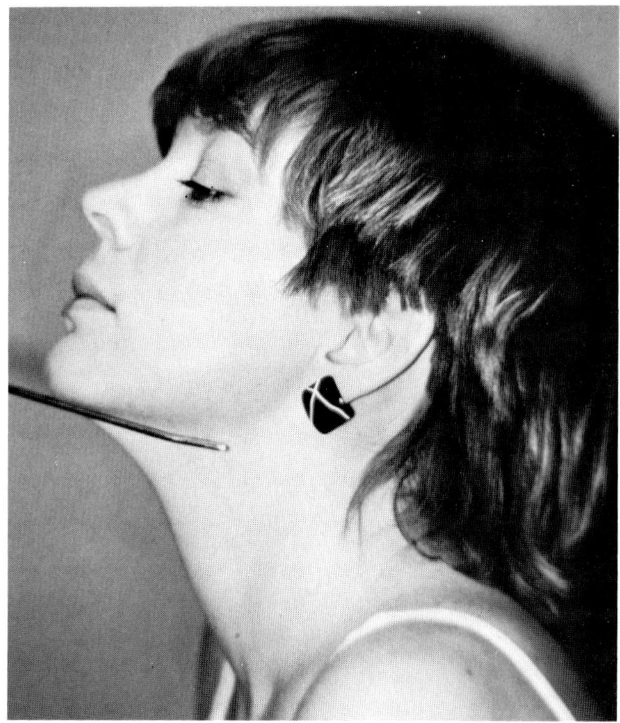

A

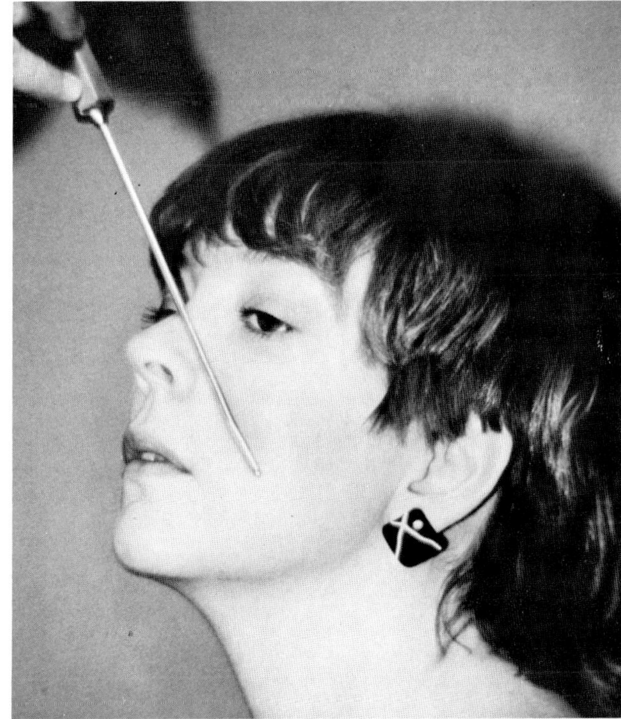

B

Fig. 16-15.
A. A #4 cannula demonstrated on a model for removal of submandibular-submental fat.
B. A #4 demonstrated on a model for removal of preantral fat.

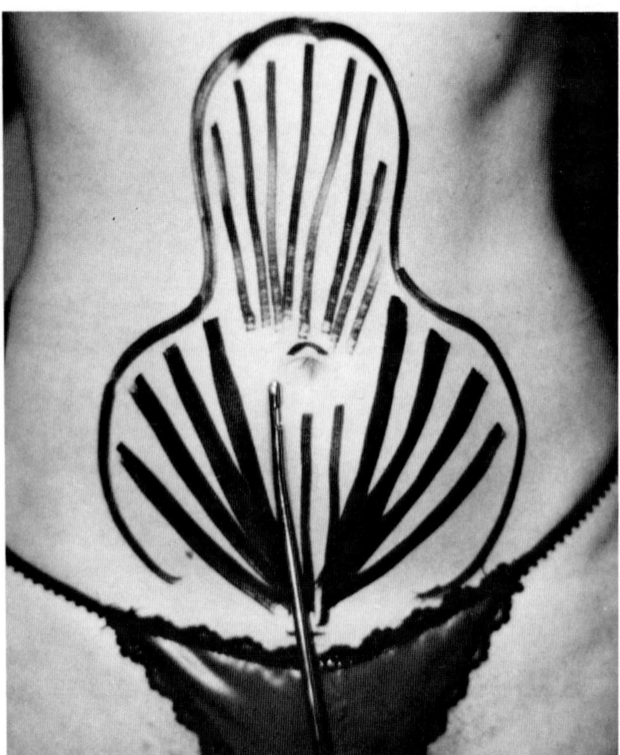

A

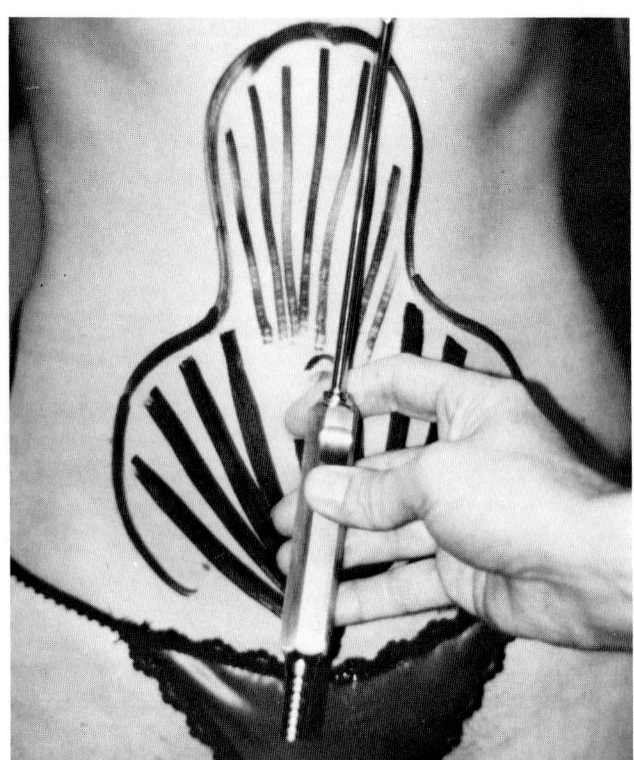

Fig. 16-17. The epigastrium is more fibrous and a #6 is more easily pushed through this area through a periumbilical incision.

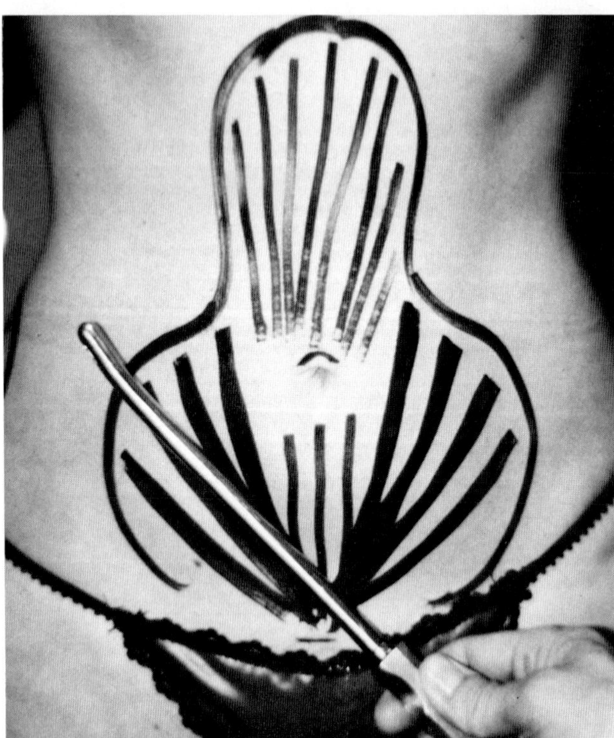

B

Fig. 16-16.
A. A #6 short Illouz cannula is useful for the epigastric extraction through a periumbilical incision.
B. A #10 Illouz cannula is used for heavy hypogastric extractions.

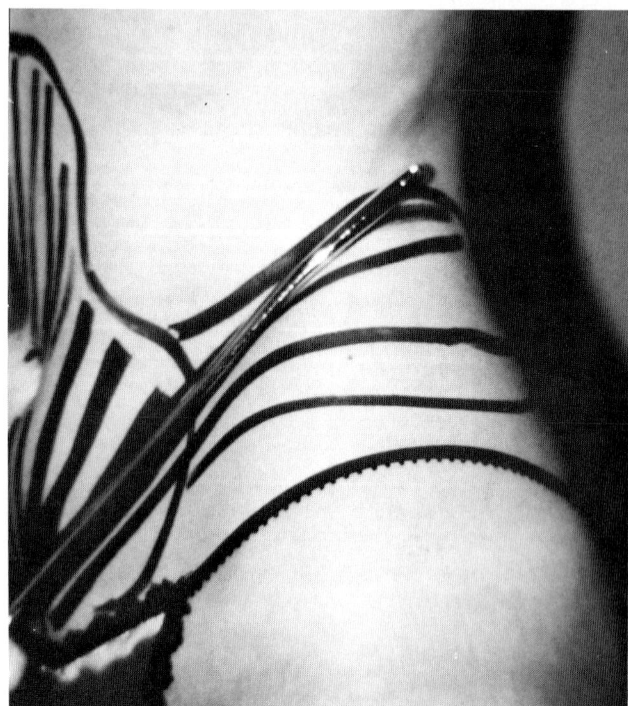

Fig. 16-18. A #10 Concorde-style Hetter-Padgett cannula reaches the iliac crest or flank fat through an escutcheon or periumbilical incision.

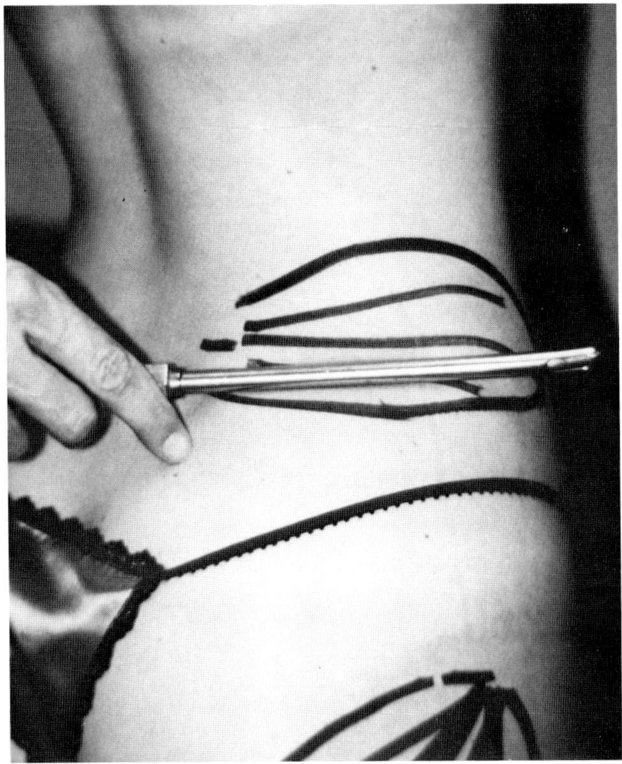

Fig. 16-19. A direct approach to the iliac crest with short cannula is shown.

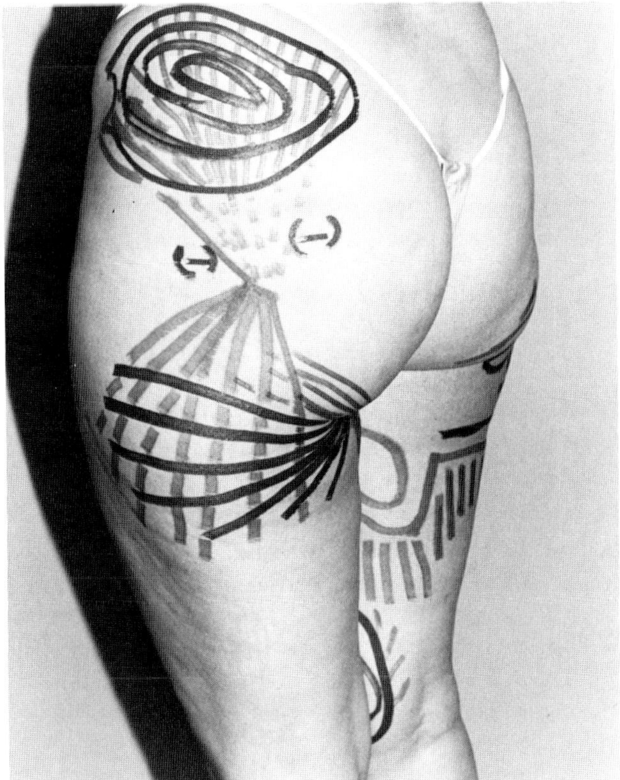

Fig. 16-20. A lateral buttock incision is hidden by bathing attire and also allows access to the lateral thigh.

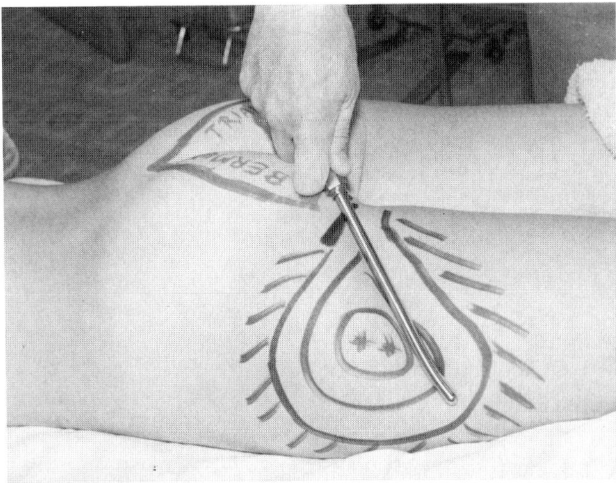

Fig. 16-21. A #10 regular reaches almost to the periphery but easily reaches the major deposit.

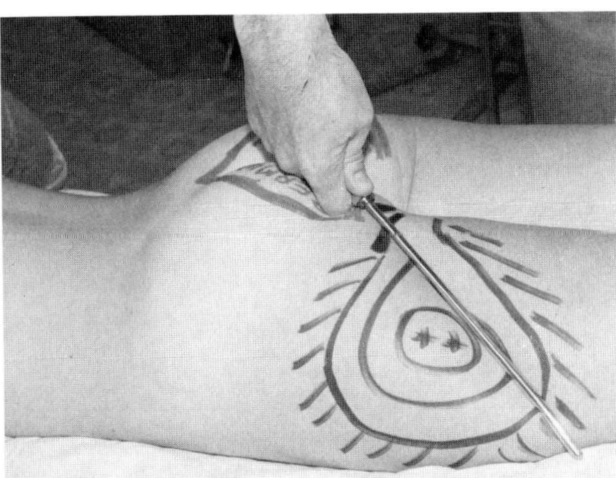

Fig. 16-22. A #8 down curve reaches beyond the periphery and into the crosshatched area to "mesh undermine."

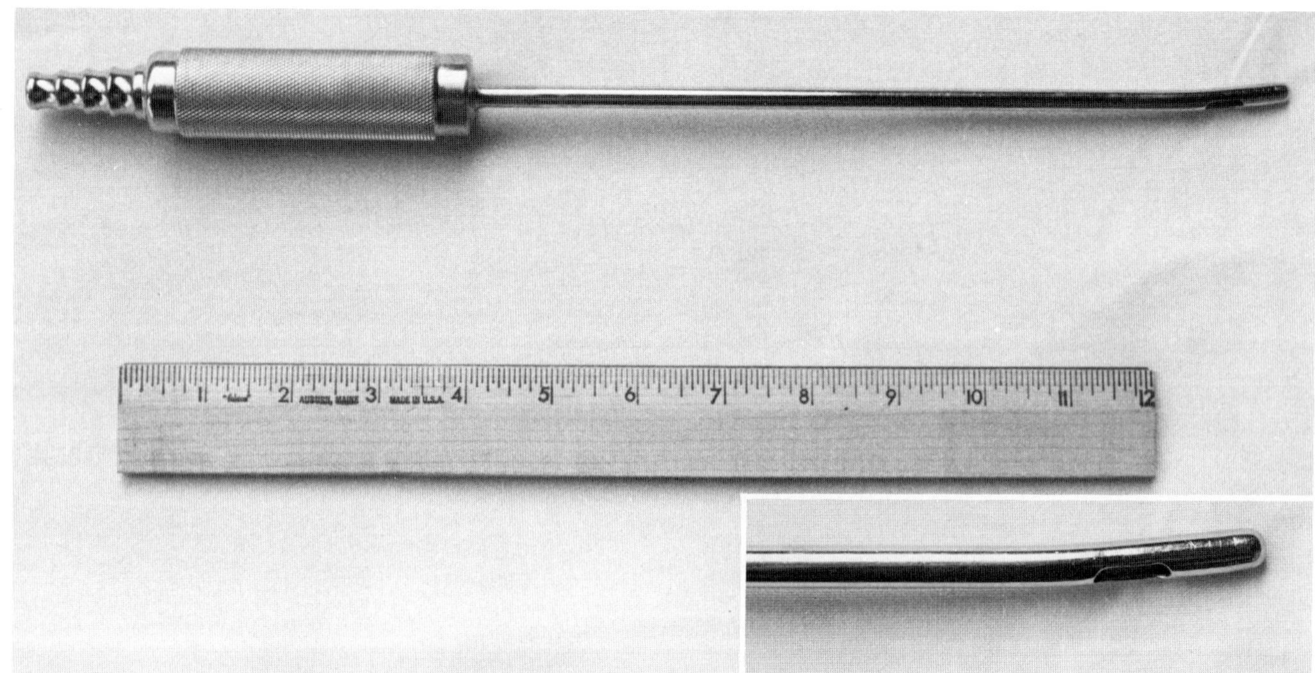

Fig. 16-23. The Padgett #7 long cannula with upturning tip.

without extracting fat. The long #8 without suction will serve the same purpose.

For subtle infragluteal contouring, the short #6 is highly useful in preventing massive extraction toward the end of the case.

The long #7 by Padgett with an opening 1 inch behind the tip allows adequate reach from the ankle to the whole posterior calf or from the olecranon to the whole posterior brachial area (Figs. 16-23, 16-24, and 16-25). The diameter lessens the risk of overextraction and the 1-inch extension prevents subdermal extraction (Fig. 16-26) and feathers the edges.

The total number of cannulas as a basic setup to perform competent lipolysis procedures are (1) 3 to 4 mm for head and neck procedures, (2) 5 to 6 mm short and long for knees, calves, and arms, and (3) 8 mm short and long for abdomen, thighs, iliac crest, and pectoral area (Fig. 16-27). These five cannulas certainly provide enough versatility to do all the usual procedures.

The cannulas are commercially available in Europe, Canada, South America, and Asia from Medicalex, 39 Rue Croulebarbe, 75013, Paris, France.

American-made cannulas are available through Padgett Instruments, 2838 Warwick Twy., Kansas City, MO 64108.

Other instrument makers may have models available from time to time. A fine instrument should be made of very high-grade stainless steel, which is expensive to

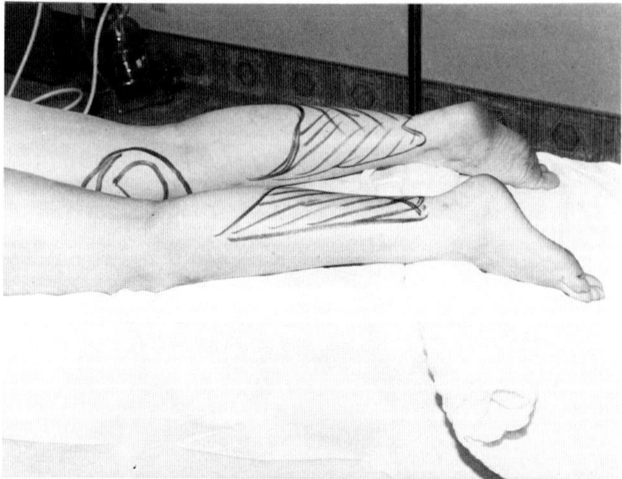

Fig. 16-24. Ankles and calves marked for extraction.

machine; #304 stainless is desirable. If softer steel is used, it will pit and stain during autoclaving. Ask the manufacturer before purchase. Beware of plastic, brass, or aluminum cannulas unless a written replacement warranty is provided and a certification of product liability insurance is provided.

THE PUMP

The pressures necessary for the original Illouz technique have been discussed. It requires vaporization of

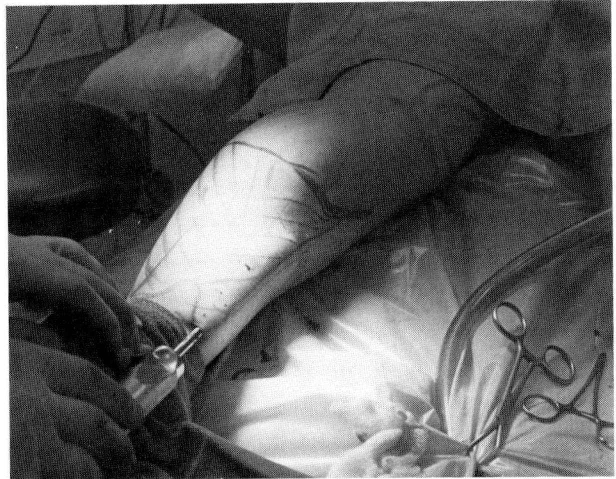

Fig. 16-25. Cannula tenting up skin of lower calf.

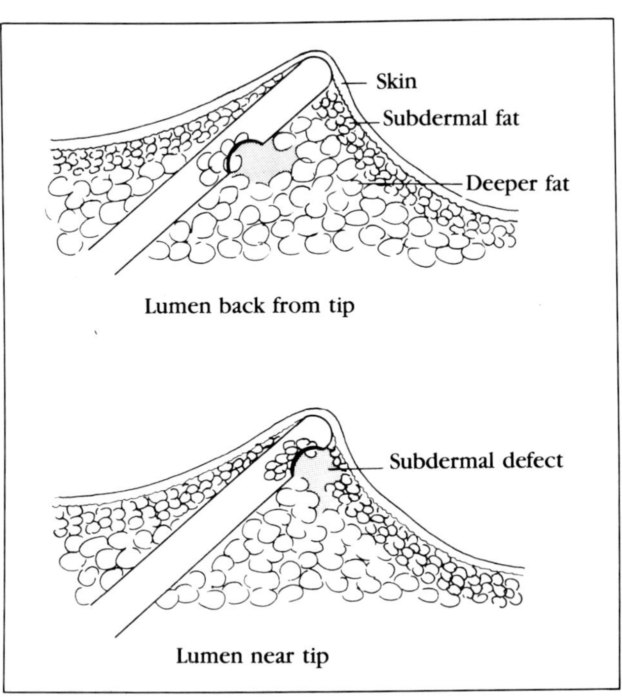

Fig. 16-26. Diagram shows how lumen too close to opening risks extraction of subdermal fat.

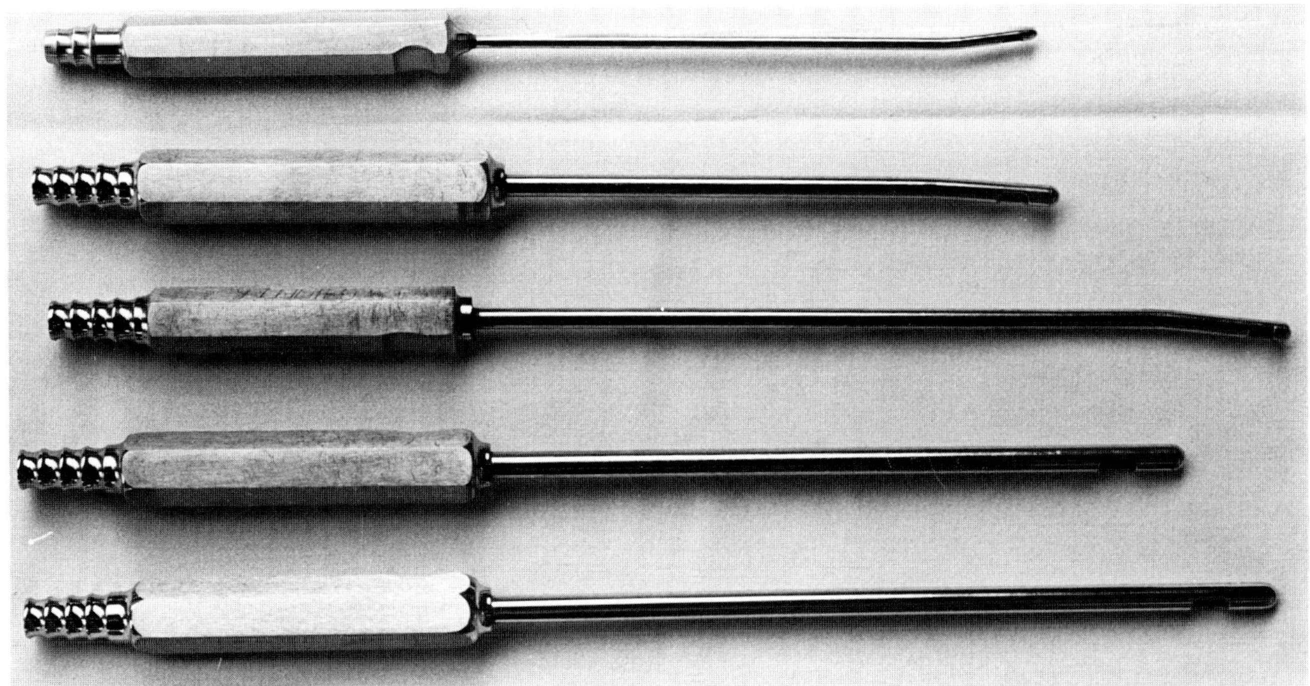

Fig. 16-27. Set of Illouz-type cannulas sufficient for facial and body contour procedures.

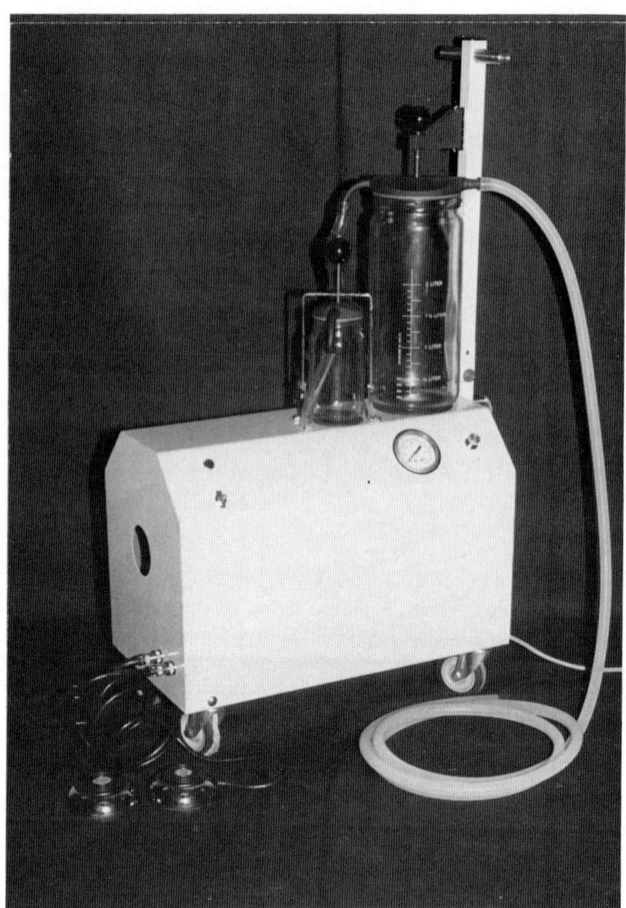

Fig. 16-28. High-vacuum machine (Power Source PS-1) used for suction lipectomy.

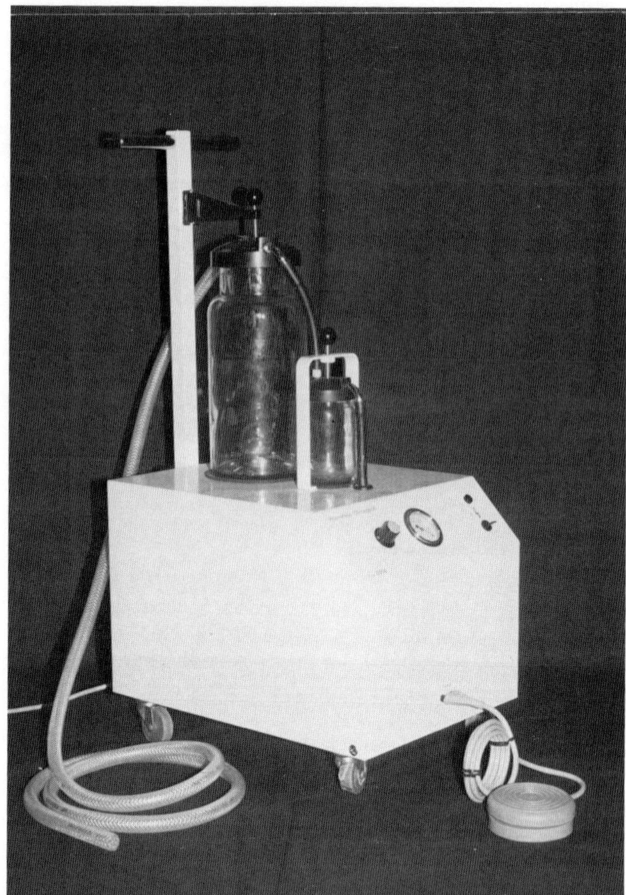

Fig. 16-29. Original suction pump manufactured in France for Dr. Illouz.

tissue fluids at or near room temperature. This process requires a vacuum pump producing 20 torr or less.

With a 3- or 4-liter collection bottle, a pump must exhaust the air quickly to raise the vacuum to the working level. It has been found that pumps providing in excess of 50 L per minute air movement work adequately, and 100 L per minute work well.

Vacuum pumps fall into two main categories: reciprocating and rotary. The reciprocating pumps can be subdivided into piston pumps and membrane pumps. Neither approach absolute vacuum but both will come close to 25 torr—at least while new.

The most common vacuum pump in hospitals today is the Berkeley pump used for terminating pregnancy and manufactured by Cabot Medical. This is a membrane pump of good quality and reliability. Recent models all produce about 30 torr (or 30 mm Hg less than absolute vacuum). This pump is sufficient to perform blunt suction lipectomy in the Illouz manner and more than sufficient for those other techniques that have air leak or use air leak cannulas. Most so-called portable machines will be membrane pumps since they have no oil reser-

voir to spill, are light in weight but cannot produce very high vacuum, and are noisy. A number of small manufacturers have turned out shoddy products in this category in a rush to saturate the suction lipectomy market. A Berkeley pump is still the best buy in this type of pump. Cabot Medical has a good record for reliable machines, has single-use plastic accessories available, and has been in business many years.

The very high vacuum machines are rotary vane pumps with two or more stages. There is no need for more than two stages to produce 5 torr or less. These machines require close tolerances and must be oil lubricated. The exhaust therefore contains oil particles which require a filter to remove the oil. These filters may be retrofitted to a pump, as on the Grazer-Grams machine, or may be a built-in filter that traps the oil and recirculates it back to the oil reservoir (Power Source PS-1, Fig. 16-28). This machine has a high air flow (100 L per minute) and is very quiet in the operating room. Such machines provide close to absolute vacuum.

The original pump manufactured for Illouz (Fig. 16-29) by Medicalex SA France was a single-stage rotary vane pump and has been used all over the world by Illouz's trained surgeons. It produces about 25 torr, has a high air flow (approximately 100 L per minute), and is easy to use. It has been reliable but is noisy due to power transfer from motor to pump via a belt drive. It has been retrofitted with an oil filter because of American objection to the fumes.

The characteristics to look for in the choice of a suction machine are as follows:

1. Reputation of the distributor or manufacturer in the plastic surgery field
2. Availability of service arrangements for the power train (i.e., motor and pump)
3. Suction pressure = 20 torr or lower
4. Free air flow of approximately 100 L per minute
5. Noise level of <60 DBA as measured in a standard operating room
6. Mobility in the operating room
7. Ease of cleaning (wide-necked jars)
8. Availability of single-use supplies, including collection jars and tubing

Discuss each of these requirements with the salesperson. Obtain written verification about each characteristic. A good quality pump should last a surgeon's working lifetime. It is a good idea, however, to have a second unit available should a mechanical or electrical failure occur in the midst of an operative procedure.

References

1. Illouz, Y. G. Communication à la Société Français de Chirurgie Esthetique, Juin 1978 et 1979.
2. Illouz, Y. G. Une nouvelle technique pour les lipodystrophies localisées. *Rev. Chir. Esthet. Lang. Fr.* 4:19, 1980.
3. Illouz, Y. G. Réflexions apres quatre ans et demi d'experience et 800 cas de ma technique de lipolyse. *Rev. Chir. Esthet. Lang. Fr.* 6:27, 1981.
4. Illouz, Y. G. Body contouring by lipolysis: A 5-year experience with over 3000 cases. *Plast. Reconstr. Surg.* 72:591, 1984.
5. Hetter, G. P. Experience with "lipolysis": The Illouz technique of blunt suction lipectomy in North America. *Aesth. Plast. Surg.* 7:69, 1983.
6. Kesselring, U. K. Regional fat aspiration for body contouring. *Plast. Reconstr. Surg.* 11:610, 1983.
7. Courtiss, E. Videotape presentation at the American Society for Aesthetic Plastic Surgery Annual Meeting. Century City, Calif. April 1983.
8. Teimourian, B., Adham, M., Gulin, S., and Shapiro, C. Suction lipectomy: A review of 200 patients over a six-year period and a study of the technique in cadavers. *Ann. Plast. Surg.* 11:93, 1983.
9. Chajchir, A. Suction curettage lipectomy. *Aesth. Plast. Surg.* 7:195, 1983.
10. Hetter, G. Optimum vacuum pressures for lipolysis. *Aesth. Plast. Surg.* 8:1, 1983.
11. Kesselring, U. K. Suction curette for removal of subcutaneous fat. (Letter to the editor.) *Plast. Reconstr. Surg.* 63:560, 1979.
12. Teimourian, B., and Fisher, J. B. Suction curettage to remove excess fat for body contouring. *Plast. Reconstr. Surg.* 68:50, 1981.

CHAPTER 17

Surgical Technique

Gregory P. Hetter

The goal of the lipolysis technique is to bring unaesthetic localized fatty bulges into a more harmonious relationship with the surrounding areas. Treatment is therefore directed at areas that have an excess of fat in relation to their surroundings. The evaluation of the thickness of each area is carried out at the preoperative examination. Then a diagnosis and a treatment plan is established, discussed, and agreed on by the patient, as discussed in Chapters 12 and 13.

Preoperative Preparation

MARKING THE PATIENT

The markings are done the day before or the day of surgery with a broad, felt-tipped indelible marking pen such as El Marko (a Flair product). I mark the patient immediately before going to the operating room in my own ambulatory plastic surgery facility.

Photographs with the markings in place may be valuable in defusing a later dispute about what was planned and agreed on. If so, the markings should be the actual operative markings, not markings at the time of consultation. I recommend a series of photographs as outlined in Chapter 10 on photographic documentation. Documentation of the operative markings may be taken in the operating room or in the "holding area" with a Polaroid camera (if done in a hospital setting where the photo-room is not adjacent).

The patient's fatty deposits should be evaluated by both sight and touch in the standing position before marking. Turning the patient slowly in side lighting and in light from above will reveal areas of irregularity, high spots, waviness, and depressions. These areas should be marked and pointed out to the patient.

The area of greatest deformity is marked in a topographic fashion like a military map. The surgeon should decide (1) where to use the largest bore cannula and place " + " marks here, (2) where to switch to the smaller one, and (3) where to merely mesh undermine (Figure 17-1).

Occasional dells or valleys should be noted with " − " signs and should be avoided in order to avoid worsening such areas. When on the operating room table, such an area may no longer appear as a depression due to shifting of the fat. Such notations are seen in Figure 17-2.

THE PINCH TEST

Before completing the marking, an appraisal of surrounding subcutaneous thickness should be made by pinching the tissues. On the lateral thigh usually 3 to 4 cm can be pinched above and below a "saddlebag." The

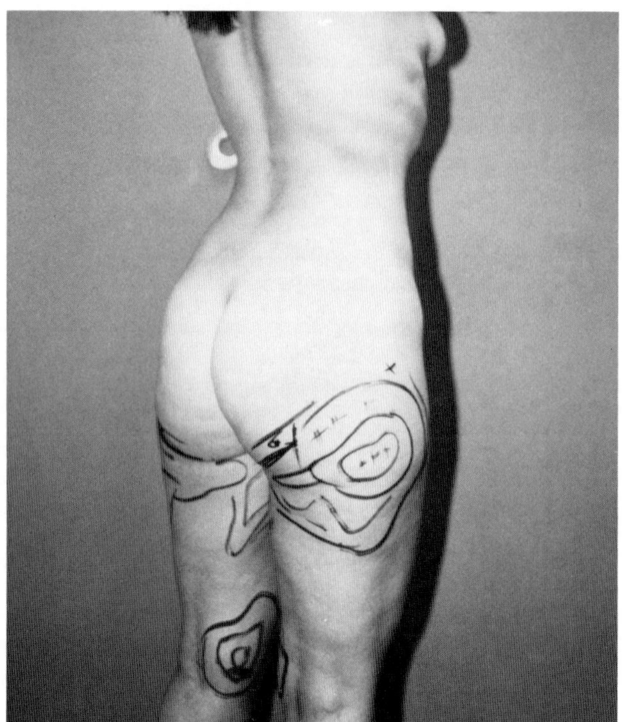

Fig. 17-1. Markings of lateral thigh area showing high areas and concentric rings of lesser thickness.

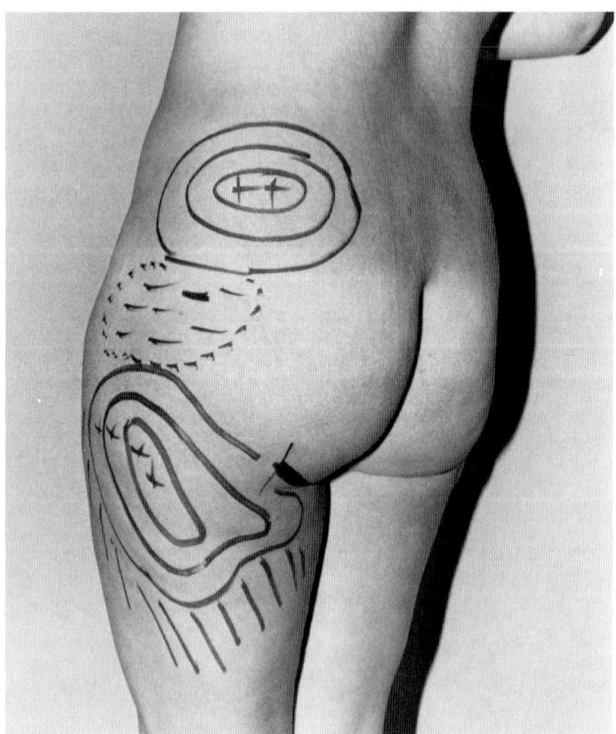

Fig. 17-2. Declivities are marked with a (−) to indicate avoidance of these areas. When on the operating room table, this area may not be visible in the horizontal position.

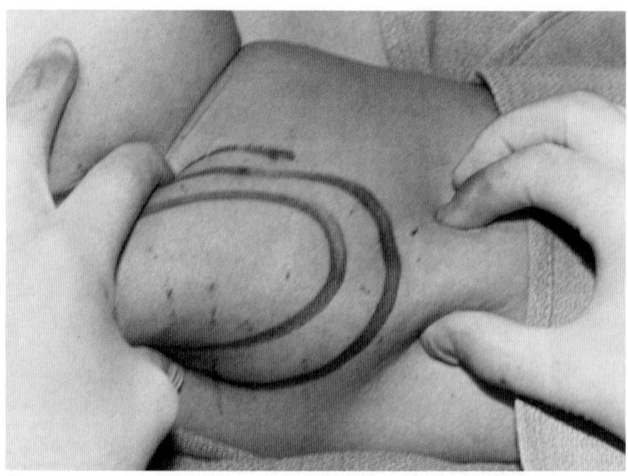

A

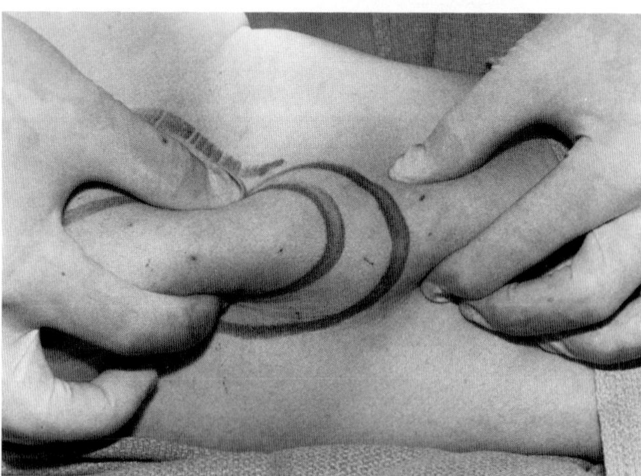

B

Fig. 17-3.
A. Photograph of lateral thigh illustrates a 6- to 7-cm thickness of fat but only 3 cm below the affected area.
B. After fat extraction. Both areas are now similar in thickness.

localized fatty deposit, however, may range from 5 to 8 cm in most patients. The extraction process reduces this to the surrounding 3- to 4-cm thickness (Fig. 17-3A,B).

For the initial defatting, the largest cannula is used in the major areas of concern, followed by the next smaller size for the periphery (Fig. 17-4). Lastly, a small, long cannula without suction or a Fournier solid rod is used to break up the peripheral edge to allow the tissues to redrape at the margin (Fig. 17-5).

When finished, the tissues should be fairly consistent from untreated to treated areas. Any residual thick islands are treated with a small bore cannula to even them out.

Examples of marking are shown for various areas to illustrate the information gained. Once the patient is in a recumbent position all topography changes completely, and therefore no further changes should be made (Figs. 17-6 to 17-10).

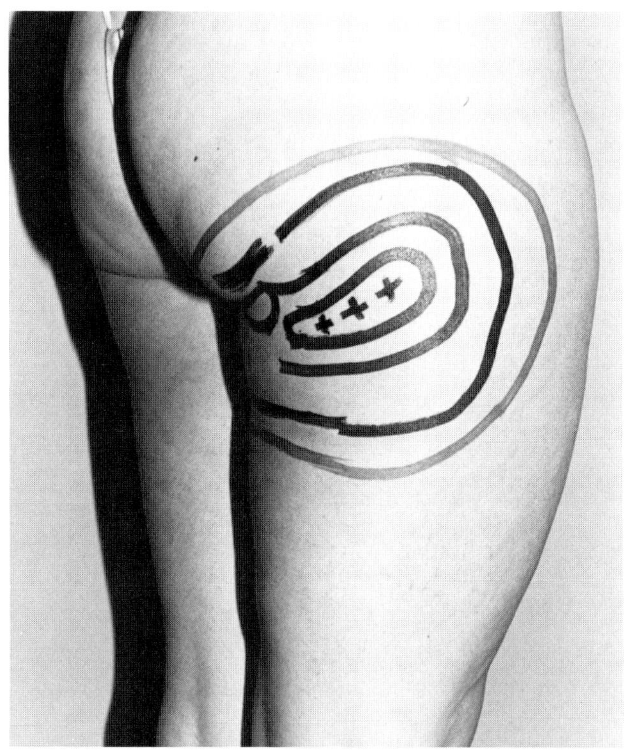

Fig. 17-4. The central rings are treated with the #8 cannula, the outer ring with the long #6.

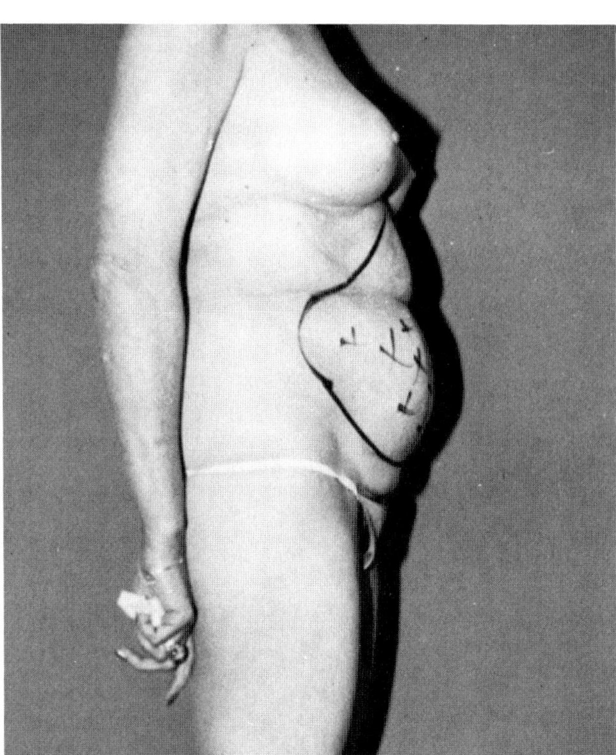

Fig. 17-6. Abdominal markings in a 64-year-old female with extensions toward flanks and upper abdomen; 950 ml was extracted.

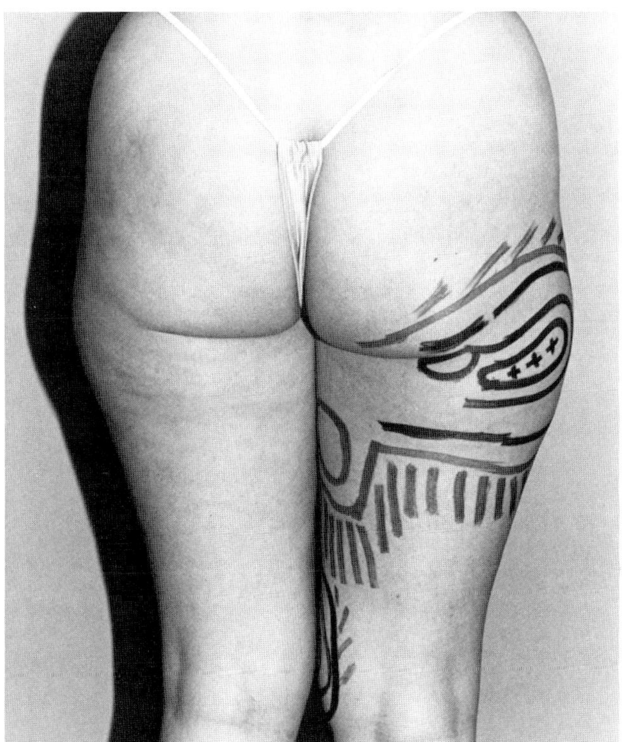

Fig. 17-5. Mesh undermining is carried out in the cross-hatched area to finish the procedure after extraction is complete.

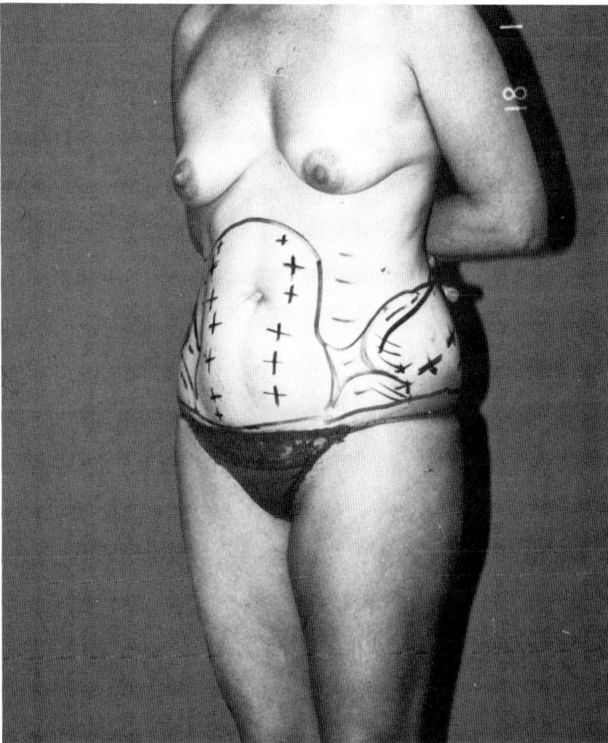

Fig. 17-7. Abdominal markings in a 42-year-old female confluent with marked iliac crest rolls; 1200 ml was extracted. Note (−) areas marked where fat is very thin.

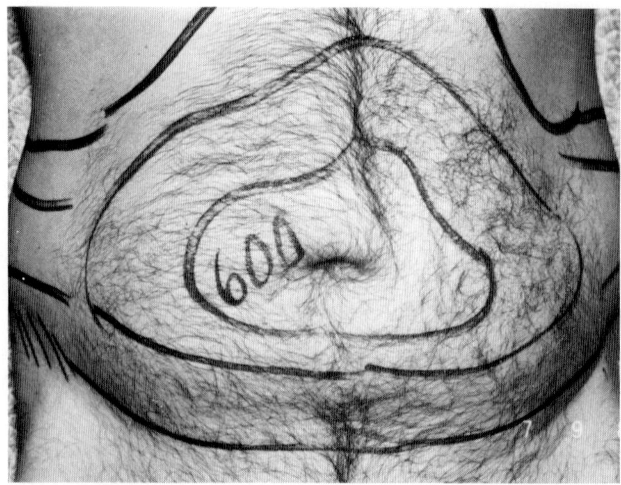

A

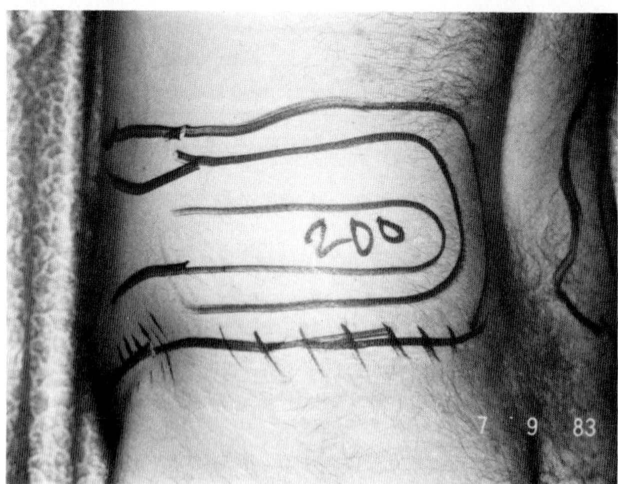

B

Fig. 17-8.
A. Abdominal markings in a 34-year-old male. Preoperative estimate was 600 ml, but close to 950 ml was removed.
B. Significant flank extensions ("love handles") estimated accurately at 200 ml per side.

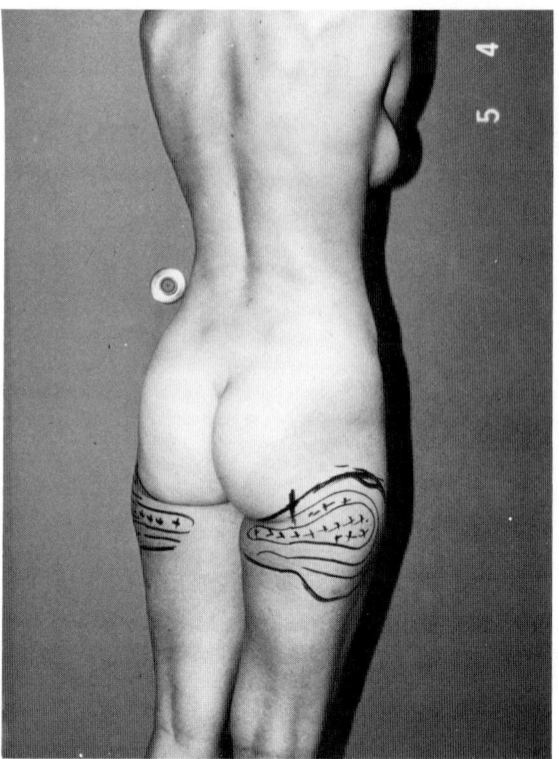

Fig. 17-9. Lateral thigh markings in a 27-year-old female; 475 ml was extracted.

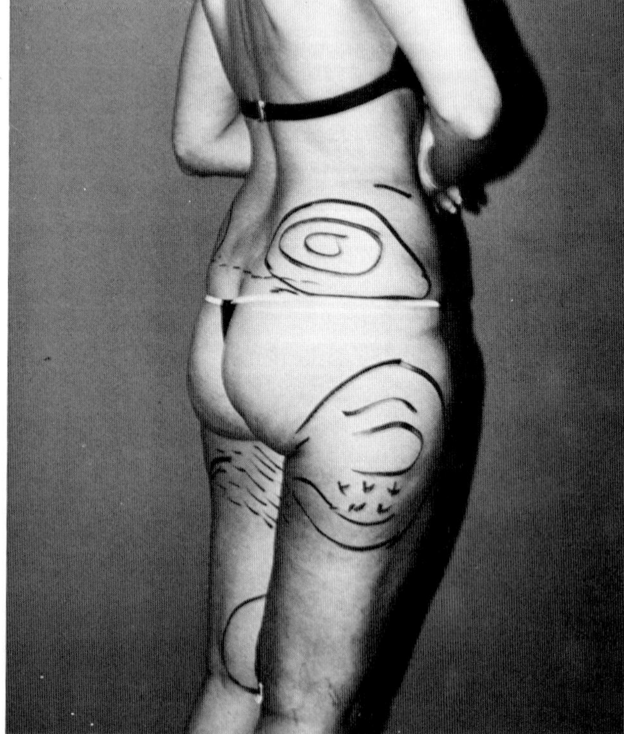

Fig. 17-10. Markings for a violin deformity of a 33-year-old female involving iliac crest and lateral thigh; 1000 ml was extracted.

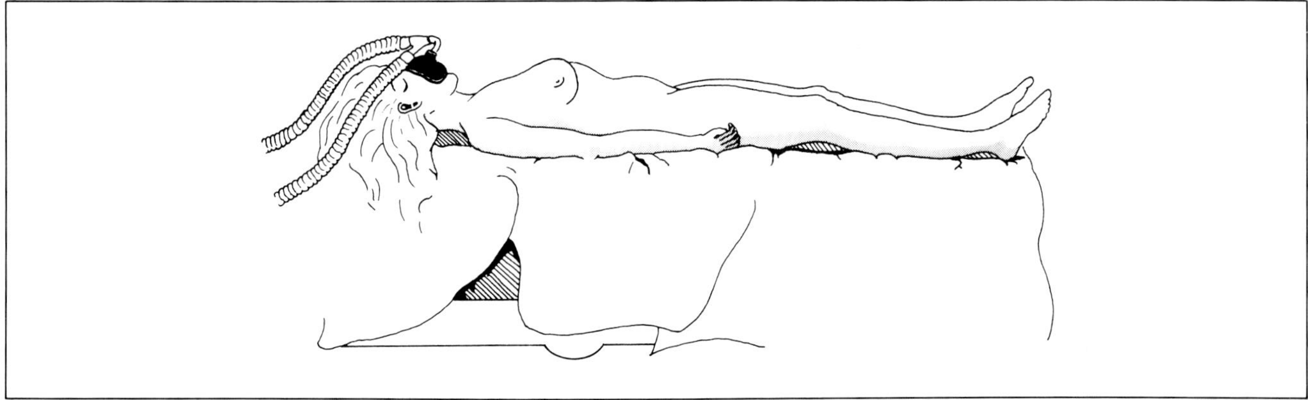

Fig. 17-11. Mask anesthesia in supine position for anterior torso procedure including pectoral area, abdomen, flanks, anterior and medial thighs, and anterior knees.

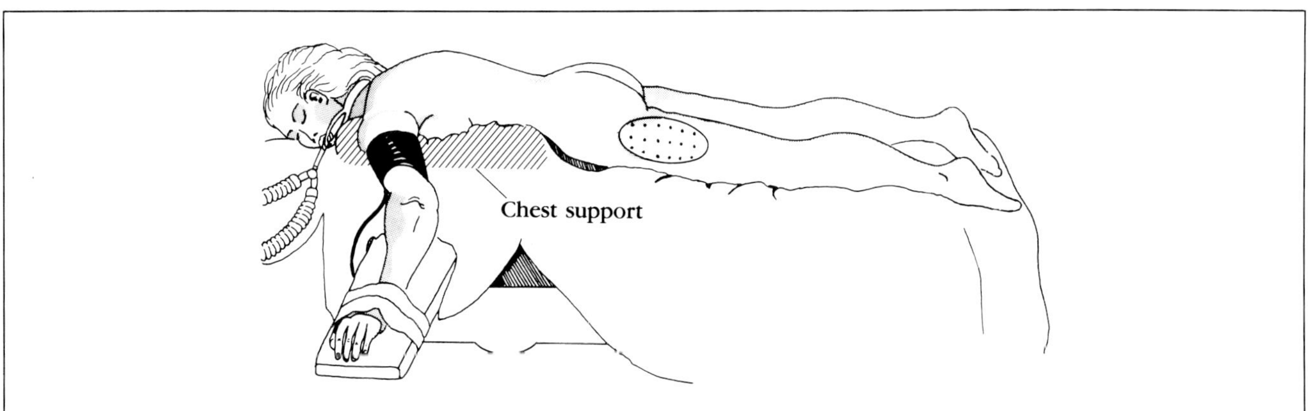

Fig. 17-12. Intubation in prone position for posterior torso procedures including iliac crest, lateral, posterior, and medial thighs, medial knees, and calves.

ANESTHESIA AND POSITION

For body contour procedures of any magnitude, general anesthesia is recommended. For anterior torso procedures, the supine position and mask anesthesia is common (Fig. 17-11). For posterior torso procedures, intubation and prone positioning is the most common (Fig. 17-12). To change or create a gluteal fold this is far and away the best position. It allows immediate comparison of the two sides for this as well as all posterior procedures. The patient is anesthetized and intubated on the transport stretcher (Fig. 17-13) and turned prone onto the operating room table. Supports are used on either side of the chest to allow good excursion of the chest (Fig. 17-14). Extubation occurs after returning the patient to the transport stretcher in the supine position. Since these maneuvers require intubation plus four persons to turn the patient, this may present a staffing problem in some situations. If so, an alternative method of keeping the patient in the supine position for posterior torso procedures is presented in Chapter 18.

PREPPING THE PATIENT

Patients are advised to shower and shampoo daily for the week before the surgery with whatever products they normally use. For the actual preparation of the patient, any of the usual solutions, if colored, are adequate. Betadine is difficult to remove from the creases and crevices and may cause occasional reactions with exfoliation. For that reason, I prefer Hibitane Tincture, a pink alcohol-based solution that evaporates quickly to leave a dry, clean surface. The solution is painted on, with no attempt to scrub the patient. None of my patients has had an infection since I began performing lipolysis in 1982. This product may be removed from the market because of slow sales; any prepping solution for surgical procedures is adequate.

HEAT LOSS AND DRAPING

For torso procedures patients have large surface areas exposed and may lose heat rapidly. To reduce this heat loss, the following steps are taken. The operating rooms are maintained at 24° to 26°C for these procedures. I have installed a 3-inch thick sponge plastic "eggcrate"

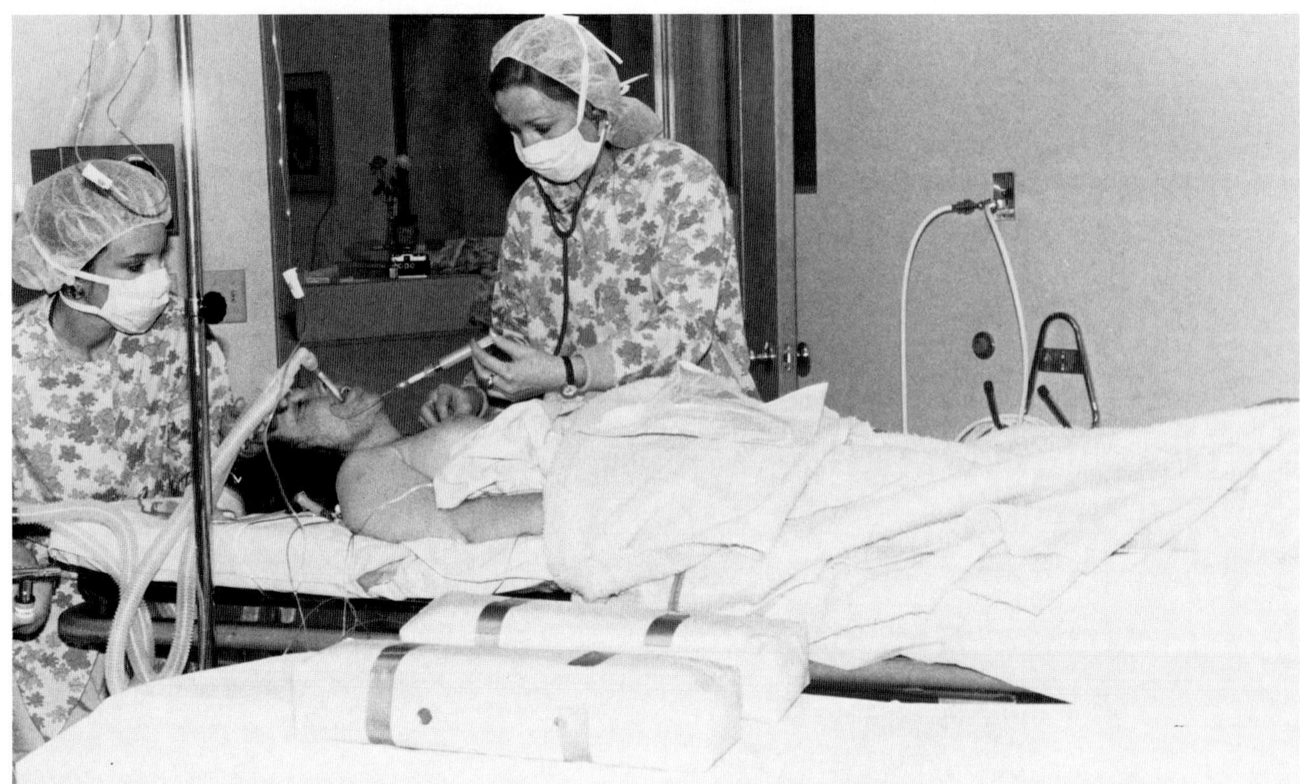

Fig. 17-13. Anesthesia is induced on the transport stretcher. Note supports on operating room table for shoulders and lateral chest.

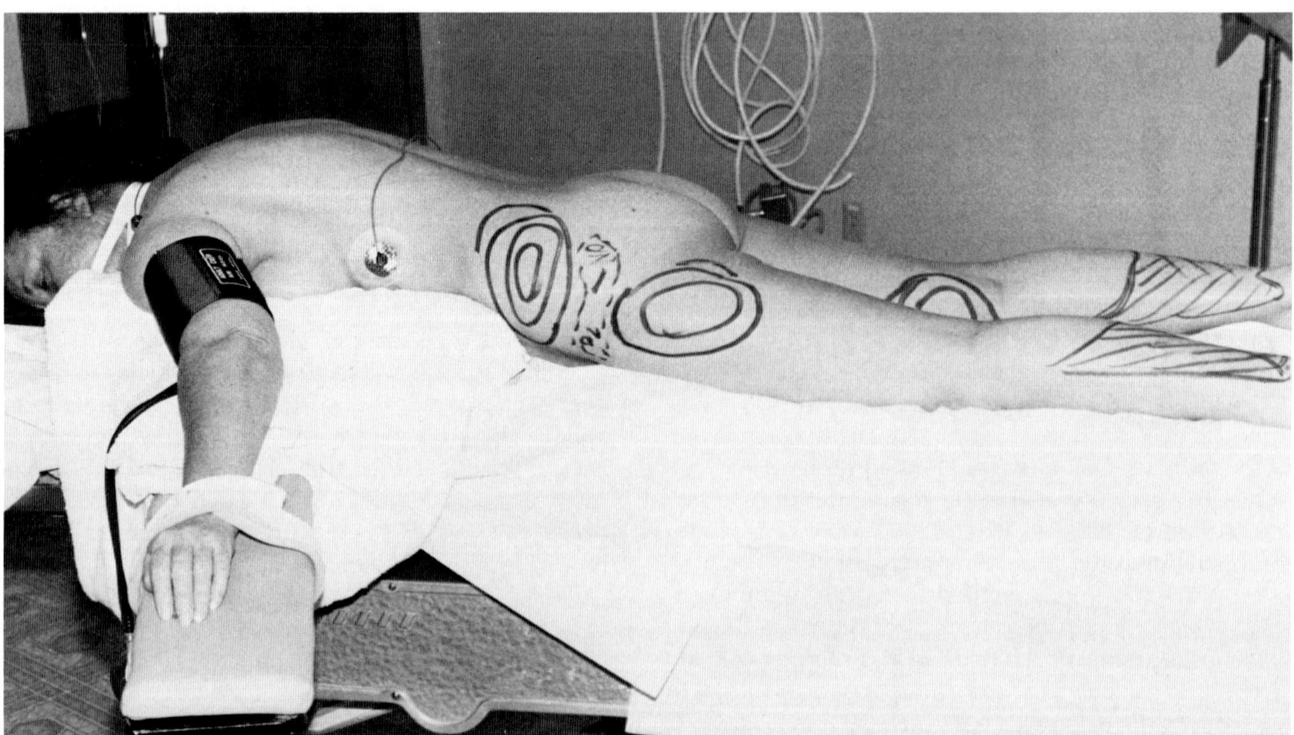

Fig. 17-14. The patient is turned from the stretcher into the prone position with shoulders and sides of chest supported by cushions to allow for thoracic excursion.

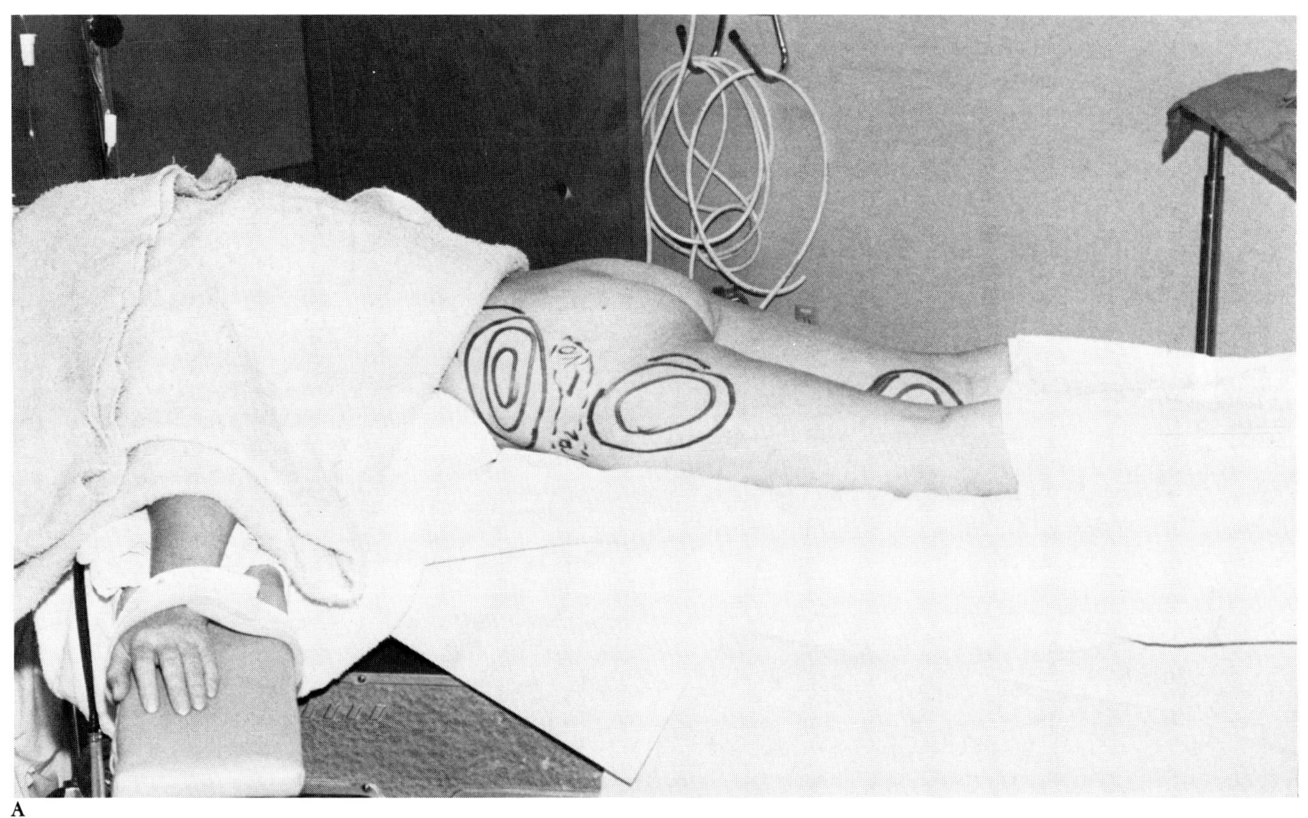

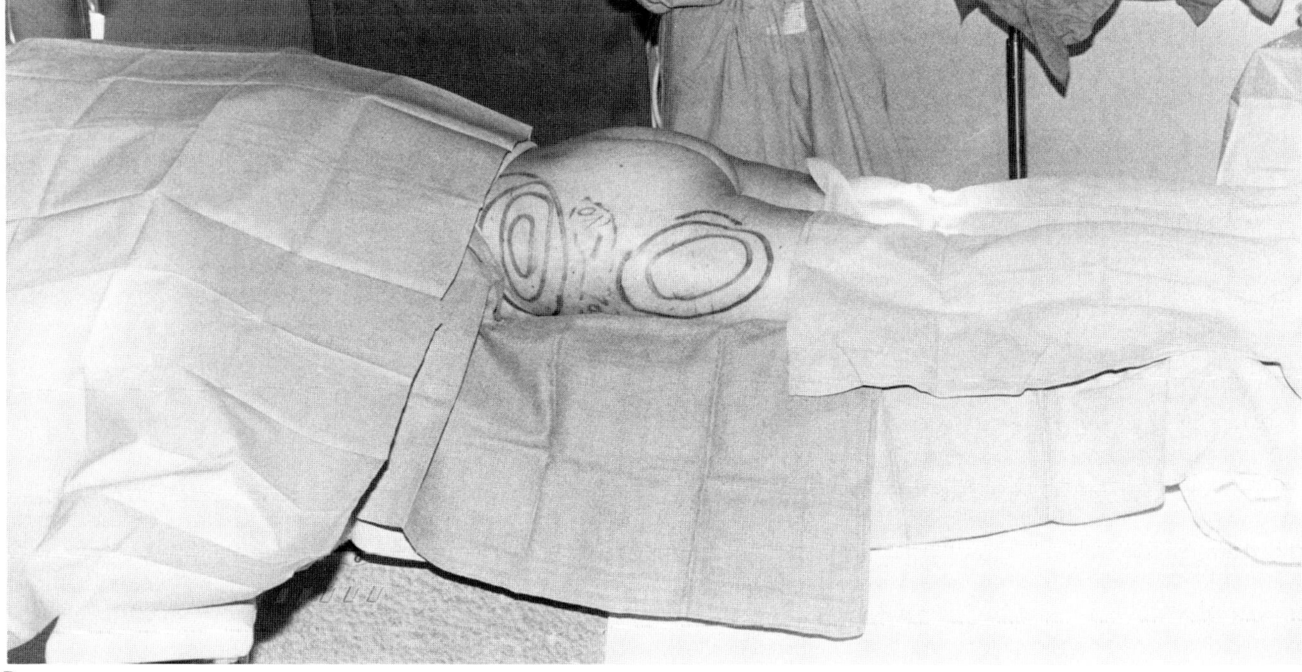

Fig. 17-15
A. Note blankets and towels supporting arms and covering
   all areas not in operative field.
B. Patient draped for posterior torso procedure.

pad on the operating room table to reduce both heat loss and pressure points. A sterile plastic, waterproof drape is placed beneath the patient to shield against liquid penetration.

The patient's anatomy that is not in the field is covered completely with cotton blankets, including arms and legs, beneath which are also placed cotton blankets or towels to insulate the patient further (Fig. 17-15A). Towels are draped as convenient, and half sheets are used to drape off the area and cover the cotton blankets (Fig. 17-15B).

These steps to insulate the patient and reduce heat loss have resulted in much less shivering and postoperative discomfort and have reduced the need for medication and recovery time. A fall of core body temperature of 1° to 2°C during the procedures was common before beginning this routine. Temperature drop is now usually less than .5°C.

PRETREATMENT WITH SUBCUTANEOUS INJECTIONS

Lipolysis clearly can be performed with or without pretreatment of the area by subcutaneous injections. The original Illouz hypotonic solution has been replaced by my isotonic formula (with or without Wydase), or a variant thereof. Such a solution contains low-dose epinephrine for minimizing blood loss, Xylocaine, or some other amide local anesthetic for minimizing postoperative pain, and Wydase to improve the dispersion of the drugs throughout the subcutaneous tissue. Wydase may also aid in the rapid resorption of the sequestered postoperative edema or "fourth space" sequestration. Any physician who has reservations about the use of Wydase should contact Wyeth Laboratories for a bibliography. The fears among plastic surgeons about this drug appear to have been engendered by an unsubstantiated allegation by the author of the American Society of Plastic and Reconstructive Surgeons (ASPRS) Blue Ribbon Committee's Report on Lipolysis after their in depth 3-day visit to Paris in December 1982.

The original Illouz technique was to inject 5 ml every 5 cm in a grid pattern with a 1.5-inch #22 needle. Spinal needles may, of course, be used to minimize puncture sites. If an area were 20 cm by 20 cm, there would be 25 puncture sites and, at 5 ml per site, approximately 125 ml would be used. The average removal for a lateral thigh excess is about 400 ml. I generally use 75 to 125 ml preinjection for these areas and 300 ml for a complete upper and lower abdomen with flank extensions. The Hetter Formula is

250 ml saline
75 ml Xylocaine 1% with epinephrine 1:100,000
300 units Wydase

The reason for these amounts is one of convenience: one 250-ml pack of sterile I.V. solution, one 75-ml bottle of Astra Xylocaine, and two bottles of 150 IU of Wydase. This formula wastes nothing and gives the volume needed for most cases. If I run short, I finish with Xylocaine diluted to 0.25% with epinephrine 1:400,000 rather than mix a new batch when only a few milliliters is needed. I draw back on the syringe to observe for blood before injecting to prevent giving an intravenous bolus of solution. The medial knee and paramedian abdomen are more vascular than the lateral thigh, but care should be taken in all areas to prevent this occurrence.

Surgical Technique

THE INCISION

The incision should be as short as possible to admit the cannula, usually no longer than the diameter of the cannula. The placement of the incision is dictated by the need to hide it in a crease, fold, dimple, stretch mark, or hidden area such as the umbilicus.

The most common sites are marked out in Figure 17-16. The length of cannula must be calculated so that the surgeon can reach all areas. A second incision may be better than trying to go too far. An incision should not be placed over a bony prominence such as the ischial spine or where pressure from sitting or lying down would cause unnecessary pain.

If a wound edge appears dirty or tattered by the piston motion of the cannula, the edges may be freshened before closure. Closure is often complete with the placement of several buried dermal sutures of 4–0 Vicryl, but I often place a superficial layer of 6–0 nylon sutures and remove them in 5 to 7 days.

Dr. Fournier has suggested using an awl which, like an ice pick, merely spreads the dermis and allows #3 or #4 cannulas to be inserted without cutting dermal fibers, eliminates sutures, and heals with a minute point not usually discernible after 2 months. This suggestion may be useful as we progress to smaller cannulas.

USE OF THE CANNULA

Depending on the size of the area and the amount of fat to be removed, a cannula is chosen. The incision is made as small as is necessary to admit the cannula tightly. Very small incisions are possible for #4 or #6 cannulas. For 2-mm cannulas, a minute stab incision with an #11 blade is more than adequate. A hemostat or scissor may be spread to deepen the opening in the fat toward the muscle fascia.

The cannula is initially inserted into the deep fat near the muscle fascia. It is then passed into the marked areas at this level with the opening down (Fig. 17-17). The first tunnel should be made at one edge of the deformity

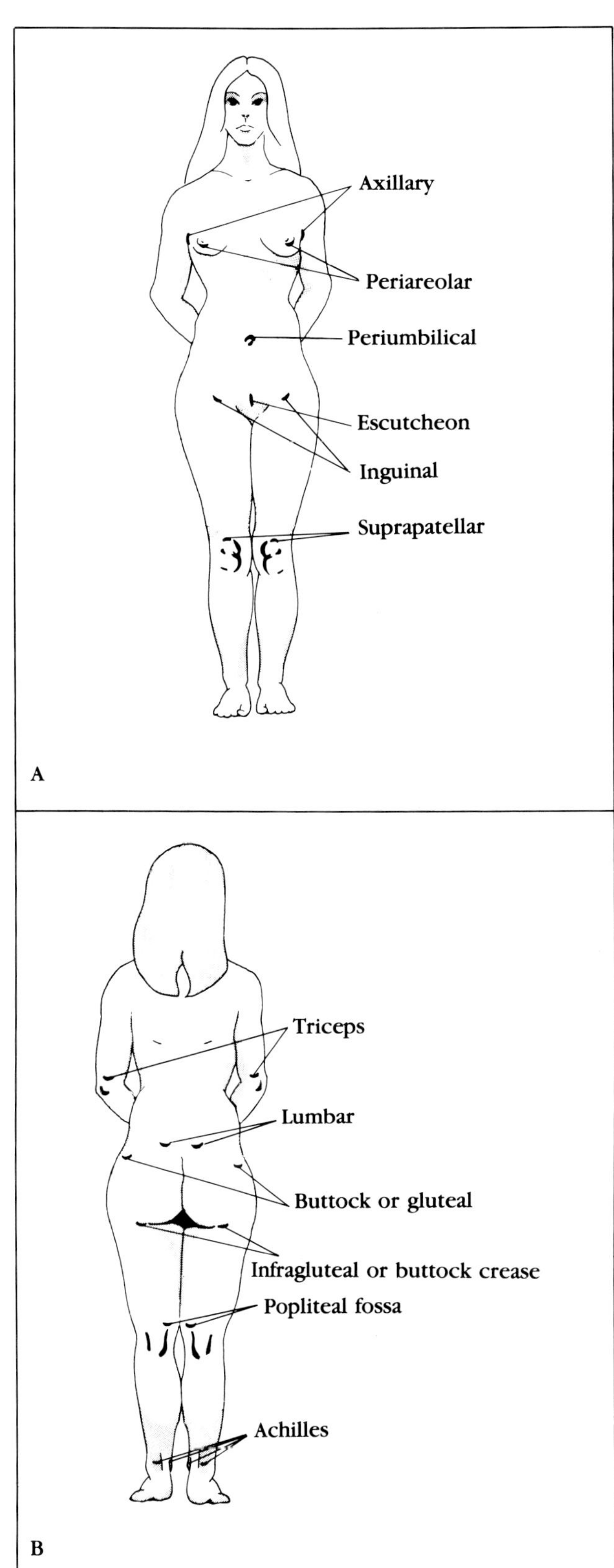

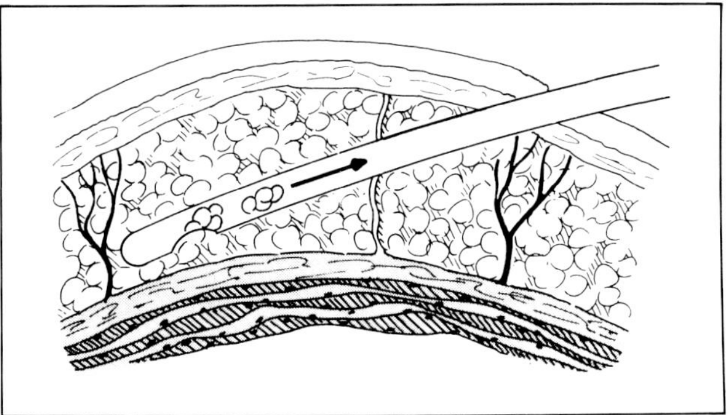

Fig. 17-17. The opening of the cannula is directed toward the muscle fascia to prevent extracting subdermal fat.

and systematic tunnels performed (Figs. 17-18 and 17-19).

Each tunnel is worked for 10 to 15 strokes in a piston-like motion, keeping in mind where the lumen is. *Avoid a side-to-side motion like a windshield wiper, which might destroy vascular septa.* The dangers of the loss of the septa and the creation of a cavity by sharp dissection are illustrated in Figure 17-20. This problem may progress to prolonged seroma, pseudoepithelialization, and a ptosis of the whole undermined area, as seen in the catastrophic result of a French nonplastic surgeon using the Kesselring sharp technique (Fig. 17-21). This is the so called golf bag deformity.

The rapidity of the stroke is related to the power of the suction and the size of the cannula. With the cannula resting deep in the fat with the lumen down, the operator waits for 15 to 30 seconds for the vapor pressure to drive the fat harvest out of the cannula into the clear tubing. The texture, amount, and color of that tunnel's harvest are then observed (Fig. 17-22, see color plate). If bloody, Dr. Illouz recommends going immediately to the next tunnel. If not, more fat could be removed if in the heaviest area of fat.

By working systematically and evenly in a clockwise or counterclockwise fashion, a regular and even work can be accomplished leaving vascular septa intact between skin and fascia. If, on the other hand, an island or peninsula of fat is created by tunneling irregularly, it may be most difficult to enter that island or peninsula, which tends to "float" about in the surrounding meshwork of defatted tissue freed from surrounding attachments. This peninsula must be held with the opposite hand and speared with the cannula. Pretunneling aids some surgeons in achieving this regularity and is recommended for beginners. By being able to see and judge each tunnel's harvest, a more predictable and even work is possible.

When the major area has been defatted, a smaller cannula is selected and the periphery is defatted in a systematic fashion. Lastly, the area 3 to 5 cm beyond the defatted areas undergoes "mesh undermining."

Fig. 17-16.
A. Common anterior incisions.
B. Some common posterior incisions.

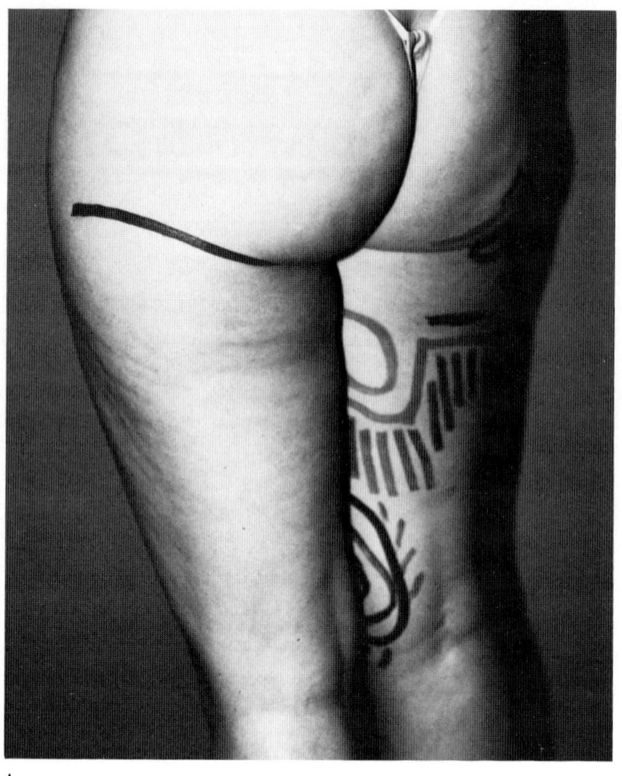

A

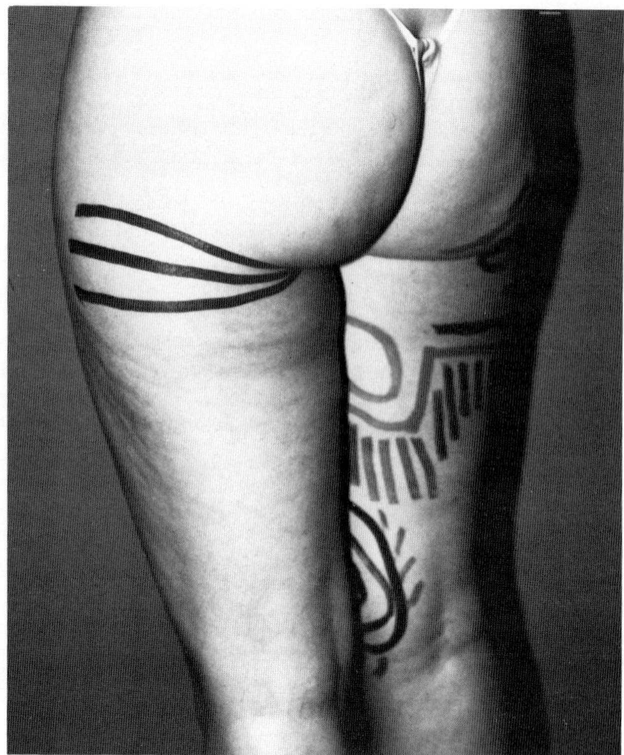

B

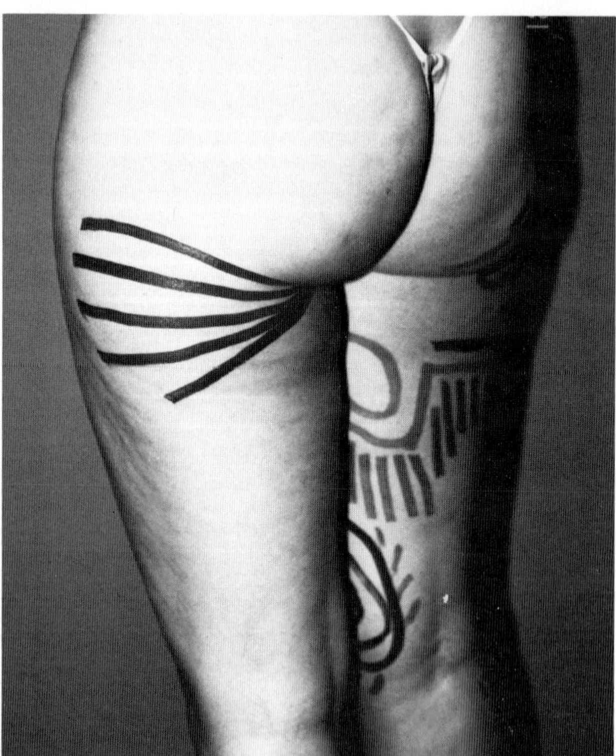

C

Fig. 17-18. A,B,C. Systematic tunnels are depicted on the model to indicate that each is discrete from the other.

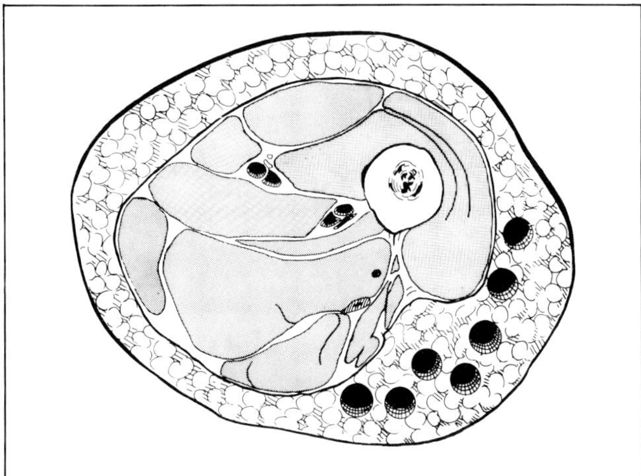

Fig. 17-19. Cross section through the upper thigh (4–6 inches down the femur) illustrating the individual tunnels.

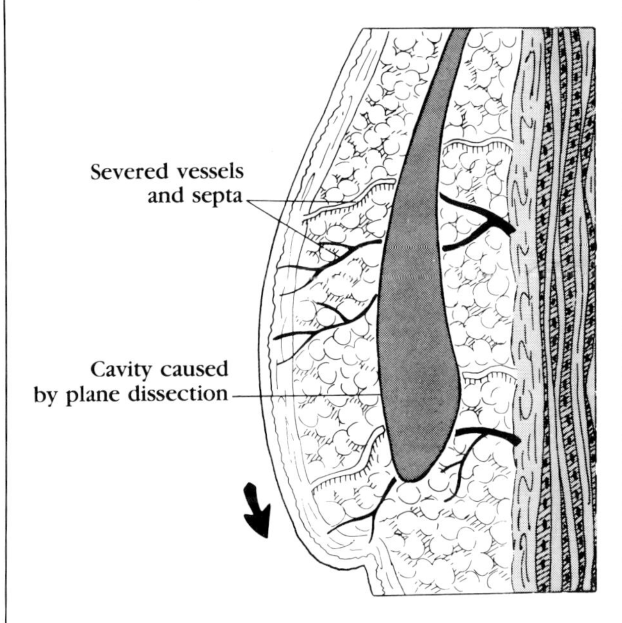

Fig. 17-20. If the fibrous and vascular connections to the skin are lost, a large serous cavity is created, which requires drainage similar to a "wringer injury."

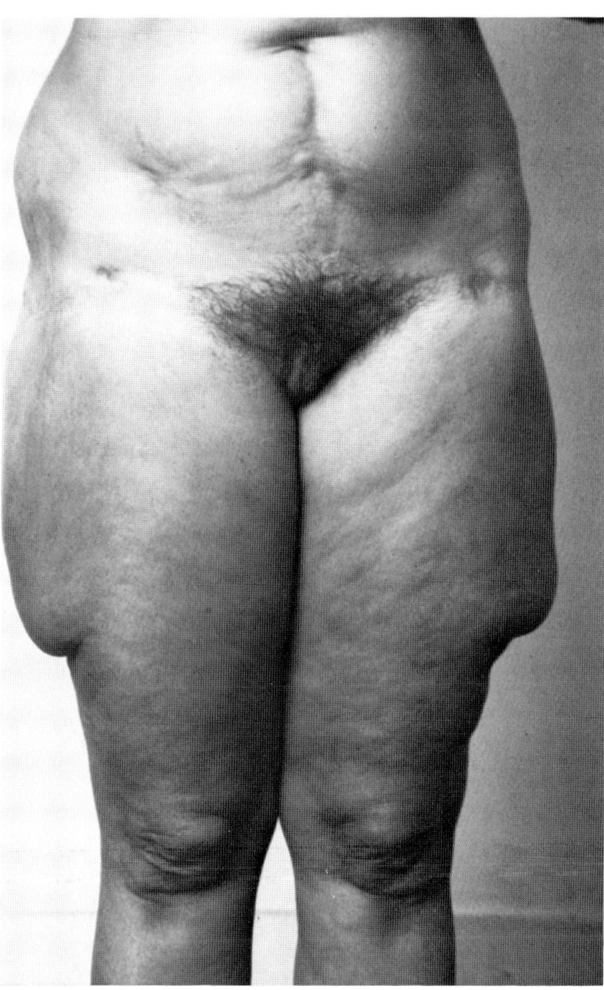

Fig. 17-21. Results of the sharp technique on a large deformity with resultant ptosis of undermined tissues performed by a nonplastic surgeon. (Slide courtesy of Dr. Pierre Fournier, after patient consulted him for reconstructions).

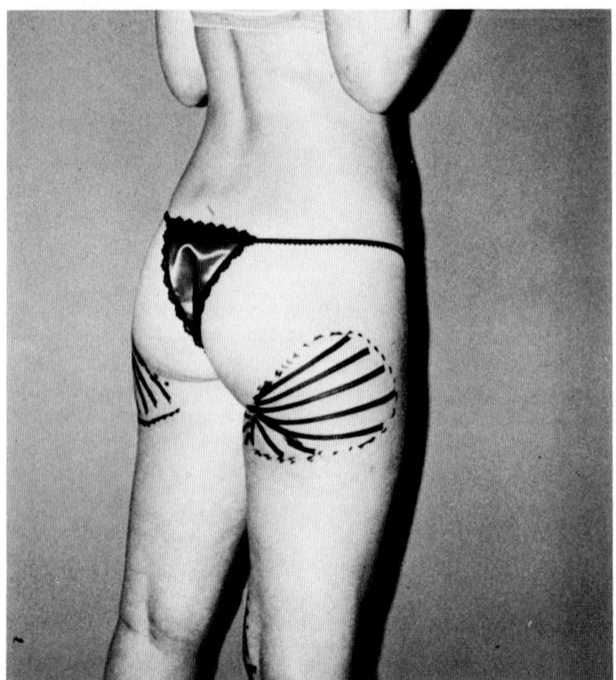

A

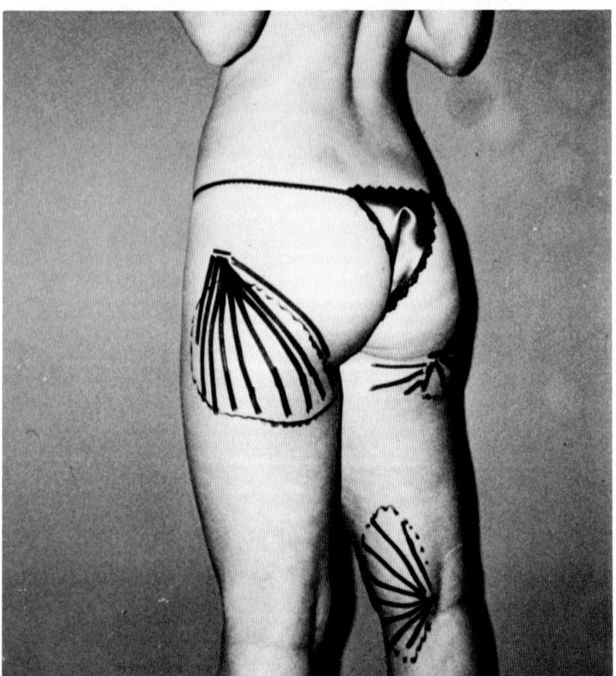

B

Fig. 17-23.
A. Infragluteal approach to the lateral thigh on a model.
   Note horizontal direction of many tunnels.
B. Buttock approach to lateral thigh. Almost all tunnels are
   vertical. This approach is useful when no infragluteal
   component exists or if the iliac crest also needs treatment.

MESH UNDERMINING

Mesh undermining is the term coined by Dr. Fournier
to describe the breaking up of the solid fat at the edge of
a resection. He uses a solid rod of varying size to achieve
this. By passing it repeatedly into the edge of the resection for 4 or 5 cm, the tendency toward a step at that
point seems to palpably disappear. I simply use a #7 or
#8 long cannula without suction attached to break up
the edge, and a smoother transition results.

CRISS-CROSS TECHNIQUE

There has been some discussion of whether horizontal
tunnels, as occur with an infragluteal approach to lateral
thigh fat or with a periumbilical approach to hypogastric
fat, might produce undulations (Figs. 17-23A and 17-
24A) more pronounced than more vertical strokes, as
seen in a supratrochanteric approach to the lateral thigh
fat or in an escutcheon approach to hypogastric fat
(Figs. 17-23B and 17-24B).

The idea of creating tunnels that were perpendicular
to each other, originating from two separate entry sites
using smaller cannulas, was put forward by Dr. Fournier
early in 1983. Since the fat extractions would be a grid
pattern (Fig. 17-25A and B, see color plate), in theory at
least, it makes sense that fewer undulations might result.
Of course, undulations also occur because of skin tension lines and are often seen preoperatively.

This proposal is easily applied to the lateral thigh,
entering from the infragluteal crease 2 to 4 cm lateral to
the ischial spine and from a point high in the gluteal
depression (easily hidden by a bathing suit). The tunnels are almost at right angles to each other in the
heaviest deposits of fat.

Experience with this technique has convinced me
that it does create smoother results when #8 cannulas
and smaller are used. This technique will not make up
for the use of a #10 cannula in a small deformity, however. An island or peninsula difficult to pierce from one
entry point may often be entered easily from the other
entry point.

In the abdomen I routinely enter at the superior hairline of the escutcheon and through a concurrent umbilical incision (Fig. 17-26, see color plate). The tunnels in
much of the hypogastrium (lower abdomen) will be at
right angles to each other. As the deposit thins, one
should drop to a #6 cannula from either site. The #6 is
also used in the paramedian area around the major per-
forators, and bleeding is negligible. It requires a little
more time and persistence but reduces pain, ecchymosis, and blood loss and gives a smoother result.

There is little advantage in criss-crossing in very small
areas since very small (2mm or 3mm) cannulas are used
and the risk for undulations is minimal.

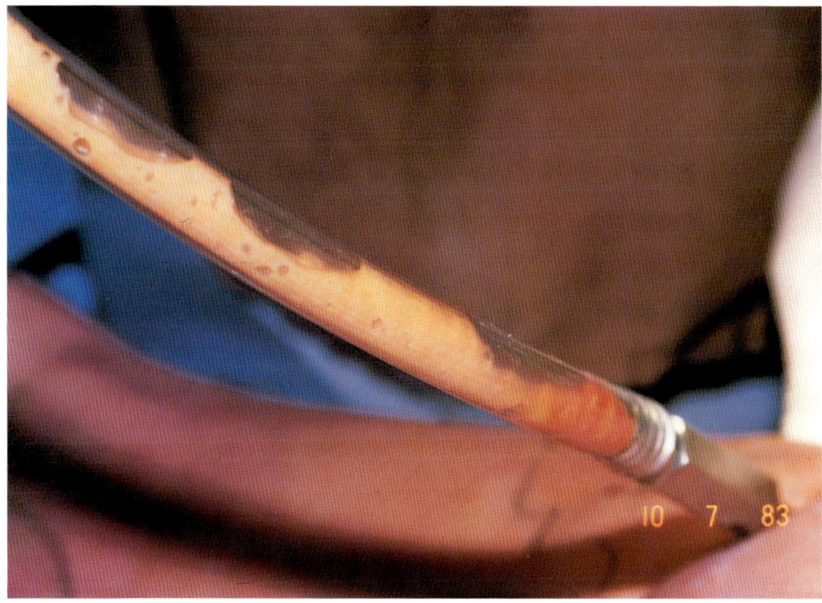

Fig. 17-22. Fat is extracted from a lateral thigh by a Power Source PS-1 vacuum pump capable of producing 1 torr or nearly absolute vacuum. Note absence of blood.

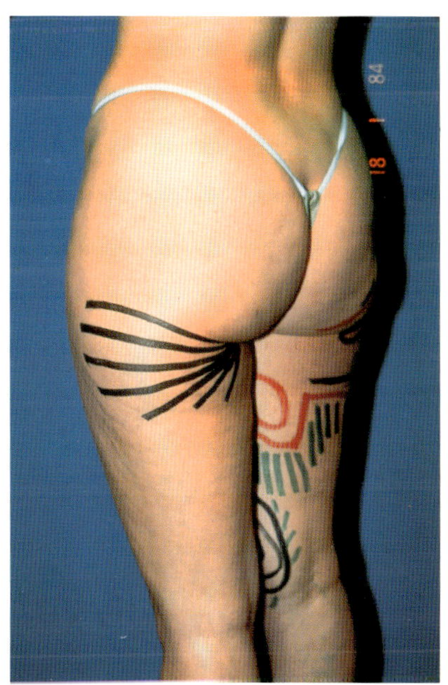
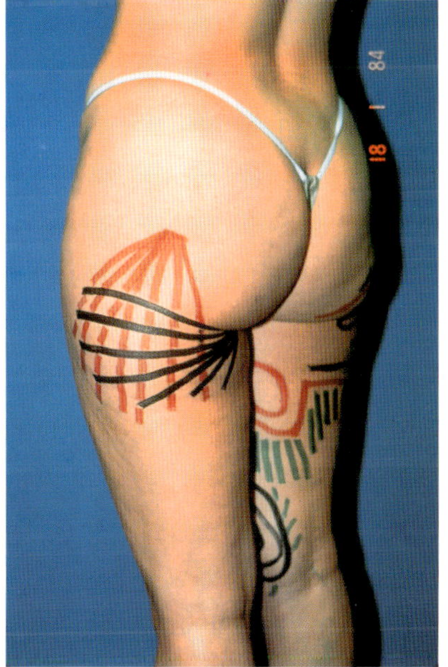

A   B

Fig. 17-25.

A. The criss-cross technique begins by performing the tunnels from one approach as shown on the thigh of this patient marked in black.

B. Then the second entry site is used to cross the previous tunnels almost at right angles, creating a grid pattern marked in red.

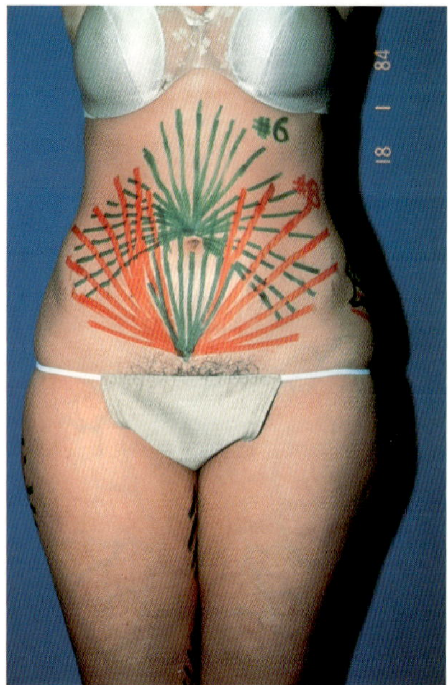

Fig. 17-26. The criss-cross technique is applied to the abdomen via a hairline and periumbilical incision. Many tunnels cross at right angles to each other. The #6 cannula is used in the paramedian area and epigastrium (colored green). The #8 is used for most of the hypogastrium and flank extensions (colored red).

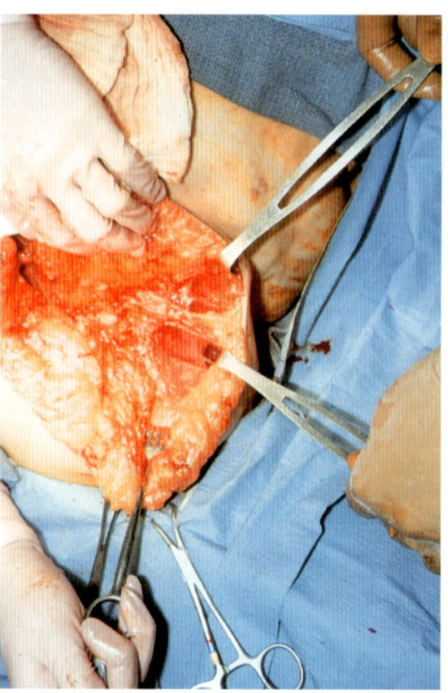

Fig. 17-29. Lateral view of incision of left breast tissue that had undergone lipolysis before performing a standard reduction mammoplasty. Note intact structures, extracted tunnels, and lack of blood stain on tissues.

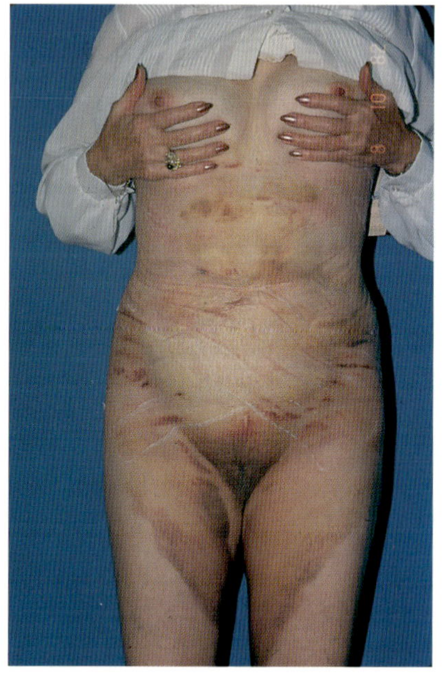
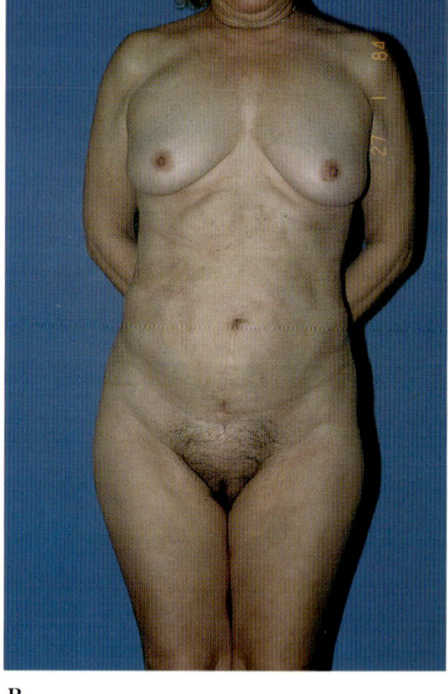

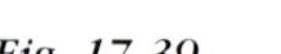

A   B

Fig. 17-39.
A. Ecchymosis in a 64-year-old female at eighth postoperative day. A #10 cannula was used. No epinephrine was used, and ecchymosis did not clear for 3 weeks.
B. Lack of ecchymosis in a 65-year-old female at twelfth postoperative day. Both #6 and #8 cannulas were used through two sites of entry. The Hetter formula was used containing epinephrine.

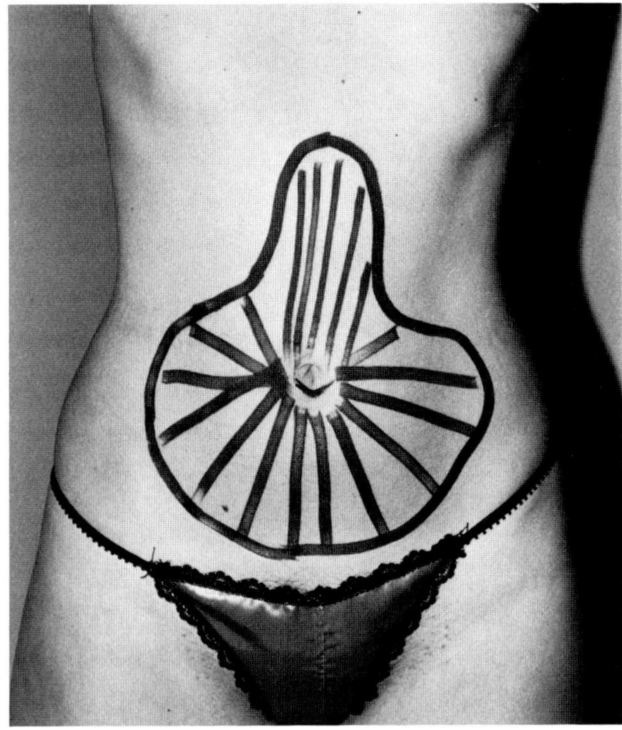

A

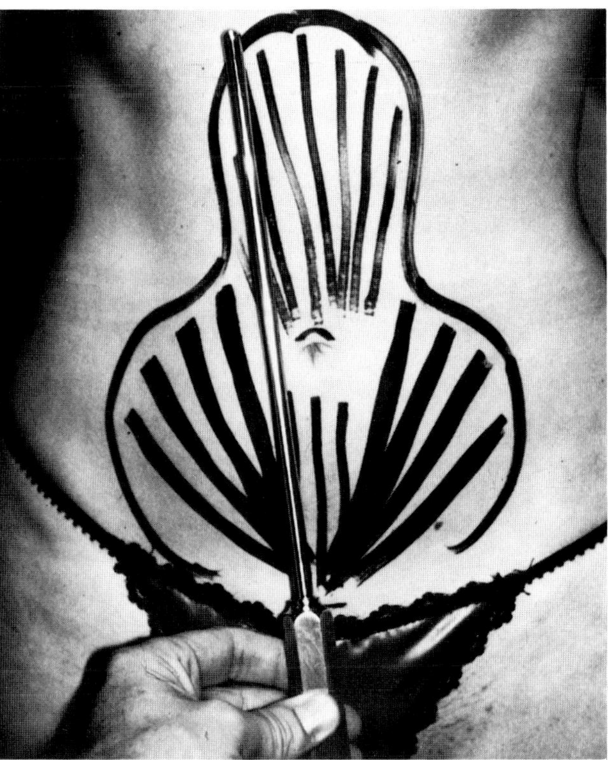

B

Fig. 17-24.

A. Periumbilical approach to the hypogastrium. Note horizontal direction of many tunnels.

B. Escutcheon approach to hypogastrium and epigastrium through a hairline incision. Note number of almost vertical tunnels.

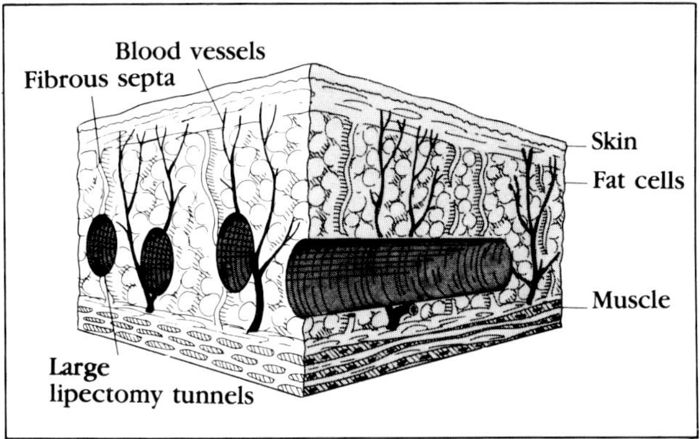

Fig. 17-27. Large tunnels in subcutaneous fat.

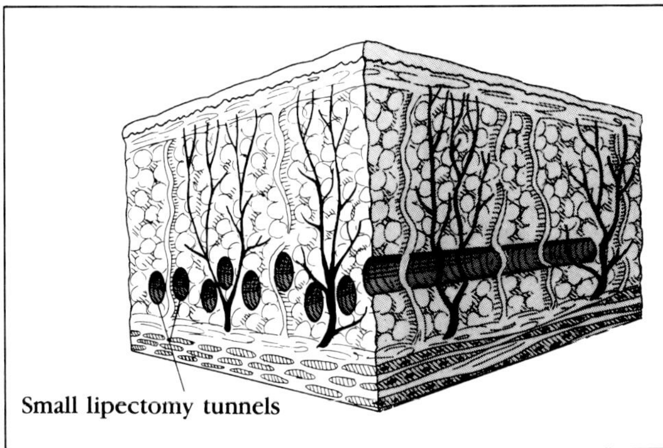

Fig. 17-28. Smaller but more frequent tunnels with less chance of vascular injury.

DEPTH OF TUNNELS

The tunnels should be made in the lower two-thirds of the fatty tissue next to the muscle fascia. The subdermal fat should be respected since it is more vascular and its loss creates obvious dents, waves, and irregularities. Figure 17-27 shows a cross section of integument where the tunnels have been made with a large bore cannula. As the skin contracts, it forces the unextracted fat into the spaces created by the tunnels, and the volume decreases. Figure 17-28 shows a similar cross section with smaller and more frequent tunnels, which lessens the chance of irregularities showing through the more superficial layer of subdermal fat. Figure 17-29 (see color plate) shows a defatted area with the vessels, nerves, and septa stretching between the skin and fascia. A layer of subdermal fat should be left untouched to provide cover for the collapsing deeper tissues.

The hand opposite the cannula is critical for the accuracy of the tunneling. Some helpful hints are in order. At the start when the fat is block-like, the lateral thigh area may be flattened out (Fig. 17-30) as the cannula is

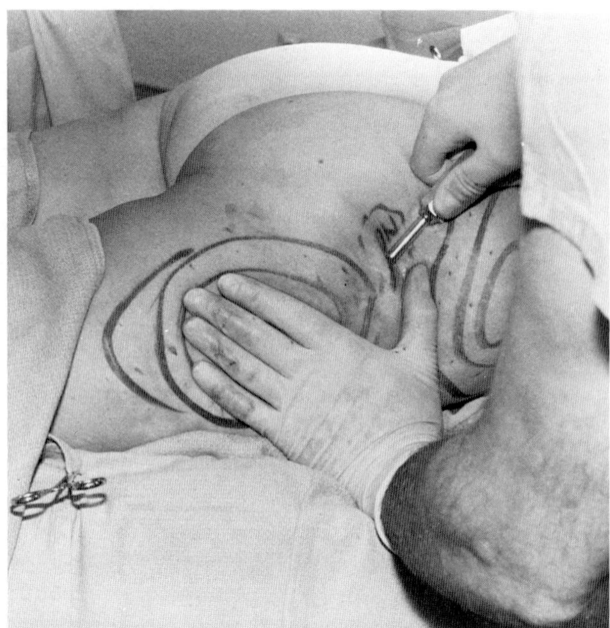

Fig. 17-30. The opposite hand pushes the lateral thigh fat flat, helping the cannula to stay deep in its trajectory.

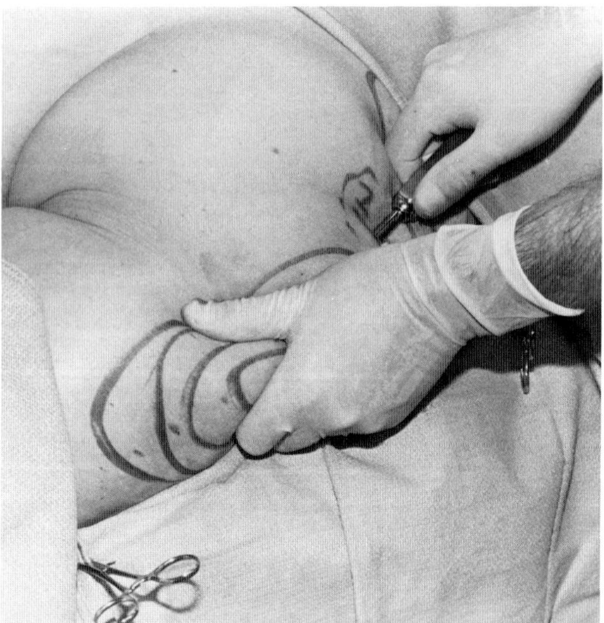

Fig. 17-31. The opposite hand holds a now-loose "peninsula" of fat for spearing by the cannula. So-called pinch and roll technique.

driven into the fatty deposit to minimize the curve of the thigh. Later in the procedure, when the fat is less cohesive, the opposite hand controls the fat by grasping it like a large sausage, and the cannula is driven down the center of this sausage (Fig. 17-31). This maneuver is particularly common when treating the iliac crest and abdomen and not used at all in the knees or calves.

RAISING OR ACCENTUATING THE GLUTEAL CREASE

The infragluteal fold may be poorly defined (Fig. 17-32) or tend to fade downward, creating a "sad buttock" (Fig. 17-33).

The desired crease is marked out in the standing position. The fold should only go two-thirds of the width of the thigh so it is the middle third that normally must be treated (Fig. 17-34). Care must be taken not to take the fold into the lateral third where it is not normally present.

The technique with the #10 "shark mouth" cannula is exactly the opposite of all the rules. It is used with the lumen up and forced along beneath the skin so tightly that it tears the subdermal fat away. The dermis is rasped in this fashion. Next, the cannula is turned and the superficial fat immediately beneath the skin is tunneled out to create a superficial furrow into which the rasped skin will drop and adhere (Fig. 17-35). The opening of the lumen can be seen through the skin in Figure 17-36A. Properly performed, this maneuver, developed by Dr. Illouz, is highly successful. It is more easily learned by observation than by description, however, and I know several competent practitioners of lipolysis who insist they cannot achieve good results when attempting this.

The dressing of this area is critical. The fold should be taped precisely with two layers of Elastikon to force the dermis into the furrow. This tape is left on for 7 to 10 days (Fig. 17-37). Pressure garments can be used after other procedures (see Chap. 18). Advocates of pressure garments, however, have trouble raising gluteal folds, and taping is still necessary to complete this procedure.

DRAINS

Since beginning the use of low-dose epinephrine and smaller cannulas (mainly #8 and #6), I have not used drains. Even in abdominal procedures that previously were very bloody and in which I routinely used drains, the present blood loss is negligible when the paramedian vessel area is treated with a #6 cannula.

If necessary, a suction drain may be placed, but the opening must be near the confluency of the tunnels. When large cannulas were used, 400 ml might be obtained from two drains placed bilaterally in an abdominal extraction after 24 hours. Bleeding was obvious and

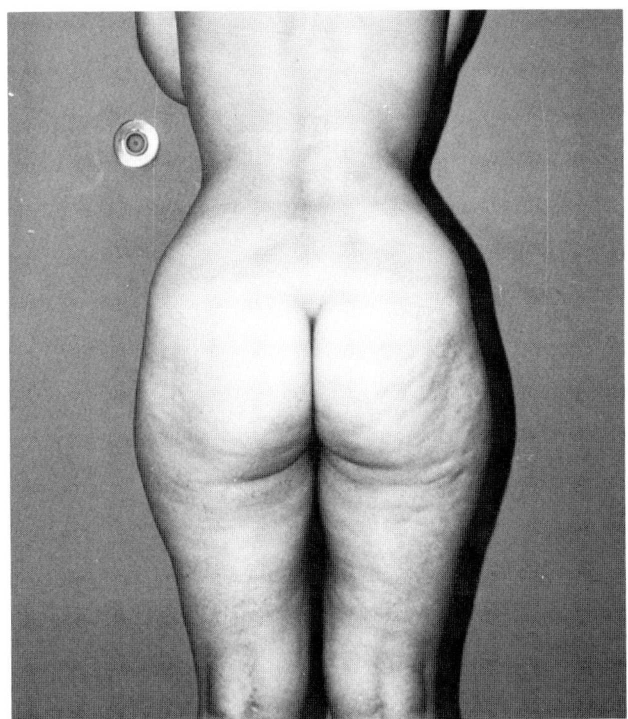

Fig. 17-32. Gluteal fold fades into confluency of buttock and upper thigh with no definition.

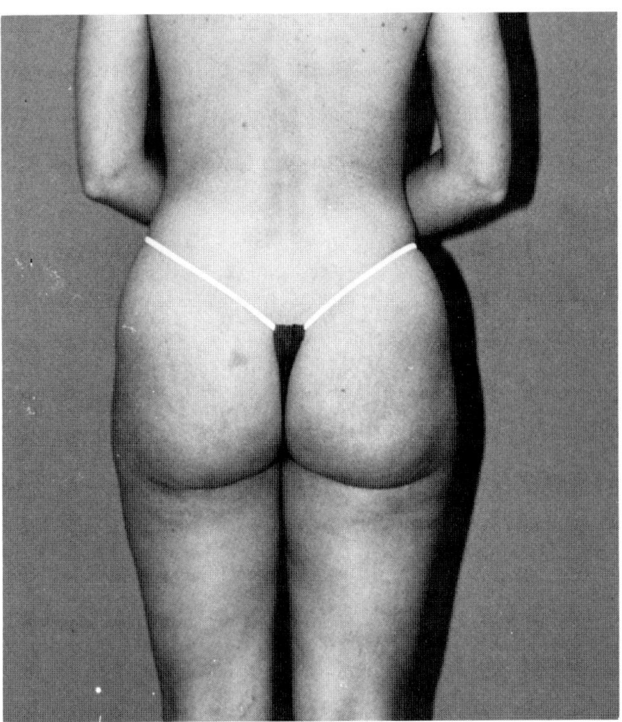

Fig. 17-34. Postoperative view of 32-year-old patient in Fig. 17-33 with newly created "smiling buttock" 3 months postoperatively.

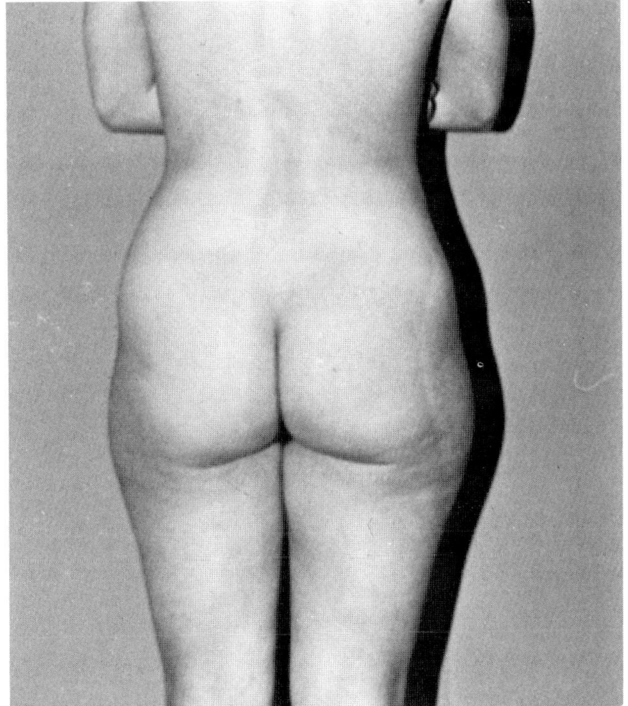

Fig. 17-33. "Sad buttock" due to down-curving gluteal fold.

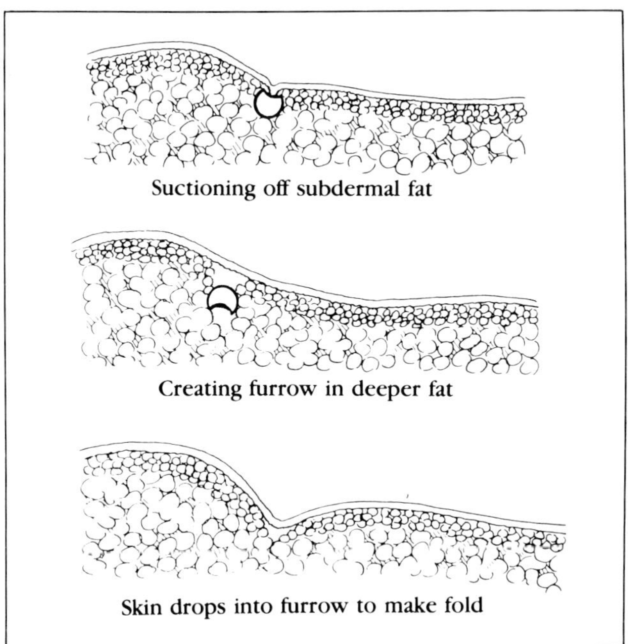

Fig. 17-35. The subdermal fat is stripped from underside of dermis. A furrow is created in the intermediate fatty layer, then taped to form the new crease.

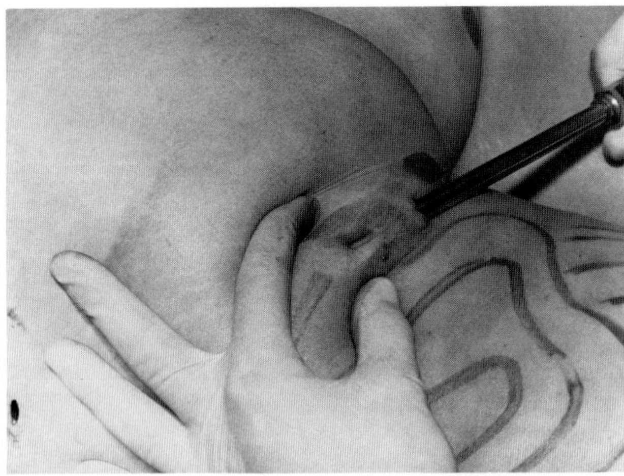

A

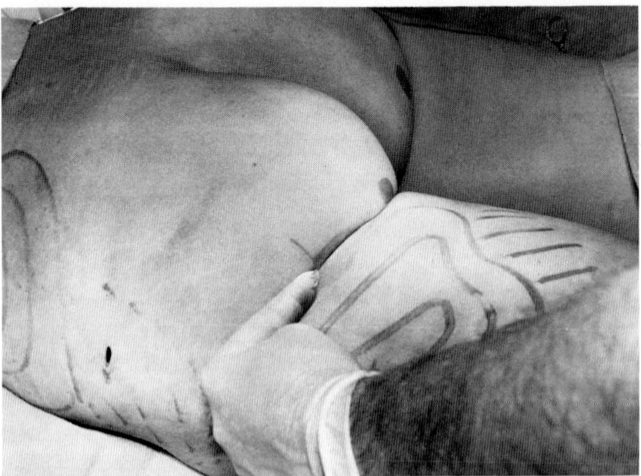

B

Fig. 17-36

A. "Shark Mouth" #10 Illouz cannula used to strip subdermal fat in the creation of a new gluteal crease. Note lumen seen through dermis.

B. The fold just created on a patient. Note large dot to indicate ischial tuberosity, gluteal depression incision for criss-cross technique, and limit mark for fold.

a drain seemed natural and worked in these cases. Only if bleeding appears to persist when the area is rolled with a sponge toward the site of entry is a drain necessary. If the technique is harsh because of a low-pressure machine that requires many more thrusts than necessary, there will be more bleeding.

ANTIBIOTICS

The controversy about preoperative, intraoperative, and postoperative antibiotics goes on without obvious winners. The procedure as I perform it is not a sterile procedure. Working around the perineum obviously prevents this. It is a clean procedure, however. Many surgeons do not feel it necessary to gown for this procedure. Their

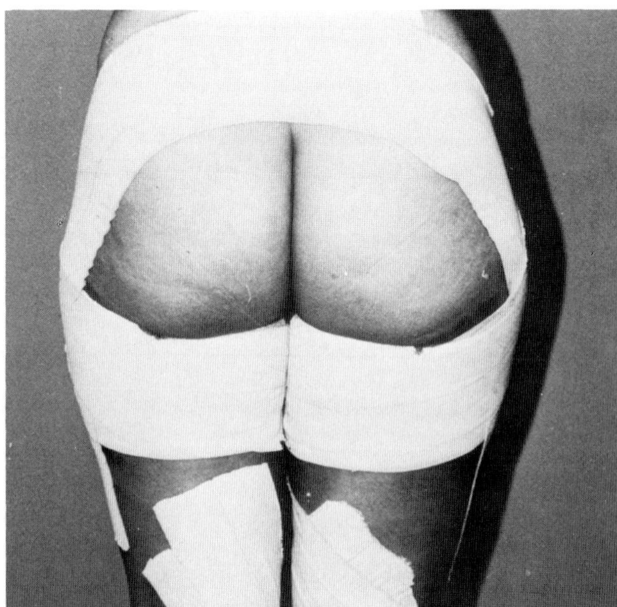

Fig. 17-37. Taped gluteal fold forcing rasped dermis into the furrow during healing phase of patient.

lack of complications speaks clearly for their point of view. It requires attention to detail and a team used to working together to maintain the clean procedure routine.

I never allow the gloved hand to touch the cannula barrel. If it does, the barrel is wiped with saline containing G.U. irrigant (Neosporin). I give the nonallergic patient 1 g of cephalosporin I.V. early in the procedure and a prescription for Keflex, 250 mg q.i.d. for 5 days, or other equivalent oral cephalosporin. The rationale for the use of antibiotics is to have the drug in the tissues while they are damaged in case an outside organism is carried by the cannula into the damaged tissues. These operations are entirely elective, and I feel this regimen is justified to reduce the risk of infection. Other choices of antibiotics and the choice not to use antibiotics may be equally defensible based on the literature and on local infectious disease opinion.

The choice must ultimately be based on what the surgeon feels is best for the patient, who has entrusted not only his or her appearance but very life to the surgeon's judgment and skill.

Complications of the Technique

IMMEDIATE COMPLICATIONS

Blood loss and serum loss are a major concern. Removals up to 6 L have been performed on outpatients. However, I believe that ambulatory discharge is safe—when

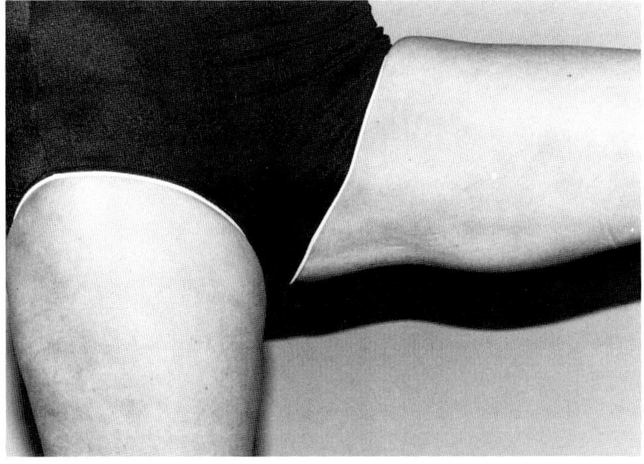

A

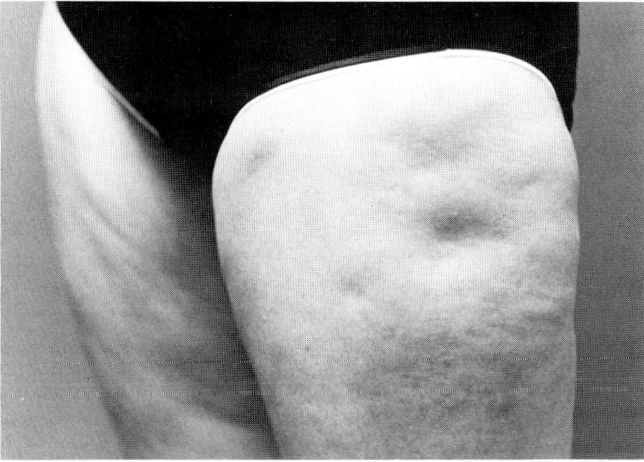

B

Fig. 17-38.
A. Unattractive result from overzealous removal of crural and infragluteal fat.
B. Dent in lateral thigh from subdermal fat removal, resulting from cannular lumen too close to or turned toward skin or from poorly designed cannula (opening at tip).

using low-dose epinephrine—with removals up to 1500 ml if clinically warranted.

Removals from 1500 to 3000 ml are best observed for 24 hours for tachycardia and evidence of hypovolemia. I do not wish to use blood or blood products (see Chapter 14 on anesthesia and fluid replacement for details).

I do not recommend removing more than 2500 ml at one session but rather staging sessions if more tissue needs to be removed. I do this at 3-month intervals whether in the same site or in different sites.

Perforation of the abdomen, which is alleged to have occurred in Indonesia, is treated by laparotomy for diagnosis and indicated procedures. The rare unexpected complications of any surgical procedure, including thromboembolic phenomena are treated according to the current state of the art in the surgeon's community.

DELAYED SEQUELAE

The single most frequent cause of postoperative patient concern is inadequate preoperative counseling. The properly informed patient must be willing to accept the following normal results of this operation:

1. Minor irregularities
2. Minor bulges
3. Minor dimpling
4. Minor skin hyperpigmentation
5. Minor asymmetries
6. Minor sensation change including dysesthesia and hypesthesia
7. Edema for 2 to 6 months, depending on the area

MAJOR IRREGULARITIES

When the irregularities are not minor but noticeable enough that the surgeon feels they are outside the range of the usual and customary result, he or she should consider further treatment. Overvigorous resection of fat leaving a true deficiency cannot be treated except by open surgery with dermofat flap advancement. Figure 17-38 shows a patient of Dr. Illouz in whom too much fat was removed in the high medioposterior thigh area, leaving a real trough and a dent on the lateral thigh. Only a crural thigh lift with shift of lower thigh tissue into this area will provide improvement. These problems are best avoided by not removing too much.

Dimples as well as bulges and waves are normally improved by careful analysis, marking, and a touchup under local infiltration anesthesia using the Hetter formula. Wait 20 minutes for good local effect. A #4 or #6 cannula used either through the original entry point or, sometimes better, at right angles to the original tunnels, provides modest improvement but not perfection. The patient must always be made aware that we are searching for improvement and not perfection. As Dr. Regnault of Montreal has so aptly counseled: "The enemy of *good* plastic surgery is perfectionism."

HYPERPIGMENTATION

Hyperpigmentation is minimized by reducing the attendant bleeding at the time of surgery to a minimum. This is accomplished by the use of as small a cannula as practical along with the use of epinephrine-containing solutions. The difference can be seen in Fig. 17-39 (see color plate).

I believe massage helps mobilize the ecchymosis earlier and decreases the amount of hemosiderin deposit, but I cannot prove it to the skeptical. The foregoing regimen has prevented any significant hyperpigmentation to date. I recommend staying out of the sun for 3 months but believe few young women follow this advice.

Postoperative Follow-up

Lastly, showing the patient a preoperative and a 3-month postoperative photograph usually puts many small dissatisfactions to rest. The Polaroid Polaprinter has proved very valuable in postoperative follow-up with the patient who forgets his or her earlier deformity. Often the staff handles this before I even see the patient. The concern for a minor irregularity has been transformed to thankful awe at seeing the improvement demonstrated by the two photographs. The visit is short, pleasant, and gratifying to both surgeon and patient. I neither discuss nor perform a touchup before 3 months and wait no longer than 6 months. The financial arrangements for touchups should be included in the informed consent, clearly understood, and require no discussion during a period of potential dissatisfaction.

This discussion of technique is meant to complement and not replace alert observation, competent instruction, and guided hands-on experience. Before attempting the procedure, the novice plastic surgeon should visit a plastic surgeon proficient in lipolysis. A list of these plastic surgeons is available from the Lipolysis Society of North America, P.O. Box 28534, Las Vegas, Nevada 89126-2534.

CHAPTER 18

Alternative Patient Positioning and Pretunneling

Richard A. Mladick
Richard L. Morris

French surgeons have performed lipolysis on many patients with endotracheal anesthesia in the prone position; however, anesthesia professionals expressed concern that prone position general anesthesia was not an accepted standard of care for outpatients in our community. It was felt that endotracheal anesthesia in the prone position requires (1) greater depth of anesthesia to achieve a surgical plane, (2) careful positioning to allow for expansion of the lungs and prevention of abdominal compression, and (3) close observations for complications such as laryngeal trauma or edema in the postoperative period.

The concerns expressed to us about prolonged recovery time and supposed increased incidence of complications made postoperative hospitalization, as in France, necessary. Thus, an alternative to the prone position was needed for us to allow lipolysis to be performed on an outpatient basis in our outpatient facility because of the anesthesia standards in our area.

The supine position was obviously ideal for access to the submental area, gynecomastia, abdomen, arms, knees, and inner thighs. Modification of the supine position led to the development of the supine lateral decubitus position (SLD) for access to hip rolls, "saddlebags," buttocks, and calves. The need for the prone position was eliminated and we could offer lipolysis on an outpatient basis.

Alternative Patient Positions

SUPINE POSITION

The normal supine position is the position of choice for lipolysis of the submental area, upper arms, gynecomastia, and abdomen. Some slight variations of the supine position are necessary for the inner thighs, knees, and calves.

Submental lipolysis is most often performed during a face-lift and uses the incision of the face-lift (see Chap. 25). However, a small incision under the chin (in the same location as used for the external approach to a chin implant) is ideal for submental lipolysis that is not in conjunction with a face-lift (Fig. 18-1).

The upper arms are reached through an incision placed on the medial aspect of the arm, either by the elbow or near the axilla (Fig. 18-2). It is preferable to have the arms abducted on an armboard with a sterile stockinette covering the hand and forearm to facilitate movement. Proper attention must be directed toward avoiding injury to the ulnar nerve when placing the incision near the elbow. A midarm incision is also possible (Fig. 18-2B).

Lipolysis for gynecomastia is performed through a small incision at the bottom of the areola. The #8 can-

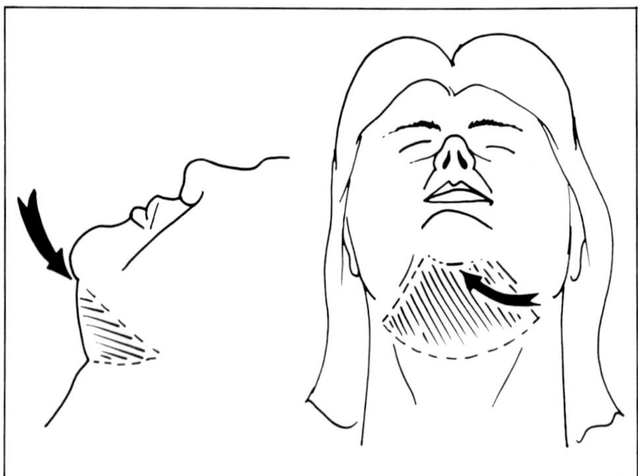

Fig. 18-1. A small 1-cm incision *(arrow)* placed under the chin can be used for submental lipolysis. A #4 or #6 cannula is used, and an effort is made to feather the fat removal out to the sides to achieve a smooth contour on the neck. The shaded area represents a typical area treated by lipolysis.

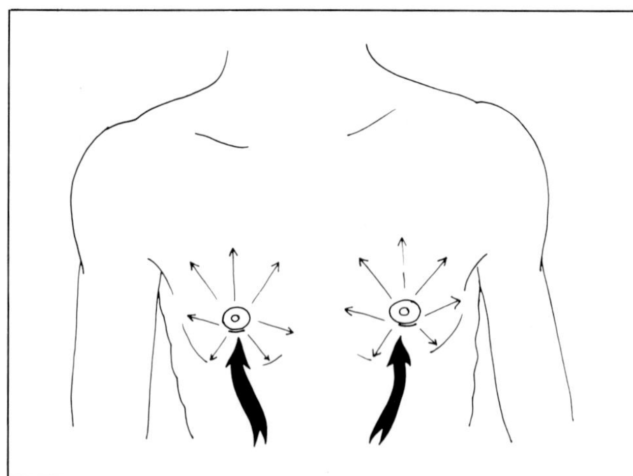

Fig. 18-3. The incision for gynecomastia is infraareolar *(arrow).* Through this incision, the cannula is passed in all directions to complete removal of all tissue except the subareolar fibrous tissue.

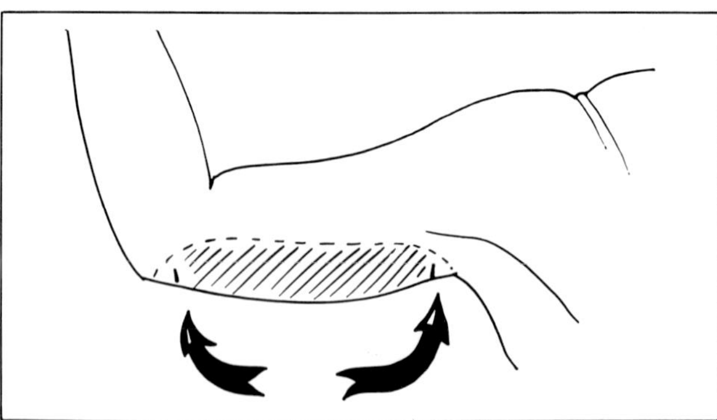

A

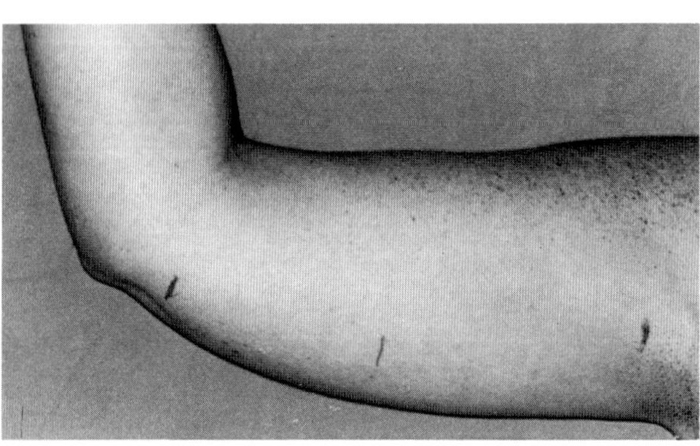

B

Fig. 18-2.
A. The incision for arm lipolysis can be made on the inside of the arm, by either the elbow or axilla *(arrows).* The elbow incision provides easy access to the entire length of the upper arm. A long #6 or #8 cannula is preferred, and the shaded area represents the area usually benefited most by lipolysis.
B. The upper arm is marked with incisions at both the elbow and the axilla. A midarm incision is also marked, which can be used simply by turning the cannula in opposite directions.

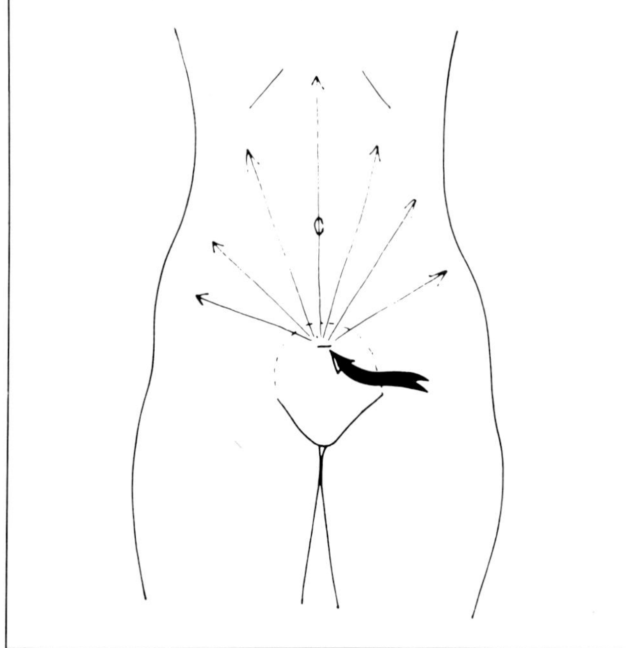

Fig. 18-4. For abdominal lipolysis, the upper portion of the pubic hair is shaved and the incision placed about ½ to 1 inch below the most superior pubic hairline. The lipolysis is extended in all directions including the epigastric fat region. Through this suprapubic incision, even the anterior portion of the hip rolls ("love handles") can be corrected. A long #8 or #10 cannula is preferred.

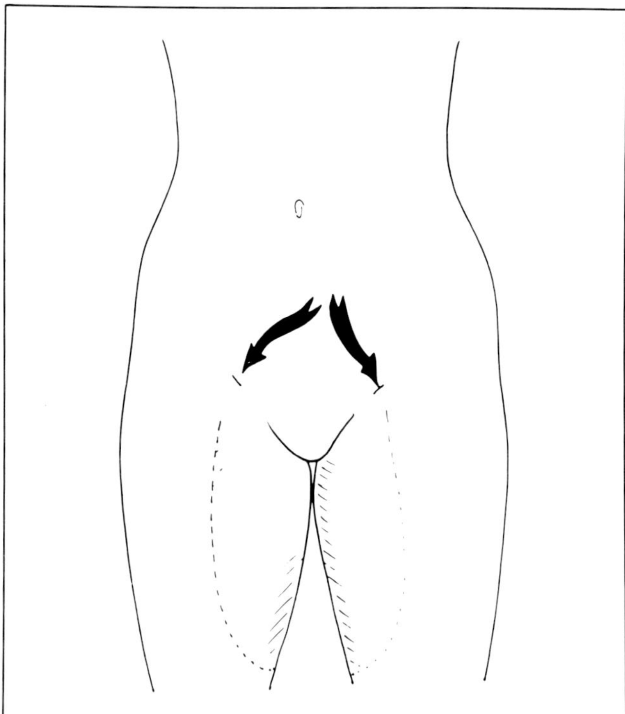

Fig. 18-5. The incisions for the lipolysis of the inner thighs are made along the groin crease *(arrows).* A long #8 cannula can reach almost halfway down the thigh. To reach the posterior aspect of the inner thighs, the legs need to be moved into the abducted ("frog") position.

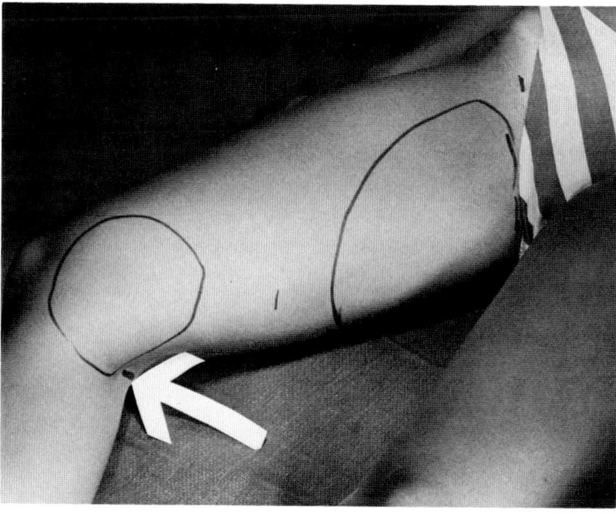

Fig. 18-6. The fat around the knee may be treated by an incision placed in the posterior popliteal area *(arrow).* This incision can be done either in the supine position or in the supine lateral decubitus position. The *arrow* points to the location of the incision behind the knee. The small midthigh mark is for a single incision that may be used for both the inner thighs and the knees.

nula is passed in all directions, and the incision is enlarged to facilitate removal of the remaining subareolar fibrous breast tissue by sharp dissection (Fig. 18-3). "Feathering" of the periphery is much easier than with the traditional sharp dissection technique.

For abdominal lipolysis, a small area of pubic hair is shaved and the incision placed 1 inch below the pubic hairline in the midline (Fig. 18-4). Through this incision a long #8 cannula enables lipolysis of the abdomen, waist, and even the anterior hip rolls ("love handles"). Reaching the posterior hip rolls necessitates a separate incision in the hip or buttock region. Abdominal lipolysis may also be performed through a periumbilical incision.

The inner thighs are accessible through an incision placed in the anterior groin crease (Fig. 18-5). The anterior inner thigh area is easily approached, but the posterior inner thigh area can be reached only after the hip and knees are flexed and the leg rotated outward ("frog" position). Lipolysis of the inner thighs is usually confined to the discernible fatty bulge in the upper one-third to one-half of the inner thigh.

Lipolysis of the medial knee region requires the hips and knees to be flexed and the legs rotated outward to accomplish the frog position (Fig. 18-6). The incision is made in the posterior popliteal area, and a short #6 and #8 cannula is used. While the legs are in the frog position, a single incision in the mid inner thigh region allows lipolysis of both the knees and the inner thighs by changing direction of the cannula (Fig. 18-6).

SUPINE LATERAL DECUBITUS POSITION

The supine lateral decubitus (SLD) position is an effective alternative to the prone position for performing lipolysis of the saddlebags, buttocks, and hip rolls. The head and shoulders are essentially supine, but the trunk is turned acutely with one hip rolled upward and the hip underneath in the lateral decubitus position.

Proper positioning of the patient in the supine lateral decubitus position is shown in Figures 18-7 to 18-10. To accomplish this position, the patient is placed supine and the legs are angled toward the side of the table nearest the surgeon (Fig. 18-7). Then the closest knee is flexed (Fig. 18-8). The assistant maintains this position from the opposite side of the table by placing a hand on the knee and another hand on the back of the patient's waist. While the hip is upright in the lateral decubitus position, the shoulders, head, and neck areas remain supine, permitting the anesthetist to administer general anesthesia by mask without difficulty.

The SLD is a useful position for lipolysis of the saddlebags, hip rolls, and buttocks. The incision is placed high on the posterior lateral buttock in an area covered

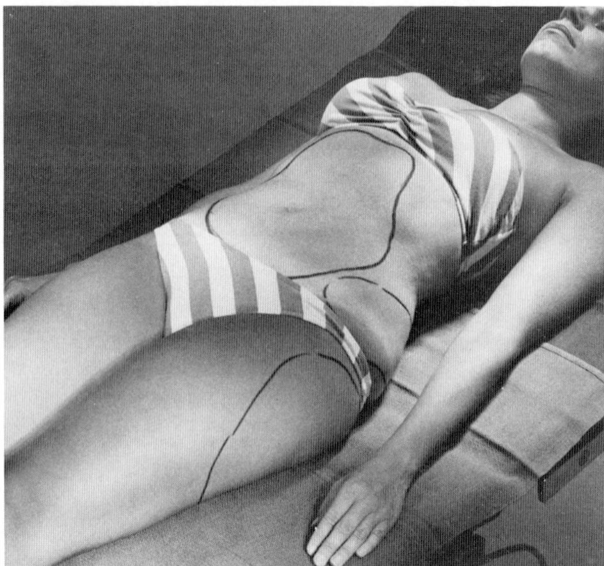

Fig. 18-7. The first step in positioning the patient for the supine lateral decubitus (SLD) position is to start with the patient in the supine position and slide both legs toward the surgeon.

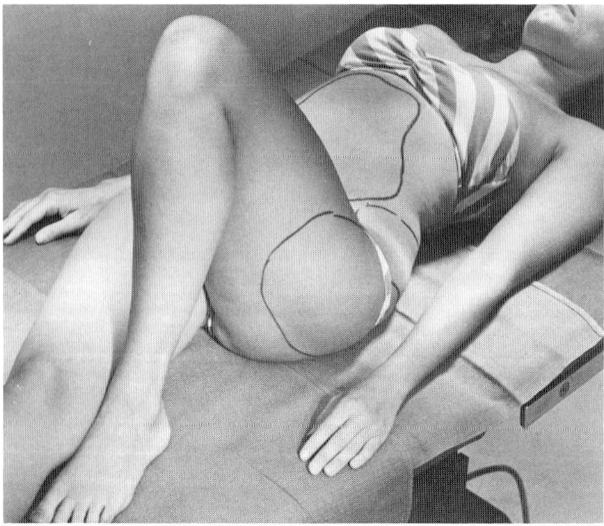

Fig. 18-8. The knee closest to the surgeon is now flexed, allowing the knee to be used as a lever to twist the torso.

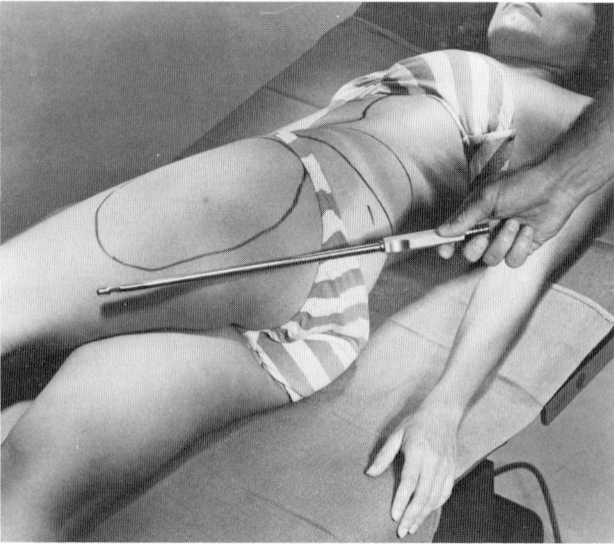

Fig. 18-9. The knee is pulled away from the surgeon, bringing the hip upright into the lateral decubitus position. However, the patient's shoulders and face are supine, allowing general anesthesia by a mask. The incision is marked on the posterior lateral buttock area. The cannula can easily reach below the lower limits of the "saddlebag," anywhere on the buttocks including the buttock crease and upward into the hip rolls (saddlebags). In this position, an incision can also be made in the buttock crease to reach the saddlebag area.

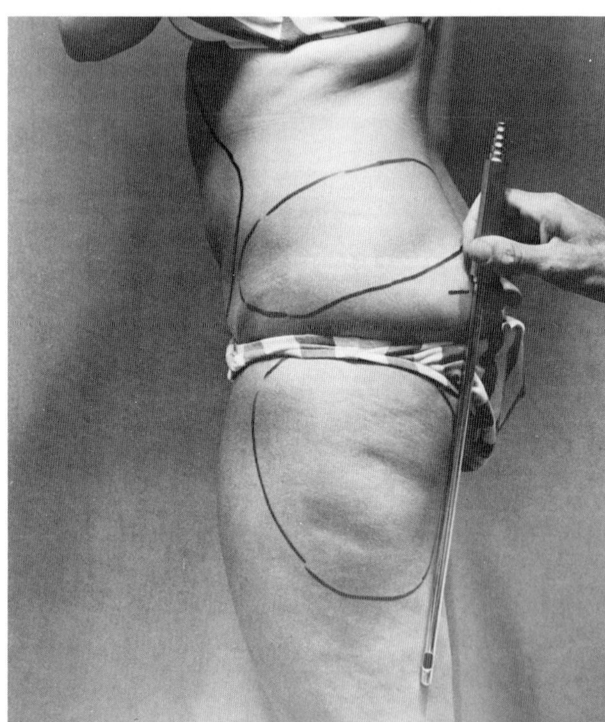

Fig. 18-10. In this standing view, the abdomen, hip rolls, and saddlebags are marked. The small incision in the posterior lateral buttock area will be covered by a bikini. The cannula easily reaches below the lower limits of the saddlebags.

by almost every bikini (Figs. 18-9 and 18-10). A long #8 cannula easily extends downward to the saddlebag area, backward to the buttocks, and then upward to reach the hip rolls. Pulling the knee too far over toward the opposite side results in very marked flexion, which tightens the iliotibial tract, making the tunneling difficult. Decreasing the flexion of the hip and knee immediately releases the tension, allowing the loosened subcutaneous tissue to be suctioned.

One theoretical advantage of the posterior lateral buttock incision is that the direction of the tunneling for saddlebags is vertical, and the pull of gravity is along the longitudinal (vertical) direction of the tunnels. It is not known whether this incision actually decreases rippling of the skin as compared to the technique of using a posterior gluteal fold incision with horizontal tunnels. In an occasional case, cross-tunneling, or tunnels at 90-degree angles from two sites, may more evenly contour the fat from the saddlebag area. Cross-tunneling requires two incisions, one high in the posterior lateral buttock area and a separate incision in the gluteal fold, both easily performed in the SLD position.

The buttocks are accessible for lipolysis through the same incision used for the saddlebags or through an incision in the buttock crease made while turning the hip even more upright. The buttock crease is easily developed by performing lipolysis while rotating the orifice of the cannula upward toward the skin of the crease through either incision.

Lipolysis of the calves requires two incisions. The lateral calf is treated through an incision in the lateral popliteal or in the lateral ankle region, made while the patient is in the SLD position. The medial calf is reached through an incision in the medial popliteal area or medial ankle, made while the patient is in the supine frog leg position.

SUMMARY

In our total experience of more than 300 outpatient lipolysis procedures, only the supine, supine lateral position, and modifications thereof have been used. General inhalation anesthesia by mask was adequate in all but one very large, obese male with a short neck who was intubated solely for airway maintenance.

Early procedures were less complex than those now regularly performed. The supine position was used for abdominal procedures, and the supine lateral decubitus position was used for hip rolls and saddlebags. Patients recovered rapidly and the results were pleasing. Lipolysis has been extended to more areas of the body and many patients now request treatment of multiple areas. Cautious scheduling is required, however, to allow for a prolonged recovery period with adequate colloid and electrolyte replacement. When removing very large

volumes of fat, patients are admitted overnight into an intermediate skilled nursing center. Patients from out-of-town also use this facility.

There is no claim made in this chapter for developing unique positions or approaches, as similar ones have been used in France for years. The simple modifications outlined, however, have facilitated safe and effective outpatient surgery with reduced costs.

Pretunneling

BACKGROUND

Since the introduction of the Illouz technique for lipolysis in the United States, the technique has become widely accepted and the list of enthusiasts grows daily. My experience is probably typical—initial skepticism, followed by enthusiastic application, followed by some frustration in trying to achieve perfectly smooth results with just the right amount of resection. Most surgeons experienced in the technique would probably agree that there is room for refinement of the technique or equipment or both.

One such refinement, which has been a great aid in my practice, is extensive pretunneling before using the suction cannula. This addition is especially helpful to those less experienced in the technique, but also should be useful even to experienced surgeons.

RATIONALE

Early experience was fraught not only with some uncertainty, but also with difficulty in making the cannula passages on an even plane beneath the skin. Since the hole in the cannula is directed downward and fat is removed from below, the passages should be made on a plane that is even with the deepest point in the fat surrounding the prominence to be removed (Fig. 18-11). It would seem that the more evenly and finely the tissue is penetrated with tunnels, the smoother the result (Fig. 18-12).

This technique proved difficult with full suction applied. Ultimately, some passages are made in areas not desired, and fat is being resected all the while. The same often occurs when the cannula becomes trapped around either a dense band or a firm accumulation of fat. These problems are easily avoided by pretunneling in a precisely controlled plane.

Most surgeons performing lipolysis have occasionally seen more bleeding than desired and perhaps some temporary postoperative numbness. The technique is based on the principle of passage of a blunt instrument that spares the larger vessels and nerves. These structures would seem to be more vulnerable when splinted by surrounding fat and connective tissue on the initial

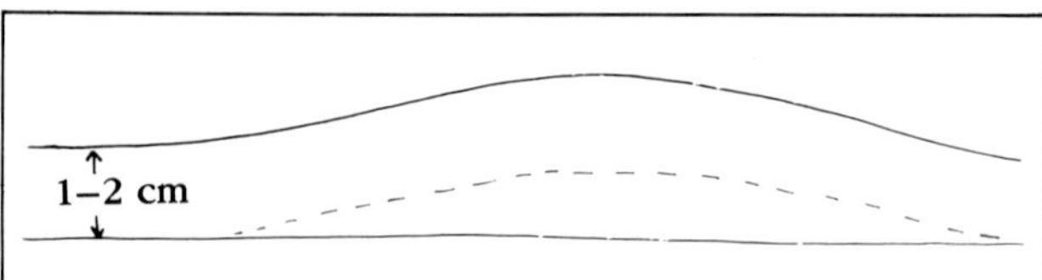

Fig. 18-11. The dotted line represents the approximate level at which the tunnels are created. The fat resection is done below this level.

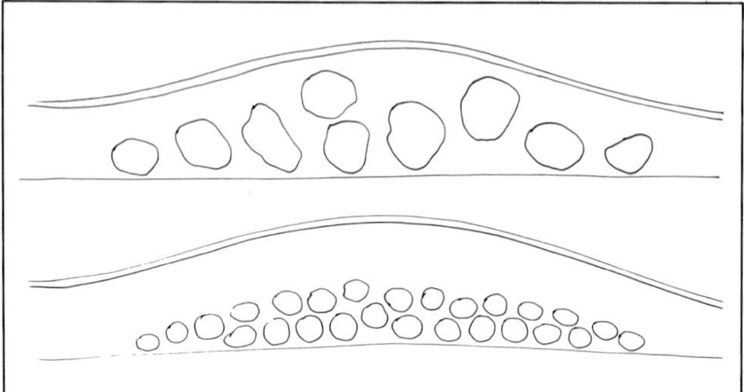

Fig. 18-12. Top. Random tunneling with a large cannula tends to create areas of adjacent over- and underresection. Bottom. The goal is to finely and evenly perforate the tissue, resulting in a smoother resection.

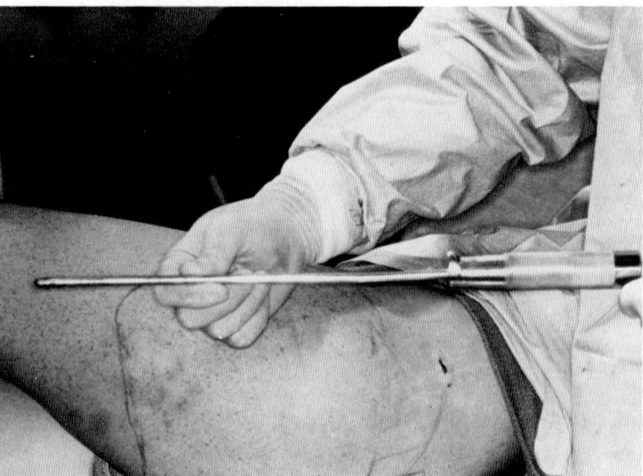

Fig. 18-13. Custom-made 6-mm pretunneling instrument.

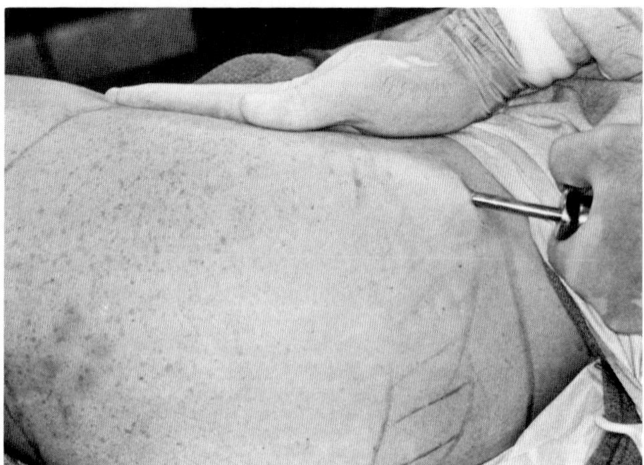

Fig. 18-14. Note the even passage of the pretunneler. Passage is facilitated by stretching the tissue tightly over the curvature of the area being worked on.

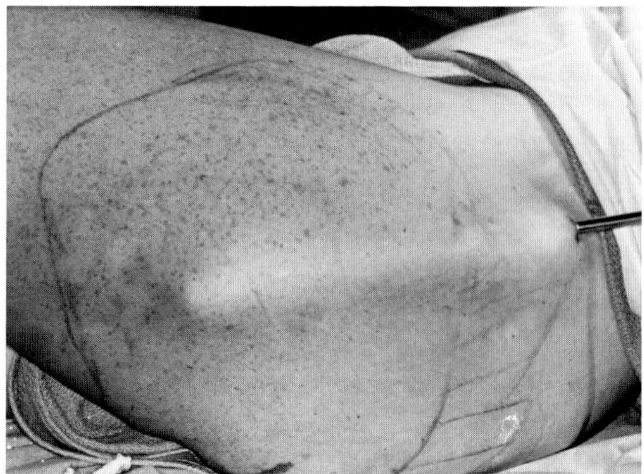

Fig. 18-15. When the instrument is lifted, the overlying layer of fat is shown in relief. Irregularities become obvious.

thrust of a suction cannula. Pretunneling with a smaller, highly polished smooth instrument frees these structures before they are subjected to the cannula. In my opinion, there has been a decrease in bleeding associated with pretunneling.

Another difficulty with the Illouz technique has been the surgeon's physical exhaustion. It is typical to develop a soaking sweat and tremor that interferes with any kind of delicate work following the performance of a lipolysis procedure. The pretunneling procedure is done slowly, carefully, and with minimal exertion. If the pretunneling is performed adequately, the lipectomy is done with less effort.

TECHNIQUE

After making the incision, usually a stab wound with a #15 blade, a 6-mm pretunneler with a hemispheric tip (Fig. 18-13) is introduced to the desired level (usually between 1 and 2 cm deep for the abdominal, iliac, and lateral thigh areas). The instrument is slowly and carefully worked along, controlling the depth by stretching the tissue away from the tip with the free hand (Fig. 18-14) and raising or lowering the instrument tip. After the instrument is advanced the desired distance, it is elevated (Fig. 18-15); showing the thickness of the overlying fat and revealing any irregularities. If there are thin or thick spots, the instrument is withdrawn and read-

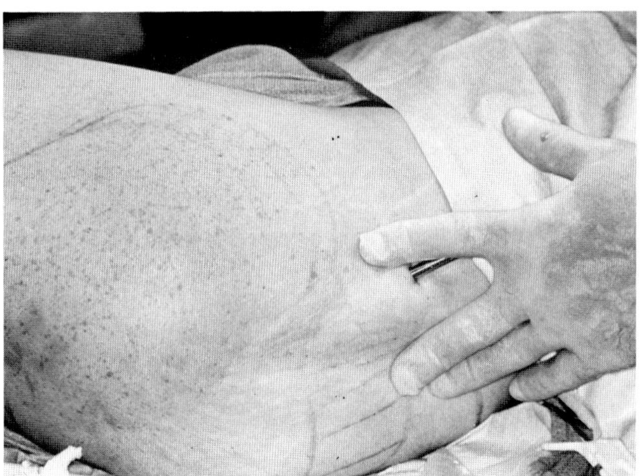

Fig. 18-16. Note the fine dimpling commonly seen when the instrument is at the correct depth.

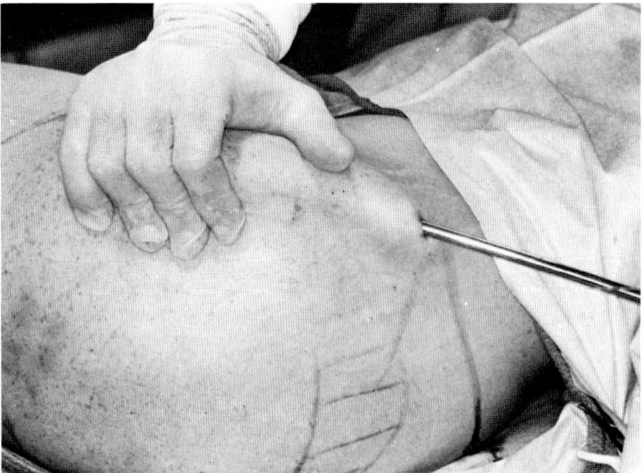

Fig. 18-17. Firm or dense accumulations of fat may be splinted as shown to allow penetration by the pretunneler.

vanced in a manner compensating for the deficient areas. There will usually be a faint dimpling over the instrument as it is advanced when it is at the correct level (Fig. 18-16). This procedure is repeated in adjacent tissue carefully and repeatedly.

Once the whole area has been treated, the instrument is passed repeatedly in the plane until there is very smooth passage over the entire area with no resistance. Occasionally, some stubborn areas are encountered. These areas may be broken up by pinching up the area between the fingers and the palm and by passing the tip directly into the tissue that is now firmly trapped (Fig. 18-17).

The suction cannula (usually 8 mm) is then introduced and the suction extraction is performed with ease, control, and rapidity. With practice, even difficult areas such as the area immediately around the navel or near the infragluteal fold become quite easy to deal with. In my experience, pretunneling has reduced bleeding and provided more uniform, smooth results. The procedure has been more gratifying than the Illouz technique since there is a greater sense of control and much less effort is required.

CHAPTER 19

Dressings and Garments

Carson M. Lewis

Lipolysis is different from any other surgical procedure. In conventional surgery, we make incisions and under direct visualization perform sharp dissection with ligation or cauterization of bleeding points. In contrast, in lipolysis we insert a blunt cannula through a small incision. With force the cannula is pushed through the subcutaneous tissues, avulsing fragments of fat. Bleeding is minimal as the vessels are generally preserved. Fat is pulled into the cannula by a high-powered suction apparatus and avulsed by the vigorous stroking maneuver. The procedure is similar to sawing wood; the inexperienced surgeon is often surprised at how much energy is required. The passage of the cannula through the subcutaneous tissue is traumatic. Fat cells are removed leaving tunnels, and many of the remaining cells are injured. The result has been described as a *crush-type injury.* A pathological phenomenon causes increased permeability of the capillary wall and massive transudation and extravasation of plasma- and electrolyte-bearing fluid [1]. The comparison of the pathological condition varies from the type of crush injury caused by a person being partially buried, as described by Bywaters and Boyer [2], in that there generally is no associated muscle injury or renal dysfunction produced by lipolysis.

Compression dressings are applied to the operative site to minimize the egress of tissue fluid and to decrease morbidity. In addition, the other benefits from dressings include the splinting of the part to reduce pain, an absorbent surface for any oozing fluid, and the dressings provide a barrier against infection.

Compression may be applied by elastic tape to the operative site. A second method of dressing is the use of a compression garment, providing circumferential pressure around the part and theoretically, at least, advantages over the tape.

The type of dressing applied varies among surgeons and includes (1) elastic tape, (2) compression garment, or (3) a combination of the two.

Elastic Tape Dressing

HISTORY

From the beginning, the French pioneer operators have used a 4-inch elastic dressing applied to the operative site while the patient was still on the operating table. Their tape is French Elastoplast Hypoallergique.* American tape is available as Elastikon (Johnson & Johnson) and Elastoplast.

---

*Available from Laboratories Fisch, Rue De La Riviere 72320 Vibraye, France.

TECHNIQUE

Taping of the operative site is performed in the following manner:

1. The skin is washed with saline to remove any dried blood or other debris and dried.
2. A solution of acetone or ether is applied to remove any oil from the skin.
3. A tape adherent—Mastisol, tincture of benzoin, or Aeroplast spray—may be applied to the skin. Allow the substance to dry before applying the tape. Be aware of any allergies to such skin substances.
4. The tape is applied to the operative site, extending for several inches beyond the operated area in a criss-cross or a figure-of-eight fashion. An experienced operative team will precut tape so the surgeon can apply the strips rapidly. The tape is applied and placed under modest tension, contouring the part as desired.
5. No adhesive tape is placed at the edges of the elastic tape; otherwise, blisters and skin burns result.

SPECIFIC AREAS

Lateral Femoral and Iliac Crest Roll

The lateral femoral and iliac crest roll are the most common areas treated and are frequently treated in combination. The dressing recommended initially by Yves-Gerard Illouz (Fig. 19-1A, B) has not been changed appreciably. With the patient in the prone position, 2 to 3 short strips of 4-inch tape are applied, beginning at the gluteal crease and continuing down the posterior aspect of the leg beyond the area of dissection. On the lateral thigh, beginning below the dissection, a long strip is applied and carried up cranially over the lateral femoral area, above the buttocks, and connected in the midline of the lower back. Contouring of the operative site can be performed by this maneuver to elevate the skin and subcutaneous tissue in a cranial fashion. Other short strips of tape over the iliac crest can be brought together in the midline, providing one continuous support dressing. It is important to tape the gluteal area if a new gluteal crease has been created.

Abdomen, Chest Wall, Lower Extremities, Knees, and Ankles

Taping can be performed in a criss-cross fashion, one to two layers extending beyond the dissection and *not* circumferentially. Circumferential dressings have the danger of restricting venous return and producing edema.

Neck and Face

The neck can be taped with a 2- to 3-inch tape contoured over the central neck extending up onto the cheeks. Areas of the face can be taped away from the midline in an upward pull similar to the pull from the face-lift.

Upper Arm

If tape is applied to the upper arm, it is done over the operative area and not circumferentially. The area is covered with a Kling or Curlex dressing not tight enough to restrict venous return.

Axillary Breast and Lateral Chest Wall

This area is commonly done in combination with reduction mammoplasty. Elastic tape of appropriate width is applied to the operative site to provide compression of the tissue.

REMOVAL OF TAPE

The tape is removed on approximately the seventh day. Some substances have been used to aid in tape removal:

1. Mineral oil. The patient is instructed to obtain a pint of mineral oil from the drugstore, lubricate the tape well while resting in the bathtub, and remove the tape. Another person present is most beneficial to help the patient to remove the tape and to get out of the bathtub because it is quite slippery from the oil. The patient must use extreme care to avoid injury.

2. Acetone or ether. Patients have successfully applied acetone or ether to help dissolve the adherence of the tape. The problems involved are that acetone and ether remove fingernail polish, and if any drops of liquid contact the genital area, they will cause considerable burning. Smoking and fire must be avoided.

3. Several patients have removed the tape satisfactorily without the use of substances, particularly if the areas are small and the tape is minimal.

DISADVANTAGES OF ELASTIC TAPE

The use of bulky tape prevents movement of the patients in a standing, sitting, and walking position. Discomfort is also associated with the use of tape, caused by the pulling and bulkiness of the dressing. In addition, removal of the tape is a tedious and somewhat painful procedure. Tape is recommended in the following circumstances:

1. After the creation of a gluteal crease, tape should be applied to cause adherence of the tissue and to maintain this crease.

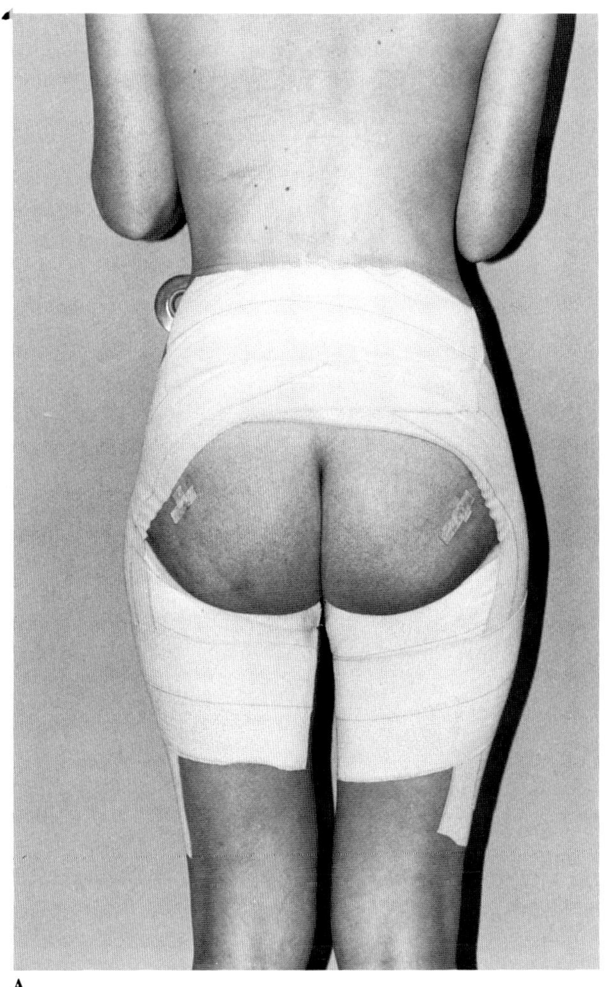

A

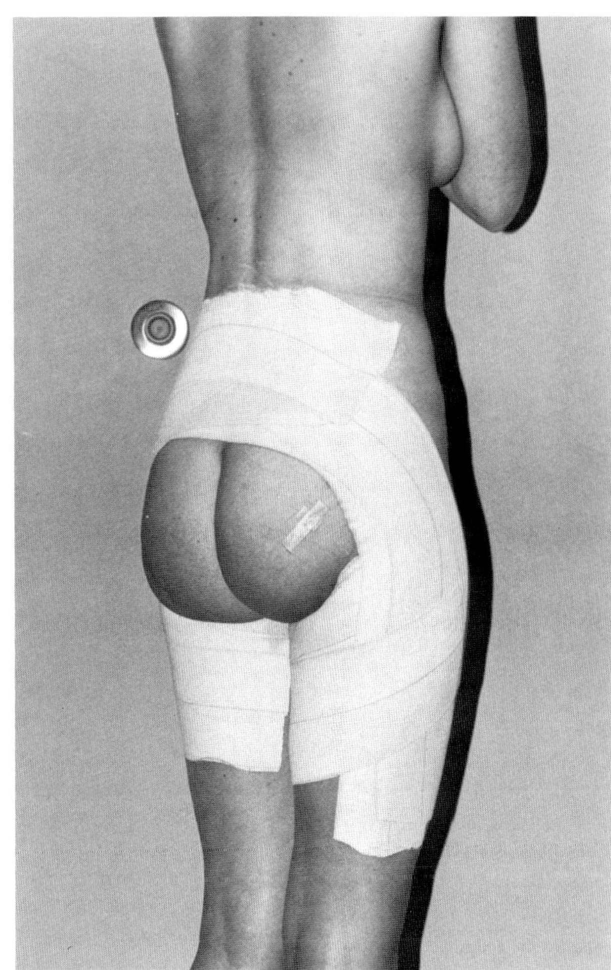

B

Fig. 19-1. A, B. Elastic tape dressing recommended initially by Dr. Illouz.

2. In the presence of laxity of the skin, tape is used to help contour [3]. Obviously, tape can only do so much. Major skin excesses require excision of skin.
3. When no garment is available.
4. At the surgeon's preference.

Compression Garments

HISTORY AND TYPES AVAILABLE

Shortly after the introduction of the lipolysis procedure in the United States, several surgeons, including Drs. Robert Winslow from Raleigh, North Carolina, and Richard Morris from Virginia Beach, Virginia, began using compression garments, seeing advantages over elastic tape. Girdles as elastic garments were available through stores such as Sears and J. C. Penney. These garments have the advantage of low cost (approximately $15 each), and patients can select their own garment preoperatively. The garment should fit, but not too snugly to allow for postoperative swelling. One disadvantage of these store-made garments is a closed crotch. Some means must be found to facilitate urination and defecation, either by pulling down the garment or cutting out the crotch area. Another difficulty has been placing the patient in the garment while still asleep. Some surgeons wait until the patient can assist in its application, and others apply the garment immediately in the operating room. An innovative idea is to place the garment over the feet or knees before beginning the operative procedure [4]. Then the garment is pulled up over the operative site at the completion of the procedure before transferring the patient from the operating room table.

GARMENTS MANUFACTURED SPECIFICALLY FOR LIPOLYSIS

Garments specifically for lipolysis procedures are made by three companies. Two garments were designed by nurses working with plastic surgeons, and one garment was designed by a surgeon. The companies are

Name of Company	*Location*	*Originator*
Caromed Company	4105 Yadkin Drive Raleigh, NC 27609	Barbara Beck, R.N.
Circumpress	1625 Godfrey Lane Virginia Beach, VA 23454	Kathy Morris, R.N.
Electric Enterprise	Scurlock Tower Suite 1730 6560 Fannin Houston, TX 77030	Joe Agris, M.D.

There are an array of garments to fit various areas. Primarily the garments are used for the abdomen, lateral femoral, and iliac crest rolls. The garments vary in size, from small to extra large, and in their length, some above the knee and others below the knee. Closures vary from garment to garment. Some use Velcro, others hooks and eyes, and others zippers. Some garments have a combination of closures. A typical lipolysis garment is seen in Figure 19-2A, B, C.

ADVANTAGES

1. Circumferential pressure. Theoretically, it is an advantage to apply pressure from all directions instead of just over the operative site.

2. Less restricting than elastic tape.

3. More comfortable. Some patients report more comfort and security from compression garments. The garment can be removed as needed.

DISADVANTAGES

1. Fit. Apparently, most manufacturers' garments do not fit well despite multiple sizes. The garments fail to fit uniformly in all areas and often are loose about the knee and upper abdomen. Although manufacturers have attempted to provide multiple sizes, proper fit still remains a problem in many patients. Solutions include (1) rolling down the garment, (2) cutting the garment and fashioning it for the individual, or (3) the use of accessory garments (upper abdomen and chest) to provide supplementary support.

2. Open crotch. Many patients voice problems with urination and defecation with the garments in place despite the presence of an open crotch. The openings are not well placed or are too small. The store-made garments, of course, have no crotch opening. Several alternatives have been used in the past including opening the crotch wider or pulling the garment down to perform bodily functions. Another innovative suggestion used by one patient was the use of a funnel to urinate [4].

3. Discomfort. Some garments were reported as producing an itching sensation, which was reduced with washing, or of being very hot during the warm summer months, particularly in the southern part of the United States.

4. Cost. Store girdles are approximately $15; special lipolysis garments are between $20 and $45.

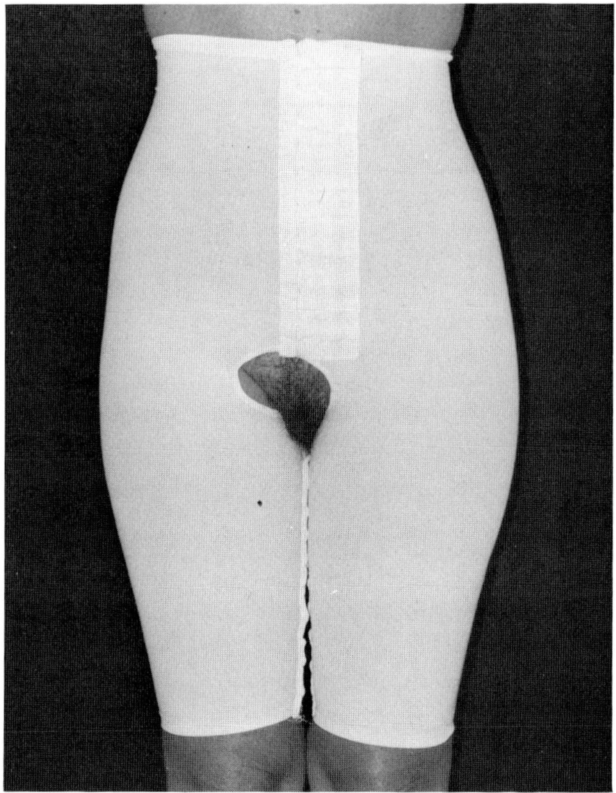

A

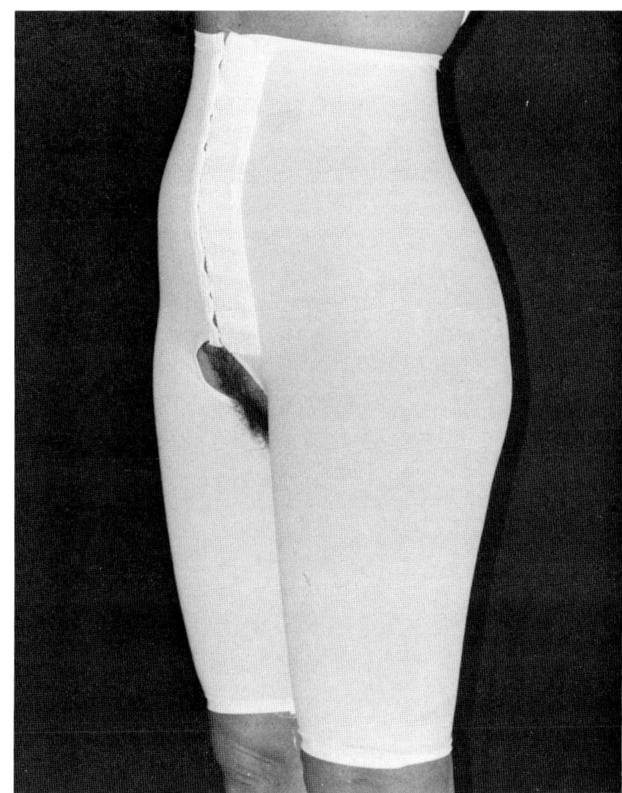

B

Fig. 19-2. A, B, C. Typical garment specifically for lipolysis procedures.

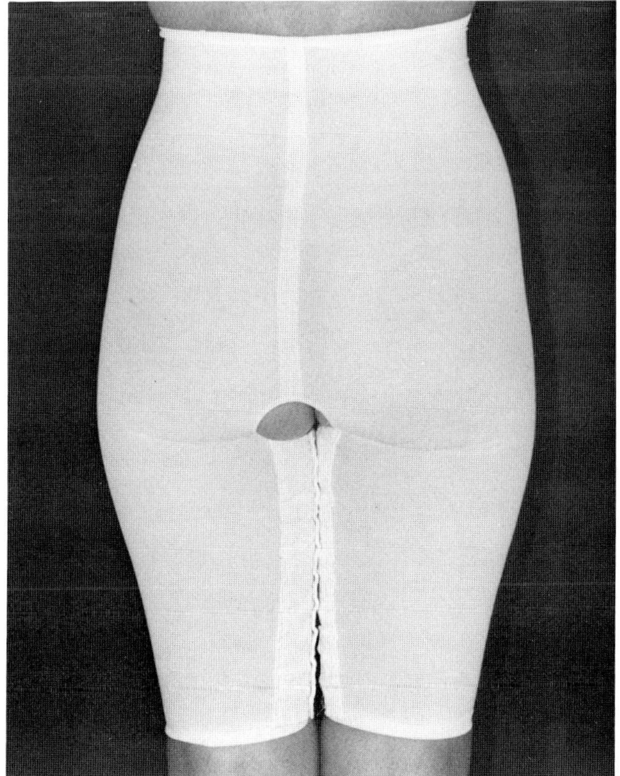

C

Combination of Tape and Compression Garment

Some surgeons have combined the two dressings, applying the tape then the garment. Some apply a few strips of tapes; others apply the standard taping.

VARIATIONS

1. Micropore tape is sometimes used instead of the elastic tape [5]; some surgeons believe the micropore tape is as effective and softer and allows skin to breathe.

2. ABD. Placed under compression garment over operative areas that have increased height or tissue reaction. Used to apply added pressure [5].

3. Massage and ultrasound. Used in the postoperative period beginning 10 to 14 days after the operation (see Chap. 22).

ACCESSORY GARMENTS

Accessory garments designed for the upper abdomen and lower chest are available in combination for support to these areas. Garments are also available for the face and neck. Accessory garments for the male for the upper abdomen can be used in conjunction with the standard garments for the abdomen and thigh.

Opinions About the Garments and Dressings

In questioning patients regarding garments, opinions vary widely. Some patients choose to wear their garments after the required time, feeling the garments provide support. Others discard them as soon as possible. The use of two garments, one clean while the other one was worn, appeared to be better than the use of a single garment.

There appears to be a great deal of variation in opinion as to what is the best dressing. Some believe that compression is superior, and others feel that tape offers more support and advantages. There appears to be no best way. A certain amount of trial and error is necessary to arrive at the method that is best for the surgeon and the patient.

References

1. Weeks, S. R. The crush syndrome. *Surg. Gynecol. Obstet.* 127:369, 1968.
2. Bywaters, E. G. L., and Beall, D. Crush injuries with impairment of renal function. *Br. Med. J.* 41:4185, 1941.
3. Herhahn, F. T. Third Teaching Symposium of the Lipolysis Society of North America. Albuquerque, New Mexico. November 1983.
4. Burkhardt, B. R. Personal Communication. March 1984.
5. Wall, S. Third Teaching Symposium of the Lipolysis Society of North America. Albuquerque, New Mexico. November 1983.

CHAPTER 20

Blood Chemistry Changes After Lipolysis

Frank T. Herhahn

The first international symposium on lipolysis was presented in Paris, France, in June 1982, under the guidance of Drs. Yves-Gerard Illouz and Pierre Fournier. The information gained during that symposium was presented in a clinical atmosphere with relatively brief mention as to physiological changes occurring in patients undergoing this procedure.

To allay our own fears of the unknown of such a technique, especially when applied to major fat resections, Dr. Gregory P. Hetter and I felt that certain laboratory parameters needed investigation. These concerns were reinforced by the research and education committees of the involved hospitals when seeking privileges for a new technique in North America. While verifying the French indications for this technique, safety in patient selection was felt to be of paramount importance. With the assistance of other specialties, that is, general surgery, pulmonary, and internal medicine, a protocol was developed to study the first 50 patients undergoing this procedure.

With the assistance of these disciplines, the protocol established relatively conservative guidelines for patient selection. This protocol included limiting patients to 40 years of age or younger who were in good general health and possessed only moderate contour deformities. Criteria were expanded as experience was gained in the safety of this procedure in patients with underlying organic disease such as mild to moderate obesity and hypertension.

Laboratory Parameters

After interdisciplinary discussions, the following laboratory parameters were felt to be necessary: urinalysis, complete blood count, and a SMAC chemistry panel consisting of total serum protein evaluation, electrolytes, triglycerides, cholesterol, and serum liver enzymes. In addition to these basic laboratory tests, a smaller group of patients was selected on whom arterial blood gases were obtained, as well as a lipid profile. The basic laboratory determinations were obtained preoperatively, 24 to 48 hours postoperatively, and approximately 7 days postoperatively. Arterial blood gases were obtained at 3 to 5 hours postoperatively in an attempt to determine subclinical changes in arterial profusion that might indicate early or subclinical evidence of pulmonary fat embolization.

Of all of these laboratory studies, significant changes were noted in the hemoglobin and hematocrit and lesser changes in the total serum protein, serum albumin, calcium, and lactic acid dehydrogenase (LDH). No changes were noted in the urinalysis either pre- or postoperatively.

Table 20-1. Comparison of hemoglobin and hematocrit changes after lipolysis with and without epinephrine

	Without epinephrine		With epinephrine	
	Preoperative	Postoperative	Preoperative	Postoperative
Hgb	14.0	11.0	14.2	12.4
Hct	42%[a]	36%	42%[b]	37%

Hgb = hemoglobin; Hct = hematocrit.
[a] 1180 ml average emulsion removal.
[b] 1263 ml average emulsion.

Table 20-2. Comparison of changes in total serum protein fractions after lipolysis with and without epinephrine

	Without epinephrine			With epinephrine	
Protein fraction	Preoperative	Postoperative	Normal	Preoperative	Postoperative
Protein	6.7	6.0	5.5–7.5	7.0	6.5
Albumin	4.2	4.0	3.0–4.6	4.4	4.0
Globulin	2.4	2.3	2.0–3.6	2.5	2.5
Calcium	9.4	9.0	8.5–10.6	9.3	9.0

Table 20-3. Comparison of serum enzyme levels after lipolysis with and without epinephrine

	Without epinephrine			With epinephrine	
Enzyme	Preoperative	Postoperative	Normal	Preoperative	Postoperative
Alkaline phosphatase	40.0	42.0	20–90	34.0	35.0
SGPT	8.0	11.5	0–24	11.0	9.9
SGOT	5.0	20.0	0–24	14.2	14.7
LDH	94.0	123.0	50–150	83.0	109.0

SGPT = serum glutamic pyruvic transaminase; SGOT = serum glutamic oxaloacetic transaminase; LDH = lactic acid dehydrogenase.

Blood counts showed a slight increase in the white cell count and a differential that was consistent with the degree of tissue trauma and therefore unremarkable. Red cell mass loss was more significant and reflected this relationship: a hematocrit drop of 1% was seen for every 90 ml ± 30 ml of fat emulsion removed by the lipolysis technique in those patients undergoing a fat removal of greater than 500 ml. This hematocrit drop was significantly reduced in 1983 when the basic Illouz formula for lipolysis was modified by Hetter (see Chap. 15). This change in solution incorporated the use of a solution of Lidocaine 0.25% with epinephrine 1:400,000. Laboratory data gained with this modified formula revealed that 140 ml ± 30 ml of fat emulsion could be removed before reducing the hematocrit by 1% in those patients undergoing a fat removal of greater than 500 ml (Table 20-1).

Total serum proteins dropped slightly in both groups, with the major drop reflected in the serum albumin fraction (Table 20-2). A concomitant drop in the serum calcium was noted and was readily explained by the parallel drop of serum albumin. Serum calcium is bound to the albumin fraction; consequently, a drop in the serum albumin is accompanied by a concurrent drop in the serum calcium. At no time did the serum calcium level drop to a degree to become clinically significant.

Serum cholesterol and triglyceride levels rose and fell in the two series in an unpredictable fashion. These data were not felt to be significant by the evaluation of the multidisciplinary team assessing the laboratory results.

Serum enzyme studies were likewise unaffected, except for a slight rise in the LDH fraction, which again was felt to be related to the degree of tissue destruction (Table 20-3). Similarly, in a smaller series of patients

Table 20-4. Measurement of arterial blood gases

	Postoperative	Normal
pH	7.44	7.32–7.48
PCO_2	33.79	28–38
PO_2	76.20	64–80
HCO_3	22.40	17–25
O_2SAT	93.20	86.0–96.5

undergoing lipid profile studies, no significant changes were seen between the pre- and postoperative results. These studies were abandoned as a necessary laboratory parameter early in the investigation.

Arterial blood gases drawn in the recovery room between the third and fifth postoperative hour were found consistently to fall within a normal range. No patients, either in the original series or subsequently, have shown evidence (either clinical or subclinical) of fat embolization (Table 20-4).

Crude measurements of the hematocrit of the fat emulsion during the earlier series demonstrated a 20 to 25% red cell mass in the fat emulsion. After Dr. Hetter modified the Illouz solution by adding dilute epinephrine, this figure dropped to below 15%. This drop was felt to be a significant improvement and became the single most important argument for the wet technique of lipolysis.

After these data were presented to the research committees, along with an evaluation of general patient results and satisfaction, the technique was released from investigational status in January 1984. The results of this review by members outside the field of plastic surgery favorably supported the basic technique as advocated by Dr. Illouz, including his general recommendations for fluid, colloid, and blood replacement, as well as indications for hospitalization.

Summary

Patients undergoing lipolysis in 1982 and early 1983 underwent a number of laboratory tests in an attempt to determine physiological changes secondary to moderate amounts of fat removal. Significant drops in the hematocrit and hemoglobin values reflect the marked degree of red cell loss that may occur with this procedure. This occurrence could result in a shock syndrome, leading to significant complications if the surgeon is not prepared and not looking for it.

Minor changes in the serum albumin and serum calcium have been noted but have not been prolonged problems. Postoperative arterial blood gases have remained normal and have lent support to the claim by others that fat embolism does not seem to occur with this technique.

CHAPTER 21

Nutritional Support of Surgical Recovery

Patrick Quillin

Research in the past two decades has shown a definite relationship between the well-nourished patient and a rapid recovery from surgery [1,2]. Conversely, the malnourished patient heals slowly, with an elevated risk of infection [3]. Studies have shown extensive malnutrition of hospital patients [4]. The typical American diet is lacking in various nutrients [5]. This chapter summarizes the relationship between rapid recovery from surgery and an optimal nutrition program.

There are at least 45 known essential nutrients required by the human body. Each of these dietary essentials contributes, at least indirectly, to the healing processes. Some of these nutrients, for example, ascorbic acid, protein, and zinc, have a direct influence on the anabolic phases of tissue repair. These three nutrients are discussed in some detail in this chapter, yet keep in mind that *all* other nutrients must be present for anabolism to occur at a maximal level.

The continuum concept illustrates the limitless shades of gray between black and white. Likewise, there are numerous degrees of well-being between death and optimal health. There are also various degrees of nourishment between total deprivation and optimal nutrition. Many patients are marginally nourished [4]. Their current intake of nutrients allows them to function in their normal activities, yet is insufficient for rapid recovery following the physiological stress of surgery. Most patients will recover eventually; with optimal nourishment, however, they will recover more rapidly and with a lower risk of infection.

The physiology and biochemistry of wound healing indicate that certain nutrients are more important than others. Tissue repair requires the proper ratio of free amino acids and pyridoxine (B_6) for their transamination, ascorbic acid for the hydroxylation of proline and lysine ("adhesive" proteins found in high levels in collagen), and zinc as a critical cofactor in enzymes that activate protein synthesis [6]. Surgical patients are also at risk for infections, although the risk is minor with proper aseptic conditions. Body defense mechanisms include (1) mechanical (intact epithelial surfaces, mucous barriers, digestive enzymes), and (2) humoral (gamma-globulins) [4]. Each of these defense mechanisms requires protein, ascorbic acid, and zinc as precursors. These nutrients are involved both in wound healing and in preventing infections.

Protein

As the primary constituent of regenerating tissue, elevated intake is recommended for pre- and postsurgical patients. Protein requirements for the average healthy adult are calculated at 1 g/kg of body weight/day [5].

Increasing this amount by 50 to 100% for optimal wound healing enables anabolism to proceed unimpeded by amino acid deficiency [2]. A 160-pound (73 kg) healthy adult normally requires 73 g of protein per day to maintain balance. The additional 50 to 100% adds 36 to 73 g per day for a total pre- and postsurgical diet of 109 to 146 g per day (depending on the extent of tissue regeneration necessary). Grams of protein should not be confused with grams of foodstuffs.

Ascorbic Acid

Although healthy adults receiving large supplements of vitamin C usually excrete most of it, the surgical patient has been proved to need significantly elevated levels of ascorbic acid [7]. Studies show that 500 to 3000 mg per day are effective supplement levels for rapid tissue regeneration [7]. With minimal contraindications, and good evidence that additional vitamin C speeds recovery time, ascorbic acid supplements before and after surgery are highly recommended.

Zinc

Zinc is found in at least 60 different enzyme systems in the human body and plays a significant role in healing and in natural immunity from infection [5]. The recommended daily allowance (RDA) for zinc is 15 mg per day. Dietary surveys have shown a common deficiency in the American population. Zinc supplements of 50 to 660 mg per day have been shown to be effective in accelerating wound healing [8]. Excess zinc (400 mg/day) for more than a few weeks has been shown to alter blood lipid profiles (lowers high-density lipoproteins) [9]. Therefore, zinc supplements (as zinc sulfate) should be monitored by the physician. Studies indicate that the efficacy of zinc during healing is highest in the second half of the healing phase (epithelialization phase).

Iron

At least half of all female lipolysis candidates show a low or borderline serum iron and all show a postoperative iron deficit. Therefore, iron supplements begun before surgery and continued after surgery will shorten the anemic phase.

Foodstuffs

The patient should always attempt to obtain nutrients with a "fork and spoon" if at all possible. Ideally, the physician refers the patient to a dietitian/nutritionist before surgery. The patient can prepare his or her body for surgery by consuming the proper quality and quantity of nutrients. Patient compliance in following dietary instructions is sporadic, however. For this reason, food should be encouraged as the primary source of nutrition. Supplemental pills can be prescribed for their auxiliary effect during the healing phase.

Studies have shown that people with ideal nutrition heal in as much as 50% less time than control groups of the standard North American food and life style. Optimal nutrition includes:

1. Presurgical dietary consult for proper dietary recommendations.
2. Pre- and postsurgical prescription for:
   a. 500 to 3000 mg per day extra ascorbic acid (divided doses with meals)
   b. 50 to 660 mg per day extra zinc sulfate in divided doses
   c. Iron supplement as sulfate or gluconate, 325 mg twice a day with meals
   d. 50 to 100% extra protein from food sources
   e. A broad-spectrum, low-potency vitamin-mineral supplement

The lipolysis patient started on this regimen 2 weeks before surgery and continued for 4 weeks after surgery should have a more rapid healing process and less sense of fatigue (see Chap. 23).

References

1. Goodhart, R., and Shils, M. *Modern Nutrition in Health and Disease.* Philadelphia: Lea & Febiger, 1976.
2. Mitchell, Rynbergen, Anderson, and Dibble, *Nutrition n Health and Disease.* Philadelphia: Lippincott, 1976.
3. Butterworth, C. The Skeleton in the Hospital Closet. *Nutrition Today.* March 1974, pp. 4–8.
4. Butterworth, C., and Blackburn, G. Hospital Malnutrition. *Nutrition Today.* March 1975, pp. 8–18.
5. Guthrie, H. *Introductory Nutrition.* St. Louis: Mosby, 1983.
6. Lehninger, A. Biochemistry. New York: Worth Publishing, 1975.
7. Ringsdorf, W., and Cheraskin, E. Vitamin C and human wound healing. *Oral Surg.* March 1982. P. 231–236.
8. Liszewski, R. The effect of zinc on wound healing: A collective review. *J.A.O.A.* 81(2):104.
9. Hooper, Visconti, Garry, and Johnson. Zinc lowers high-density lipoprotein-cholesterol levels. *J.A.M.A.* 244(17): 1960, 1980.

CHAPTER 22

Massage and Ultrasound

Carson M. Lewis
Margaret Pruitt

Although patients are informed preoperatively that satisfactory results after lipolysis require 6 weeks or longer, it is not uncommon for them to become anxious in the immediate postoperative period. With the removal of the elastic support dressings at the end of 1 week, the patient sees a bruised, swollen postoperative site and feels soreness. With this traumatized appearance, the circumference may be larger than preoperatively and becomes a focus of concern on the part of the patient. Coupled with this "ugly" appearance, the patient may experience fatigue and depression, particularly when large quantities of fat have been removed. The patient may ask, "Was I wise to have this operation?"

What can we do to help the patient in the immediate postoperative period? Concern and reassurance are helpful. Other therapeutic modalities are beneficial at this time. We have used forms of physical medicine to enhance healing and to provide psychological support for the patient. Treatments used are massage and ultrasound. Their use by experienced personnel provides multiple benefits to the patient.

Benefits

The physical benefits of massage and ultrasound include a reduction in soreness. Most patients are stiff and sore after the operative procedure. This soreness is frequently described as similar to using a muscle not exercised recently. With the use of massage, the soreness disappears during the massage treatment and may not return for several hours. The swelling in the tissue can actually be measurably reduced during a treatment. The tense tissue may be softened and more pliable at the completion of the massage. Bruising and ecchymosis are improved noticeably after treatment by the movement of the bloody and lymphatic elements from the tissue. Subcutaneous knots that occur due to the traumatized fat can be softened and reduced by a series of treatments.

Of equal importance to the physical benefits are the psychological rewards. Simply touching the patient has a therapeutic value. The patient senses a caring and concern on the part of the physician and the staff. Patients are seen frequently in order to perform these treatments, which enhances the feeling of caring. A great benefit is that the therapist provides frequent opportunity for patients to communicate with someone with knowledge. They can express their feelings, including their frustrations and any disappointments, which, in itself, is therapeutic. The benefits from the treatment are immediate and provide a psychological boost. At this time, the patient is encouraged repeatedly not to be critical of the results until at least 6 weeks postoperatively.

The physician benefits indirectly by the use of massage and ultrasound. Mundane questions are answered by the therapist, thereby freeing the physician of this time-consuming task. This is not to say that the doctor should be unavailable to his or her patients during this period. The physician should see these patients approximately once a week. By using physical treatment, the physician will find that patient visits are shorter and the patients are in a good mood, sensing that something is being done to promote their recovery.

Massage

Massage is a term used to signify a group of systematic scientific manipulations of body tissue that are performed with the hands. It is probably the oldest of all remedies. The oldest written record was made some 3000 years ago by the Chinese. Other societies, including ancient Hindus, Persians, and Egyptians, recorded some form of manipulations for ailments. Hippocrates wrote important papers about massage. Two centuries ago, Chinese books on massage were translated into French, which accounts for the French terminology used in massage texts [1]. The physiological effects of massage occur in two ways. First, by reflex action through the nerves, the brain causes relaxation of muscle, dilation of arterioles, decrease in sensation, and a reduction in mental tension. Second, the mechanical effects include the increase in circulation of blood and lymph and an increase in body heat. Techniques should be performed with the patient in a relaxed and comfortable position, without tight clothing. The therapist should be relaxed and comfortable in a position where he or she can easily perform the service. The technique requires skill rather than strength. Training is important. It should not be done by an inexperienced or untrained person. The lubricating creams consist of a mineral oil base, which facilitates a good technique. The types of massage used include various forms of effleurage and pétrissage. Effleurage consists of (1) a superficial stroke of extremely light pressure, using the entire palmar surface of the hand, and (2) a deep stroke with sufficient pressure to produce mechanical as well as reflex effects. For deep stroking, the palmar surface of the whole hand, finger, or thumb is used in the direction of venous circulation.

Pétrissage includes kneading and friction. Kneading is primarily used and is described as a motion in which the soft tissues are picked up between the fingers or hands and manipulated in an alternating fashion. It does not need to proceed in a particular direction but must be followed by effleurage, which is always in a centripetal direction. Friction is especially used on adhesions, scar tissue, and nodules. It is a rapid circular motion performed by placing a small part of the hand, usually the thumb, on the area with steadily increasing pressure [2].

Ultrasound

Ultrasound is the use of acoustic vibrations (sound waves) as a therapeutic modality. These sound waves are propagated as longitudinal compression waves. The waves are not audible to most people at 17,000 hertz (Hz). The sound passing through the tissue is converted into heat.

Ultrasound equipment consists of a generator, which produces a high-frequency alternating current from 0.8 to 1.0 MHz. The transducer converts the electric current into a mechanical acoustic vibration by means of a crystal that is inserted between two electrodes. The instrument is held in contact with the skin and moved about in motion with the skin lubricated. Reactions are due to a production of heat, which increases peripheral blood flow, and to an increased permeability in the biological membrane. This increased permeability results in a reduction of edema due to the absorption of intercellular tissue fluids [3]. Physiochemical effects include the diffusion of ions across the biological membrane.

If the instrument is placed in close proximity over bone, pain may develop. The absorption of heat in the tissue near bone is about ten times greater than in soft tissue. Our technique for the use of ultrasound is as a complementary modality prior to the use of massage. It appears that the ultrasound warms the tissues more rapidly than massage alone. When ultrasound is applied over the healing incisions, it aids in the reduction of adhesions formation. The incisions must be at least 10 to 14 days postoperative. We believe ultrasound has some beneficial effects in dissolving subcutaneous nodules.

When ultrasound was added to our therapy, we used a control to test its validity. We tested a patient whose surgical area included her knees. Both knees had subcutaneous knots and were thickened. The left knee received both ultrasound and massage. The right knee received the control massage only. Before the second treatment, the patient complained of greater sensitivity in the right knee control. By the third and fourth treatment, there was a noticeable decrease in the thickening of the left knee versus the right. The right knee remained sore. At the completion of therapy, the right knee control still had a subcutaneous knot with considerable thickening, and the left knee had no knots or thickening. We are convinced of the efficacy of ultrasound.

Regimen

The regimen of treatments is administered by a physical therapist with a positive mental attitude and enthusiasm for the procedure. In our office, the physical therapist has special knowledge and can relate well to the patient because she is a former lipolysis patient. The procedures of massage and ultrasound are started between the tenth and fourteenth postoperative days and are performed in the office. A total of eight to ten treatments are given over a 3-week period—ideally, six massages during the first 2 weeks, two the third week, and possibly two the fourth week. The treatments vary in length, depending on the number of operative sites. If two or three major areas were operated on, the treatments will last from 45 minutes to 1 hour. If fewer or smaller operative sites are involved, the treatment will require less time.

The patient undresses in a separate room, comes into the massage room, and is placed on a table in a comfortable position with the aid of pillows. Patients with lipolysis of the abdomen lie in a supine position, with a pillow supporting the head and a pillow under the knees to alleviate tension of the abdominal muscles. If multiple sites are treated, treatment begins with the patient lying in the supine position. For lateral hips and femoral areas, the patient changes from side to side with pillows between bent knees and under the head. For posterior hips and thighs, the patient lies prone with pillows under hips and lower abdomen to relieve tension of the lower back. A pillow must support the ankles and feet to reduce tension in the thighs. This position is also used for treating the posterior and medial aspect of the knees.

After positioning the patient, the areas are lubricated and ultrasound is begun at an intensity of 1 watt/cm^2. The duration is 10 minutes per side for most patients who have had surgery on two or three major surgical sites. The lubricating cream, Albolene, is a mineral oil–based coupling agent. It is used to facilitate a smooth transition from ultrasound to massage. (A water-based coupling agent transmits sound waves more efficiently but cannot be used for massage. It is not compatible when an oil base is later applied, without thoroughly rinsing the patient's skin. This has a detrimental cooling effect and causes loss of time.)

The massage follows immediately and the technique varies from the first treatment to the last. Initially, due to excessive swelling, bruising, and soreness, the patient can tolerate only two forms of effleurage, beginning with a superficial stroke that progresses into a full-handed vigorous stroke. To decrease the patient's tension, massage is initiated and completed with a superficial effleurage stroke. Effleurage is always applied in a centripetal direction to facilitate venous and lymph flow. As the patient progresses, ultrasound application is localized to only those areas that are thickened, bruised, hard, and sore. Massage time is then increased to compensate for a decrease in the ultrasound duration.

As the patient's pain threshold increases and healing progresses, pétrissage and friction are added to the regimen. After the initial effleurage, two forms of pétrissage—kneading and friction—are used. Kneading is performed intermittently with deep, vigorous, full-handed effleurage strokes to all thickened subcutaneous areas. At the onset of the fifth or sixth treatment, the patient begins to tolerate the pressure of friction to break up subcutaneous nodules. This friction must be followed by a vigorous centripetal effleurage stroke. To keep the patient relaxed, it is very important to maintain contact with the patient, even on the return strokes. This contact must be very light. At the completion of therapy treatments, the therapist may take pictures or record measurements to document the patient's progress.

The patient pays for a specific number of treatments, and this payment is included in the operative fee. If the patient misses treatments without warning, no replacement treatment is allowed. If a replacement treatment is desired, the patient pays for this as in any physical therapy regimen. Most patients preoperatively understand the procedure and the cost. They approach their physical therapy treatments enthusiastically. Many feel that this therapy is a most beneficial part of their operative experience.

Patients who have never undergone massage or ultrasound are often apprehensive at first, but they respond well and usually express that they had relief of discomfort. A comment by one patient after her first treatment: "I imagined therapy to be horribly painful since I'm so bruised and swollen, but instead it's soothing and the soreness disappears for a little while." Another patient, near the completion of therapy, stated, "I asked my daughter to hold off going shopping until today so we could go right after my massage. I couldn't make it through the afternoon otherwise. I feel less tired and irritable." The patients experience an increase in energy as well as a boost in their spirits. At the initial visit, they are very bruised and swollen. By their second or third treatment, the bruising has diminished by 50%.

Some patients who initially are skeptical about massage in the immediate postoperative period subsequently become enthusiastic about the use of massage and ultrasound and about the procedure as a whole. There is a marked reduction in soreness. Patients have diminished morbidity and are able to return sooner to activities without discomfort. The psychological benefits of providing patients with these services is immeasurable. They continue to feel cared for and any sense of neglect is prevented.

Summary

The effect of massage and ultrasound in the postoperative period has been to enhance physiological and psychological aspects of treatment after lipolysis. The effects have been gratifying to the patient and to the physician and staff. The massage and ultrasound procedures represent an integral part in the overall treatment for the patient undergoing blunt suction lipectomy.

References

1. Kottke, F. J., Stillwell, G. K., and Lehmann, J. F. *Handbook of Physical Medicine and Rehabilitation* (3rd ed.). Philadelphia: Saunders, 1982.
2. Wood, E. C., and Becker, P. D. *Beard's Massage* (2nd ed.). Philadelphia: Saunders, 1974. Pp. 9, 45, 46.
3. Summer, W., and Patrick, M. K. *Ultrasonic Therapy.* New York: Elsevier, 1964. P. 96.

CHAPTER 23

Convalescence

Gregory P. Hetter

Different surgeons in different cultural climates establish their own routines to help smooth out the postoperative course of the body sculpture patient. Even cultural differences within the United States play a role. For example, the more tradition-bound, small-town Southeast, where families have historical roots as well as a greater respect for the surgeon and his or her role, may allow for less patient "attention." On the other hand, the many transient, lonely, and alone patients without local roots, characteristic of the large Northern and Western urban centers, require physician attention to psychological and physical support normally provided by family and friends. Cultural differences outside the United States also result in variations of care regimens best adapted to the social-cultural bias of each population. Some behavioral patterns, however, recur when observing body sculpture patients. This chapter addresses these recurring patterns of behavior during convalescence.

Selection

Once again, it must be stressed that selection is the single most important step: selection of the proper patient and selection of the proper operation!

The patient who has a body image disturbance (see Chap. 7) will *never* be happy no matter what you do or how long you do it. The patient who has magical thinking and great expectations of life changes (see Chap. 12) will also never be happy. The patient must have a normal psychological makeup first and foremost.

Informed Surgeon

What is the satisfaction rate for a particular operation for a localized deformity? What do we know about the results of lipolysis applied to various body areas from the point of view of both the surgeon's and the patient's rate of satisfaction? Are some operations better accepted than others? To examine these questions, Dr. Herhahn and I developed a questionnaire that patients filled out 6 months after surgery. Approximately 150 patients were sent questionnaires and about 100 were returned. These data are the basis for a future paper, but the basic trends are clear:

1. The operation producing the greatest satisfaction and fewest postoperative complaints is lateral thigh removal.
2. The operation producing least patient satisfaction is arms, followed by calves and ankles.

3. Lipolysis of the abdomen (because of irregularity and waviness) falls in between.
4. Patients in their early twenties and older than 55 are more satisfied in general than patients between 30 and 40 years of age.

In a study of 370 patients by the board of directors of the Lipolysis Society of North America, the surgeon's evaluation of the results closely paralleled the subjective responses of the patients:

1. The lateral femoral area, iliac crest, and knees were felt to give good results most often.
2. The abdomen was an intermediate area where results were less predictably good.
3. The arms and calves were a disappointing area (remember these patients have quite a different body configuration and body image than those in group 1).
4. Combined procedures often enthused the surgeons because of the improvements they recognized as compared to their classical dermatolipectomies.

Informed Patient

The postoperative patient who has been well informed by the surgeon has a lower level of anxiety, a greater sense of confidence, and a better disposition toward the postoperative phases of discomfort. For most people, 4 to 6 weeks is a long time to wait to see results. This waiting period, as well as the time for final evaluation of, and financial arrangements for, touchups must be clear to the patient.

Informed Staff

The surgeon's staff must create a knowledgeable, supportive atmosphere regarding the phases of recovery. A staff member's round-eyed look of surprise at excessive ecchymosis on an abdomen may undermine more than just the preoperative consultation. The surgeon is obligated to train his or her staff to know the phases of recuperation that can be recognized in the postoperative lipolysis patient and how best to deal with them.

Phases of Convalescence

The phases of convalescence seen in most patients occur in a sequential fashion. They may be brief or more prolonged than outlined here, but each patient usually passes through each one. Sometimes staff or physician intervention and support may be necessary. Do not neglect the patient's nutritional status since many of these patients will have low serum iron or zinc (or both), subsequent to constant or desultory dieting as prescribed by various women's magazines. Both the physical and psychological convalescence of the patient is shortened by good nutrition, as outlined in Chapter 21.

The identifiable phases of convalescence are (1) bandage phase, (2) fatigue phase, (3) disappointment phase, (4) relief phase, and (5) satisfaction phase.

BANDAGE PHASE (DAYS 1 THROUGH 7)

The bandage phase is the result of acute injury to the tissues and is characterized by acute sequestered edema (fourth space phenomenon), drop in both hematocrit and serum protein, and a rise in enzymes of injury such as lactic acid dehydrogenase (LDH). By the fourth day, the fluid shifts normalize and the patient diureses most excess fluid. By the fourth day, the scavenger system begins to clear up the damaged area. Cytoplasmic and nuclear breakdown products from dying adipocytes are excreted. During this period the patient *expects* to be stiff, tired, sleepy, uncomfortable, and *expects* to be able to play the role of a sick person with due family attention to his or her needs. Whether a girdle, pressure garment, or elastic tape is used, its use indicates to the patient that he or she is in the "bandage" phase of the postsurgical course. The patient has few questions during this phase. Pressure garments are worn 24 hours per day, and exercise consists only of walking.

FATIGUE PHASE (DAYS 8 THROUGH 15)

The removal of the tape dressing, pressure garment, or surface stitches (if any) marks the end of the patient's relative immobilization. Patients often return to work or other duties during this time. They may note easy fatigability, mild shortness of breath, and an inability to concentrate. Rather than work a half day, they often overdo. They find they cannot keep up with their anticipated schedule.

Serum iron and proteins are low during this time, reflecting the metabolic impact of the surgery. Collagen begins to be laid down in the injured areas and interstitial edema is lessening. It is in this stage, at 10 to 14 days, that I recommend beginning massage twice a week for 2 to 4 weeks (see Chap. 22). Protein, vitamin C, zinc, and iron requirements should be met during this time. During the fatigue phase support-type pantyhose is worn while the patient is awake. Exercise consists of walking and swimming.

DISAPPOINTMENT PHASE
(DAYS 16 THROUGH 25)

After 2 weeks patients have resumed their normal duties or feel a strong obligation to do so. They begin to look for results and expect to be vigorous. Instead they may see persistent swelling and ecchymosis. Their pants or jeans may still feel as tight as they did preoperatively. These patients are somewhat stiff and feel clumsy. They are usually encouraged to continue wearing a pressure garment or support hose, which adds to their sense of "heaviness." This period may be brief or prolonged, depending on the amount of removal and how quickly results become apparent. The presence of the masseuse, who the patient knows has seen and cared for many others, is a great comfort psychologically. The physical massage also produces a sense of tranquility and security in the patient. Most patients report that massage is one of the most positive parts of their treatment program.

I believe that swelling is lessened by the pressure garments, which the patient wears while awake, and also by the massage, which mobilizes the edema. Investigations are in progress to quantitate these clinical impressions. Interestingly, our patients receiving massage therapy have had no cases of hemosiderin staining of tissue, while those not using massage have occasionally reported this problem. Regardless, psychological support at this time is needed and valued by the patient and should not be neglected or deferred.

The patient must be reminded that collagen repair is only 50% complete 17 days after the operation and is 100% complete first by day 42. Furthermore, remodeling of the collagen bundles takes about 1 year.

Patients should be aware that the fat extraction and remodeling occurs in three stages. The first stage is the immediate loss due to the gross fat extraction. The second stage is the fat cell death during the week or two after the removal due to injury sustained at the time of the procedure. The third phase is the laying down of collagen, retraction, and remodeling of the fat layers, which occur over many months and which are just beginning at this point in their convalescence. During the fatigue phase, support-type pantyhose is worn while awake. Exercise includes walking, swimming, and cycling (stationary), and the patient can begin general fitness exercise.

RELIEF PHASE (DAYS 25 THROUGH 42)

As the anticipated result begins to show in the mirror or, more usually, as excess cloth in their clothes or jeans, patients begin to lose their sense of anxiety about the result. Perhaps against a friend's good advice, they had spent a good deal of money on their vanity and they have been worrying that they would have little to show for it. When the improvement shows, these worries melt away. Between 4 and 6 weeks after surgery, the patient benefits by shopping for new clothes. The desire for new clothes indicates the patient is ready to accept the new body image. It marks the transition from the "old me" to the "new me." Patients who do not mark this change by some change in attire are uncommon. Those patients who do not acknowledge the change or do not feel the change is sufficent are going to be problem patients. I encourage all patients to get new clothes to document for themselves that they are indeed a size or two smaller or can fit into clothes previously impossible to wear. Support-type pantyhose is worn while the patient is awake. Exercise includes walking, swimming, cycling, general fitness, beginning aerobics and dance *(no jogging)*.

SATISFACTION PHASE (AFTER 6 WEEKS)

The results continue to mold and change, at least for 3 to 6 months for most body areas and 6 to 9 months for calves and ankles. Continued small amounts of bulk loss are expected if the patient is not in caloric surplus. If patients have passed through the "relief phase" normally and accepted their new look as their true body image, they will be happy—pleased with themselves and pleased with the surgeon and staff. If they have body image disturbances of a mild to moderate degree of severity, however, the patient may become a chronic complainer: They want a touchup here or there. Was this bulge really there before the surgery? Would some other procedure help? For these patients, good photographs are invaluable, and recurrent reality reinforcement is a must. Giving in to questionable or unwarranted touchups may seem to be the easy way out but does not address the real problem, which is not amenable to surgery. If the patient has a severe body image disturbance, he or she will see little or no improvement. No amount of confrontation with reality or surgery or consultations will make up for the fact that a patient who should have been dismissed was operated on.

No specific garments need to be worn, except patients who have had calf surgery. These patients should continue to use a support-type garment. Any tolerated exercise and all sports are permitted.

Follow-up

I request that patients return at 3, 6, and 12 months for measurements, photographs, and interviews. At 6 months, the patient fills out an evaluation questionnaire about the surgery, which is used to evaluate patient satisfaction. Ninety percent of my patients are satisfied and would have the procedure again.

Touchups

Contour irregularities are evaluated 4 months after the operation. If there is a small bump or wave that is annoying to the patient and *can be improved,* there is no sense in delay. These touchups are easily done under local anesthesia with a #4 or #6 cannula. The financial understanding about touchups should have been discussed before the operation. Abdomens may continue to improve for up to 6 months and a delay is acceptable in that case. Calves and ankles should be evaluated at 1 year.

Diet, Exercise, and Life Style

If patients can be appropriately referred and will accept nutritional counseling, this may be a time when they may be motivated enough to really benefit. Likewise, the motivation derived from looking better may give surgeons the chance to benefit their patients by putting them in touch with appropriate exercise programs, stop smoking clinics, or other group therapies. Many patients are expressing a desire not only *for* change but also *to* change when they seek consultation for body contouring procedures. Whereas their dietary efforts were never successful previously and their interest waned, their new-found pride may go farther in sustaining their will to alter their habits. Appropriate referral in these areas rounds out the surgeon's role to that of a caring physician.

PART II

Clinical Applications

Adjunctive or Isolated Lipolysis of the Face and Neck

Facial Lipolysis
Gregory P. Hetter

As Dr. Illouz pointed out in Chapter 3, from its localized beginnings, lipolysis was gradually extended to cover more areas. Inevitably, the face and neck became areas to which suction extraction of fat was applied. Illouz and Fournier found lipolysis useful in their French cases [1]. American plastic surgeons and some otolaryngologists interested in plastic surgery began using the technique for facial extractions in 1982 [2,3,4].

The facial areas of most concern, as a result of fatty excess (in order of frequency), are submental, submandibular (and jowl), preantral (nasolabial fold area), preparotid, and malar (Fig. 24-1).

Originally, the #6 cannula was used by Illouz for both open and closed extractions. Larger cannulas were also used but appeared too gross as seen in Dr. Teimourian's photographs [2].

CANNULAS

Surgeons interested in more finesse worked with machinists to obtain cannulas of smaller caliber. These smaller cannulas pass between the SMAS and skin or between the platysma and the skin with greater ease. The French firm of Medicalex* first made small cannulas available. Later many American manufacturers marketed various designs. Figure 24-2 shows a 2.0 mm and a 3.7 mm next to a standard Illouz #6 cannula.

I have found the 4-mm or 5-mm size highly useful for the submental-submandibular area, using a single submental incision (Fig. 24-3).

The 3- or 4-mm size is good for the preantral and preparotid areas, where one wants to stay close to the skin (Fig. 24-4). The 2-mm cannula is best for the "malar bag."

Because these cannulas are lighter and more delicate, a smaller, more flexible tubing is desirable, which allows a better feel and a more controlled motion. This tubing is connected to the regular tubing near the suction bottle (Fig. 24-5).

PRESSURE

I use the suction machine at or near absolute vacuum for these procedures (0–25 torr). There is no advantage to using less pressure.

---

*Medicalex, 39 Rue Croulebarbe, 75013 Paris, France.

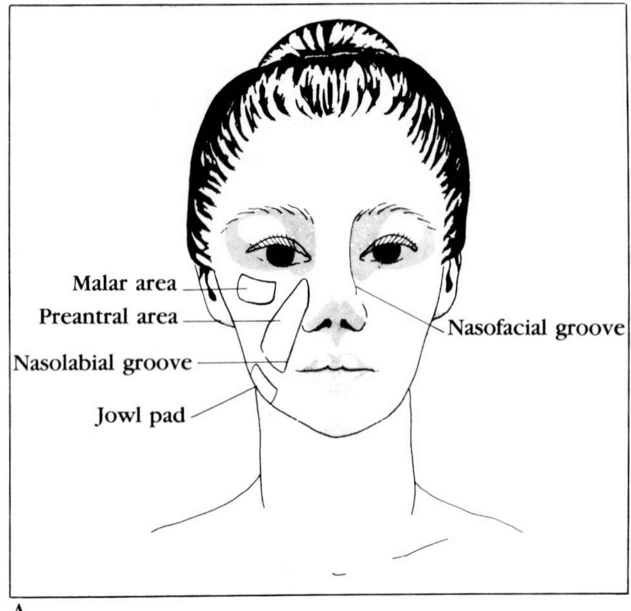

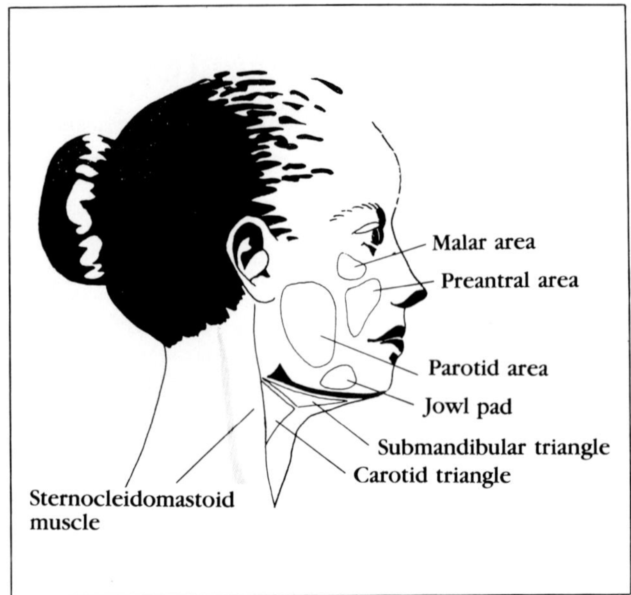

Fig. 24-1.
A. Frontal view showing the areas in which lipolysis may be useful.
B. Lateral view showing the most common areas for isolated facial lipolysis.

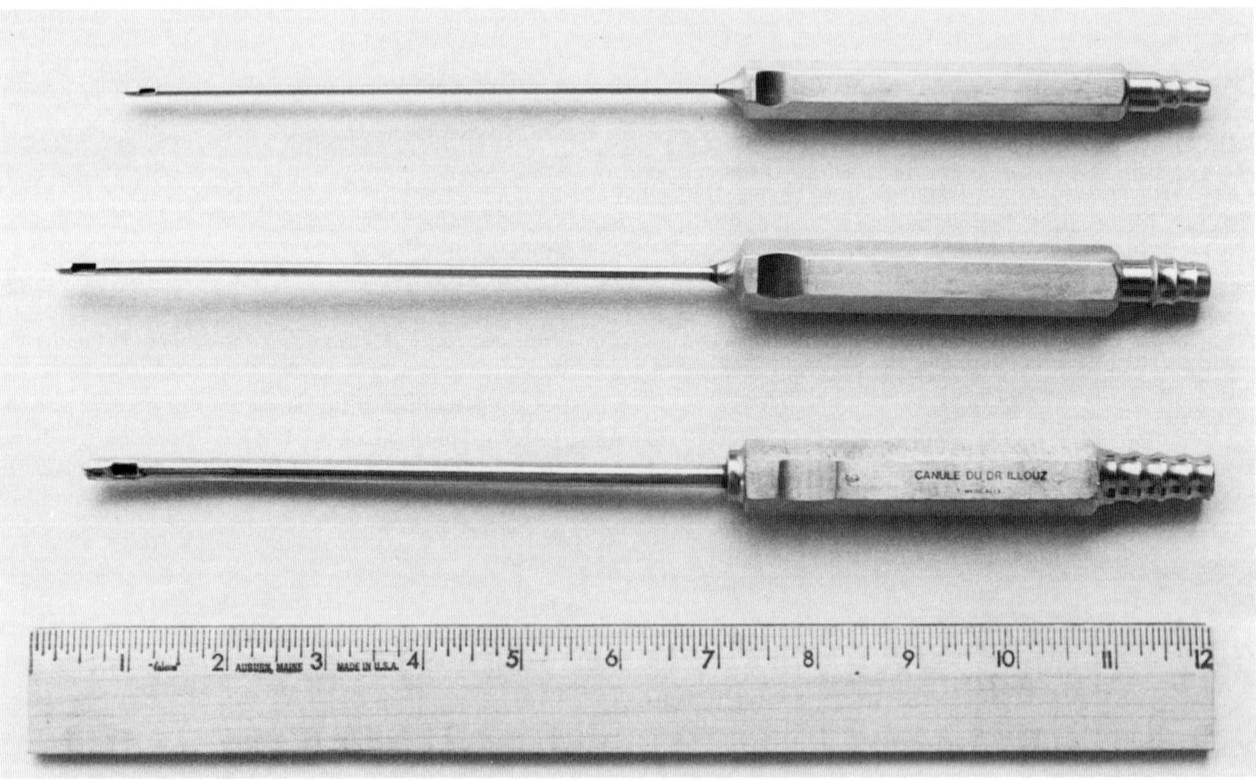

Fig. 24-2. A 2-mm and a 3.7-mm facial cannula next to the smallest of the original Illouz cannulas. (Manufactured by Guenter Grams, 2443 Norse Avenue, Costa Mesa, California 92627.)

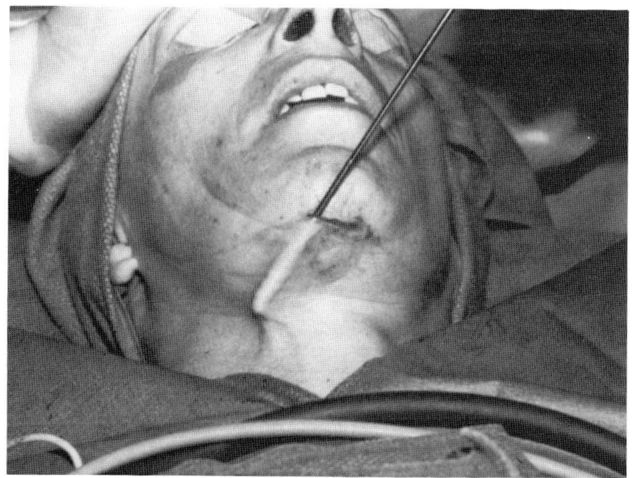

Fig. 24-3. A #4 cannula inserted into submental-preplatysma space for fat extraction through a single submental incision.

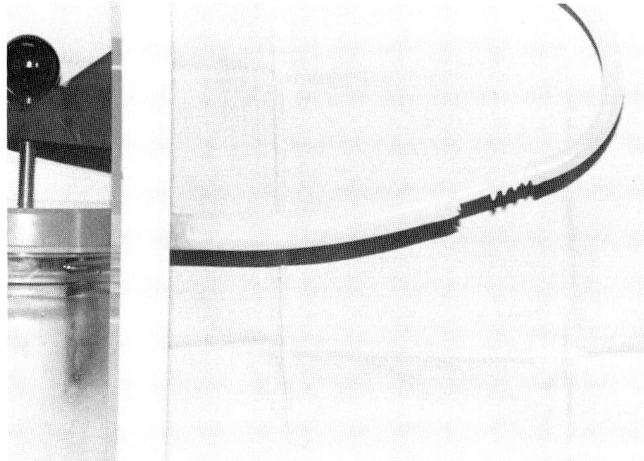

Fig. 24-5. Lighter, ¼-inch silastic tubing joined to ⅞₁₆-inch tubing near collection bottle.

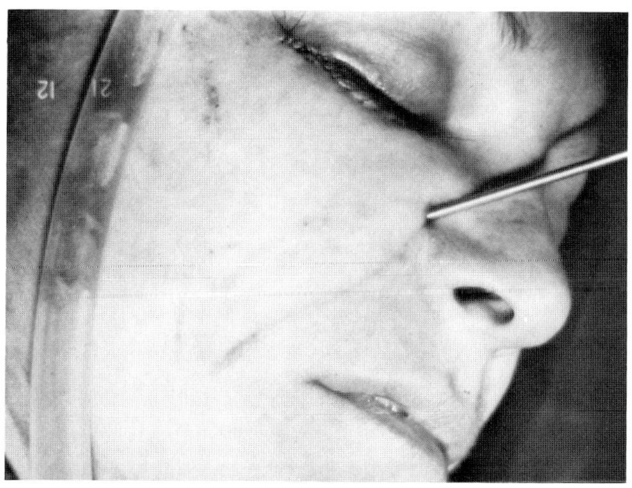

A

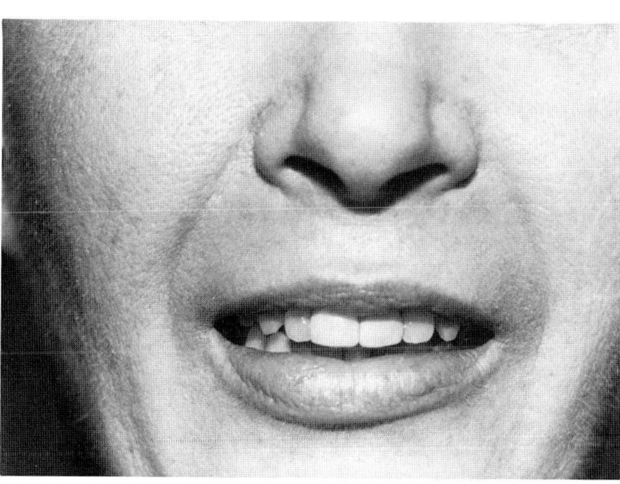

B

Fig. 24-4.

A. A #4 cannula inserted through an alar groove incision for extraction of preantral fat.

B. Alar incision healed 6 weeks postoperatively.

ANESTHESIA

Submental and infraorbital nerve blocks are performed through the buccogingival sulcus with either Xylocaine 2% with Epinephrine 1:100,000, Duranest 0.5% with Epinephrine 1:200,000, or Marcaine 0.25% with Epinephrine 1:200,000. Thereafter, thorough infiltration of the area is carried out. It appears that Marcaine infiltration provides better pain relief postoperatively, especially for the submental-submandibular defatting. Ten minutes is allowed to elapse before beginning the fat extraction. The adrenaline effect is noticeably better after 10 minutes than after 5.

Short-acting drugs for intravenous sedation are used such as thiopental, fentanyl (Sublimaze), or low-dose ketamine.

MARKING THE PATIENT

The patient is marked with Magic Marker or Sharpie in the upright position (Fig. 24-6). Occasionally, transverse lighting is necessary to throw the involved area into relief (Fig. 24-7). No change is made in the predetermined treatment plan for any differences that may occur when the patient is in the supine position.

TECHNIQUE

A small skin incision is made in any appropriate crease. A tunnel is started with a hemostat, and closely adjacent tunnels are made with the small-bore cannula. Pretunneling may be performed and is useful for the beginner. *The lumen of the cannula should be kept away from the skin.* Otherwise, tracks will appear on the surface from the removal of the immediate subdermal fat. These

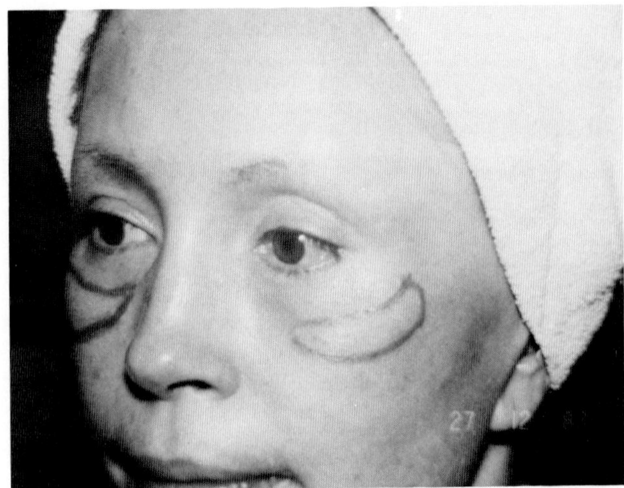

Fig. 24-6. Markings made in upright position defining malar bags.

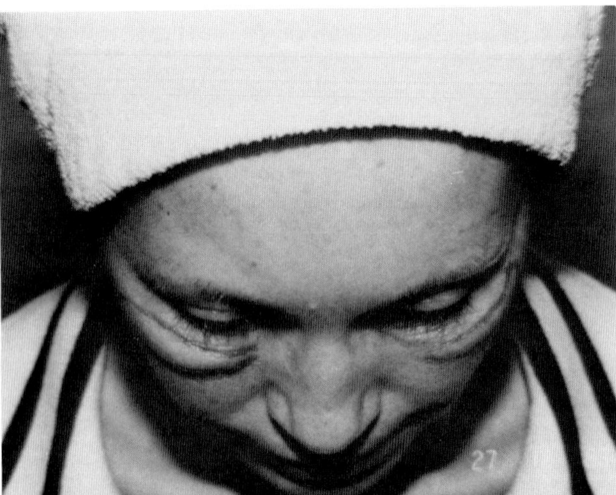

Fig. 24-7. Cross-lighting makes the malar bags more evident and allows more accurate marking.

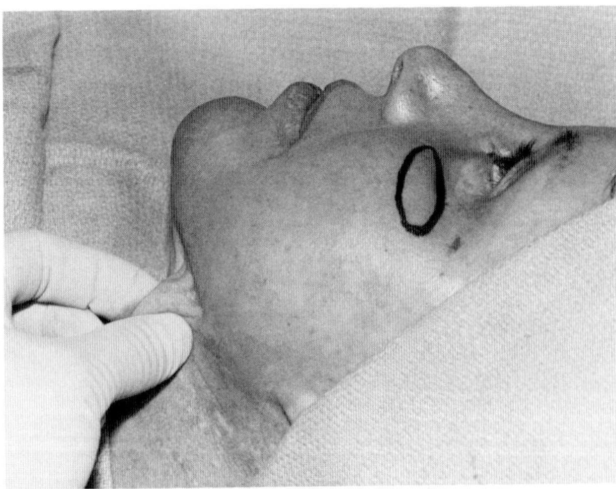

Fig. 24-8. During and after extraction, the skin and remaining subcutaneous fat is pinched and rolled to determine evenness and thickness over the whole area of extraction.

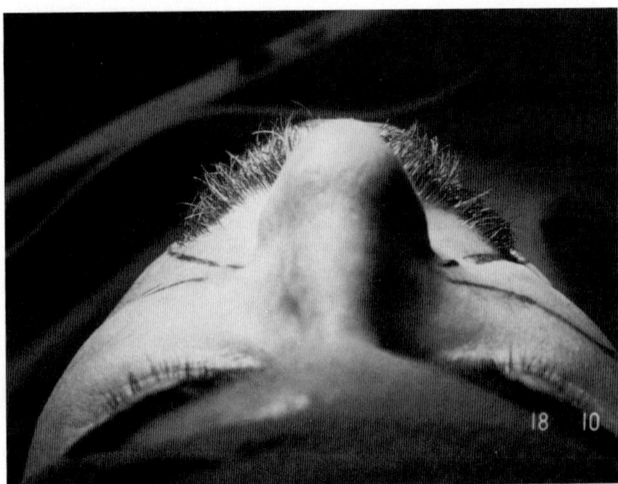

A

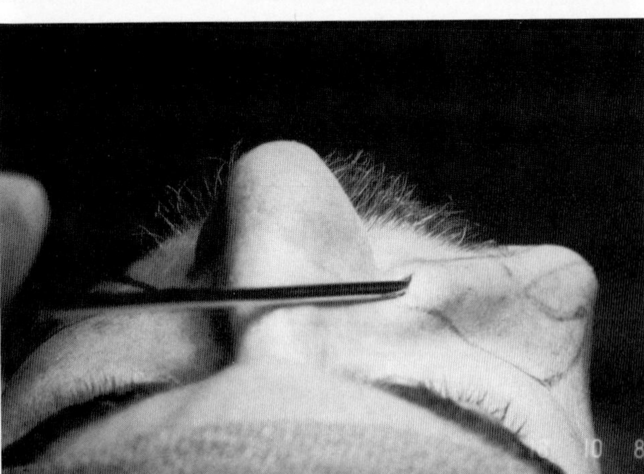

B

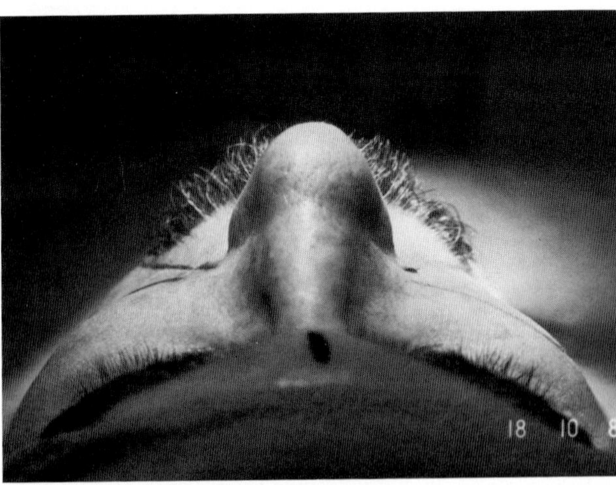

C

Fig. 24-9.
A. View from above after extraction from left cheek but before extraction from right cheek.
B. View during extraction from right cheek.
C. View after extraction from both sides.

surface tracks take many months to only partially re-solve, as shown by Newman at the Dalinde Seminar in February 1984 in Mexico City [4].

Stroking in the usual manner is carried out with eight to ten strokes per tunnel. In the neck the "pinch and roll" technique is useful (Fig. 24-8). In the preantral fat and malar area, however, visual inspection is usually the only guide to adequate removal (Fig. 24-9). *Do not overdo!*

Malar Area

A small stab incision is made laterally in a "crows foot" line and the cannula passed medially into the malar bag (Fig. 24-10). A light Elastikon pressure dressing is sufficient for 24 hours. Full resolution of swelling takes 3 to 6 months in this fibrous area.

Preantral Area

The fatty overhang above a deep nasolabial fold throws a dark shadow that accentuates the appearance of aging. This condition is largely hereditary but is worsened by the aging process (Fig. 24-11). Before the use of suction extraction, no excisional procedure gained a significant following because of the residual scars (Fig. 24-12).

Entry can be through an alar crease incision, a nasal vestibular incision (the same incision as for a lateral osteotomy in rhinoplasty), or a buccogingival sulcus incision next to the periform aperture.

Extraction with superficial adjacent tunnels may be followed by somewhat deeper tunnels. Stay cranial (superior) to the nasolabial fold. Forewarn the patient that symmetry is impossible to obtain. A typical postoperative dressing is seen in Figure 24-13 and is kept on for 3 days. Considerable immediate swelling is usual and resolves rather more slowly than excisional procedures. A typical result is shown in Figure 24-14.

Jowl Fat

The jowl fat is reached through a submental incision, an alar crease incision, or a lobular incision. Generally, jowl fat is removed in conjunction with a face-lift but may be approached on an isolated basis.

Preparotid Fat

The preparotid fat is reached most easily by a lobular or pretragal incision. As with the jowl fat, preparotid fat is generally removed by the "open sky" technique during a face-lift. The closed technique is used in unusual cases (Fig. 24-15).

Submental-Submandibular Area

The submental-submandibular area for defatting is marked out as shown in Figure 24-16. An intraoperative supine pre- and immediate postoperative view is seen in

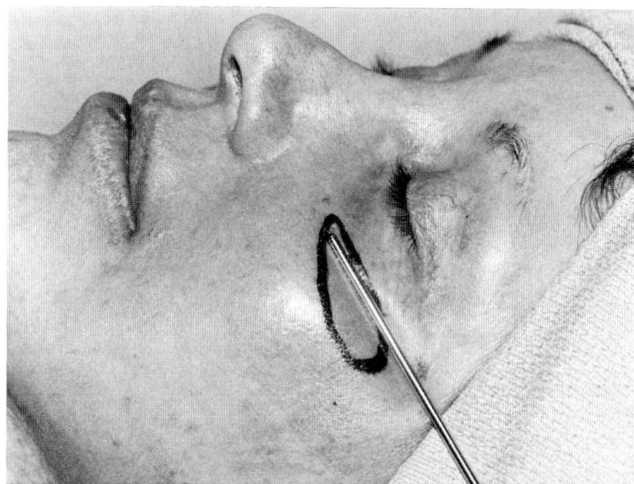

Fig. 24-10. A #2 cannula shown next to malar bag. Entry point is in one of "laugh lines" or "crows feet."

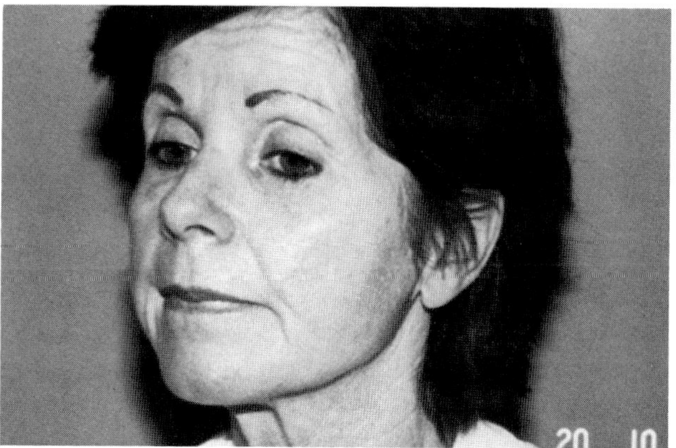

Fig. 24-11. Deep nasolabial grooves make the patient look older.

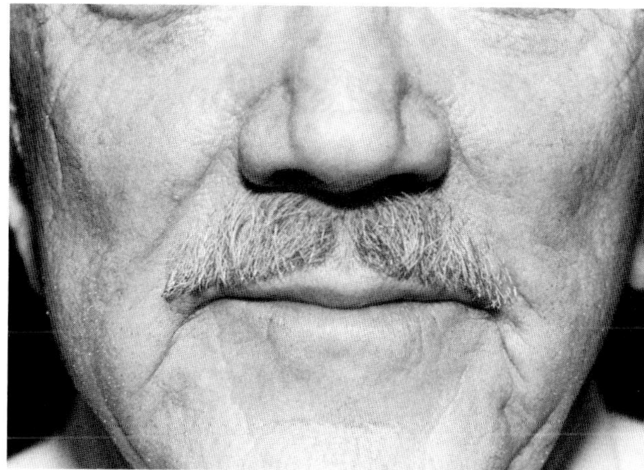

Fig. 24-12. Good nasolabial scars from long elliptical excisions of excess skin after failure of skin contraction after adequate lipolysis of the preantral fat. No underlying fat resection at time of skin excisions. Compare to Fig. 24-4B.

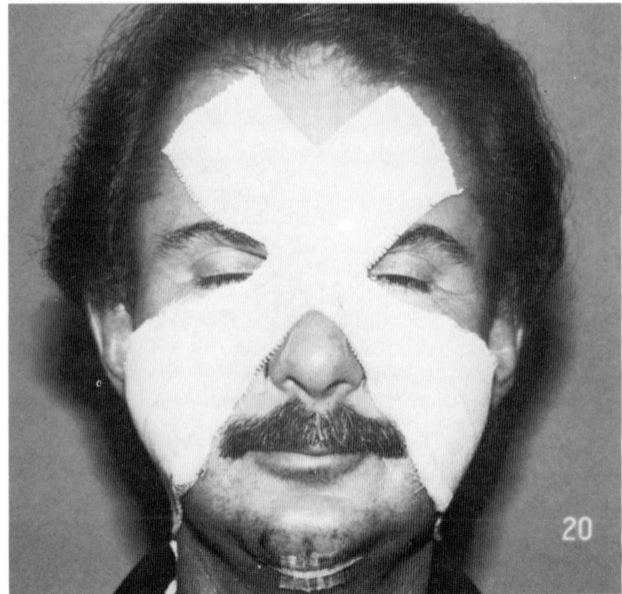

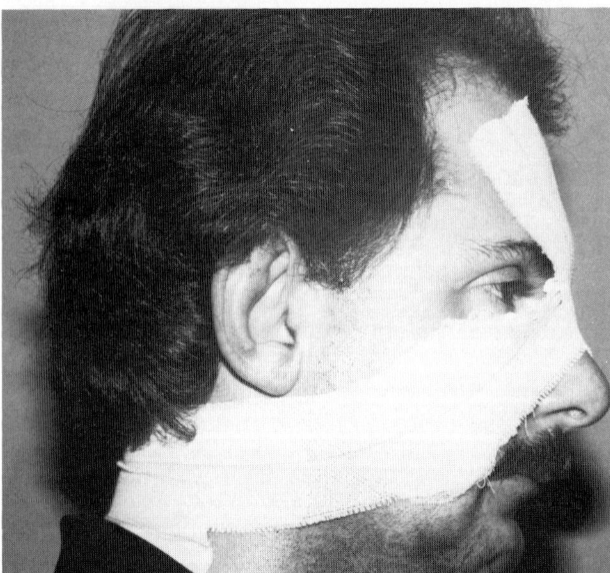

Fig. 24-13.
A. Frontal view of dressing for preantral fat extraction.
B. Lateral view of same dressing.

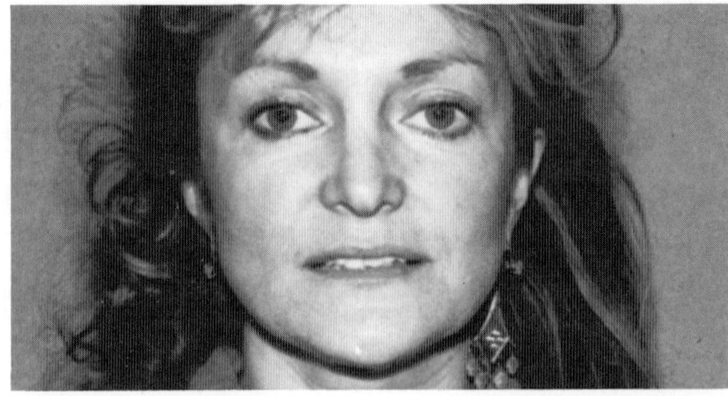

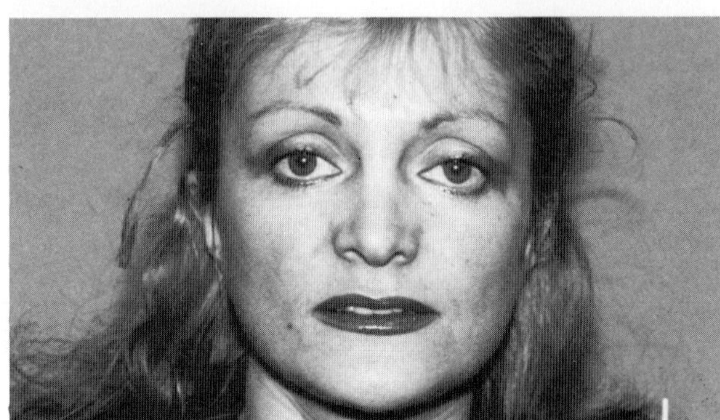

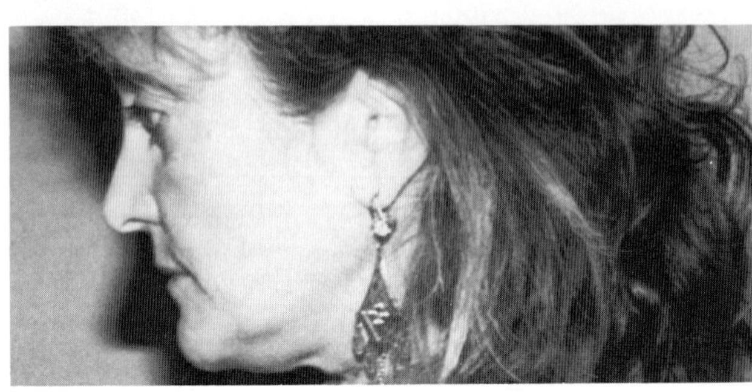

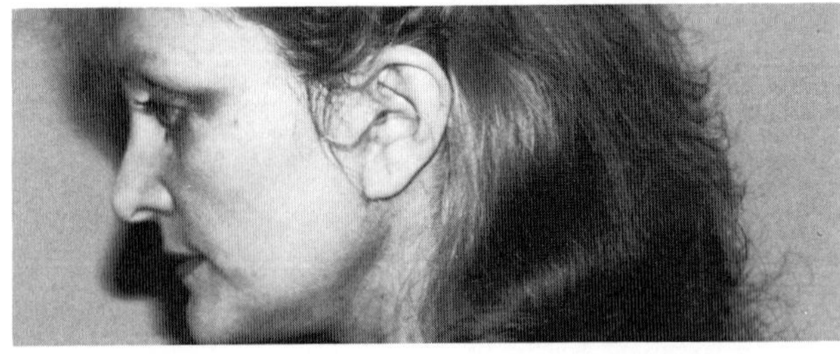

Fig. 24-14.
A. Preoperative frontal view of 42-year-old female with deep shadows. Camera-mounted flash actually diminishes this feature.
B. Postoperative frontal view 1 month later showing more feminine appearance achieved with modest fat extraction.
C. Left lateral preoperative view with head flexed.
D. Left lateral postoperative view with head flexed.

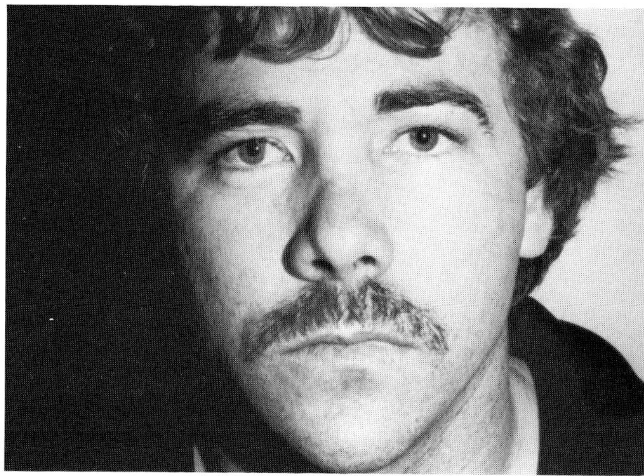

A

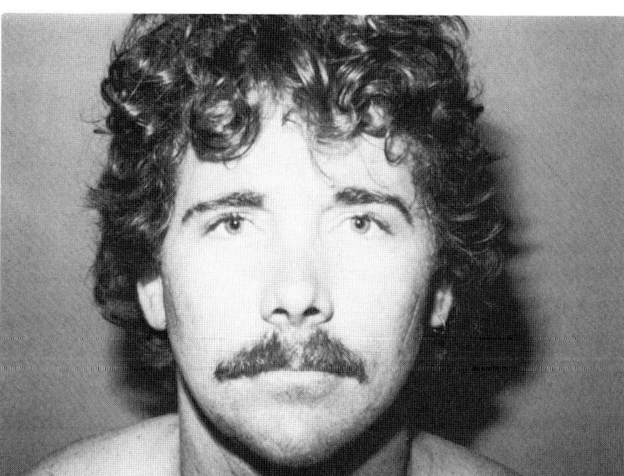

B

Fig. 24-15.
A. Preoperative view of preparotid excess.
B. Postoperative view after closed extraction.
(Photographs courtesy of A. Aiache, M.D.)

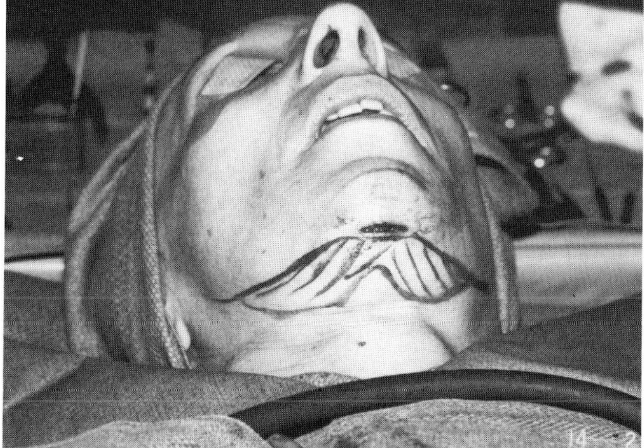

Fig. 24-16. Submental-submandibular marking is outlined in upright position. Patient is in supine operative position.

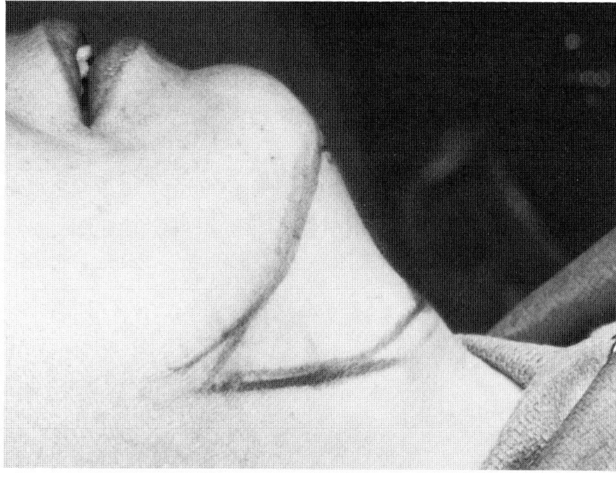

A

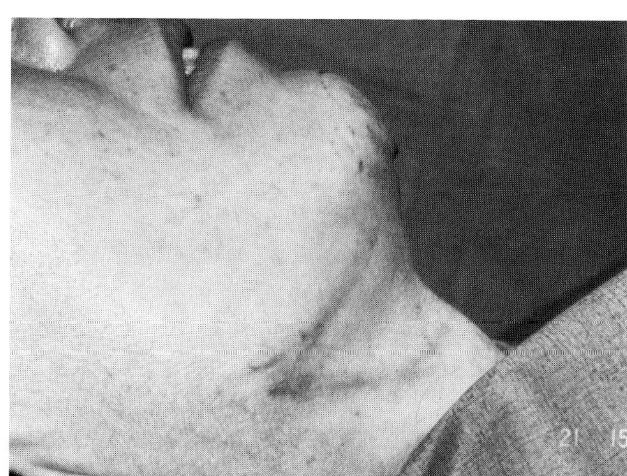

B

Fig. 24-17.
A. Submental area bulges before extraction.
B. Same area immediately after extraction.

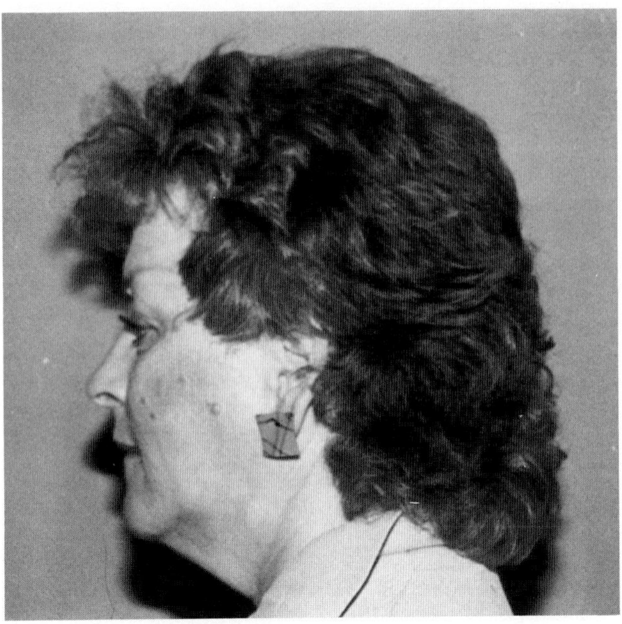

A

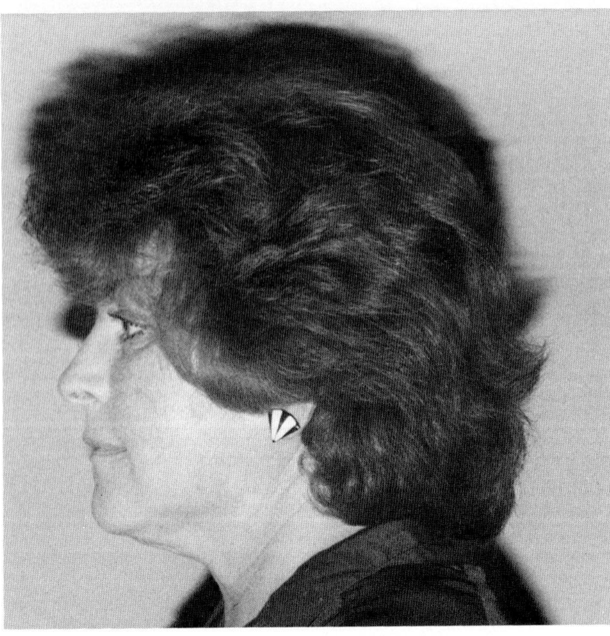

B

Fig. 24-18.
A. Preoperative lateral view of 49-year-old female with blunted cervicomental angle.
B. Three-month postoperative view after isolated submental-submandibular lipolysis.

Figure 24-17. An upright pre- and 3-month postoperative view of a middle-aged patient is seen in Figure 24-18.

The submental-submandibular and the nasolabial areas are the most frequently performed isolated lipolysis procedures. For the young person with a hereditary submental fat accumulation, this procedure offers easy improvement without face-lift incisions (see Submental and Submandibular Adiposities, this chapter).

ADJUNCTIVE PROCEDURES

Isolated facial lipolysis can be combined beneficially with other procedures. The most common procedure is neck defatting combined with chin augmentation or rhinoplasty (or both). Figure 24-19 shows the results of such a combination. Submental-prehyoid fat was removed at the time of chin augmentation. Figure 24-20 shows the result after the removal of a small submental bulge at the time of chin augmentation and rhinoplasty. These facial lipolysis procedures give an added finesse that separates the really fine result from the average result.

COMPLICATIONS

Overvigorous removal of fat or the use of the cannula with the lumen up may result in the overlying skin being stuck to the underlying muscle or fascia, with a fixed point in the middle of the face or a depressed furrow or a washboard appearance (Fig. 24-21).

Ultrasound may be beneficial in the treatment of these problems. Time is helpful, but without the ultrasound to speed resolution, the patient may not tolerate waiting several months before seeking consultation with an attorney. If you do not believe in ultrasound, do not use it. Those who have used it believe it works. Studies to prove this are almost impossible to structure, so no satisfactory scientific proof yet exists for those with doubt.

The use of Zyderm injections along the track areas to fill them out and to soften scarred tissue has been helpful in ameliorating these sequelae, according to Newman [4].

A significant defect caused by overextraction cannot be repaired, and prudent avoidance of overresection is the answer. Remember, the surgeon can always extract more later. The possibility of skin resection must always have been discussed with the patient in the event that skin contraction fails, providing both the patient and the surgeon with a fallback position. When the possibility of skin resection is discussed preoperatively, it is informed consent; when discussed postoperatively, it is an excuse and an unwelcome and unexpected surprise for the patient.

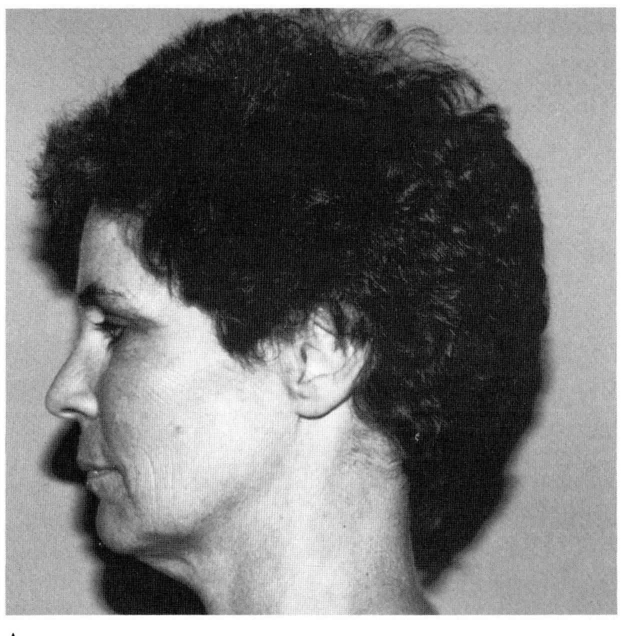

A

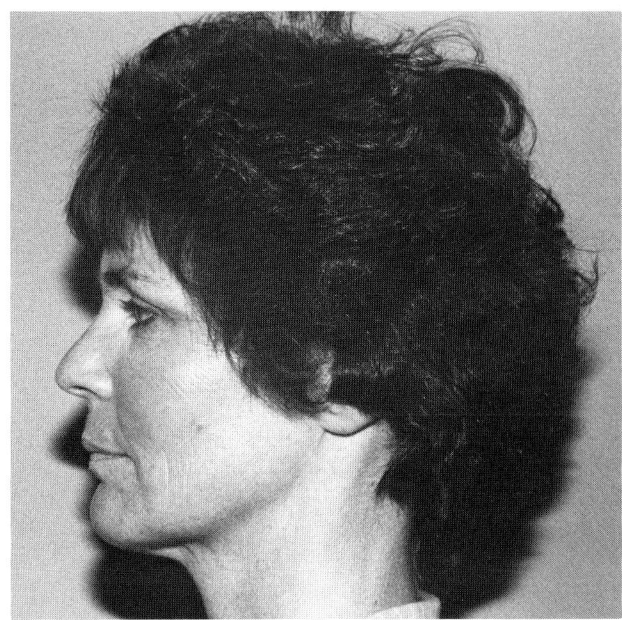

B

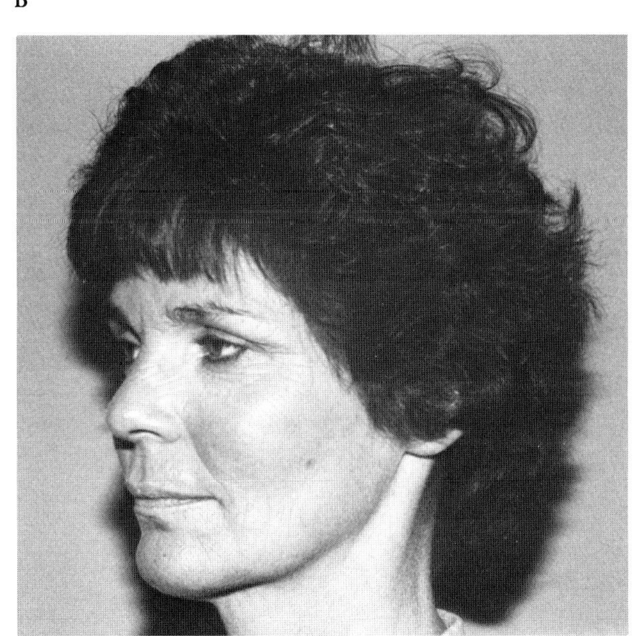

C

D

Fig. 24-19.
A. Preoperative lateral view of a 44-year-old female with low anterior hyoid and fatty accumulation. Patient did not submit to recommended face-lift surgery.
B. Postoperative view at 3 months after chin implant, and submental-submandibular lipolysis.
C. Preoperative oblique view.
D. Postoperative oblique view.

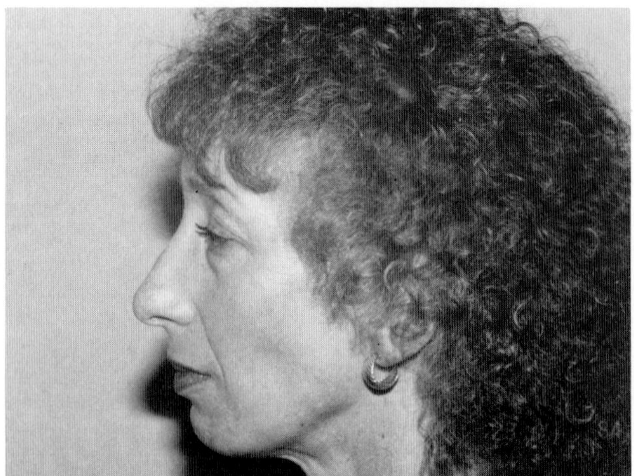

A

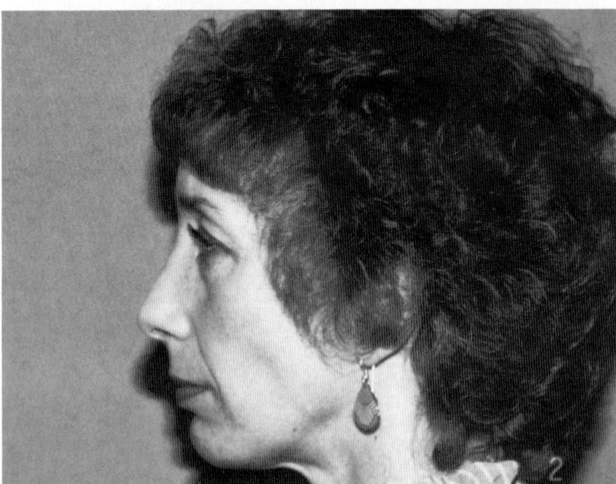

B

Fig. 24-20.
A. Preoperative lateral view of a 39-year-old female presenting for rhinoplasty. Discussion of profile led to adding
   chin implant and small submental lipolysis to rhinoplasty.
B. Postoperative result at 3 months.

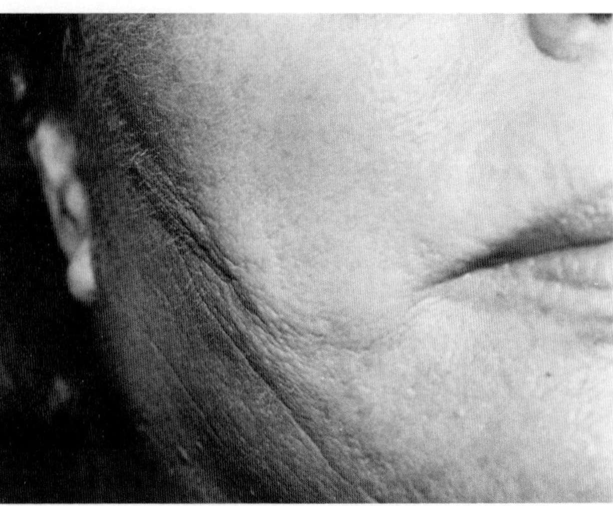

Fig. 24-21. Early adhesion (3 weeks) from fixation of skin to
fat-denuded preparotid fascia. Responded well to ultrasound.

Submental and Submandibular Adiposities
Frank T. Herbahn

Submental and submandibular adiposities have been
found to respond well to lipolysis, especially in the
younger patient who has good skin turgor. This condition is relatively common and is usually related to a
familial pattern. This particular area also lends itself well
to lipolysis when combined with skin resection procedures such as a face-lift. In the future, this procedure
may well become the standard treatment for submandibular and submental lipectomies where there is no
platysma problem present (Fig. 24-22).

THE INTERVIEW

Many men and women seek plastic surgeons, complaining of a localized fatty deposit in the submental region.
Frequently they are in the 20-to-30-year age group and
state that they do not want to develop a turkey neck as
one of their parents had. Many believe they will need a
surgical face-lift to get correction. Other candidates
present for a rhinoplasty or other facial profile problems. Some may mention this area during the course of
an interview for other body contouring procedures.

During the examination, the patient must be evaluated for beginning loss of skin turgor and facial extensions of the submandibular fatty deposits. The latter is
difficult or perhaps hazardous to correct because of the
underlying vital structures. I have seen several temporary facial nerve (mandibular branch) palsies associated
with face-lifts combined with lipolysis. No permanent

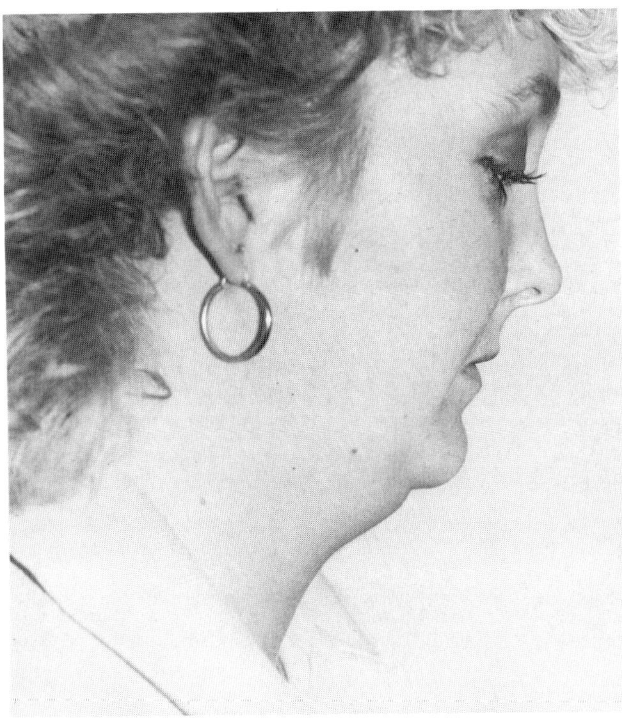

Fig. 24-22. Typical hereditary anterior neck fatty accumulation in a 34-year-old woman.

nerve injuries have been noted. The longest temporary palsy lasted 1 week.

Important areas to clarify during an interview with these patients, besides temporary weakness, include temporary anesthesia, lumpiness, persistent edema, and even small seromas. Excessive periods of lumpiness may require ultrasound and massage. Minor asymmetries are probably the only long-term sequelae. The obvious advantages of lipolysis over "lipectomy by direct vision" are the absence of the submental scar, the reduction in the occurrence of hematomas and seromas, and a quicker return to work.

PREOPERATIVE PLANNING

Before the patient is positioned for surgery, the limitations of the adiposity are marked with the patient in a sitting position with the neck extended and flexed. The area of skin incision is also marked at this time for improved symmetry of scars. After marking the skin, the area to be treated is demonstrated to the patient, using a mirror so he or she may appreciate what the surgeon is planning to treat. Current instrumentation for this procedure remains somewhat awkward, especially in the treatment of the lower extension of an early jowl deformity. Limited experience with the trilumen cannula has led me to feel that the single lumen cannula is just as effective and perhaps safer.

TECHNIQUE

After skin marking, the patient is placed on the table in the supine position. Adequate skin preparation and draping is carried out. Frequently no sedation is necessary or, at most, only mild sedation. For a local anesthetic, I use a modification of the wet technique: 20 ml of 2% lidocaine with adrenaline 1:100,000, diluted with 40 ml of saline for injection, and 75 units of Wydase. In most instances, the area can be adequately anesthetized with 20 to 30 ml of this solution. When infiltrating the area to be treated, remember to infiltrate not only the superficial fat but also down to the fascia overlying the platysma muscle.

A lateral skin incision is made, most commonly predetermined, and marked in the upper cervical skin crease, approximately 2 cm from the ear lobe. A curved 3-, 4-, or 5-mm cannula is introduced after the initial 2 cm of tunneling has been started by spreading with a hemostat. The standard method of stroking is carried out, using the pinch and roll bimanual concept as described by Dr. Illouz [1]. At the conclusion of the procedure, the submandibular region is rolled laterally to determine the amount of bleeding, followed with an incision closure in a standard technique. No drains have been used in this area.

There has been a lot of discussion about using a single midline submental incision. I believe my approach is safer in that directed trauma to the anterior facial and external jugular vein is avoided. Another concern is that short strokes in the immediate submental region may result in penetration of the fat pad occupying the space deep to the platysma between the digastric anterior bellies, producing a submental depression, as frequently seen after scissors excision in this area. In addition, direct trauma to the cricoid or thyroid cartilage might produce enough edema to produce stridor or temporary hoarseness.

POSTOPERATIVE CARE

In older patients with early loss of skin turgor but not severe enough to require a face-lift, I apply a 2-inch fabric elasticized tape (Elastikon) beginning from the midline, splitting the tails to terminate 2 or 3 cm behind the pre- and postauricular skin. The skin preparation before tape application should consist of degreasing only. Additional elastic support to this area, using a commercial conforming elasticized head bandage, is available. The head bandage is maintained from 48 to 72 hours, followed by nocturnal use for 7 to 10 days. The tape is usually removed on the fifth to seventh postoperative day. In the younger patient with good skin turgor, I use only the commercial elasticized head bandage.

After tape removal, the patient begins basic skin care and massage, maintaining well-lubricated skin with up-

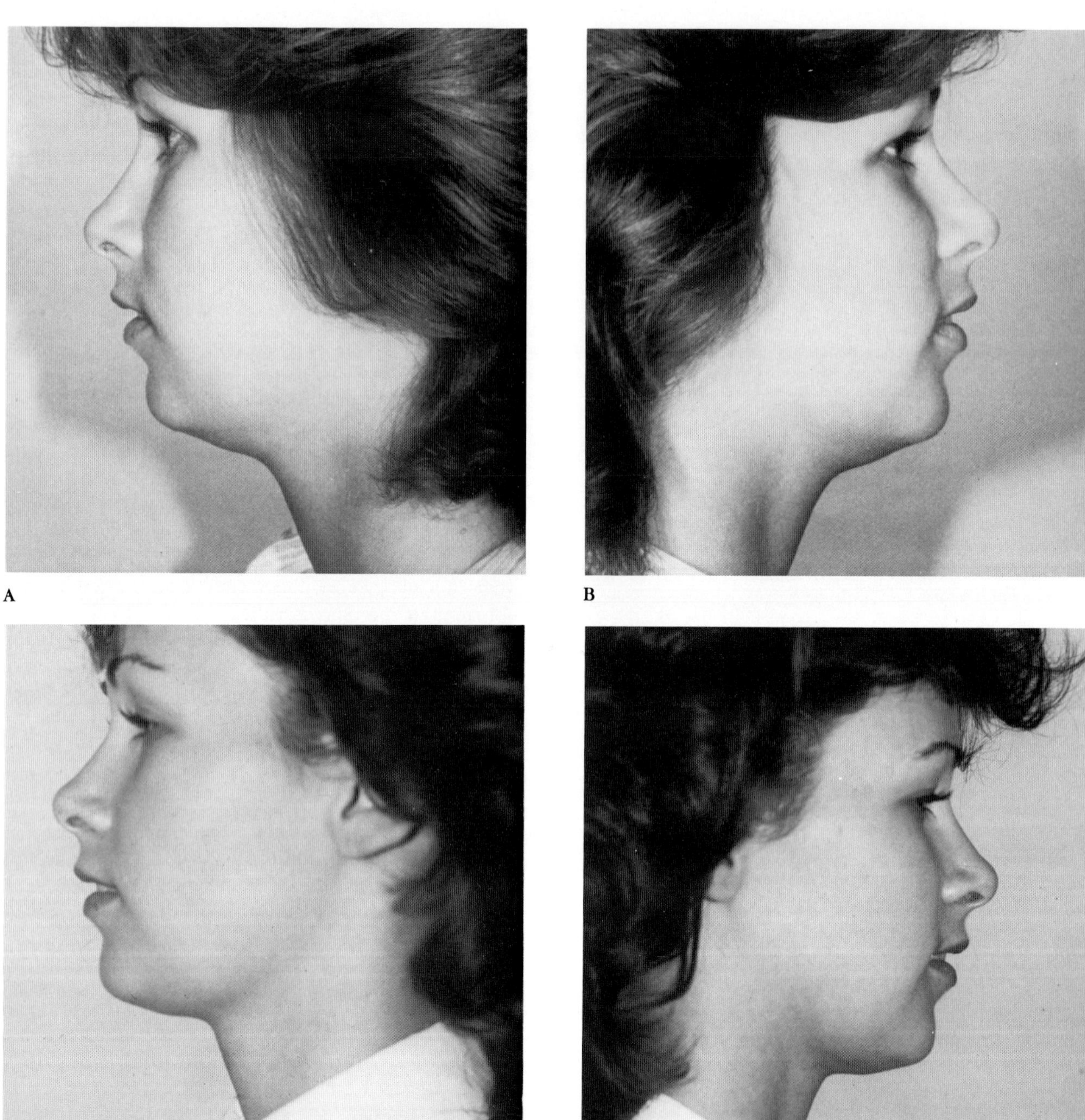

Fig. 24-23.
A,B. Preoperative views of 27-year-old woman with prehyoid adiposity.
C,D. Postoperative views 5 months after closed lipolysis.

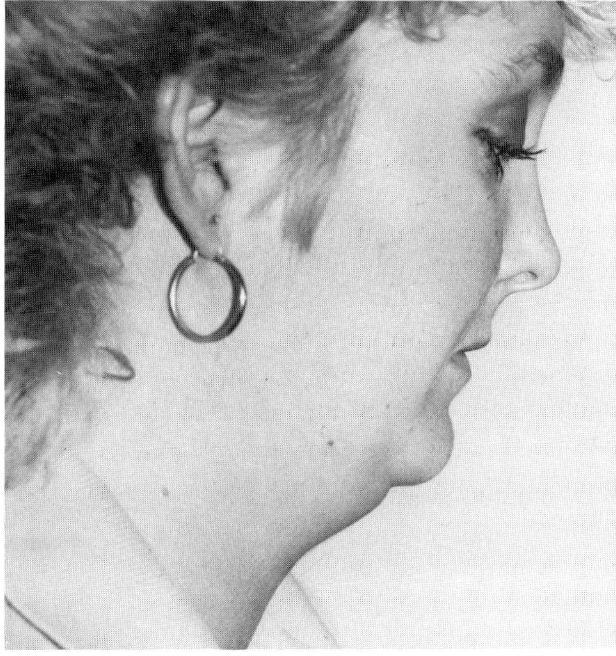

A

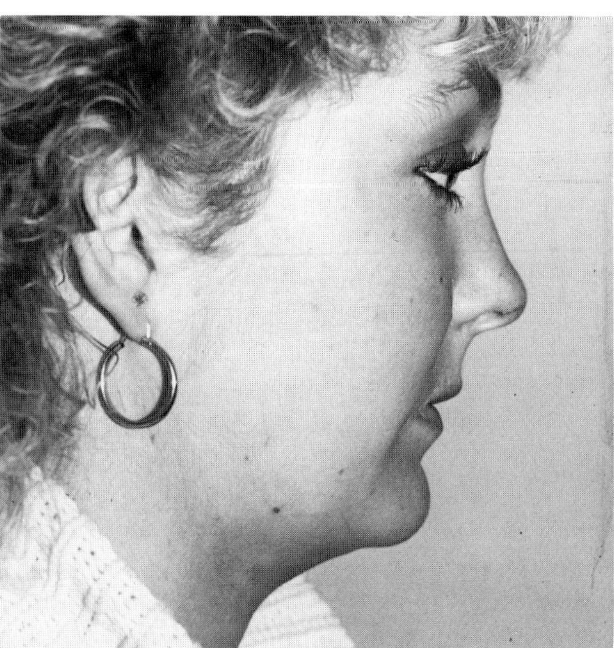

B

Fig. 24-24.
A. Preoperative view of patient shown in Fig. 24-22: low hyoid bone, submental, submandibular, and carotid triangle fatty deposits.
B. Postoperative view 2 months after closed lipolysis.

ward stroking. Patients with persistent edema are encouraged to use alternating warm-to-cool compresses in conjunction with massage. The occasional patient who exhibits an inordinate amount of subcutaneous induration (lumpiness) may require ultrasound or other formal physical therapy modalities.

RESULTS

Between June 1982, and January 1984, seventeen patients with submental adiposity have been treated using the closed technique of lipolysis. Ages of the patients range from 22 to 55 years (Figs. 24-23, 24-24).

There have been no surgical complications. Two patients experienced significant lumpiness between the second and third week; both patients had additional ultrasound and massage. These same two patients were unsure about the efficacy of the procedure until the second postoperative month. At that time, they became satisfied with the results. Bruising was minimal and disappeared by the tenth postoperative day in almost all cases. One patient has sought a touchup procedure to remove 1 cm^2 lump of fat.

Most patients return to work the day after surgery. The appearance of all patients is presentable, with no dressings and minimal makeup, between the fifth and seventh day.

SUMMARY

Submental lipolysis is an efficient, safe method for the treatment of submental and submandibular adiposities in the younger patient. Skin turgor, age, and absence of platysmal bands are important considerations in patient selection. Current instrumentation has been somewhat awkward, but the results, as judged by both the patient and surgeon, have been satisfactory. Most surgical complications are easily and quickly corrected. No excessive fat removal or depression of the submental area has occurred using the bilateral submandibular approach. The sometimes noticeable submental scar has been avoided.

Lipolysis has become a rapid outpatient procedure with minimal morbidity. When used in the properly selected patient, the results are good, and patient satisfaction is high.

References

1. Illouz, Y. G., and Fournier, P. *Illouz's Technique: Collapsing Surgery and Body Sculpture.* Paris, April 1983.
2. Teimourian, B. Face and neck suction-assisted lipectomy associated with rhytidectomy. *Plast. Reconstr. Surg.* 72: 627, 1983.
3. Nemetz, J. Presentation at the Annual Forum of the Lipolysis Society of North America. Dallas, Texas, October 1983.
4. Newman, J. Presentation at the XVI Dalinde Medical Seminar. Mexico City, February 1984.

CHAPTER 25

Lipolysis Combined with Facial Rhytidectomy

Richard A. Mladick

For many years there were few innovations in the rhytidectomy procedure. Most discussion on the subject centered around minor variations in technique such as the location of incisions and the use of drains and pressure bandages. Progress came about only after critical scrutiny of postoperative patients revealed mediocre results, especially in patients with fat necks. Plastic surgeons were also motivated to take an analytical look at the superficial fascia, platysma layer, and superficial musculoaponeurotic system (SMAS). Gradually, a new development focused (1) on tightening the subcutaneous layers (2) on defatting the entire neck, and (3) on a combination of the two procedures.

Defatting of the neck is now recognized as a most important step for some patients undergoing rhytidectomy. This step was first described in 1932 by Maliniac [1], who carried out a skin excision along with submental fat removal. In 1948 Padgett and Stephenson [2] also described removal of submental fat through a transverse incision and, at the same time, plicated the platysma muscle. In 1955 Davis [3] reported the removal of the submental fat with a curette through a small 1-cm submental incision. In 1972 Millard [4] emphasized thorough submental and submandibular defatting in conjunction with a face-lift. Then, in 1976 two Frenchmen, Mitz and Peyronie [5], described the details of the SMAS anatomy, and face-lift surgery was extended one more step. In 1978 Connell [6] discussed contouring the neck in a rhytidectomy by defatting and treatment of the platysma muscle. Today, face-lift treatment varies from those who still advocate the basic skin flap face-lift to those who carry out radical treatment of the SMAS and platysma with varying degrees of undermining and defatting. Most plastic surgeons now agree with the need for submental or submandibular defatting or both to achieve improved definition of the neck and chin in selected patients. For the past several years, some French plastic surgeons have been defatting the neck by the lipolysis technique [7]. In 1983, at a meeting of the Lipolysis Society of North America, I [8] presented my experience with 35 cases of lipolysis done in conjunction with rhytidectomies. At that same time, I performed a surgical demonstration of lipolysis contouring of the entire neck and face as part of a rhytidectomy procedure.

As more plastic surgeons are introduced to this method, their enthusiasm will lead to the refinements and innovations necessary to develop lipolysis into a routine procedure and possibly bring face-lift surgery another step forward.

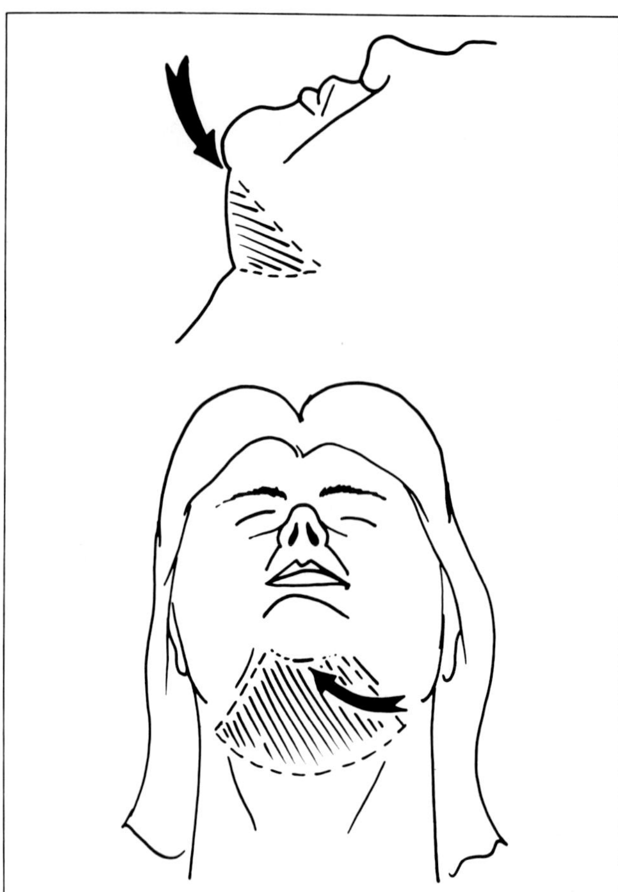

Fig. 25-1. Lipolysis for submental area. A patient who does not need a face-lift may be operated on through the small incision shown *(arrow),* often under local anesthesia or local with sedation, with a #4 or a #6 cannula. Shaded area represents the area of basic fat removal.

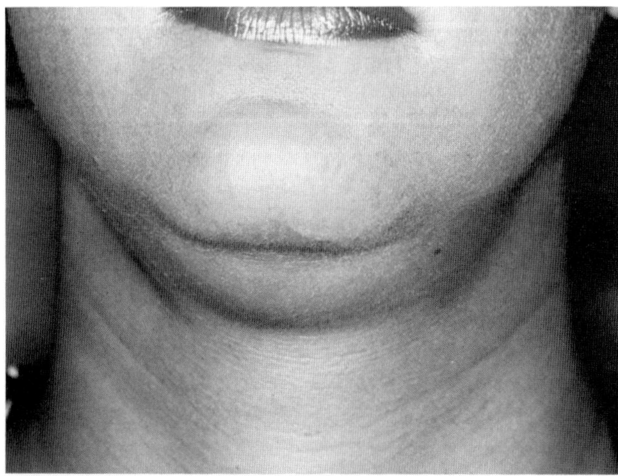

Fig. 25-2. The typical young patient with a submental bulge. Submental lipolysis alone is indicated.

Patient Selection

Approximately 50% of all rhytidectomy patients can benefit from lipolysis. The ideal candidate has a chubby neck, a large submental bulge, heavy jowls, and a fat lateral neck with poor definition of the lower border of the body of the mandible. There may also be a prominent buccal fat pad which, when decreased, creates a more aesthetic contour.

The patient is examined in repose, smiling and grimacing, with the neck flexed and extended. The neck is evaluated for fat bulges and also for the status of platysmal bands and sagging submandibular glands. The submental fat pad is carefully palpated and pinched to determine its size and to estimate the amount to be removed. The lower border of the mandibular body is marked and the extent of defatting planned for the lateral neck, parotid area, and jowls. If the patient has had a previous rhytidectomy, there may be dispersion of scar tissue throughout the subcutaneous plane of dissection, making the lipolysis procedure more difficult. Some younger patients who have a sizable submental bulge, but who have no need for a face-lift, are ideal candidates for the submental lipolysis procedure done through a small incision in the submental area (Figs. 25-1, 25-2) (see Chap. 24). The fat in male necks seems to be more difficult to remove by lipolysis than the fat in female necks.

Fat Bulges in the Face and Neck

For the purpose of discussion, the fat areas that may be treated by lipolysis during rhytidectomy are divided into three spaces: subcutaneous, subplatysmal, and buccal. The subcutaneous spaces are further subdivided into: (1) submental, (2) submandibular (lateral neck), (3) preparotid, (4) lower nasolabial fold (jowls), (5) upper nasolabial fold, and (6) malar fat pad (Fig. 25-3).

In the majority of rhytidectomy patients undergoing lipolysis, both the submental and submandibular subcutaneous spaces are defatted. In patients with a very full, large, bulging submental area, lipolysis is extended beneath the platysma. In those patients with a very full, round face, lipolysis is extended into the preauricular area to prevent the mumps-like swelling and enlargement that often ensues after the deep tissues are tightened and pulled up posteriorly. The lower nasolabial fold is also treated if the jowls remain prominent and undercorrected in spite of the SMAS and skin tightening. Defatting the buccal fat pad may create a more hollow aesthetic cheek. The malar fat pad bulge, just below the lateral eyelid, can also be removed through the face-lift incision or through a separate incision near the lateral canthus. The nasolabial fold is easily defatted through

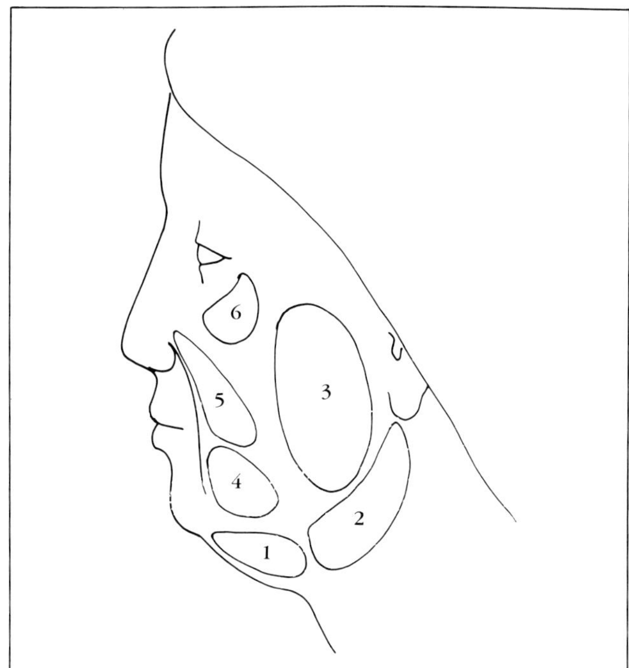

Fig. 25-3. The six areas on the face and neck that may benefit from lipolysis during the face-lift procedure: (1) submental, (2) submandibular (lateral neck), (3) preparotid (preauricular), (4) lower nasolabial, (5) upper nasolabial, and (6) malar fat pad.

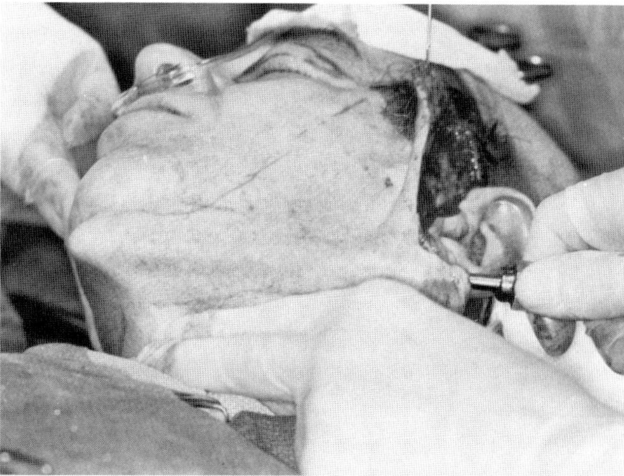

Fig. 25-4. The cannula is passed in the subcutaneous tunnel past the midline in the submental area. The hole of the cannula is kept downward away from the skin, but the cannula is passed in a very superficial tunnel. The cannula is passed repeatedly in the same tunnel to achieve the desired fat removal. The thickness of the skin flap over the cannula should be palpated repeatedly to ensure uniform removal of the fat.

the face-lift incision or by a separate incision made near the base of the alar wing.

All of these areas have been successfully treated through the face-lift incision without additional incisions.

Technique

The fat bulge to be removed is marked out preoperatively, after the preoperative marking with the patient in the sitting position. After the face-lift is under way, it is preferable to begin lipolysis in the submental area. In this area, lipolysis is confined to the subcutaneous space in most patients. Caution must be exercised to stay in the subcutaneous space because it is easy to advance the cannula accidentally through the platysma and accomplish no subcutaneous defatting at all. A #6 cannula, with a slight downward bend to the tip is good, but a #4 cannula is preferable. To achieve the exact tunnels that one desires in the subcutaneous space, it is helpful to "pretunnel" with the cannula before turning on the suction. Pretunneling achieves multiple tracks in the proper subcutaneous plane and can be done with more accuracy without the suction on. Although the smaller #4 cannula does not remove the fat as rapidly as the #6, it is much easier to pass the smaller cannula. The suction

machine should deliver as close to total vacuum as possible (less than 10 torr).

Multiple, parallel tunnels are made just beneath the skin from the lateral neck medially. When the suction machine is turned on, the operator first concentrates on cleaning out the fat in the subcutaneous, submental space. It is important to work well past the midline. Later, when the opposite side is defatted, the tunnels are again carried past the midline to overlap the first side to achieve complete removal of the fat in this area (Fig. 25-4). In any one tunnel, the cannula is passed repeatedly to achieve the desired fat removal. The thickness of the skin flap over the cannula is palpated to ensure uniform removal of fat. When lipolysis is completed, the subcutaneous space is greatly loosened, but there are numerous fibrous and vascular septa extending to the skin. Very little fat remains on the skin after thorough defatting. In some cases, however, if one stretches the skin and still sees significant accumulations of fat, it is necessary to complete the undermining to visually inspect and excise the remaining fat globules by sharp dissection. Strangely, the completion of the undermining after lipolysis is extremely rapid and bloodless in contrast to undermining or defatting with sharp instruments without lipolysis.

After submental lipolysis is completed, attention is directed to the lateral neck (submandibular area). Maximal suction is still easily maintained, even in the open wound after dissection and elevation of the skin flap, by simply keeping the opening of the cannula downward and in firm contact with the fat layer to be removed (Fig.

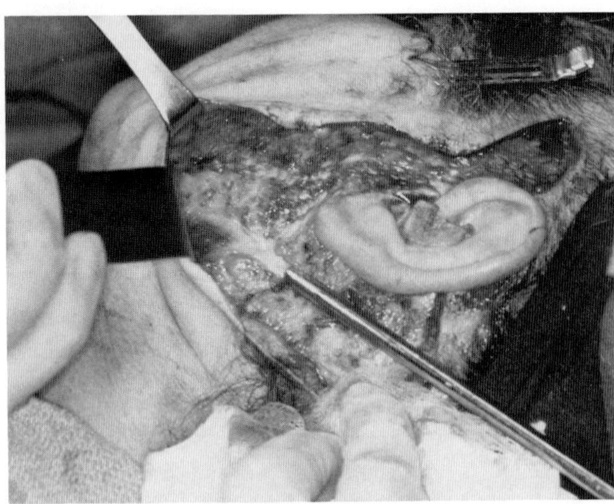

Fig. 25-5. Even though the skin flap has been elevated off the underlying subcutaneous tissue, the suction cannula easily cleans the fat off the parotid fascia simply by holding the hole downward and in firm contact with the fat to be removed. The cannula is drawn backward. The white glistening fascia devoid of fat is the white area directly in front of the tip of the cannula.

25-5). Again, caution must be exercised to stay above the platysma in the lateral neck to prevent injury to the underlying vasculature.

Note that the surgeon performing lipolysis on other areas of the body is accustomed to seeing large volumes of fat removed. By contrast, in the head and neck area, there will be very little fat appearing in the tubing when performing this procedure. The #6 cannula alone holds enough fat to produce a discernible change in the submental bulge.

After completing lipolysis on the neck from the submental region back to the angle of the mandible, attention is directed to the preparotid area. Under direct vision, the preparotid fat is suctioned with the cannula opening directed downward in firm contact with the fat. After defatting the preparotid area, the parotid fascia will be cleanly exposed for easy cutting and shifting or imbricating. Simply imbricating the exposed fascia with numerous permanent sutures is preferred by some surgeons over cutting and shifting the SMAS layer. At this point, if the imbrication and tightening of the fascia or cutting of platysma produces the contour desired, the skin is closed and attention is directed to the opposite side. If, however, a fatty bulge remains in the jowl region or in the nasolabial fold, lipolysis may now be extended to those areas. In some patients with very full submental bulges, simply carrying out subcutaneous suction is inadequate, and the cannula has to be passed beneath the musculature to obtain removal of some of the deeper fat.

Anesthesia

Anesthesia for a face-lift that includes lipolysis generally requires nothing in addition to the normal routine of the anesthetist and the plastic surgeon. In most cases, intravenous sedation is combined with local infiltration. On occasion, the motion of the cannula may arouse a drowsy patient or cause discomfort in areas where the local block is incomplete. Supplemental medication such as sodium pentathol may then be administered.

Since lipolysis allows extension of defatting into the areas of the jowls, nasolabial fold, and malar areas, the surgeon must program additional local injections to block these areas if they are not generally anesthetized during a routine face-lift. Very extensive face-lifting procedures with extensive lipolysis may benefit from general anesthesia in selected patients, but I have always used only neuroleptic anesthesia combined with local anesthesia.

Postoperative Care

The usual postoperative care for a face-lift is adequate when lipolysis has also been performed. A pressure bandage is desirable to prevent any increased swelling that might result from lipolysis. The traditional sheet cotton dressing is soaked with saline and glycerine and tightly wrapped with gauze and an Ace bandage. I use small mini-vac suction drains whether lipolysis was performed or not. The dressing is removed along with the mini-vac drains in 24 hours. The patient wears an elastic chin strap as much as possible during the next 10 days.

Postoperative Complications

In a series of 50 face-lift patients treated with lipolysis, there have been no significant complications. There were no instances of hematoma, infection, skin slough, or persisting nerve injury. There has been increased bruising of the skin, however. Two patients had a temporary induration in the lateral neck after the orifice of the cannula was directed upward to suction fat from the skin (Figs. 25-6, 25-7, and 25-8). One patient had a very minimal lower lip weakness for 3 weeks.

Illustrative Cases

Six cases illustrate the results obtainable with these techniques and are shown in Figures 25-9 to 25-14.

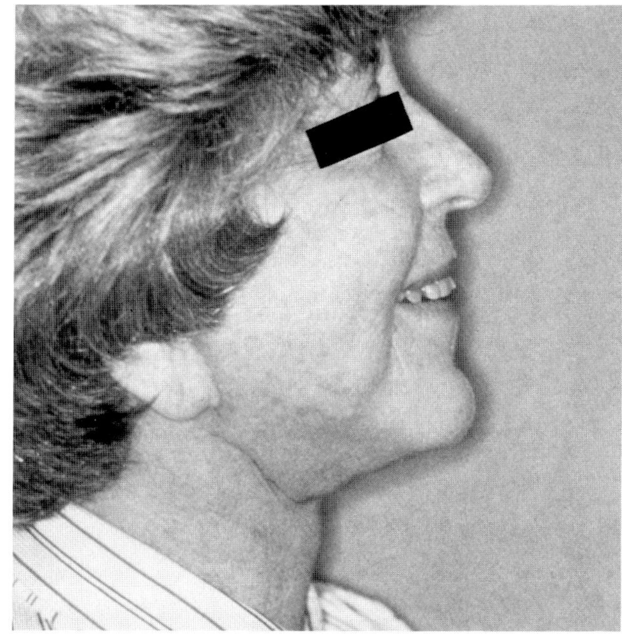

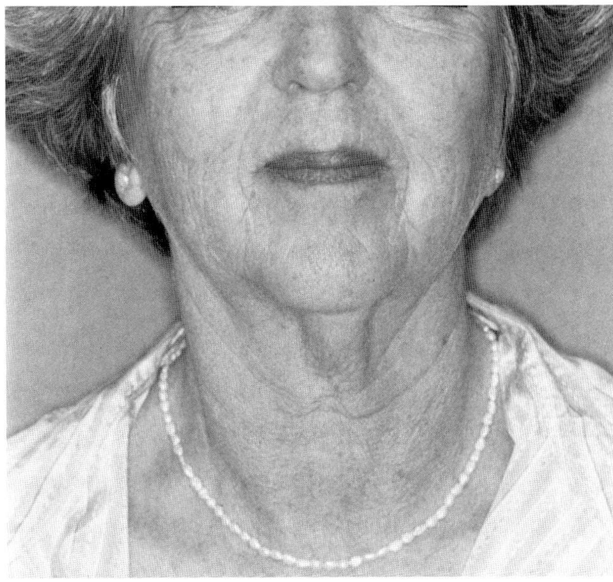

Fig. 25-7. Preoperative anterior view of patient in Fig. 25-6.

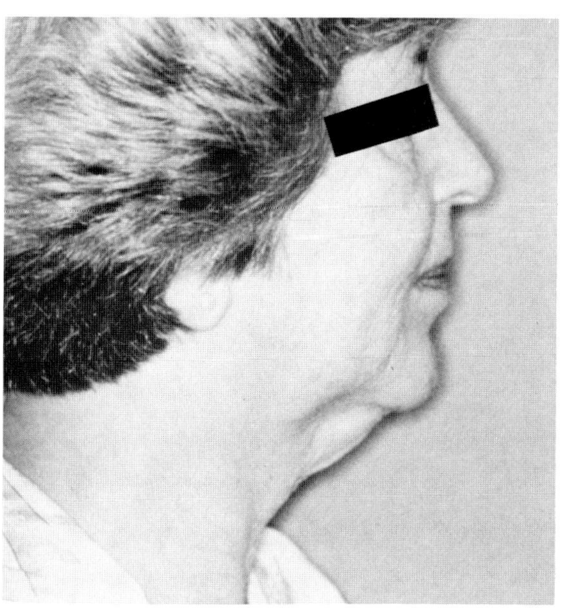

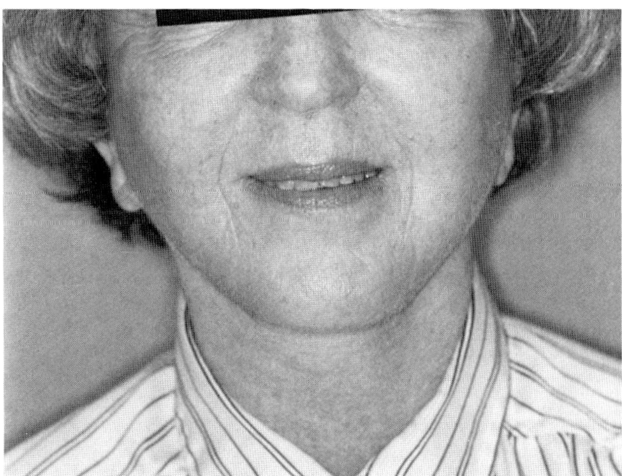

Fig. 25-8. Postoperative anterior view of patient in Fig. 25-6. The defatting has delineated the mandibular line and helped correct the lower nasolabial fold bulges of the jowls.

Fig. 25-6.
A. Preoperative view.
B. The postoperative view shows a temporary crease—an indurated band that developed in the lateral neck after the hole of the cannula was directed upward to try and clean off the fat missed by the initial pass of the cannula. Just as this technique (directing the hole of the cannula upward) will develop a buttocks crease, it will also cause a crease in the neck. This fortunately cleared after a period of approximately 6 weeks. The neck softened and the crease disappeared. One should be cautious, however, not to direct the hole of the cannula upward in the lateral neck, although it may still be a valuable technique in the submental area to help make attachment of the submental skin in the midline. This patient had full defatting of the submental area, the lateral neck region, the lower jowls, and the buccal fat pad.

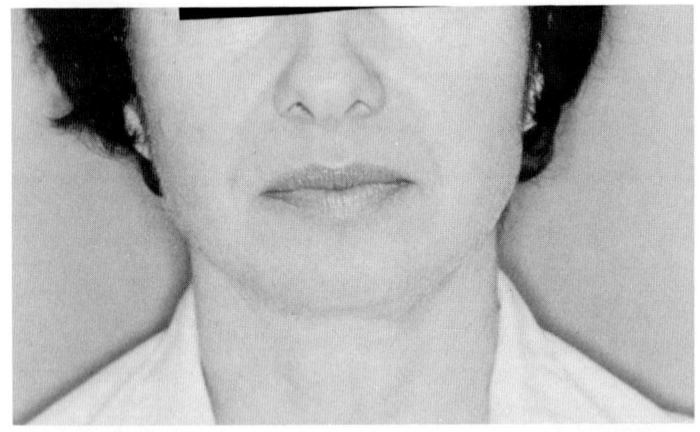

A

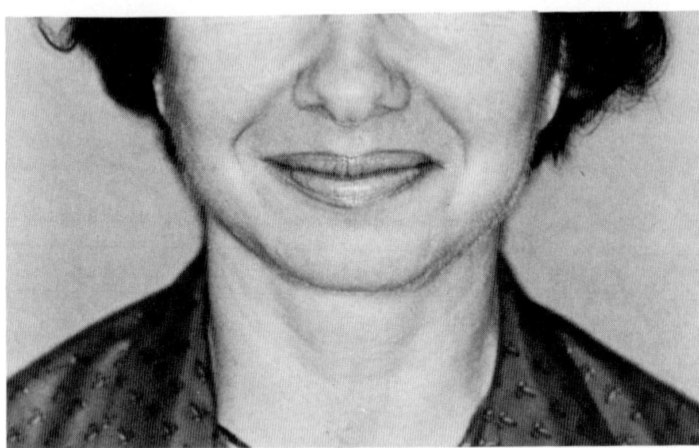

B

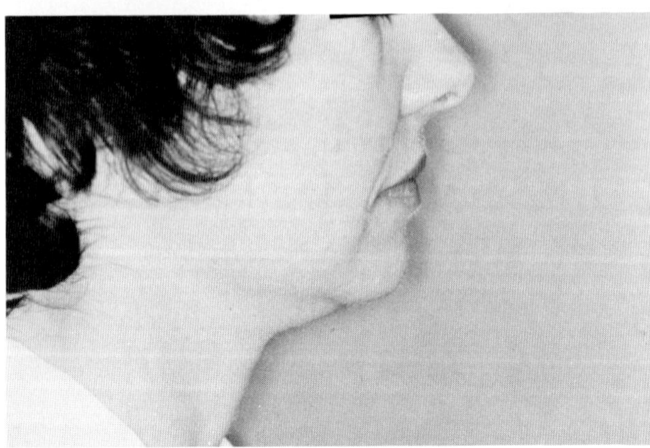

C

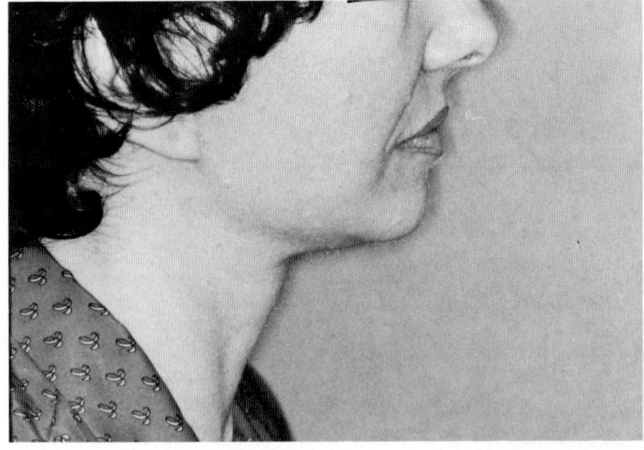

D

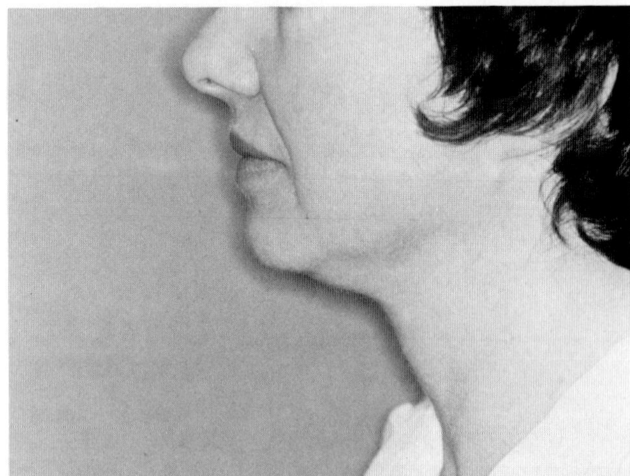

E

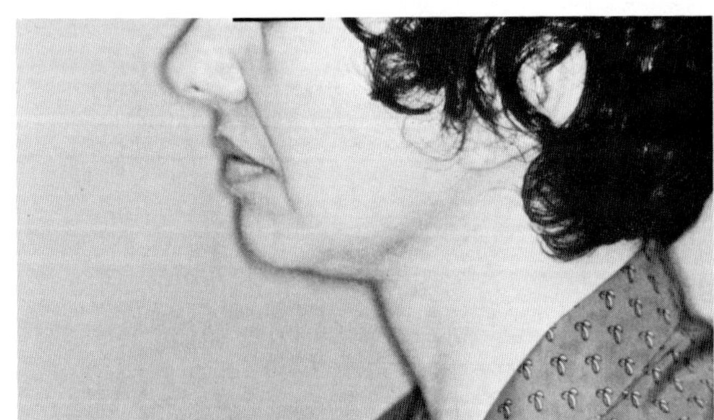

F

Fig. 25-9.
A. Preoperative view of a 44-year-old patient who had minimal but definite submental fat accumulation.
B. Postoperative view after rhytidectomy plus lipolysis in the submental area.
C. Preoperative lateral view.
D. Postoperative lateral view showing correction of submental bulge and better delineation of the mandibular line.
E. Lateral preoperative view.
F. Lateral postoperative view.

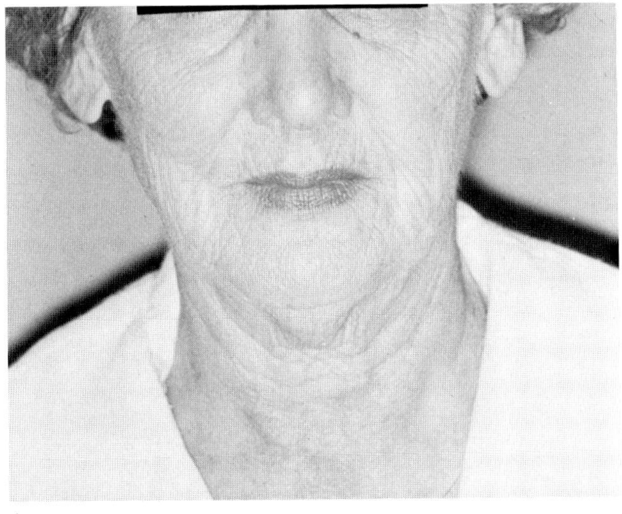

A

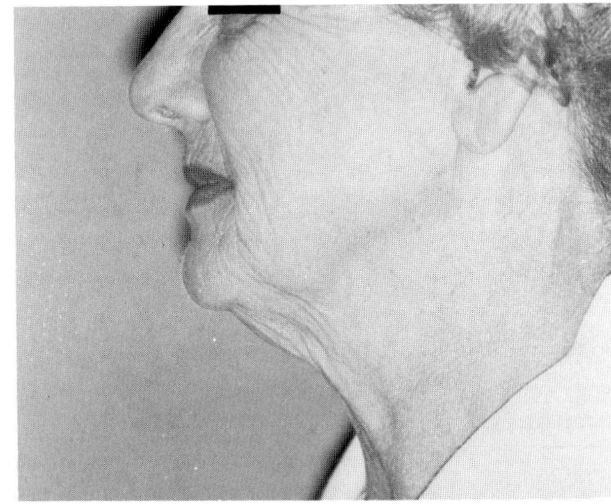

C

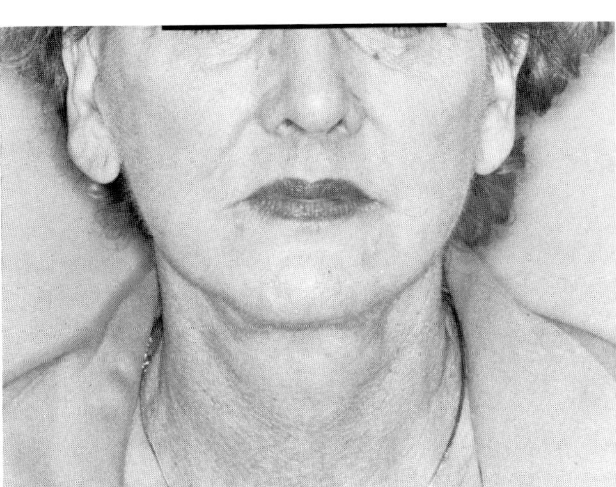

B

Fig. 25-10.
A. A 56-year-old female with submental and submandibular
   fat accumulation as well as lower nasolabial fold jowl
   problems.
B. Postoperative view after rhytidectomy and lipolysis in the
   submental, submandibular, and jowl area.
C. Preoperative lateral view.
D. Postoperative lateral view.

D

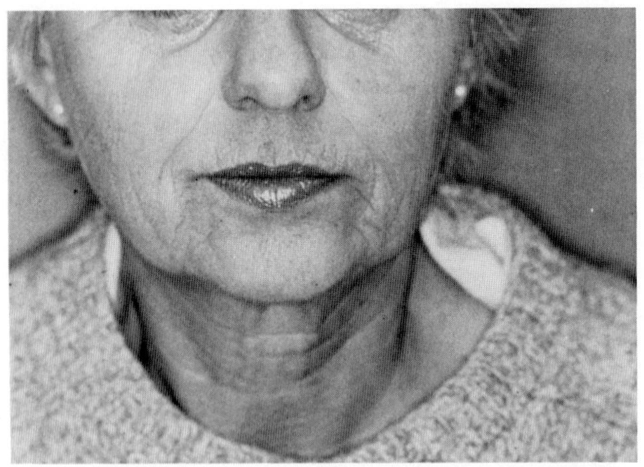

A

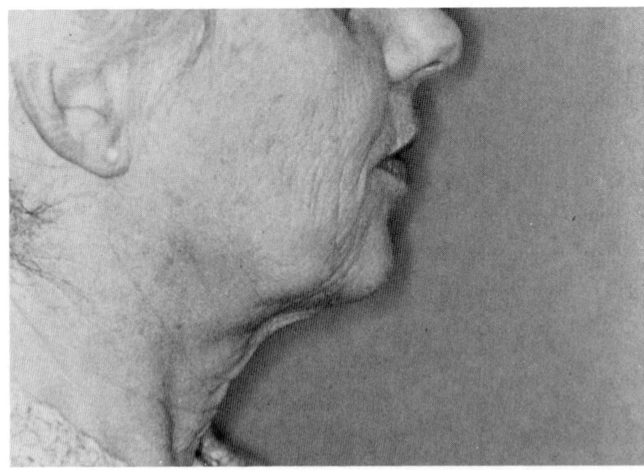

C

B

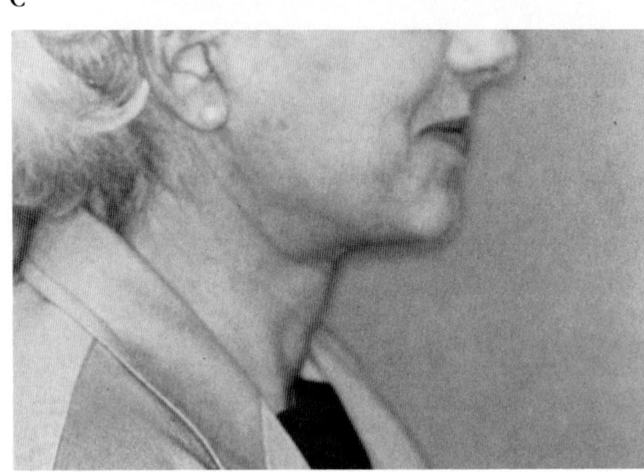

D

Fig. 25-11.
A. A 55-year-old female with the minimal lateral mandibular and preparotid and buccal accumulations. Preoperative view.
B. Postoperative view showing good neck line and cheek dimples.
C. Preoperative lateral view.
D. Postoperative lateral view.

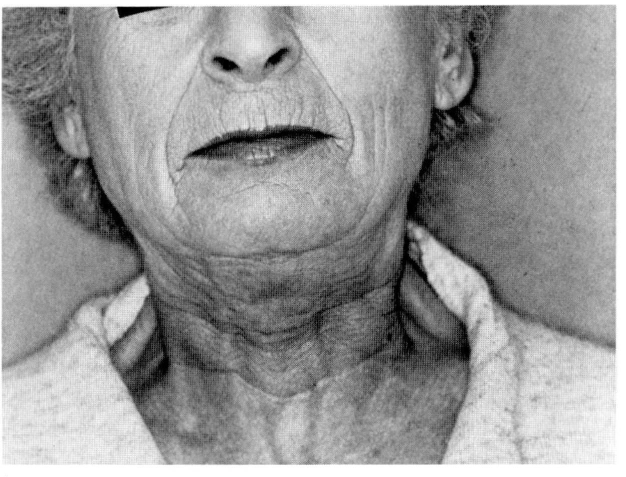

A

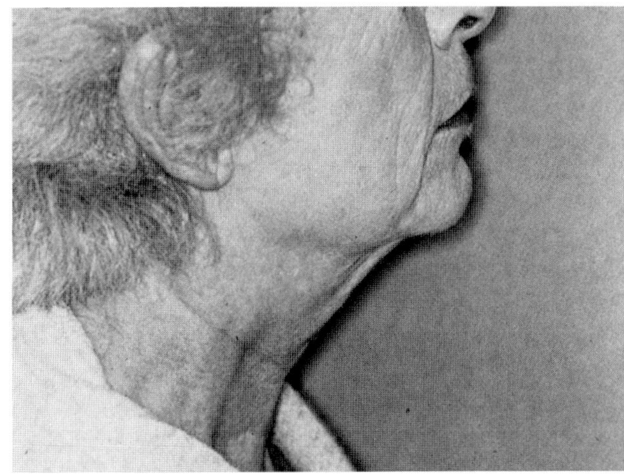

C

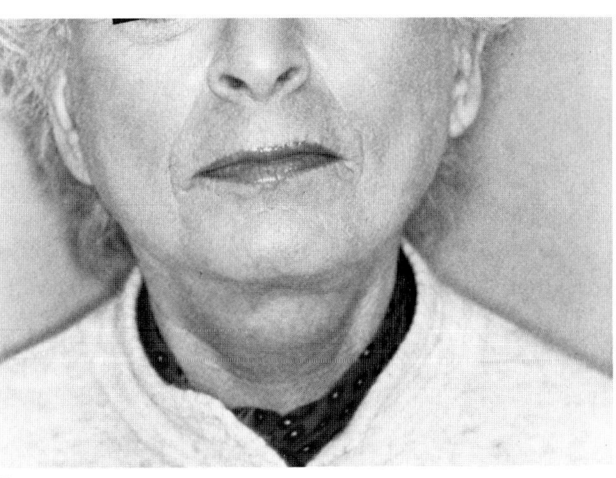

B

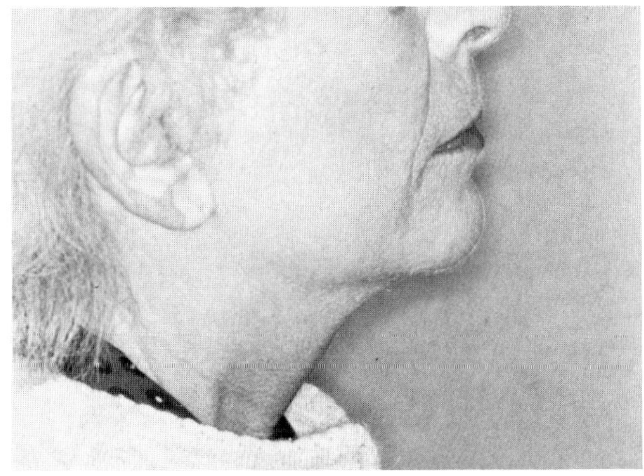

D

Fig. 25-12.
A. Preoperative view of a 62-year-old woman with submandibular, preparotid, and buccal fat accumulations.
B. Postoperative view. Slight indentation in submental area from directing hold of cannula upward in midline.
C. Preoperative lateral view.
D. Postoperative lateral view.

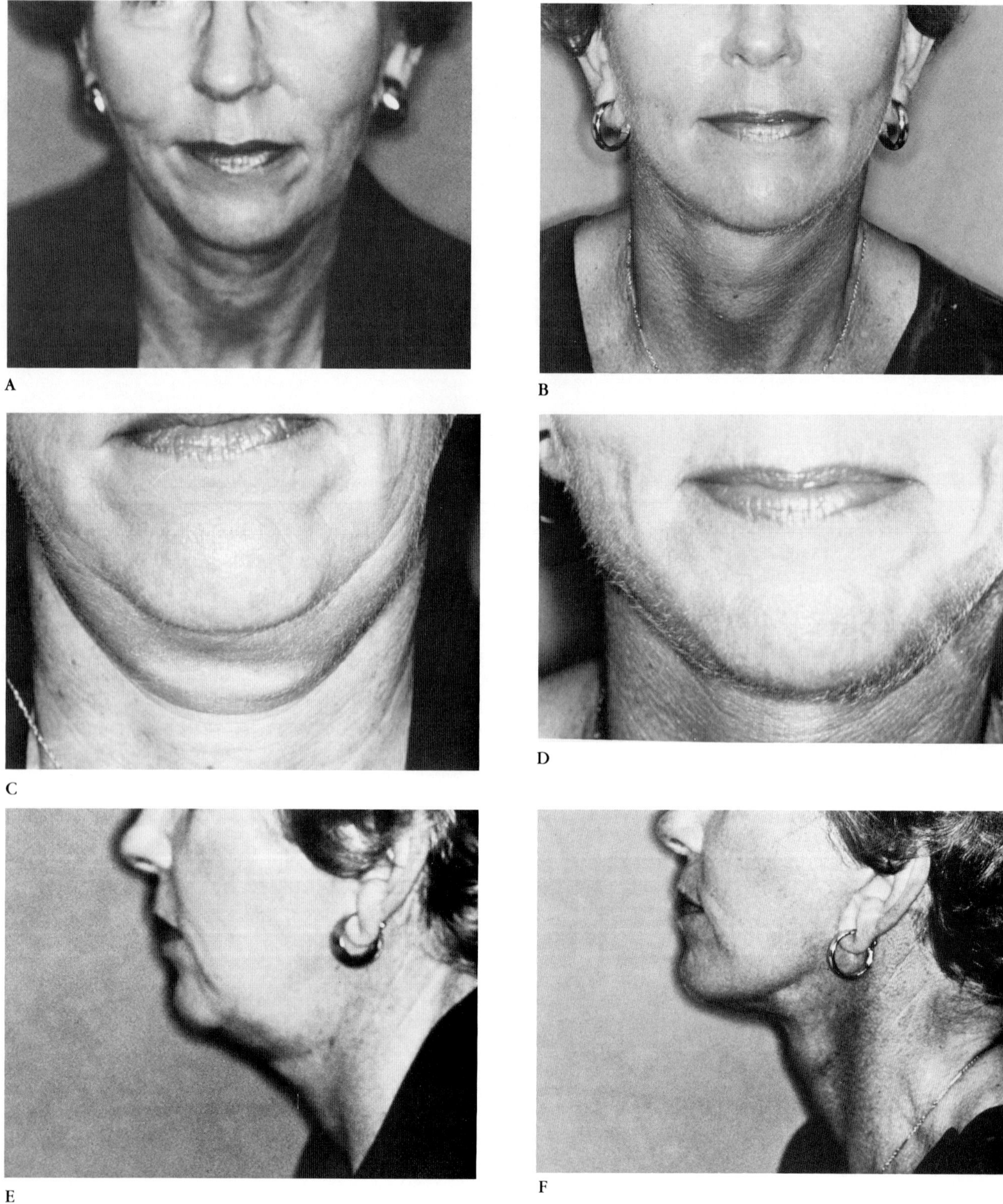

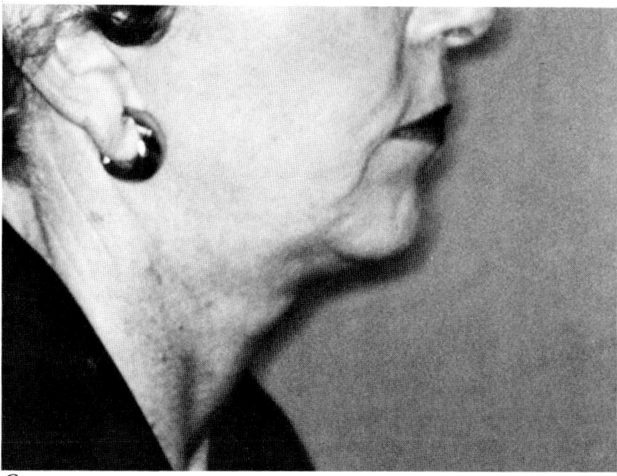

G

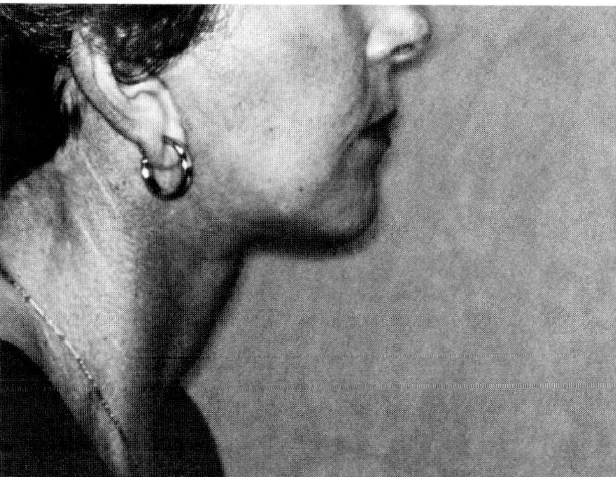

H

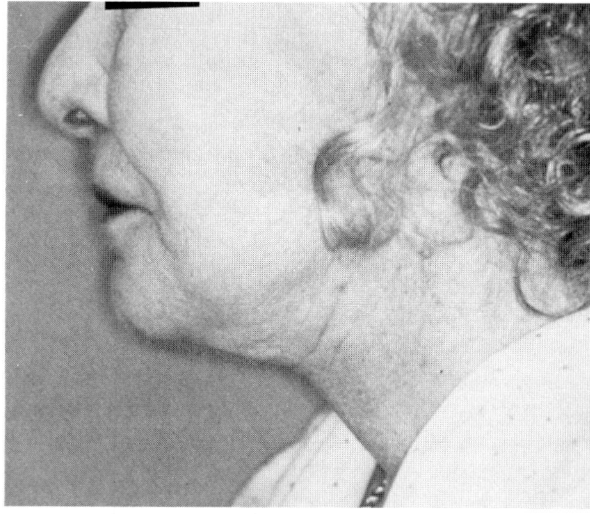

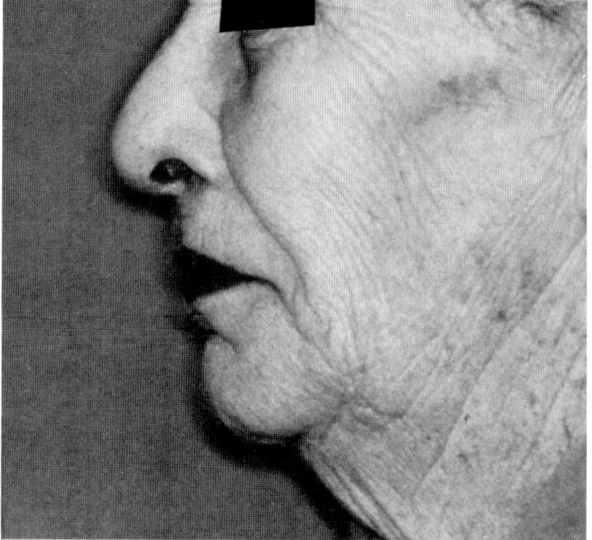

Fig. 25-13.
A. Preoperative view of a 46-year-old female requesting face-lift surgery.
B. Postoperative view after routine rhytidectomy with an SMAS imbrication and lipolysis of the submental, submandibular, and preparotid areas.
C. Close-up preoperative view. Slight flexion of the neck helps accentuate the area to be defatted.
D. Postoperative view of the neck.
E. Preoperative lateral view.
F. Postoperative lateral view shows the extent of the defatting of the submental area and lateral neck helping to accentuate a clean mandibular line.
G. Preoperative lateral view.
H. Postoperative lateral view.

Fig. 25-14. Typical preoperative and postoperative left-sided lateral views of a 64-year-old patient who had defatting of the submental and submandibular areas helping to delineate the jaw line.

Summary

Lipolysis is not advocated as a routine procedure for all face-lift patients. Like any other procedure, patient selection is essential. There can be real advantages to using lipolysis as an adjunctive procedure for the removal of fat in certain rhytidectomies. Lipolysis requires considerably less time than sharp dissection, has less need for cautery, and has less chance of hematoma or nerve injury. Also, submental scarring is minimized or eliminated since submental incisions are rarely needed.

Although the advantages of lipolysis outweigh the disadvantages, many patients still require undermining and sharp dissection to tidy up and achieve the precise contour desired in the area in which the lipolysis is performed. It is only as the surgeon gains considerable experience that he or she will be able to achieve fully satisfactory fat removal by lipolysis alone.

References

1. Maliniac, J. W. Is the surgical restoration of the face justified? *M.J. and Rec.* 135:321, 1932.
2. Padgett, E. C., and Stephenson, K. L. *Plastic and Reconstruction Surgery.* Springfield, Ill.: Thomas, 1948. P. 638.
3. Davis, A. D. Obligations in the consideration of myeloplasties. *J. Int. Surg.* 24:568, 1955.
4. Millard, D. R., Jr., Garot, W. P., Beck, R. L., et al. Submental and submandibular lipectomy in conjunction with a face-lift in the male or female. *Plast. Reconstr. Surg.* 61:376, 1978.
5. Mitz, V., and Peyronie, M. Superficial musculoaponeurotic system (SMAS) in the parotid cheek area. *Plast. Reconstr. Surg.* 58:80.
6. Connell, B. F. Contouring the neck in rhytidectomy by lipectomy and a muscle sling. *Plast. Reconstr. Surg.* 61:376, 1978.
7. Illouz, G., and Fournier, P. Personal Communication. Albuquerque, New Mexico, 1983.
8. Mladick, R. Presentation at the Annual Meeting of the Lipolysis Society of North America. Dallas, Texas, October 1983.

CHAPTER 26

Lipolysis of the Arms

Boyd R. Burkhardt

The advent of the Illouz technique of blunt suction lipectomy has influenced aesthetic surgery of the arms in much the same way as it has influenced aesthetic surgery of the trunk: Conventional dermatolipectomy is indicated less frequently. When it is done, it is often combined with adjunctive suction lipectomy to produce superior results. Even more important, some problems for which there previously was no reasonable surgical remedy can now be managed with relative ease and safety.

Indications

The indications for lipolysis of the arms are simple. If the arm is circumferentially and abnormally fat, blunt suction lipectomy is the procedure of choice. If the major problem is ptosis, but undesirable fatty accumulations are present beyond the reach of a standard dermatolipectomy (usually in the posterior arm), suction extraction of fat should be combined with conventional skin and fat excision. If the problem is ptosis without significant fatty accumulation, suction lipectomy is not indicated.

As in other parts of the body, it is difficult to predict with any precision just how much skin shrinkage will occur after suction lipectomy, so it is difficult to establish any guidelines for when skin excision is necessary. In other areas, however, the scars from skin excision often can be placed so they are easily concealed, and the aesthetic cost of the excision is consequently low. The arm is different: even well-placed incisions are difficult to conceal; and my own experience is that very rarely is a patient truly content with the scar from dermatolipectomy of the arm. For this reason, if there is any significant doubt about the need for skin excision, I prefer to do the suction lipectomy first and evaluate the patient again in 6 months for possible dermatolipectomy. It is far better to do a secondary excision for loose skin than to produce an unsatisfactory scar from a primary excision of questionable necessity.

Technique

General anesthesia is needed for all but the most minor procedures. Incisions on the shoulder should be avoided because of their proclivity for hypertrophic scar formation. Although it is technically possible to perform suction lipectomy of the arm through proximal incisions in the axilla, the operation is much more easily performed through short transverse incisions near the elbow. If there is a large posterior fat pad, it usually ends abruptly just above the elbow (best seen with the elbow extended) (see Fig. 26-5A), and one or two incisions

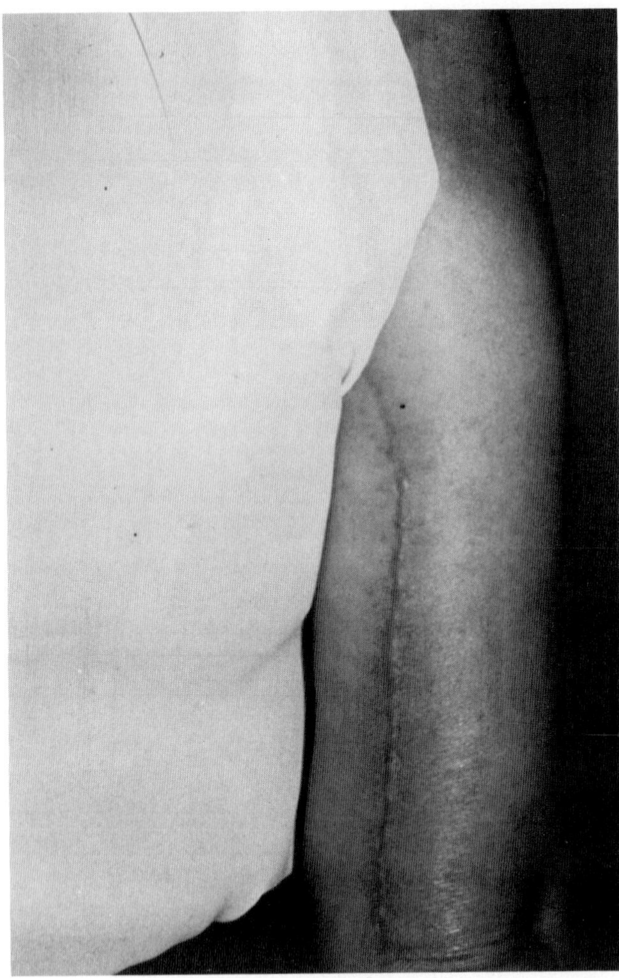

A

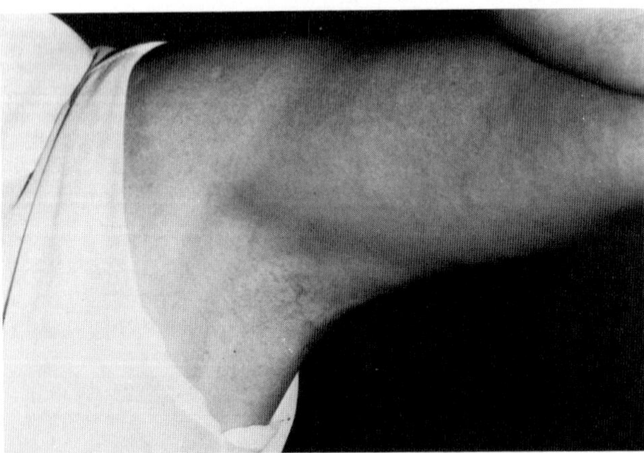

B

Fig. 26-1. A,B. Unsatisfactorily placed scars from a poorly planned dermatolipectomy. The incisions are too far posterior and extend too far up the posterior axillary fold, causing webbing.

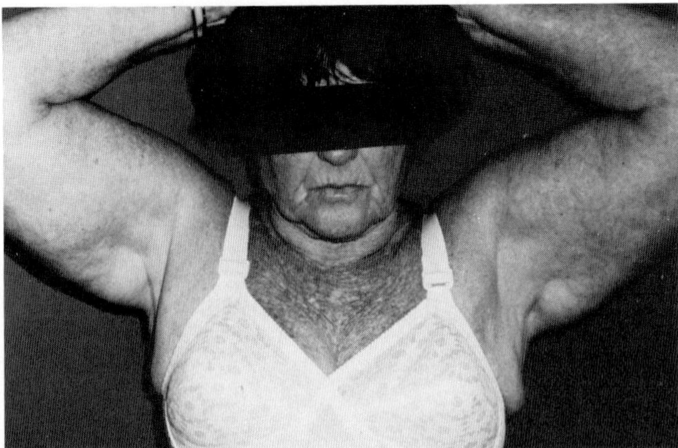

Fig. 26-2. Steatomery of the arms in a 71-year-old woman before surgery.

may be placed there. Short incisions may also be placed anteriorly. The beauty of the suction technique is that the incisions are so small as to be virtually unnoticeable.

Preoperative marking is usually not needed. I find that injections of saline, with or without enzyme preparations, are neither necessary nor helpful, while injections of 1:200,000 adrenaline solution may be useful to reduce blood loss. I ordinarily use a 6- or 8-mm straight cannula, although larger sizes may be used if there is a lot of fat. The cannula should be long enough to reach the shoulder from the elbow. The fat in this area is usually soft without much fibrous support and comes out easily. As in other areas, the subdermal fat layer should be preserved to avoid dimpling. All major structures, including the axillary sheath and contents, the ulnar nerve at the elbow, and the olecranon bursa, are deep to the fascia, and with reasonable care there should be no risk of injury. Extensive circumferential suction lipectomy has not caused cutaneous circulatory insufficiency to date, and I see no necessity to divide the operation into stages.

In doing a combined procedure, suction lipectomy is easier with the skin intact and should be done first. After removal of the fat by blunt suction, dermatolipectomy is easier (with less bleeding) and facilitates advancement of tissues for closure. Drains are not necessary. Suction lipectomy, of course, does not change the rules for dermatolipectomy.

The patient in Figure 26-1A and B has webbing of the posterior axillary fold and is greatly (and justifiably) disturbed about prominent posterior scars that cannot be moved anteriorly into a less conspicuous position. The incisions should be planned properly [1,2]. Undermine modestly if at all, and above all do not excise too aggressively or recovery will be complicated by marginal necrosis and excessive scarring. Incisions should be closed with sufficient subcuticular support so that any skin sutures may be removed at 5 to 7 days to avoid cross-hatching. Patients should be forewarned that even under the best circumstances these excisional scars remain prominent for months.

Postoperative Management

After suction lipectomy alone, I simply adjust any residual loose skin as accurately as possible and apply a light dressing, followed by a circumferential elastic bandage from the shoulder to wrist or mid-forearm for judicious compression. Although proximal compression is an anathema in hand surgery, this procedure is different, and stiffness of the hand has not been a problem. Patients are advised (1) to stay in bed most of the time with their arms elevated on pillows for 2 or 3 days, (2) to keep their hands and fingers moving, and (3) especially to loosen or even remove the compression if edema becomes significant.

Despite substantial skin redundancy immediately following major suction lipectomy, the multiple fibrous septa between the skin and fascia seem to prevent major skin displacement, and the amount of shrinkage can be truly dramatic even in older patients. Aside from a modest amount of wrinkling and irregularity, no complications have been encountered.

Case Studies

Case 1: Suction lipectomy alone (Figs. 26-2 to 26-7). V.P., a 71-year-old woman, 5′5″ tall and 170 pounds, had a massive accumulation of fat in her arms that made her upper extremities heavy and uncomfortable, made it impossible to wear normal clothes, and almost impossible to turn over in bed at night. Her forearms also had areas of excessive fat deposit, but these deposits were not functionally significant. She was legally blind, and her concerns were functional rather than cosmetic. She was willing to accept the risk of modest deformity in exchange for functional improvement.

Circumferential suction lipectomy was performed under outpatient general anesthesia, through three short transverse incisions about the elbow, removing 1625 ml from the right arm initially, and 1900 ml from the left arm 1 week later. Although the patient was placed on oral iron as a precautionary measure, blood loss was minimal: her hemoglobin was 14.1 g before the first procedure and 13.6 g one week later, just before the second procedure.

Compression by elastic bandage was maintained most of the week after the procedure. The patient then resumed normal activity and used compression and warm compresses only as needed. Two months after surgery her midpoint arm circumference had decreased from 45 to 34 cm on the right, and from 43 to 31 cm on the left. She is able to wear ordinary clothing and to turn over in bed without difficulty. Despite letters from three independent physicians attesting to the functional nature of her surgery, she has been denied coverage by Medicare. Blue Cross, her secondary carrier, has provided benefits.

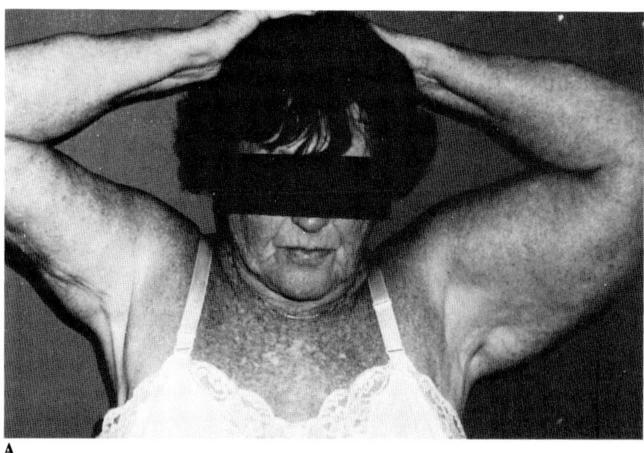

A

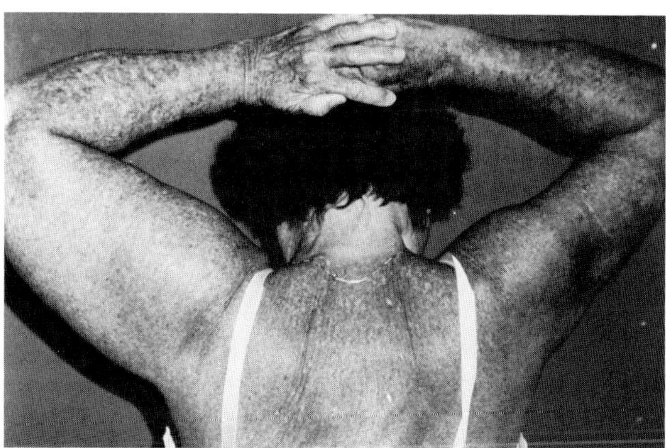

B

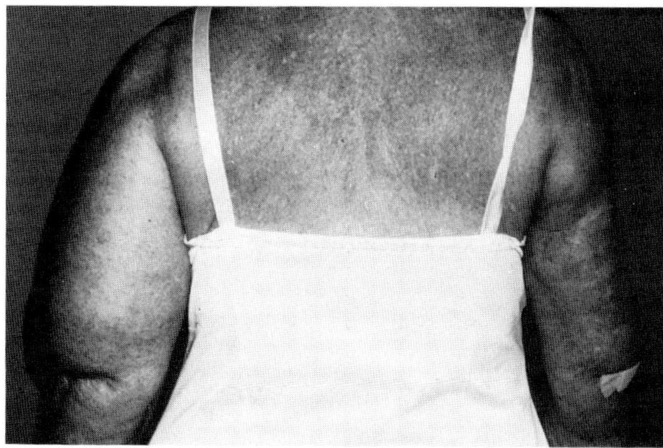

C

Fig. 26-3. A,B,C. Same patient as in Fig. 26-2 after suction lipectomy of her right arm.

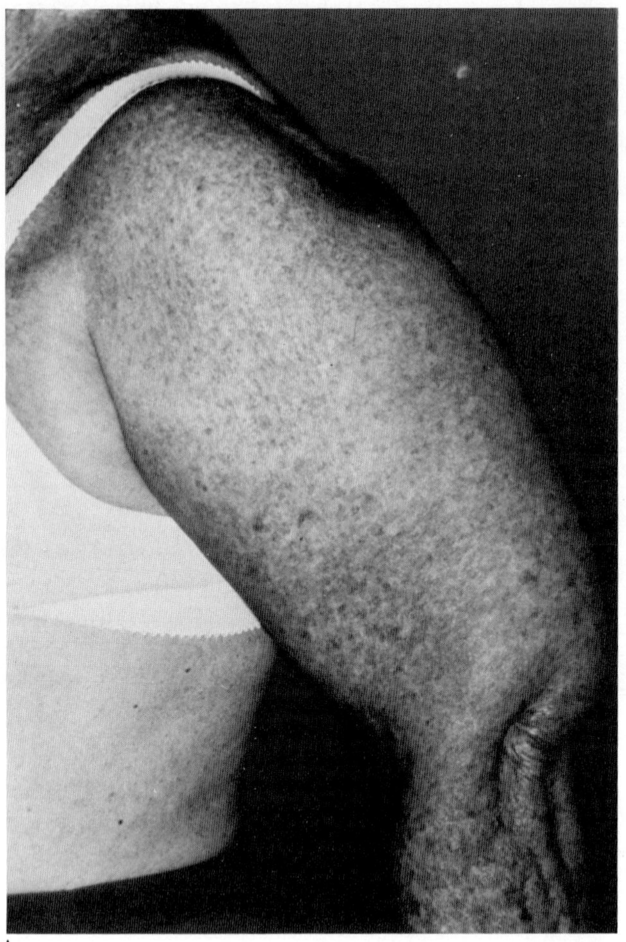

A

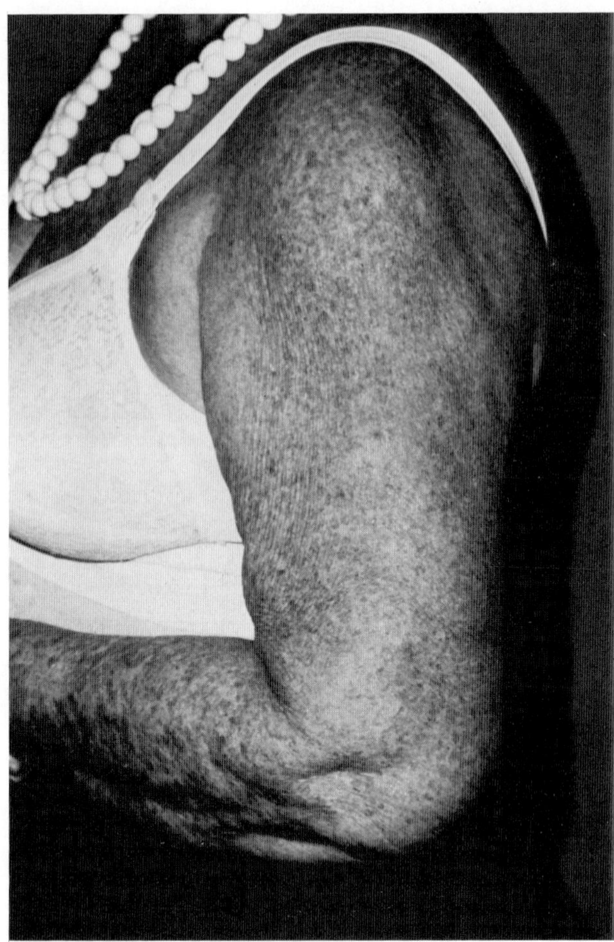

B

Fig. 26-4. A,B. Views of left arm before and after suction lipectomy (same patient as in Figure 26-2).

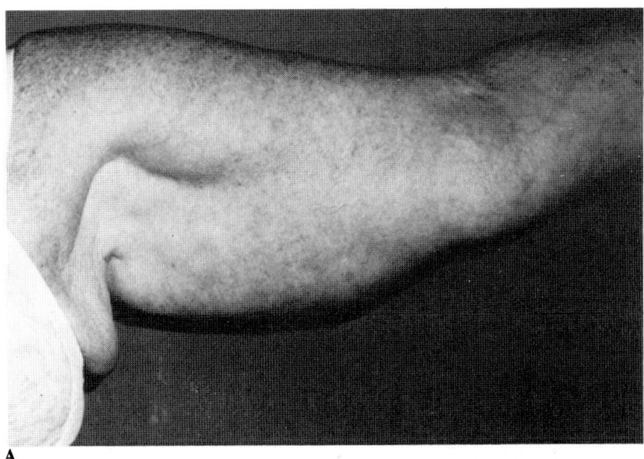

A

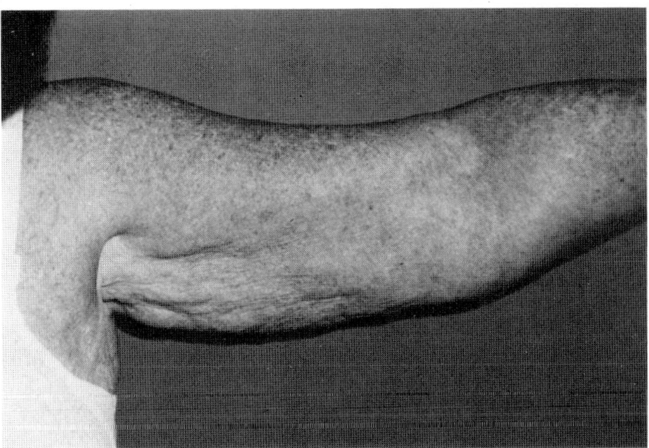

B

Fig. 26-5. A,B. Views of left arm before and after suction lipectomy (same patient as in Fig. 26-2).

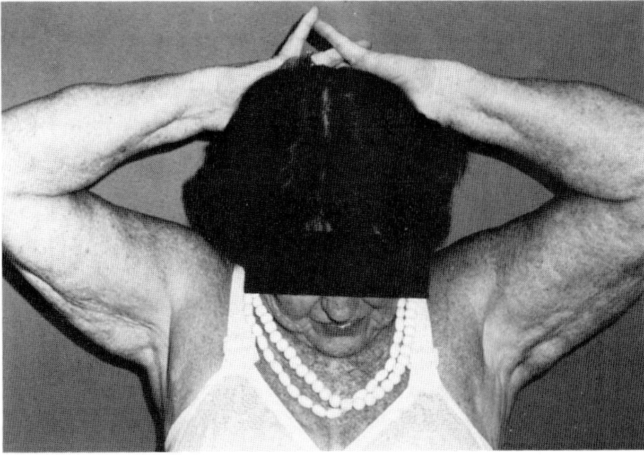

Fig. 26-6. Same patient as in Fig. 26-2 approximately 4 months after reduction of both arms.

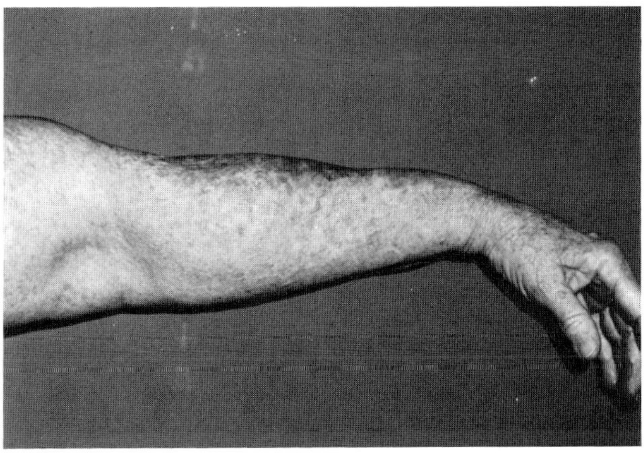

Fig. 26-7. Abnormal fatty deposits on dorsum of left forearm. The condition was bilateral (same patient as in Fig. 26-2).

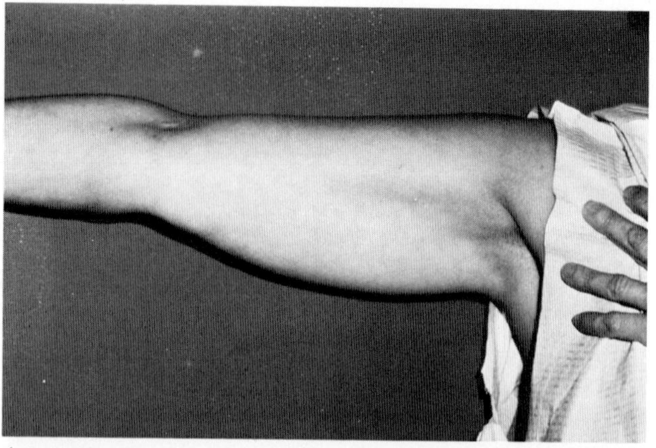

A

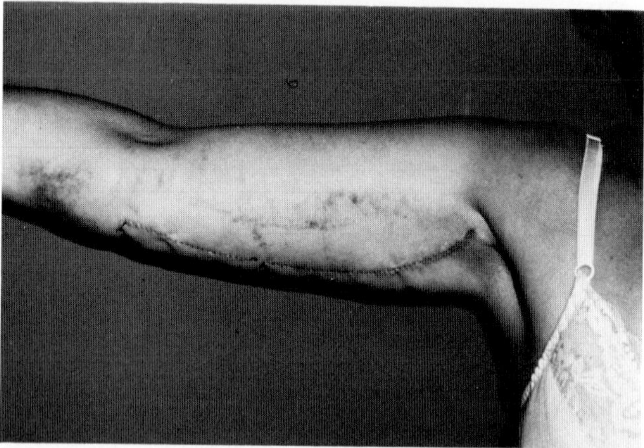

B

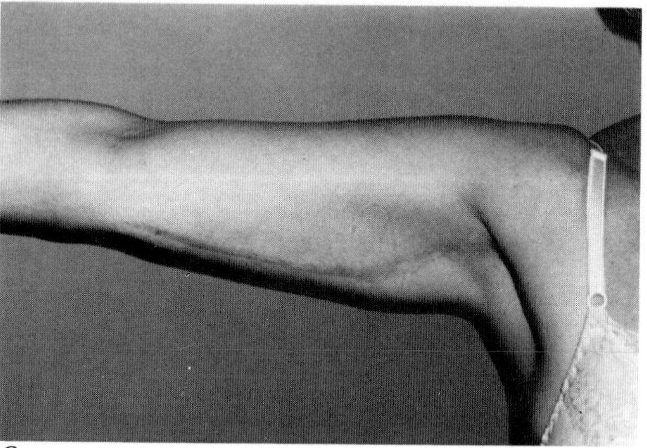

C

Fig. 26-8.
A. Right arm of patient preoperatively.
B. 1 week after combined procedure.
C. 7 months after combined procedure of suction and der-
molipectomy.

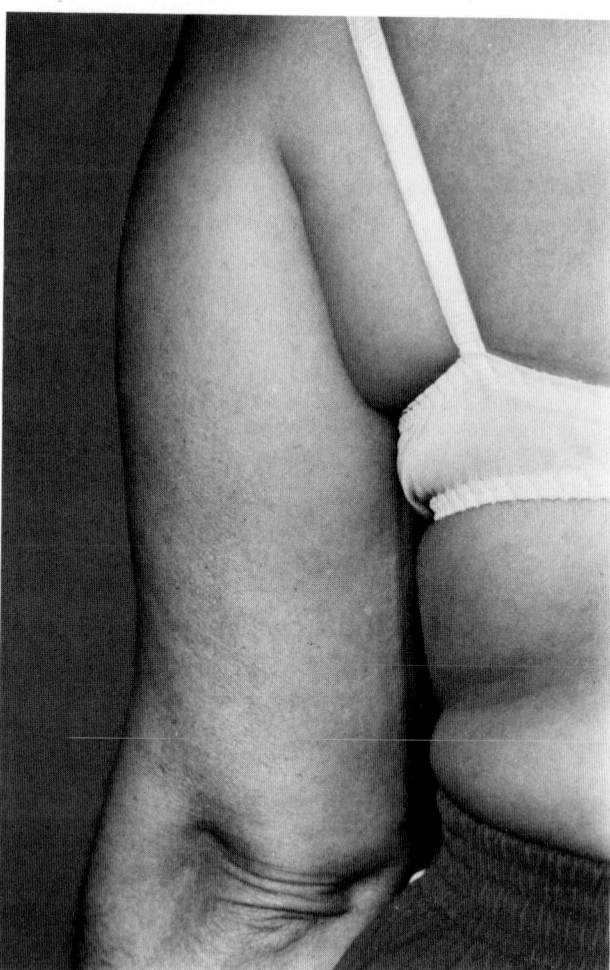

Fig. 26-9. Left arm of patient from posterior showing better
scar position, well anterior. Contrast with Fig. 26-1A.

Case 2: Suction lipectomy combined with dermatolipectomy
(Figs. 26-8 and 26-9). L.S., a 48-year-old woman in good
health, requested suction lipectomy for reduction of her arms,
knees, medial and lateral thighs, and buttocks. Her arms had
considerable ptosis in addition to adiposity over the body of
the triceps. Suction lipectomy was performed on all areas as a
single outpatient procedure, removing a total of 1500 ml. Arm
fat was aspirated through single transverse incisions proximal
to the medial epicondyle, removing approximately 100 ml
from each side and carrying the suction not only posteriorly
but also across the medial arm. Skin and underlying fat were
excised as a specimen, extending from the medial epicondyle
to the anterior axilla, and measuring 5 cm at its widest point.
Postoperative management was similar to that noted in Case 1.

Summary

If used with reasonable judgment by properly trained practitioners, blunt suction lipectomy is a safe, simple, and valuable adjunct to standard brachioplasty. The Illouz technique alone enables us to achieve reduction contouring that was previously impossible in the upper arm.

References

1. Baroudi, R. Dermolipectomy of the upper arm. *Clin. Plast. Surg.* 2:455, 1975.
2. Guerrero-Santos J. Brachioplasty. *Aesth. Plast. Surg.* 3:1, 1979.

Lipolysis as an Adjunctive Treatment for Gynecomastia

Carson M. Lewis

Before the advent of lipolysis, the surgical treatment of gynecomastia had several undesirable features. The procedure involved an excision of the enlarged breast mound, consisting of glandular tissue and surrounding subcutaneous fat. In cases of moderate to large breasts, the excision required sharp dissection and extensive undermining of tissue. Coursing throughout the adipose tissue were multiple blood vessels and nerves. Hemostasis was difficult to obtain. Postoperative hemorrhage was common. Subsequent sequelae of seroma formation, delayed healing, and prolonged morbidity with possibilities of infection and tissue necrosis occurred. On large breasts with ptosis, incisions were made outside the nipple/areolar complex to remove the excessive skin and to correct ptosis, resulting in the scar frequently being wide and poorly concealed.

More important, the postoperative appearance had noticeable flaws. Surgeons found that smoothing out the junction of resected tissue to chest was difficult. The desirable amount of tissue for removal was not accurately estimated. Along with subsequent unpredictable healing, extensive undermining, and dissection, the resultant chest wall and breast had an "operated on" look. A dished-out appearance of the chest could occur, with dents, waves, or other irregularities at the periphery; flattened, indented, or irregular nipples occur in many cases.

Many surgeons observing the results of their treatment of gynecomastia were not satisfied with their work. Although the enlarged breast tissue was successfully removed, most frequently this tissue was removed because the patient felt self-conscious about his or her appearance. Unfortunately, the patient was often left with an appearance equally bothersome due to the operated look.

Lipolysis used in combination with glandular resection offers a means to minimize or eliminate these undesirable sequelae of excision alone. Lipolysis techniques are used successfully for body contouring throughout the body. Lipolysis used in combination with excision of the glandular tissue beneath the areola has improved the technique for treatment of gynecomastia.

Preoperative Preparation

MARKING UPRIGHT POSITIONS

1. Mark the sternal notch.
2. Mark the midsternal line.
3. Mark extent of tissue to be resected with the patient in the sitting or standing position. By pressing the breast tissue toward the periphery with the other hand, the junction of breast tissue can be visualized easily and carefully marked.

4. *Topography map.* Draw a topographic map (aerial view) of the tissue to be resected. The topography map records the varying heights of tissue to be resected. This map is referred to during the operative procedure.

5. *Pinch test.* Perform a pinch test in the areas of resection by grasping the tissue, skin, and subcutaneous fat between the thumb and index finger, squeeze together, and measure the distance between the two. Record directly on the skin at the site. Perform the pinch test in normal adjacent tissue to proposed area of resection for comparison and record. The pinch test establishes a thickness of the skin and subcutaneous tissue preoperatively. As lipolysis proceeds, the operator may continue to check thickness with pinch tests to help determine the need for further fat removal.

6. *Location of incision.* Mark inferior half of periareolar junction. The site of the incision needs to be carefully placed at the junction with the skin. This junction between areola and skin is not always distinct. If unable to place exactly on the junction, for fair-skinned individuals, it is better to place the incision on the skin rather than on the areolar side. In dark-skinned individuals, it is better to place the incision slightly on the areolar side to conceal the resultant scar.

7. *Predetermine* the amount of glandular resection by palpation, and mark on the skin, frequently extending 1 to 2 cm beyond the areola.

ANESTHESIA

General anesthesia is preferred for most lipolysis procedures. Treatment of gynecomastia falls into this group. In most cases, anesthesia is carried out with a face mask, and an endotracheal tube is avoided. With the patient in the supine position, after anesthesia is induced, the breast tissue is infiltrated with approximately 50 ml of 0.25% Xylocaine, containing 1:400,000 epinephrine, with Wydase, 0.67 unit/100 ml bilaterally, using a #20 spinal needle and a 50-ml disposable syringe.

PREPPING AND DRAPING

The entire chest wall from the clavicle and sternal notch to below the umbilicus is prepped after local infiltration. Disposable towels and sheets are used, exposing the entire chest wall so the breasts may be compared.

INCISION

An 8- to 10-mm incision is made through the periareolar junction. The superficial tissue is spread by a blunt scissor to avoid surface bleeders. The #8 Illouz-type blunt cannula is inserted vertically to the chest wall and passed downward until the fascia over the pectoralis major muscle is encountered; then the cannula is turned on a horizontal plane and advanced.

Surgical Technique

A high vacuum surgical suction machine is turned on until a minimum of 25 mm of mercury residual pressure is obtained (gauge pressure of 735 mm, or 29 inches, of mercury at sea level; see Chap. 16). The strokes are begun, using 8 to 12 strokes in one tunnel, resting, and awaiting the results in the clear tubing. The operator should note the color and amount of fat coming up the tube from the cannula toward the pump. A new tunnel is made in close proximity to the first, and the procedure is repeated. The action is similar to sawing wood.

The opposite hand plays an important part in performing the operation. With the opposite hand, the operator palpates the cannula. He or she grasps the tissue to aid in the sculpting of the tissue.

EXTENT OF LIPOLYSIS

The lipolysis technique is used throughout the breast tissue, making multiple tunnels. The opening in the cannula is 1 to 2 cm proximal to its distal end, so the cannular tip must extend 1 to 2 cm beyond the periphery of the fatty tissue to be removed.

The surgeon may stop and use the pinch test to visualize thickness of the tissues to detect areas needing further suctioning.

REFINEMENTS

Feathering or removal of tissue immediately adjacent to the resection is helpful to preserve a gradual transition between the operated tissue and the surrounding tissue. The feathering technique can be done with the same-sized cannula, extending some 3 to 5 cm beyond the point of resection. This technique can be done with a cannula of the same size with no suction or with the next smaller-sized cannula with suction attached (see Chap. 4).

Final minor refinements in the fatty tissue can be performed with a #6 cannula throughout the breast tissue, grasping the tissue securely with the opposite hand and removing amounts of additional tissue as desired.

The ideal amount of resection can be checked primarily by two means: (1) direct observation; it is desirable to look at the area from several angles as we are dealing with a three-dimensional object ("skyline view"), and

(2) a pinch test, remembering the amount of tissue present when the procedure was started and how much tissue is left. Both tests are helpful in determining whether or not further resection is necessary.

GLANDULAR REMOVAL

Excision of glandular tissue is performed by extending the incision in the inferior one-half of the periareolar junction (previously marked). Small bleeders are cauterized, and resection extends beneath the nipple/areolar complex at a depth of 8 to 10 mm. Resection of the gland is done beneath this plane, leaving this thickness 10 mm beneath the nipple/areolar complex. This thickness is desirable to prevent vascular compromise and to allow adequate nipple/areolar projection.

The opposite side is performed in a similar way, performing the lipolysis first, followed by the glandular resection. Both sides are checked for any excessive bleeding by pressing the tissue in the periphery and advancing it toward the areolar incision. Bleeding is usually minimal. If there is any concern about bleeding, drains may be used. Drains for this operative procedure, however, are quite unusual.

CLOSURE

The areola is closed in layers with absorbable 4-0 sutures and a subcuticular prolene suture in the skin. Steri-Strips are used around the areola.

DRESSING

The surface of the skin is cleansed with acetone. Adhesive tape is applied, with the exception of the nipple/areolar complex. A 4-inch elastic tape is applied in a figure-of-eight fashion, covering the nipple/areolar complex with nonadherent gauze.

Postoperative Care

The patient remains in the recovery room until vital signs are stable and until fully awake; he or she is discharged to home the same day. The patient is started on prophylactic antibiotics in an intravenous solution of Ringer's lactate, approximately 1 hour before the operative procedure. Oral antibiotics are continued postoperatively for 3 days. The patient is seen on the third postoperative day.

The tape is removed by the patient at 7 days postoperatively. He or she is seen in the office in 10 days, at which time the sutures are removed and incisions reinforced with Steri-Strips. Massage and ultrasound are initiated at that time and continued for 8 to 10 treatments, if desired.

Figures 27-1 to 27-14 provide a photographic review, including pre- and postoperative views of incisions, of a 17-year-old male with gynecomastia.

Discussion

Historically, treatment of gynecomastia began with emphasis on the removal of tissue alone [1,2]. With advances in technique, more concern was placed on the aesthetic appearance of the operative result. In 1946 Webster [3] described an intraareolar incision for gynecomastia. Subsequently, to minimize the appearance of the incision, others have masked the scar either by placing the incision transareolar [4] in the axilla [5] or by using a circumareolar incision, advancing the size of the areola and excising the surrounding tissue [6].

All of these procedures attempt to refine the appearance of incisions; however, subcutaneous undermining and excision of the tissue containing vessels and nerves is not altered. Another major concern of the previous methods is the treatment of excessive skin. Previous reports indicate that incisions outside the nipple/areolar complex [7,8], with excision of skin and adjustment of the skin envelope, leave visible scarring.

The technique of lipolysis with glandular excision using the periareolar incision results in small, inconspicuously placed scars.

A limitation of the excision approach is well stated in a previous review of a reduction mammoplasty [9].

Unfortunately, it is the basic in plastic surgery as well as in tailoring or dressmaking, that in order to reduce the redundancy of skin, the surgeon must excise excessive skin or material, creating a scar. Until some clever surgeon in the future shows us how to shorten skin without cutting it, we will be condemned to leave a visible scar in such cases; the monument of our ineptitude.

Lipolysis for the removal of tissue (blunt suction lipectomy) overcomes this ineptitude. Large quantities of subcutaneous tissue can be removed through a small incision, leaving the septa connecting the skin and subcutaneous tissue, so that the tissue is pulled down as an accordion and adheres to its underlying structure. The lack of a need for skin tailoring eliminates the need for a long incision and dermolipectomy.

Postoperative hemorrhage has been a relatively common complication in the treatment of moderate to large gynecomastia. In several reported series, 4 of 17, 10 of 54, and 10 of 16 patients had hematomas [3,10,11]. Hematoma formation occurred in from 18 to 62%. No series of gynecomastia patients has been reported to

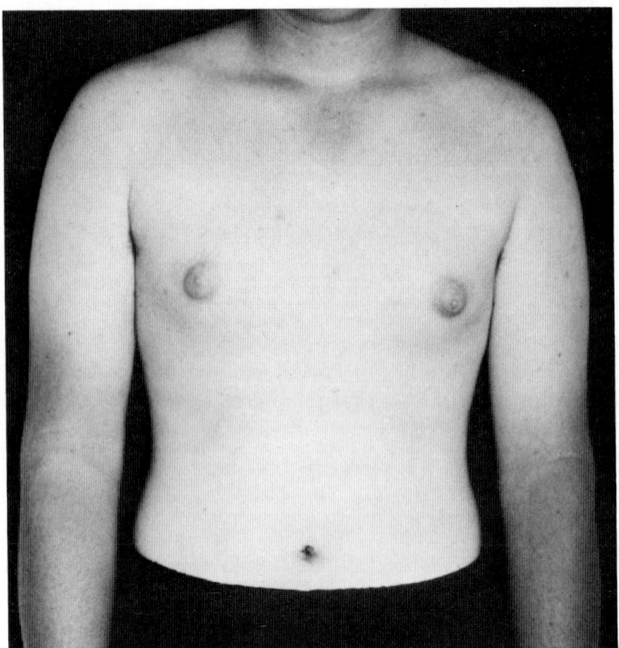

Fig. 27-1. Preoperative frontal view of a 17-year-old male with gynecomastia.

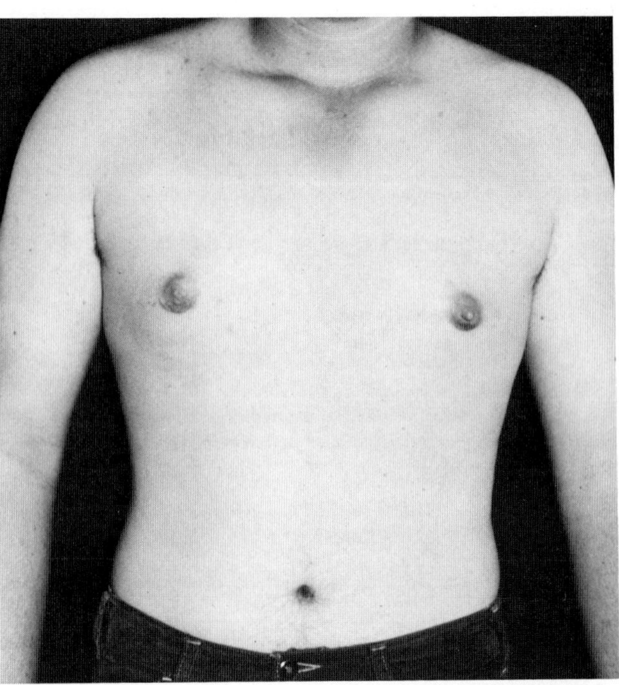

Fig. 27-2. Postoperative frontal view 2 months after removal of 300 ml of fat.

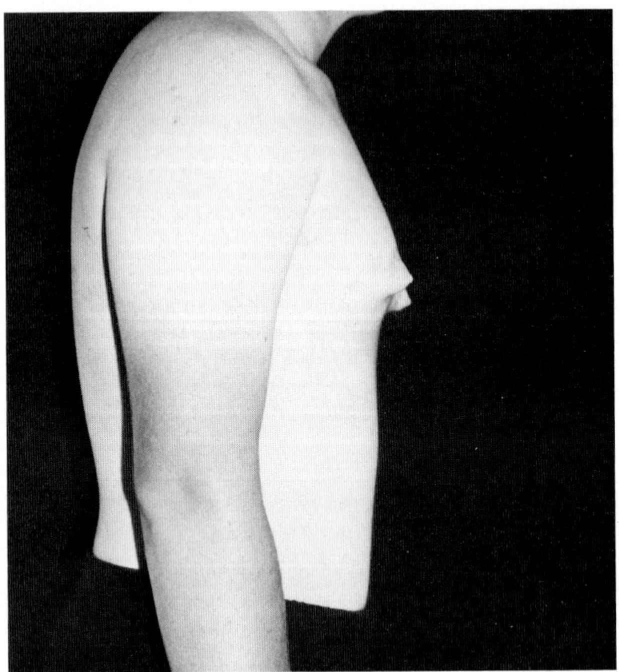

Fig. 27-3. Preoperative right lateral view.

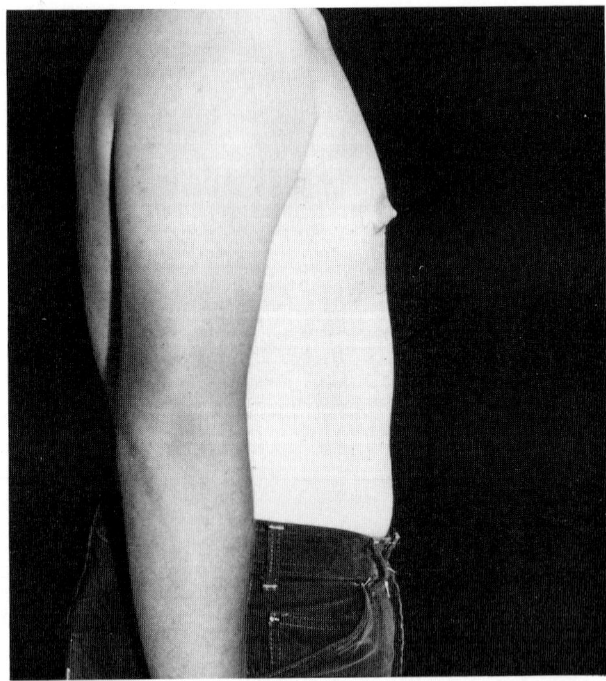

Fig. 27-4. Postoperative right lateral view 2 months after surgery.

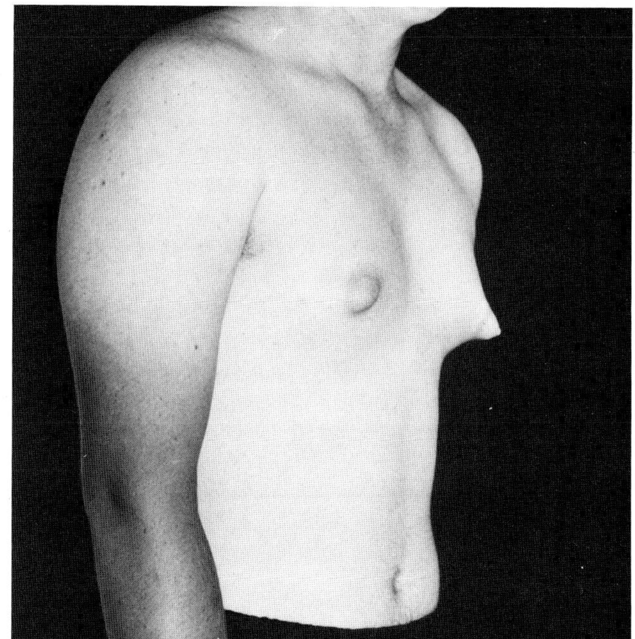

Fig. 27-5. Preoperative right oblique view.

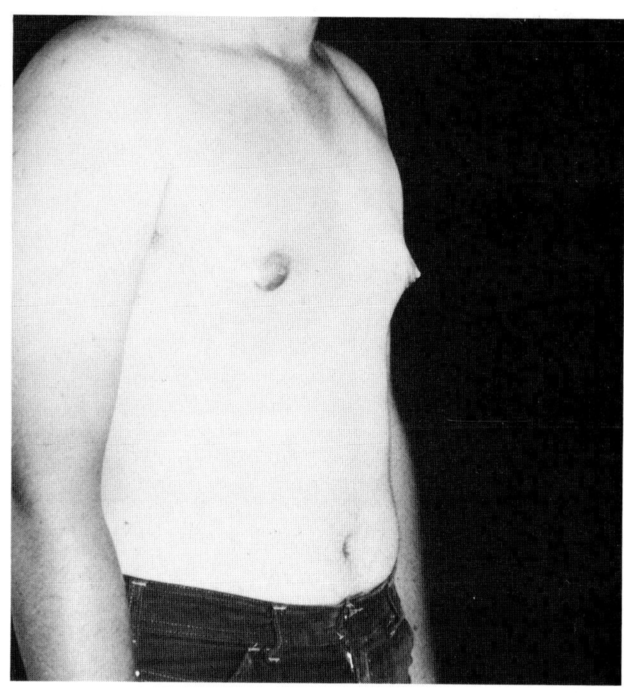

Fig. 27-6. Postoperative right oblique view 2 months after surgery.

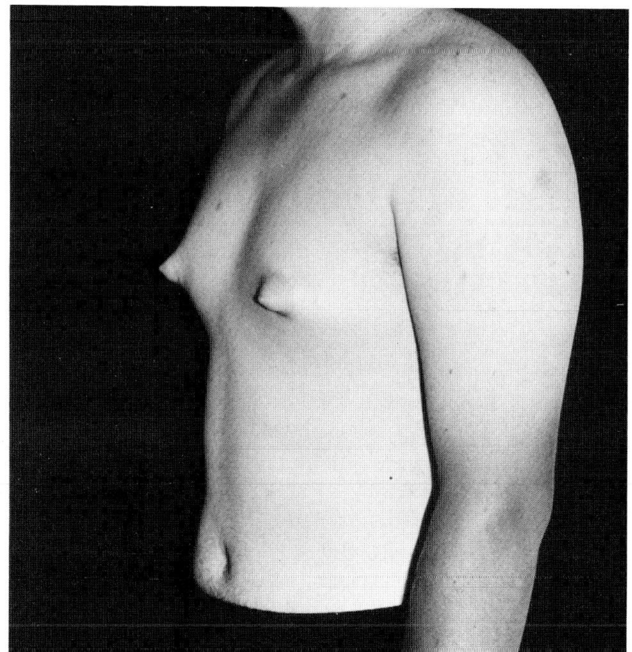

Fig. 27-7. Preoperative left oblique view.

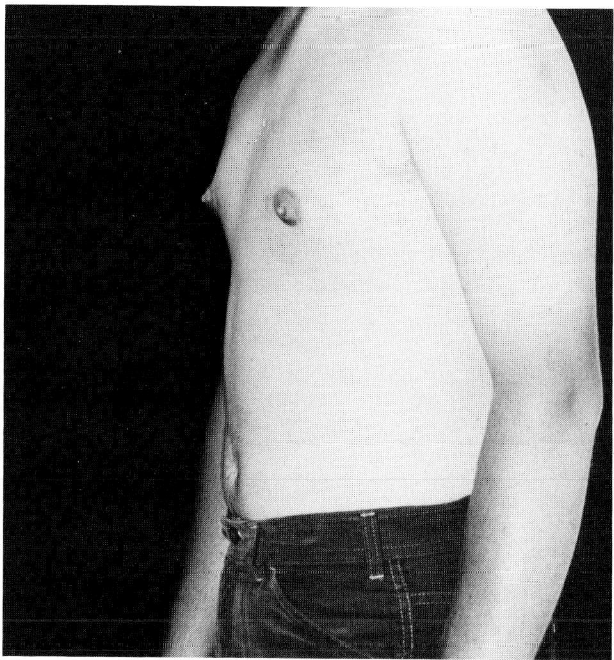

Fig. 27-8. Postoperative left oblique view 2 months after surgery.

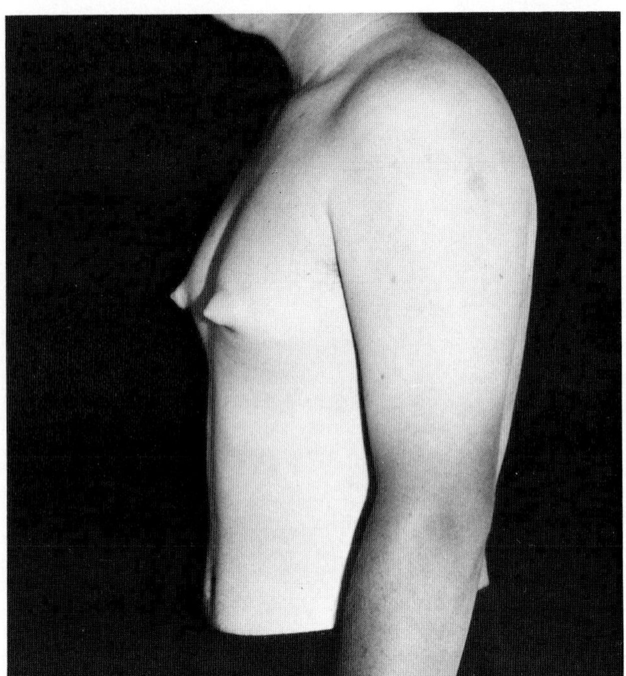

Fig. 27-9. Preoperative left lateral view.

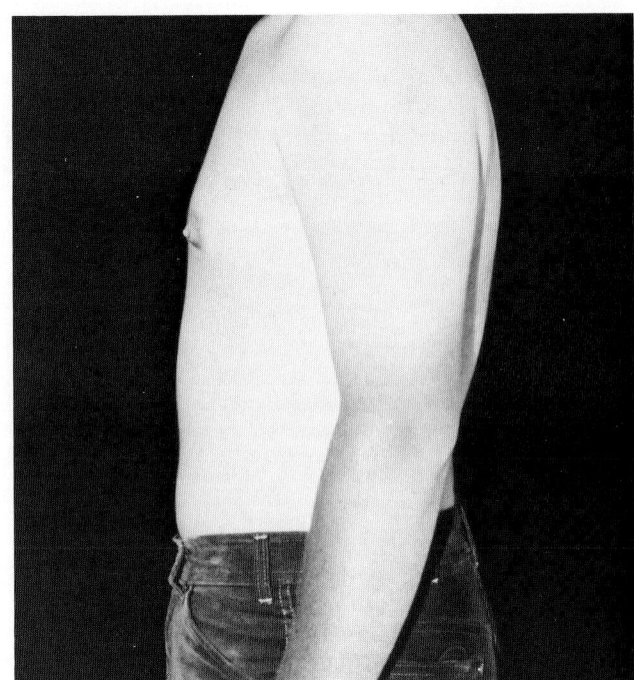

Fig. 27-10. Postoperative left lateral view 2 months after surgery.

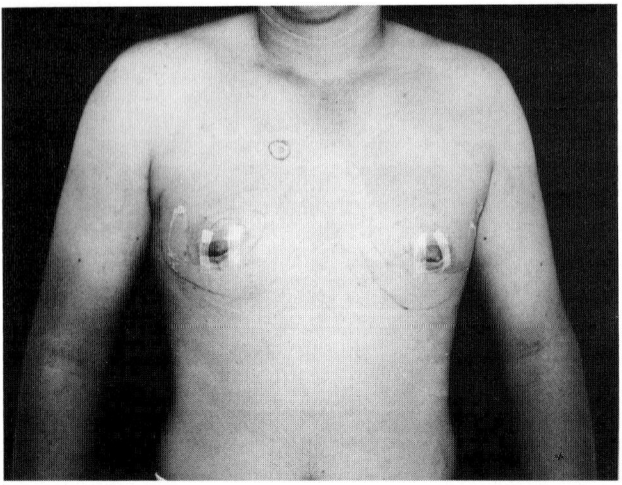

Fig. 27-11. Postoperative frontal view showing minimal bruising and swelling 1 week after surgery.

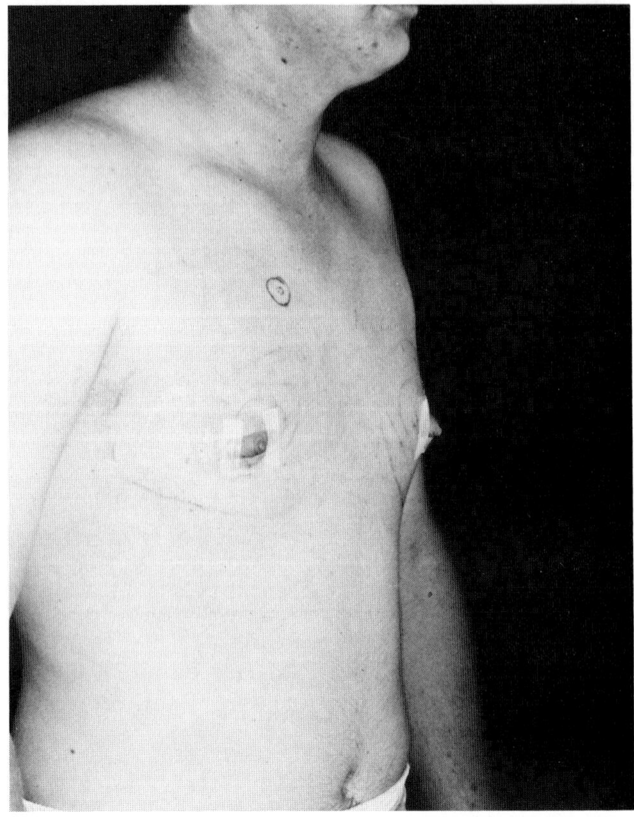

Fig. 27-12. Postoperative right oblique view showing minimal bruising and swelling 1 week after surgery.

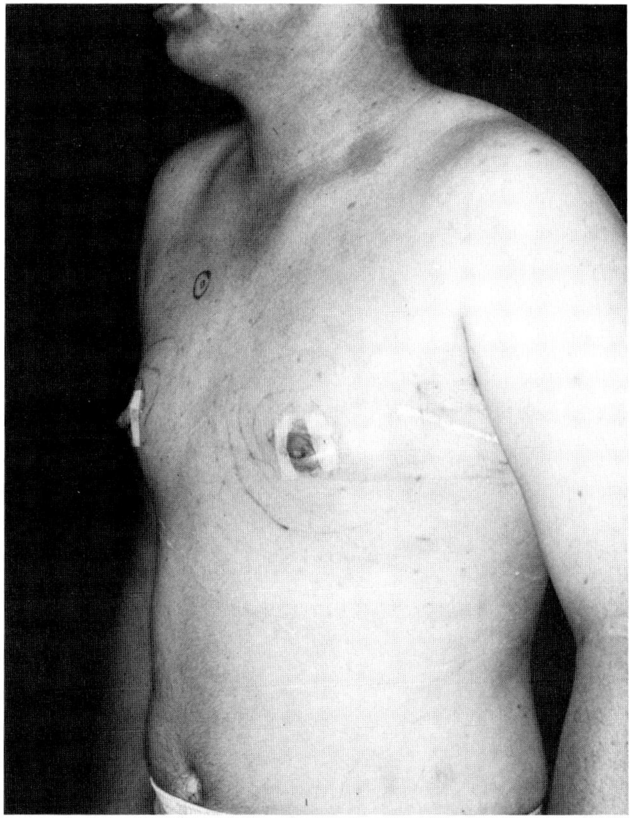

Fig. 27-13. Postoperative left oblique view showing minimal bruising and swelling 1 week after surgery.

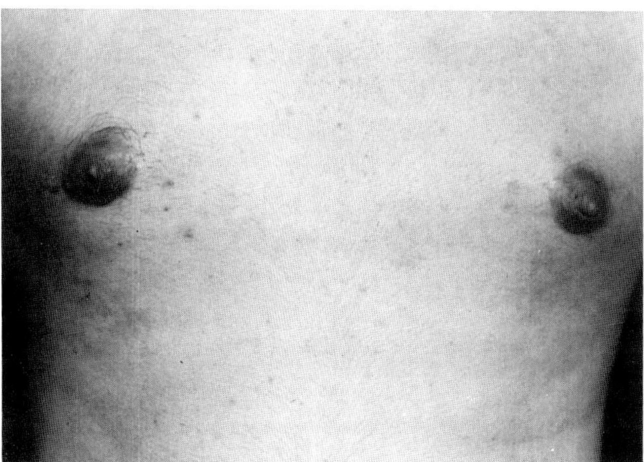

Fig. 27-14. Close-up view of incisions 2 weeks postoperatively.

give any statistical significance to the amount of postoperative bleeding. Theoretically, at least, the amount of hemorrhage and bleeding is less using lipolysis compared with using sharp dissection in the subcutaneous tissue. Lipolysis is preferred over sharp dissection for areas other than the breast since hematoma formation and hemorrhage are rare; the same results are expected to hold true for lipolysis removal of gynecomastia.

Most important, the iatrogenic deformities caused by extensive undermining and sharp dissection described in the literature [11] such as redundant skin, dishing, depressive deformity of the chest, and nipple necrosis can be minimized or eliminated with the lipolysis technique.

"An ideal method for surgical correction should be one that provides normal breast and chest contour while leaving the minimal tell-tale signs of surgery" Lipolysis, used in conjunction with excision of glandular tissue beneath the areola, fulfills these criteria expressed by Huang [10].

Summary

Lipolysis (Illouz blunt suction lipectomy) is a useful adjuvant in the treatment of gynecomastia. Resection of the glandular tissue immediately beneath the areola completes the procedure. The advantages of this combined technique over excision alone include a more desirable contour of the chest wall and breast and a lower risk of complications.

References

1. Dufourmentel, L. L'incision aréolaire dans la chirrurgie du sein. *Bull Mem. Soc. Chir.* (Paris) 20:9, 1928.
2. Menville, J. G. Gynecomastia. *Arch. Surg.* 26:1045, 1933.
3. Webster, J. P. Mastectomy for Gynecomastia through a semi-circular intraareolar incision. *Amer. J. Surg.* 124:567, 1946.
4. Pitanguy, I. *Plast. Reconstr. Surg.* 38(5), 1966.
5. Balch, C. R. A transaxillary incision for gynecomastia. *Plast. Reconstr. Surg.* 61(1), 1978.
6. Davidson, B. A. Concentric circle operation for massive gynecomastia to excise the redundant skin. *Plast. Reconstr. Surg.* 63(3), 1979.
7. Letterman, G., and Schurter, M. The surgical correction of gynecomastia. *Amer. J. Surg.* 315, 1969.
8. Artz, J. S., and Lehman, J. A., Jr. Surgical correction of massive gynecomastia. *Arch. Surg.* 113, 1978.
9. Welsh, F. Handlebar moustache breast reduction. *Plast. Reconstr. Surg.* 69(3), 1981.
10. Huang, T. T., Hildalgo, J. E., and Lewis, S. R. A circumareolar approach in surgical management of gynecomastia. *Plast. Reconstr. Surg.* 69(1), 1982.
11. Eade, G. G. The radial incision for gynecomastia excisions. *Plast. Reconstr. Surg.* 54(4), 1974.

CHAPTER 28

Lipolysis of the Female Breast

Adrien E. Aiache

Before the use of the Illouz method of suction lipoplasty, the results of mammoplasty procedures were often unsatisfactory, especially when the mammoplasty was performed on somewhat obese patients. In particular, the result was compromised by excess fat present medially, laterally, or even superiorly around the breast mound.

Breast reduction accomplished by any of the accepted techniques often improves the actual shape of the breast. When breast hypertrophy is associated with a significant degree of surrounding obesity, however, the breast appears to have extensions medially, laterally or superiorly and often ends up with a wider shape laterally and medially due to the excess of fat in these areas.

The mammoplasty procedures, whatever the specific technique being used, do not accomplish the goal of improving the area around the breast mound itself. Often it has been necessary to attempt to improve the shape of the breast medially and laterally by trying to excise as much fat as possible from these areas. Often the scar extends far onto the side beneath the axilla and becomes very noticeable. All techniques consider the length of the inframammary fold and attempt to shorten the scar within that length; however, many fail. Even in the most satisfactory techniques, there is still some deficiency in the result achieved.

The suction lipoplasty technique is particularly helpful in cases of reduction mammoplasty, by removing the excess fat present medially, laterally, and superiorly in the area of the tail of Spence. In addition, the technique allows the surgical scar to be shorter than it would have been without its use. It reduces the difficulties of postoperative bleeding encountered when a large dissection is performed in the axillary area.

Medially this technique is helpful in improving the "dog ear" that is often present after the technique of obtaining a scar medially; in addition, it allows the surgeon to obtain a shorter scar.

Preoperative Preparation

MARKING

The patient is marked in either the sitting or standing position. This marking allows the proper positioning of the nipple location. Proper positioning of the vertical and horizontal scars is important, and the surgeon must be aware that suction lipoplasty will allow the medial scar to be shortened. The markings for the excess fat are made in the form of a topographic map of all affected areas.

After the markings are made, the estimate of fat removal is accomplished by visual examination and by palpation using the pinch test. The visual examination shows the excess of fat present in each particular area of the breast, and the markings are made accordingly. In addition, squeezing by using the pinch test allows the surgeon to estimate the bulk of fat present over the chest wall. The pinch test is performed by grasping the tissue consisting of skin and subcutaneous fatty tissue between the thumb and the index finger and by measuring the distance between the two fingers. This distance is marked carefully to visualize the difference at the end of the procedure. The pinch test is useful throughout the procedure in helping to assess the excess fat, until a smooth and equal pinch test is obtained all over the treated area.

ANESTHESIA

Either local or general anesthesia is usually performed. Local anesthesia is used in cases of moderate excess, where a moderate breast reduction or lift is performed in addition to a moderate amount of fat extraction. The surgeon uses Xylocaine 1% with epinephrine 1:100,000, diluted with three equal amounts of saline to obtain a dilution of 1:400,000 of epinephrine. This solution usually provides adequate anesthesia. In an extensive breast and chest surface, however, a dose of 500 mg of Xylocaine might be exceeded. Rather than risk any untoward complications caused by a toxic effect of exceeding this dose of Xylocaine, general anesthesia may be chosen. In cases of large removals, whether of fat or breast tissue, the technique I prefer is general anesthesia in the supine position with intubation. This technique allows the surgeon to work with peace of mind. During anesthesia, the physician should inform the anesthesiologist of the amount aspirated in order to determine the amount of electrolyte, colloid, or sometimes blood that might be needed during and after the procedure.

POSITION

The procedure is performed with the patient in the supine position, with either general or local anesthesia. The patient's arms are stretched out at about 60 degrees from the line of the body to allow proper suctioning in the inframammary and axillary area. Sometimes suctioning is necessary posterior to the midaxillary line on either side.

INCISION

The incisions are particularly easy to place since they become the inframammary incision (Fig. 28-1). Two or

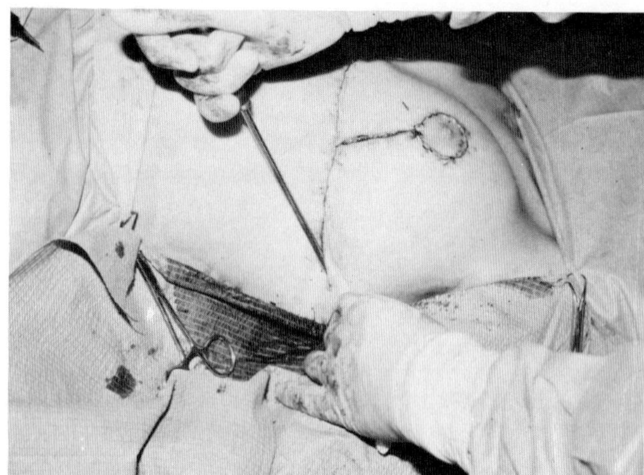

Fig. 28-1. The suction is performed from an end of the inframammary incision of mammoplasty.

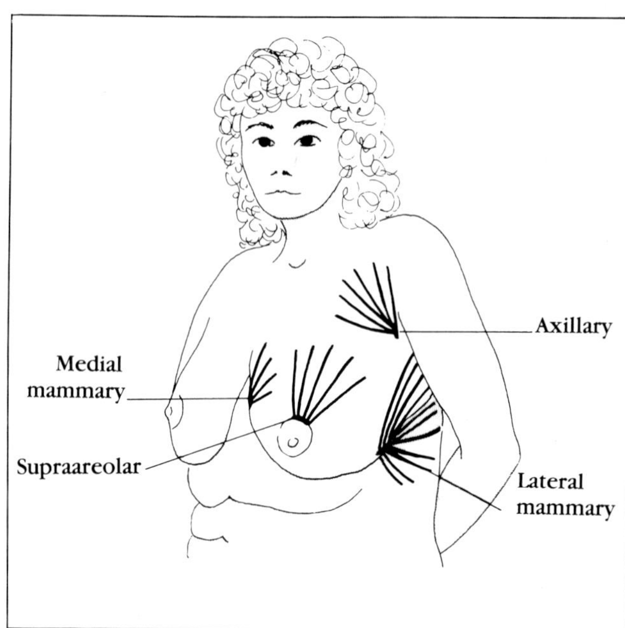

Fig. 28-2. Incisions used to reach various fatty areas.

three separate incisions are placed in the following manner: An incision is made medially at the most medial portion of the inframammary incision, which allows suctioning of both the medial and the superomedial aspects of the breast. A second incision is made in the superomedial aspect, which allows suctioning of the axillary area, the tail of Spence area, and the chest lateral to the breast. A third incision can be made in the upper part of the areola, allowing the cannula to reach the fat pad in front of the axillary fold. An axillary incision is used to reach the superior pectoral pad (Fig. 28-2).

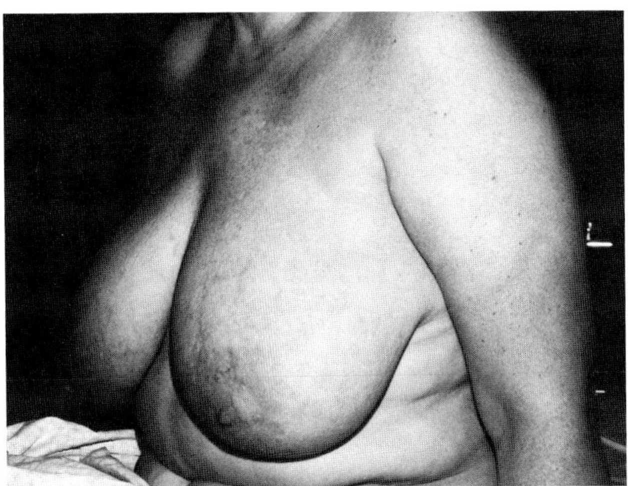

Fig. 28-3. A 54-year-old woman with gigantomastia and lateral chest wall excess.

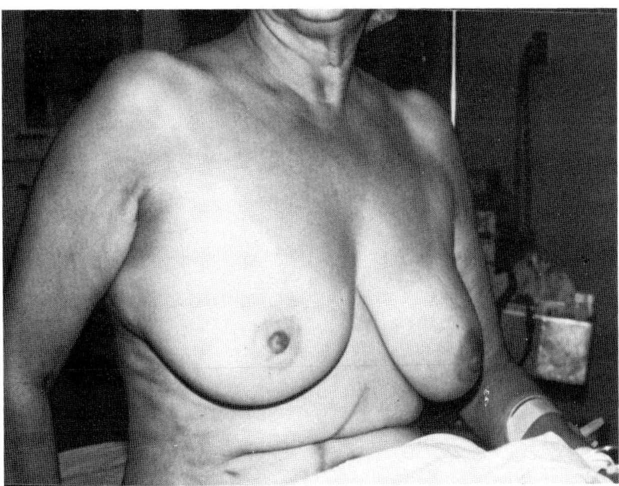

Fig. 28-5. A 52-year-old woman with gigantomastia and lateral chest wall excess.

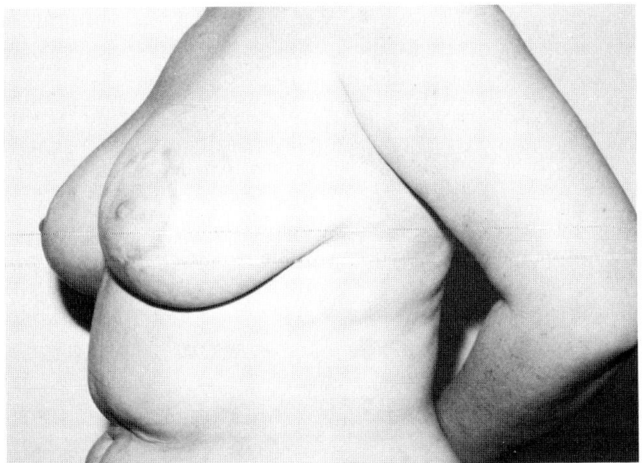

Fig. 28-4. Postoperative view of patient in Fig. 28-3.

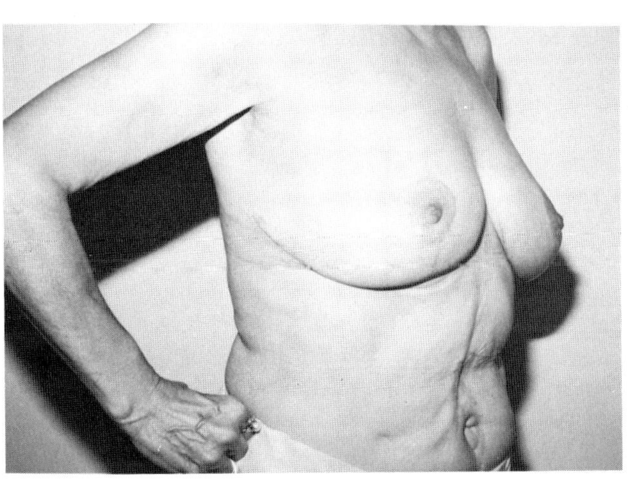

Fig. 28-6. Postoperative result of patient in Fig. 28-5.

Surgical Technique

After the incisions are made, a 6- to 8-mm cannula is introduced, and approximately 10 to 15 strokes are performed in each tunnel. The marked area is suctioned thoroughly until the appearance is adequate and until a satisfactory pinch test is obtained along the whole marked area.

The pinch test used is a pinch and roll, which consists of rolling the pinched skin to assess if there are any significant irregularities in some areas, indicating that these areas need additional suctioning. The three areas that have been marked are suctioned thoroughly until a satisfactory result is obtained. Then the aspirated area is pressed toward the exit incision. Any blood present is extruded through the incisions. Usually no blood is encountered and the wound is then closed with one or two sutures of 5−0 nylon. The suctioned area is taped at the end of the mammoplasty procedure.

It is always easier to suction the area closed to ensure good vacuum before any wide incision is made. Nevertheless, in many cases, once the area is suctioned and the mammoplasty procedure started, a suction cannula of 6 to 8 mm is used as an "open sky" vacuum cleaner. Excess fat present in the upper or lower part of the inframammary incision, as well as in the area of the breast itself, may be suctioned away by this maneuver. Once all suction maneuvers are accomplished and the mammoplasty procedure is completed, the breast is closed in a routine fashion. After the breast is bandaged, a compressive bandage is used over the medial or lateral extensions (or both) of the breast to ensure a good operative result. Figures 28-3 through 28-8 show typical patients.

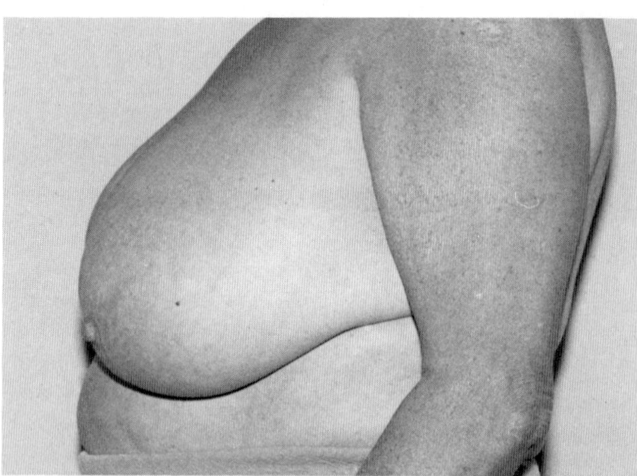

Fig. 28-7. Lateral view of a 67-year-old woman with very heavy lateral chest wall excess extending to her back. (Photo courtesy of G. Hetter, M.D.)

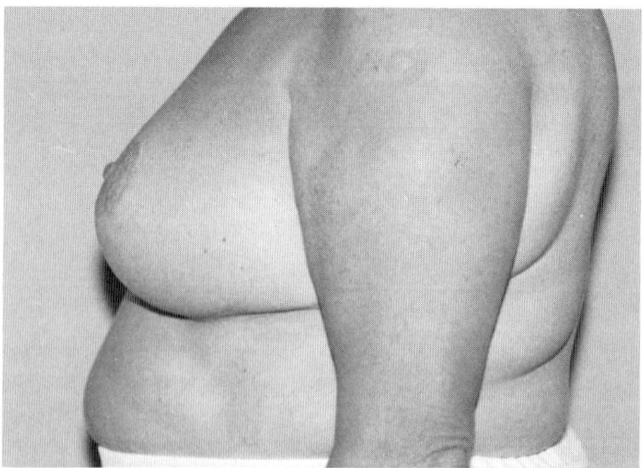

Fig. 28-8. Later view of postoperative result after aspirative defatting of lateral chest wall and lateral breast flap (same patient as in Fig. 28-7).

REFINEMENTS IN TECHNIQUE

In cases where suction lipectomy is used throughout the breast undergoing mammoplasty, the area of the chest lateral and inferior to the breast is often helped by aspiration to accomplish an even better cosmetic result. The breast may be aspirated in some instances with the open sky technique. The breast responds well as far as fat is concerned, but breast tissue is not aspirated.

Another step in refinement of the technique is to feather the edge beyond the area of aspiration by introducing a cannula without suction and freeing the tissues, allowing them to redrape. This maneuver helps prevent a step deformity encountered at the junction of the aspirated and unaspirated tissues. Continuous estimation of the amount of aspirate should be done by observation but, more particularly, by palpation and pinch test, which allow an even removal of fat from the areas surrounding the aspirated tissue.

GLANDULAR REMOVAL

No glandular removal can be performed by the suction itself. The removal is usually performed by whatever technique of reduction mammoplasty is preferred by the surgeon.

DRESSING

Dressing and closure have been mentioned. For dressing I use 4-inch elastic tape, which allows some compression in the operated area and helps reduce accumulation of hematomas.

Postoperative Management

The patient remains in the recovery room until the vital signs become stable. Once the patient is awake, he or she is transferred to home or to the hospital, depending on clinical judgment. I treat my patients with both prophylactic antibiotics and oral pain medication. No massage has been prescribed for these patients, since the involved area is localized near the breast suture lines, which presents practical problems.

Sequelae

Sequelae consisting of excess bruising and some numbness in the area of the lateral breast have been encountered, although these complications have been relatively minor. Both the surgeon and the patient should be aware of the possibility of these complications.

Postoperatively, the patient is able to wear a bra on top of the bandage and elastic tape covering the breast and axilla. This tape is removed approximately 6 to 8 days after surgery. Tape burns may occur in areas where the skin is relatively thin and should be watched for.

Discussion

Suction lipoplasty is useful in complementing many surgical procedures. In particular, it is useful in improving the aesthetic appearance of the breast obtained by reduction mammoplasty because, in many cases, the corrected breast rises from a chest wall distorted by unsightly amounts of fat. Any improvement in this area enhances the new appearance of the breast obtained after reduction mammoplasty. The technique permits the surgeon to shorten the inframammary scars and has application in most cases of reduction mammoplasty, since practically all cases present some excess fat surrounding and extending from the breast.

In summary, lipoplasty by the Illouz technique has been found useful as an adjunct to the treatment of mammary hypertrophy. Correction of mammary hypertrophy by resection of breast tissue, in conjunction with blunt suction lipectomy, has given much better results than previous resection alone.

Bibliography

Aiache, A. Mammoplasty. *Br. J. Plast. Surg.* 27:318, 1974.

Arie, G. Una nueva technica de mastoplastica. *Rev. Lat. Am. Chir. Plast.* 3:23.

Fournier, P., and Otteni, F. Lipodissection in body sculpturing: The dry procedure. *Plast. Reconstr. Surg.* 598, 1983.

Illouz, Y. G. Body contouring by lipolysis: A 5-year experience with over 3,000 cases. *Plast. Reconstr. Surg.* 72:591, 1983.

Schrudde, J. Lipexeresis for the correction of local adiposity. *Int. J. Aesth. Plast. Surg.* 1972.

Skoog, T. A technique of breast reduction transposition of the nipple on a cutaneous circular pedicle. *Acta. Chir. Scand.* 126:453, 1963.

de Souza Pinto, E. B., et al. Dermoadipose and adenadipose flaps in mammoplasty. *Aesth. Plast. Surg.* 7:101, 1983

Strombeck, J. Mammoplasty: Report of a new technique found in two pedicle procedures. *Br. J. Plast. Surg.* 13:79, 1960.

Teimourian, B., et al. Suction lipectomy: A review of 200 patients over a six-year period and a study of the technique on cadavers. *Ann. Plast. Surg.* 11:93, 1983.

CHAPTER 29

Lipolysis and Lipoplasties of the Abdomen

Francis M. Otteni
Pierre F. Fournier

Until recently, plastic surgery of the abdomen was limited to dermolipectomies and abdominoplasties [1,2]. Suction lipoplasty [3,4,5,6,7], however, has enabled us to do a pure partial lipectomy through only a tiny incision. We have gradually extended the indications for its use in the abdomen and now use suction lipectomy either alone or in combination with a dermolipectomy in almost every case [6,7].

The Classical Abdominal Dermolipectomy or Abdominoplasty

Classical abdominoplasty consists of a monoblock excision of the skin and subcutaneous fatty tissue, associated most of the time with simultaneous undermining of the flaps and a transposition of the umbilicus.

There are three main types of abdominoplasty:

1. The low horizontal, or transverse, which is the most common, with an ilio-inguino-pubic incision
2. The vertical or longitudinal, which is performed only occasionally
3. The mixed dermolipectomy, which is less common

In addition, we must add two particular types:

4. The circular, or "belt", lipectomy [8,9], which is performed on obese patients for the treatment of significant deformities; the purpose is more functional than aesthetic
5. The localized lipectomy, which is used to treat a select group of well-limited deformities; the purpose is more aesthetic than functional

In addition to significant morbidity, the dermolipectomies may have three types of aesthetic sequelae:

1. The scar may be either too high or too long to conceal beneath underwear. Unfortunately, the scar is also often widened or thickened because of excessive tension exerted on the edges of the incision.
2. There may be bulging, which is often delayed, above the scar. The bulging is due to a hypertrophy of the recurring adipose tissue or to a lymphatic problem caused by the scar.
3. The repositioned umbilicus may be aesthetically unsatisfactory.

The difficulties that arise from the transposition of the umbilicus can be compared to the difficulties that arise from the transposition of the nipple-areolar complex. But while the latter is a secondary sexual characteristic, the umbilicus is nothing more than a cicatricial residue.

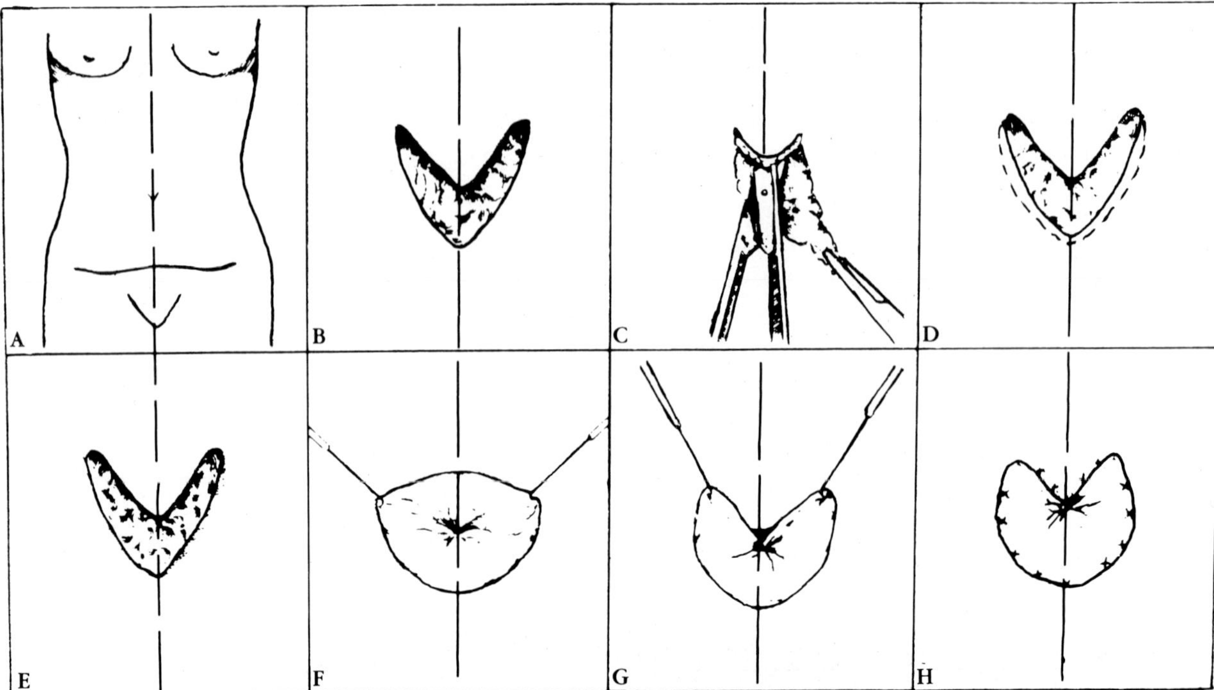

Fig. 29-1. Steps in umbilical transposition.
A. A V-shaped incision.
B. The incision gapes from tension.
C. Defatting 6 cm above and 3 cm below incision.
D. The dotted lines indicate edges to be deepithelialized.
E. Deepithelialization completed.
F. Exteriorization of umbilicus.
G. A superior radial cut at 12 o'clock to create two superior wings.
H. Suturing the tongue of the orbital incision into the V-defect and joining the deepithelialized edge to the inferior edges of the umbilicus. (Adapted from J. Juri., C. Juri, and G. Raiden, Reconstruction of the umbilicus in abdominoplasty. *Plast. Reconstr. Surg.* 63:580, 1979.)

The morphology of the umbilicus differs depending upon its shape, its dimensions, and its internal as well as external contours. Anatomically, in whites the umbilicus is situated at the point of intersection of a vertical medial line and a transverse line that is 2 to 4 cm above and parallel to a line joining the anterosuperior iliac spines. In Oriental people it may be higher. The umbilicus forms a depression, the depth of which depends on the surrounding fat deposit.

It is important to review the different surgical techniques that can be applied to the umbilicus:

1. Transposition
2. Disinsertion-reposition
3. Resection-reconstruction
4. Resection-graft

Transposition of the umbilicus is the most common technique. It often leaves a circular scar, which is rather artificial in appearance and which can sometimes shrink, resulting in a deformity. For these reasons, we recommend Juri's procedure [10] (Fig. 29-1), which aims at replacing the superior portion of the periumbilical scar in depth, giving a more natural appearance to the transposed umbilicus.

Disinsertion-reposition (Fig. 29-2) of the umbilicus is indicated when there is an excess of skin in the infraumbilical region and a lengthening of the pubo-umbilical distance. In this case, one can perform a localized, low transverse, suprapubic, crescent-shaped dermolipec-

tomy that respects the limits of the bikini (this explains why Mario Gonzalez-Ulloa named this the "bikini resection") [11]. Sometimes, when the suturing is done, the umbilicus is deformed because of the traction exerted during the lowering of the superior flap. It is then recommended to undermine upward, *disinsert* the umbilicus along the aponeurosis, carefully close the aponeurosis opening thus created with a few sutures, and suture (reinsert) the umbilicus a centimeter or two lower (see Fig. 29-2). In this manner, the umbilical morphology will be perfectly normal, the tension at the wound edges will be reduced, and the quality of the suprapubic scar will be improved.

Resection-reconstruction (Fig. 29-3) of the umbilicus (neoumbilicoplasty [12]) should be considered in certain dermolipectomies in the obese patient. It is advisable to resect the umbilicus in order to more safely correct an umbilical hernia or a diastasis of the recti

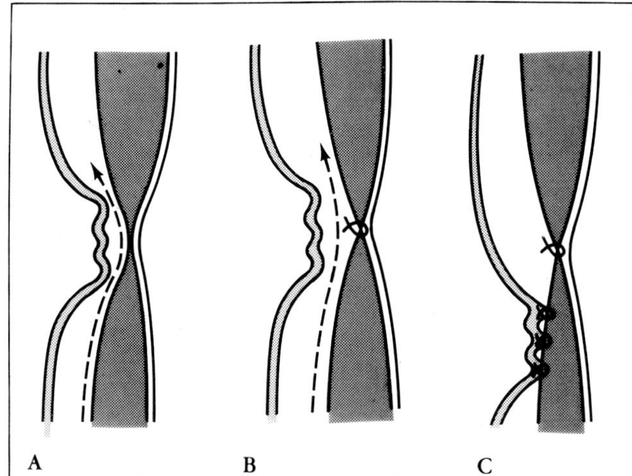

Fig. 29-2. Disinsertion-reposition of the umbilicus.
A. Transection of the umbilical stalk.
B. Suturing the resulting aponeurotic defect.
C. Resuturing the umbilical stalk at a lower level.

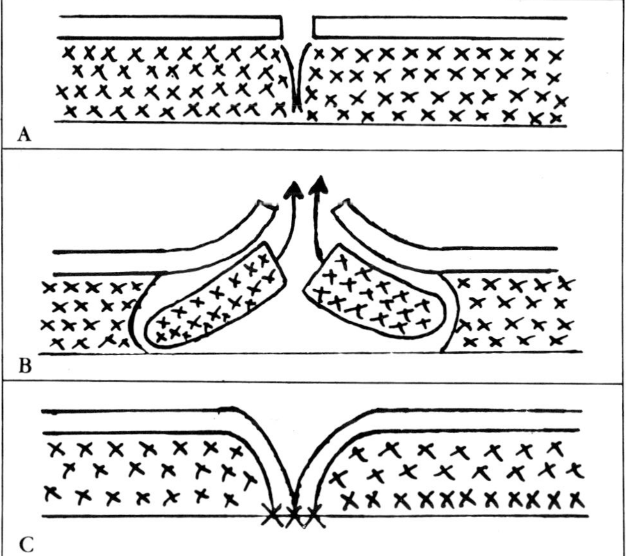

Fig. 29-3. Steps of neoumbilicoplasty.
A. Incision.
B. Defatting.
C. Suturing skin edge to aponeurosis.

muscles. The neoumbilicoplasty that we recommend is quite simple. The incision is transverse, slightly rounded, perfectly centered on the medial line, and measures approximately 3 cm. The periphery of the incision must be defatted, especially the superior flap, to create a medial supraumbilical fold. The skin edges are then deeply fixed with a few solid stitches to the denuded aponeurosis. The deepening of the neoumbilicus is maintained with a pressure dressing. This procedure of umbilical reconstruction is simple and successful in most cases.

A quadruple V-plasty [13] has also been described. Once defatted, the four flaps are sutured to the aponeurosis. However, this procedure is more complicated than the neoumbilicoplasty and does not give better results.

We do not like to graft the resected umbilicus in obese patients because of the risk of infection.

Suction Lipoplasty of the Abdomen

The abdominal subcutaneous panniculus is all too often the site of excessive fat deposits. While in women the fat deposits are essentially limited to the area around and beneath the umbilicus, in men they are often found above the umbilicus. In both sexes, the fat may extend to the lateral flank rolls.

The defatting of the whole abdominal wall is not part of classic torso surgery. We all know how dangerous it is for the vitality of a flap to defat it with a scalpel. However, this is an excellent indication for suction lipoplasty.

The preoperative marking is made with the patient in the standing position (Fig. 29-4). When marking the anterior abdominal wall, we pay special attention to the infraumbilical bulge, the often multiple supraumbilical rolls, and the periumbilical region. If necessary, we also treat the lateral flank rolls and/or iliac crests.

For the anterior abdominal wall, we usually do a medial suprapubic puncture and a medial supraumbilical puncture, and we use small caliber cannulas (Fig. 29-5). Of course, we could also make the incision in a previous scar or in a stria.

For the lateral fat, the puncture is supratrochanteric (Fig. 29-6) and more or less posterior. We use the same cannulas as used for the anterior abdominal wall (see Chaps. 30 and 31).

The usual technical principles must be respected:

1. Remain *deep* by keeping the opening of the lipodissector (cannula) facing the aponeurosis, leaving at least 1 cm of fatty tissue beneath the skin.
2. Work evenly, utilizing the *criss-cross* technique.
3. Work *symmetrically*, by removing approximately the same amount of fat on both sides of the medial line, counting the number of tunnels made, and making the same number of strokes per tunnel.
4. Free the periphery of the adiposity in order to facilitate a better repositioning of the skin. This *peripheral mesh undermining* is especially important in elderly patients with skin of poor quality.

We use suction drainage only in very large abdominal removals when the volume exceeds 1 liter. In all cases we prefer elastic tape dressing (Elastikon, Elastoplast),

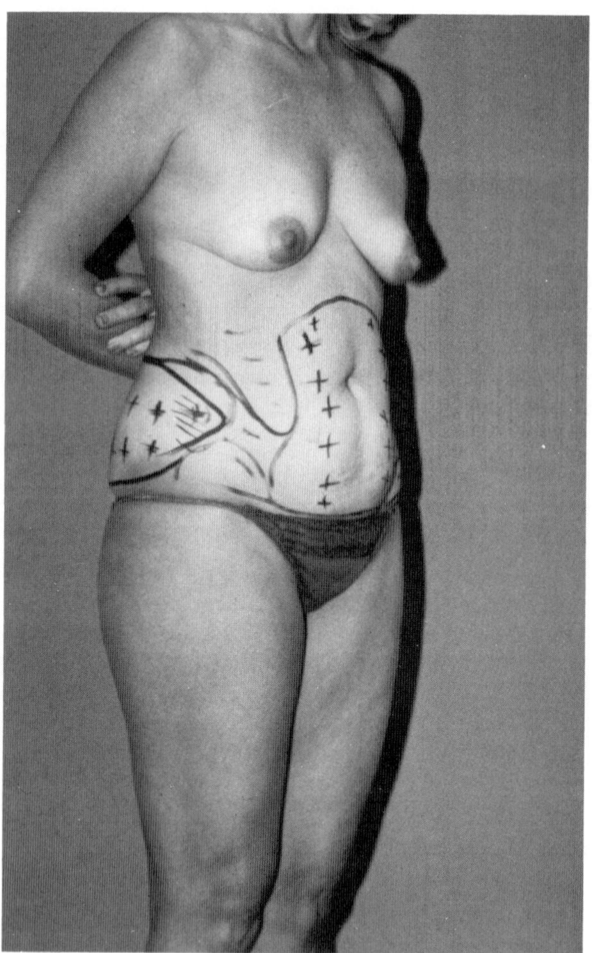

Fig. 29-4. Patient marked for abdominal lipolysis showing flank extensions and relative thickness of fat as topographical map. (Photograph courtesy of G. Hetter, M.D.)

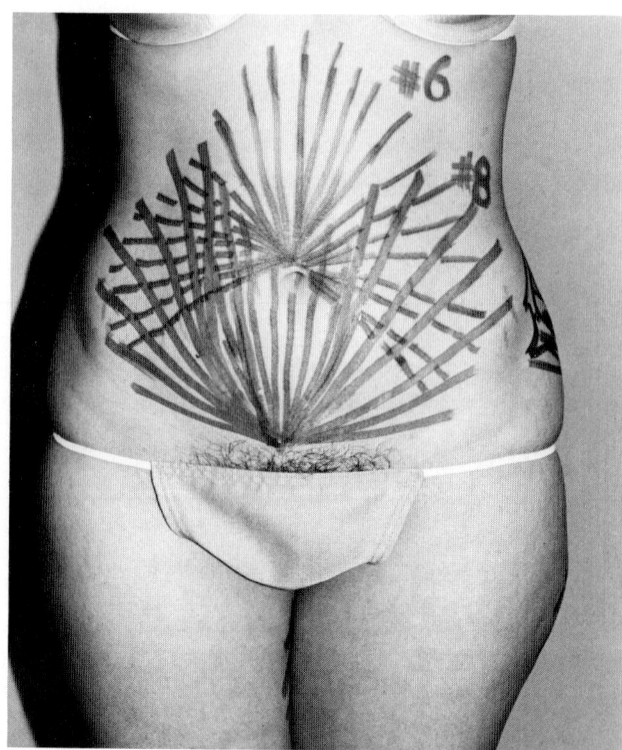

Fig. 29-5. Model marked with suprapubic and supraumbilical incision with tunnels indicated.

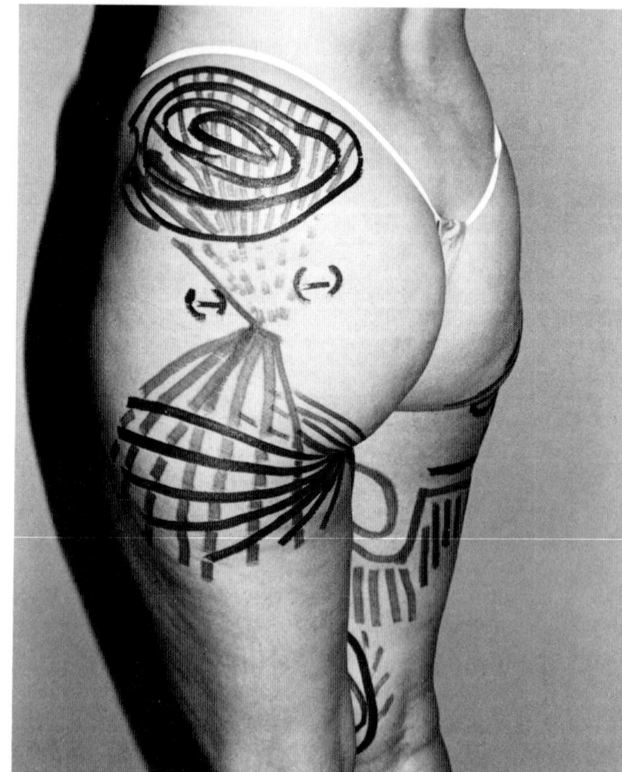

Fig. 29-6. Model marked with posterior supratrochanteric incision for approach to iliac crest fat as well as lateral thigh (if necessary).

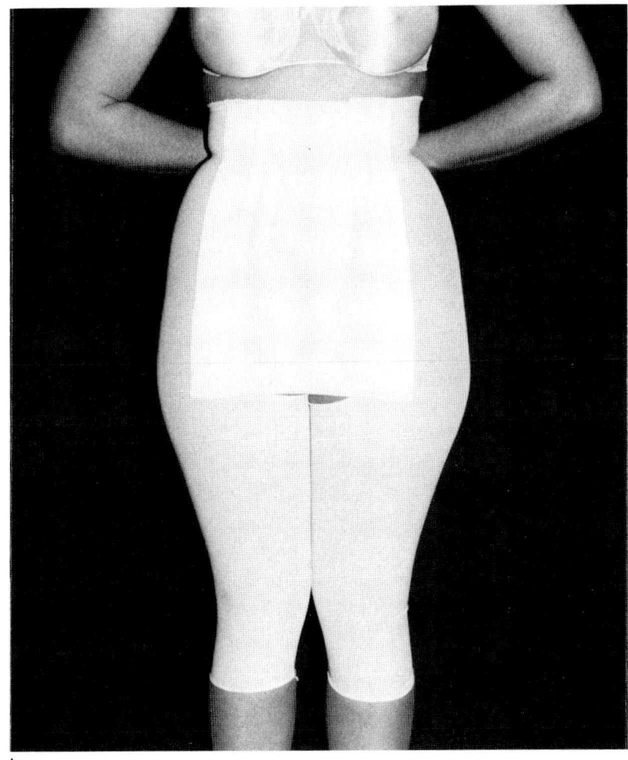

A

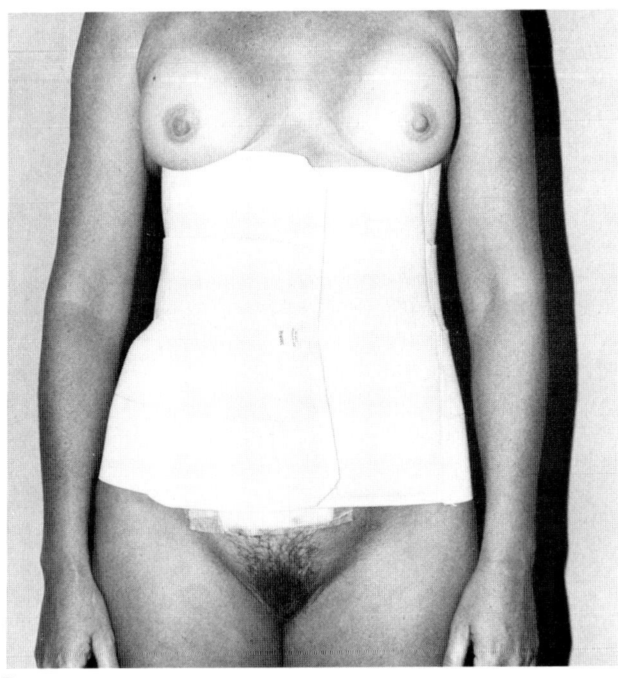

B

Fig. 29-7.
A. Girdle useful for abdominal lipoplasties as well as thigh and knee lipoplasties. Manufactured by Circumpress, 1625 Godfrey Lane, Virginia Beach, VA 23454. Crotch area is open, which eliminates need for removal during ablutions.
B. Four panel abdominal binder useful for isolated abdominal lipoplasties. Manufactured by Pro Care, San Marcos, CA 92069.

which is left on for 1 week. For 6 weeks thereafter we recommend an elastic support girdle (Fig. 29-7).

Remember, the good result must be evident immediately. One must not rely on the passage of time to correct irregularities due to poor technique. Of course, some subcutaneous irregularities may remain for 6 to 8 weeks, but they generally improve to full acceptability. However, a poor appearance at the end of the operation will remain unsatisfactory. When performed by an experienced surgeon, suction lipoplasty of the abdomen provides excellent results.

Aesthetic complications, such as permanent skin irregularities similar to "waves," seldom occur, but when they do, they usually appear in patients whose skin tone is deficient because of age, multiple pregnancies, and weight fluctuations, or in patients who presented with skin excess and needed a dermolipectomy.

Combined Procedures

Suction lipoplasty and dermolipectomy can be used together to improve the results. The suction cannula, or "lipoextractor," is a tool that we now use on a daily basis, either alone or in association with classical instruments. In the usual dermolipectomy, the surgeon treats only a well-delimited area of the abdomen. To perform a defatting of the whole abdomen, the surgeon would have to make a huge incision with wide undermining, which entails substantial bleeding, prolonged lymphorrhea, and a high risk of slough. Now we can achieve the goal of defatting the whole abdomen with a very low risk of complications thanks to the combined procedure, which consists of a dermolipectomy and a partial suction lipectomy of the remaining areas of the abdomen. This combined procedure will (1) diminish the thickness of the flaps, (2) facilitate their mobilization, (3) reduce the tension of the edges, (4) shorten the scar and improve its quality, and (5) reduce or avoid dog-ears.

The suction portion of the procedure is, of course, performed first. This enables us to limit the dermolipectomy to the clinically existing skin excess and thus avoid a lengthening of the scar. Generally speaking, *the association of the two procedures does not increase the operative risk.* Actually, suction lipoplasty performed with small cannulas is a minor, short, and only modestly traumatic procedure. This is true as long as the amount of fat removed does not exceed 1 liter. If it exceeds 1 liter, infusions of macromolecular solutions, plasma, or even blood are appropriate.

TYPES OF COMBINED PROCEDURES

We can distinguish three types of combined procedures:

1. The first includes cases where procedures are separated by a period of time, for example, suction lipoplasty followed a few months later by an abdominoplasty to correct the residual skin excess, or abdominoplasty followed later by a suction lipoplasty of the remaining subcutaneous panniculus.
2. The second includes cases where the techniques are employed during the same operation, but with only one technique employed on the abdomen. Examples are mammary reduction associated with suction lipoplasty of the abdomen, or abdominoplasty associated with suction lipoplasty of saddlebags and buttocks.
3. The third includes cases where suction lipoplasty and dermolipectomy are performed on the abdomen during the same operation. This is the technique we will now examine in greater detail.

OPERATIVE INDICATIONS, TECHNIQUES, AND RISKS

During the preoperative examination, one should look for the presence of a hernia, an incisional hernia, or a diastasis of the recti muscles.

It has to be well emphasized that, until recently, abdominal adipose excess alone was not treated. It was only treated when it was associated with a skin excess, which allowed a dermolipectomy to be performed. Today, a pure partial lipectomy or lipoplasty is possible, and may be performed with a dermolipectomy in a combined procedure.

The operative approach selected depends on the following three factors:

1. The skin excess, which can be either generalized or localized
2. The adipose excess, which can be generalized or localized
3. The size and location of scars and stretch marks

Relying on these 3 factors, one can distinguish 6 clinical types of aesthetic surgery of the abdomen (see Fig. 29-20).

1. *Fat abdomen without skin excess.* Minimal to moderate fat excess only.
2. *Fat abdomen with skin excess.* Moderate fat excess with moderate skin excess predominating in the lower abdomen.
3. *Usual case.* Skin excess and adipose excess evenly located in the whole abdomen.
4. *Abdomen pendulum* (dependent abdominal apron).

Very large skin and adipose excess causing a functional problem.
5. *Scarred abdomen.* Unsightly scars with minimal to moderate skin and adipose excess.
6. *Wrinkled or "tired" abdomen.* Skin excess with stretch marks but without adipose excess.

We will discuss each of these types in detail, suggest a surgical procedure currently in use, and show a few results since the arrival of the Illouz technique.

Fat Abdomen Without Skin Excess

This type is characterized by a minor or moderate excess of the subcutaneous panniculus prevailing in the peri- and infraumbilical region. The skin is normal and its tonicity is good. There is occasionally a slight skin excess located particularly around the supraumbilical region. There are no stretch marks or only a few localized ones.

Before the arrival of suction lipoplasty, these patients were considered inoperable. Thanks to the Illouz technique, it is now among these patients, both male and female, that we have the best aesthetic results (Figs. 29-8 to 29-12).

Suction lipoplasty of the abdomen is also an excellent temporary solution for women considering future pregnancy, since abdominoplasty should be deferred until after the last pregnancy.

Fat Abdomen with Skin Excess Predominating in the Lower Abdomen

This type is characterized by a moderate excess of the subcutaneous panniculus in association with a moderate skin excess, especially in the infraumbilical region, which produces a lengthening of the puboumbilical distance. The combined procedure, consisting of suction and a localized dermolipectomy with or without a disinsertion-reposition of the umbilicus, is indicated in these cases.

We begin by defatting the abdomen, waist, and flanks using the cannula. Then we resect a low transversal suprapubic crescent of skin in order to reduce the infraumbilical skin excess. The scar must respect the limits of the bikini ("bikini resection"). Sometimes, when the suturing is done, the umbilicus is deformed because of the traction exerted during the lowering of the superior flap. It is in this case that we recommend a disinsertion-reposition of the umbilicus.

The results are excellent among these patients since the suprapubic scar is particularly low and easy to hide, there is no periumbilical scar, and the general aspect of the abdomen is improved as a result of the lipoplasty (Fig. 29-13).

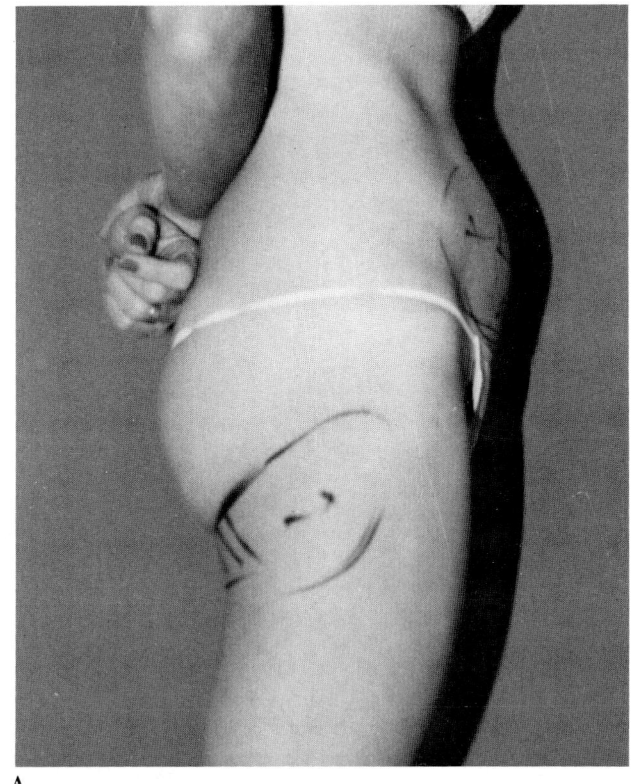

A

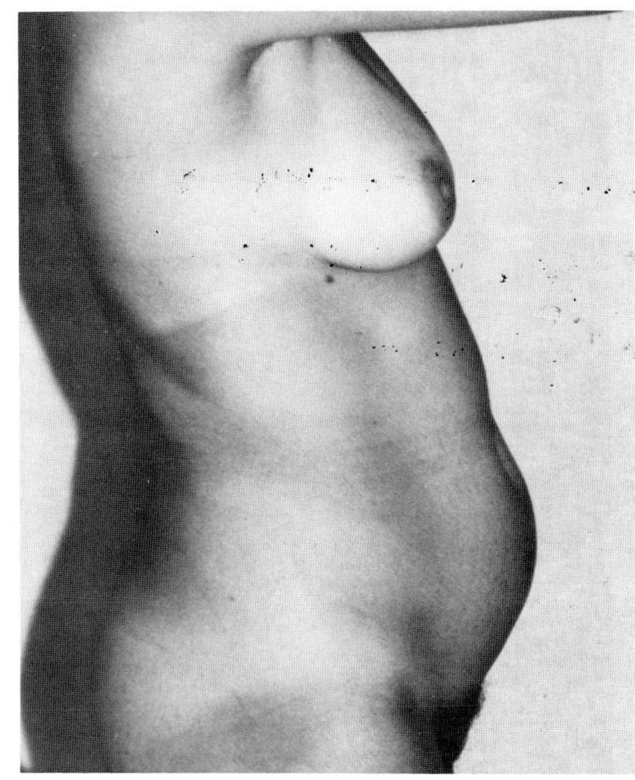

A

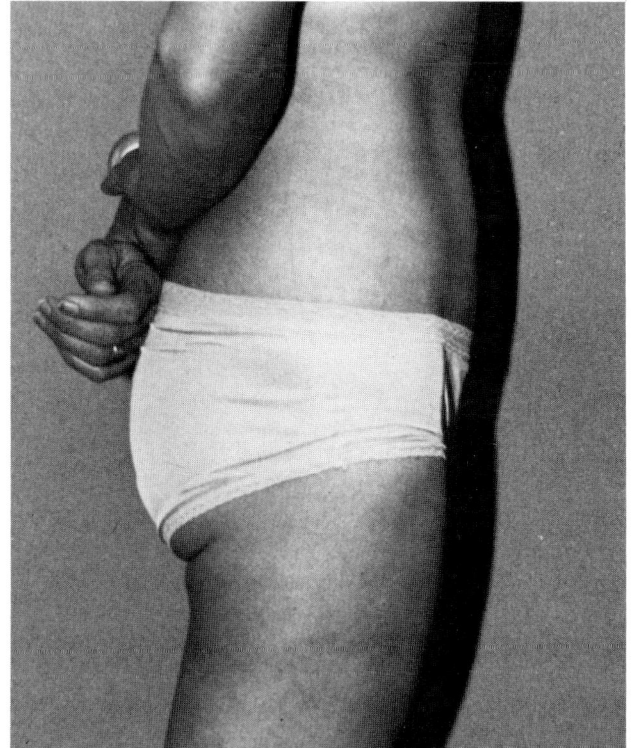

B

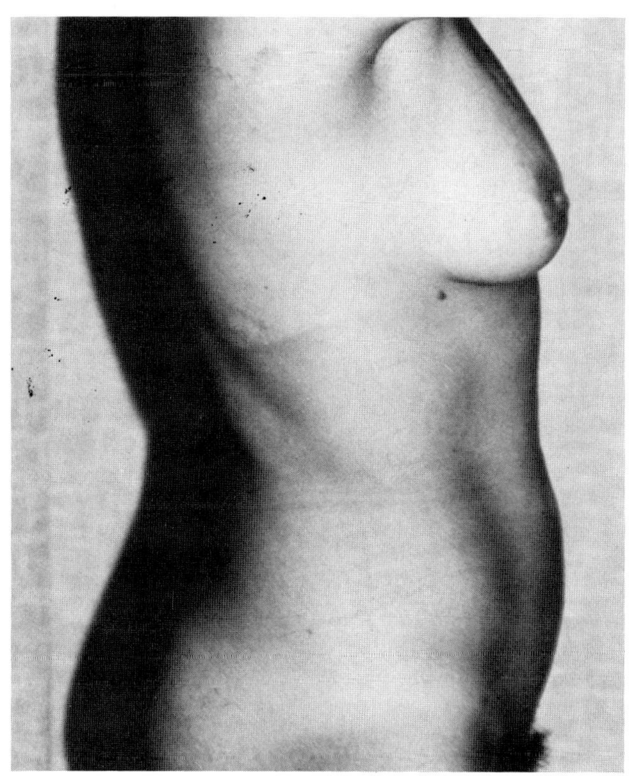

B

Fig. 29-8.
A. Lateral view of 36-year-old woman with minimal hypogastric excess.
B. Same patient 3 months postoperatively following 350 ml removal of fat from the abdomen. (Photographs courtesy of G. Hetter, M.D.)

Fig. 29-9.
A. Preoperative lateral view of 28-year-old woman with moderate hypogastric excess without generalized obesity.
B. Same patient showing marked improvement following 600 ml removal from abdomen.

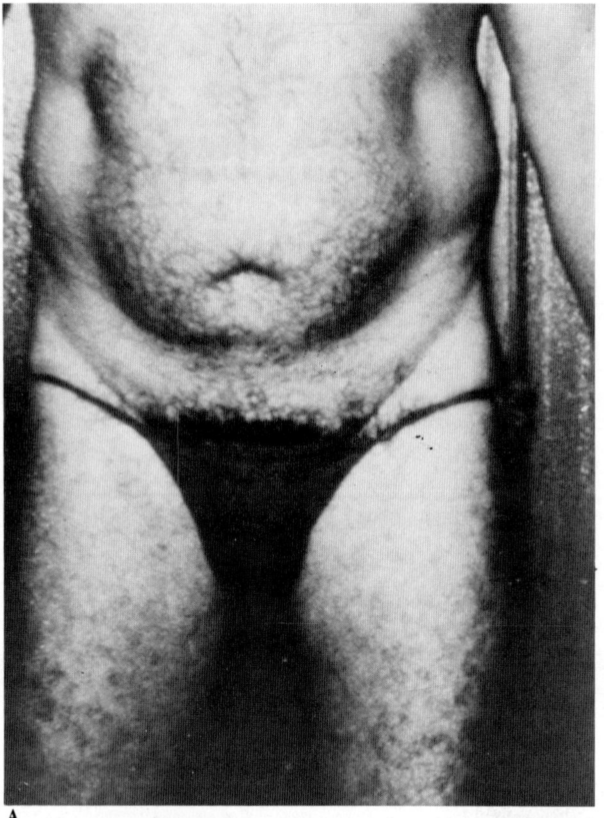

A

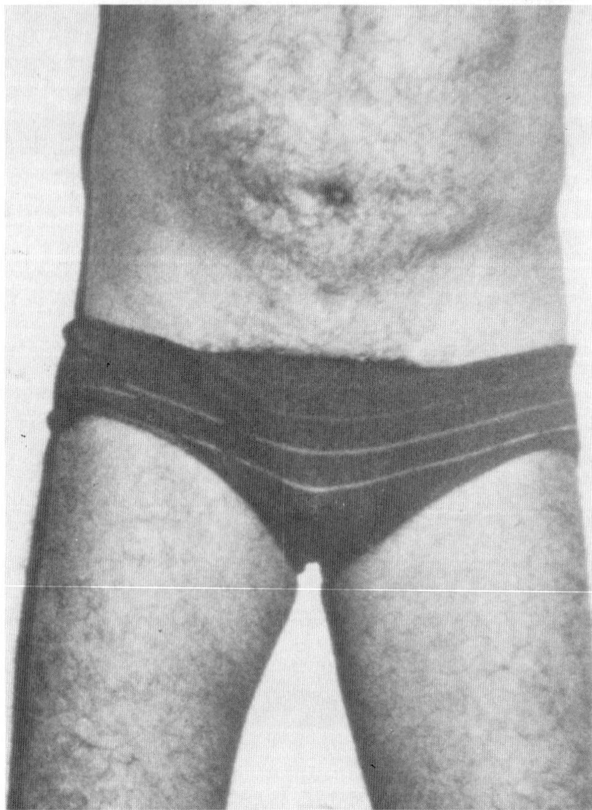

B

Fig. 29-10.
A. Preoperative anterior view of male with typical substantial android abdominal and flank excess.
B. Postoperative view showing gratifying result following 1100 ml removal from abdomen and flanks.

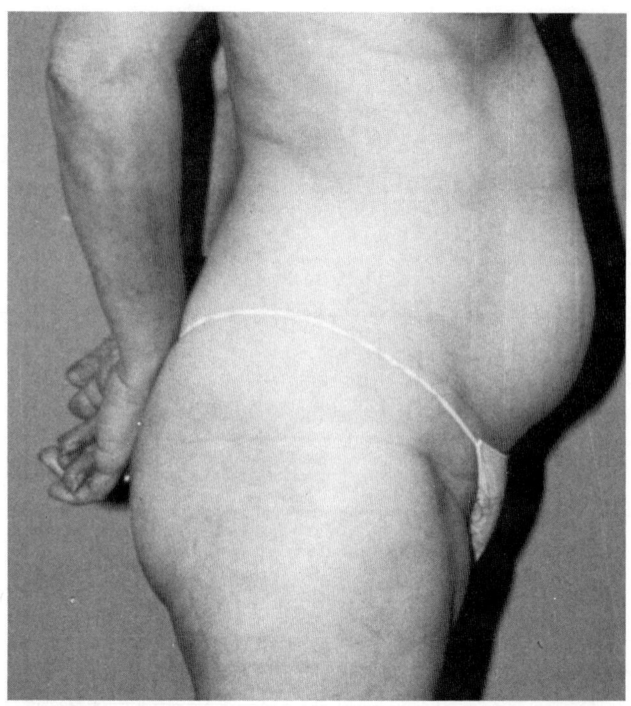

A

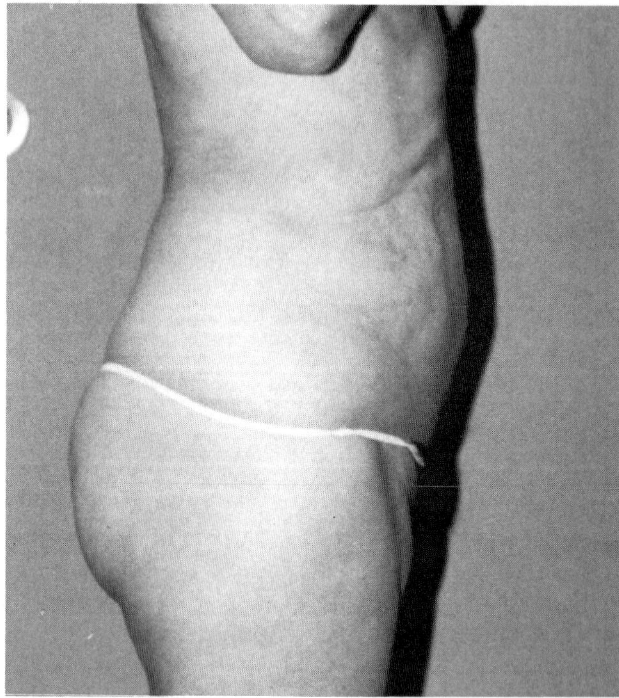

B

Fig. 29-11.
A. Preoperative view of 64-year-old female with large abdominal excess.
B. Postoperative view at 5 months following 950 ml removal as outpatient using low dose epinephrine as described in Chap. 15. (Photographs courtesy of G. Hetter, M.D.)

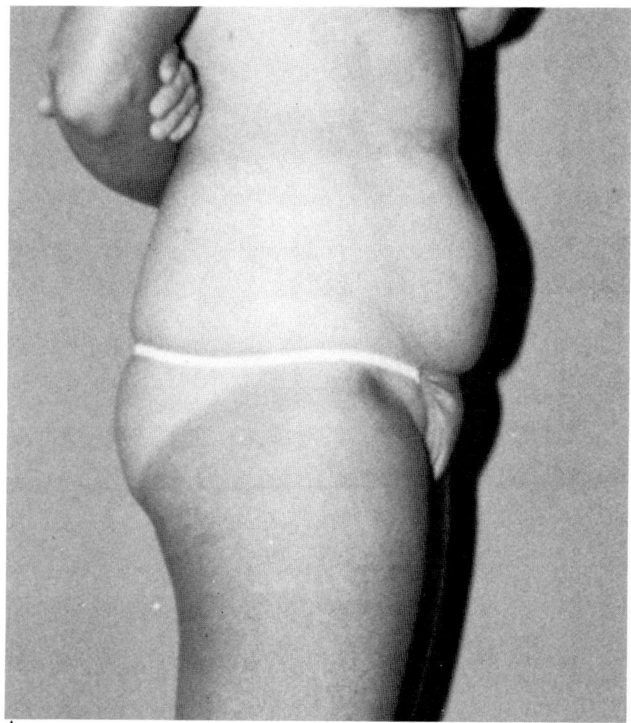

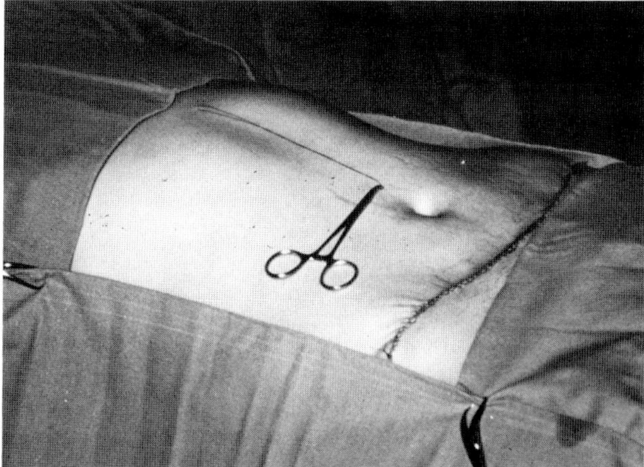

Fig. 29-13. Intraoperative picture showing repositioning of umbilicus. Hemostat marks site of umbilical stalk prior to disinsertion and repositioning.

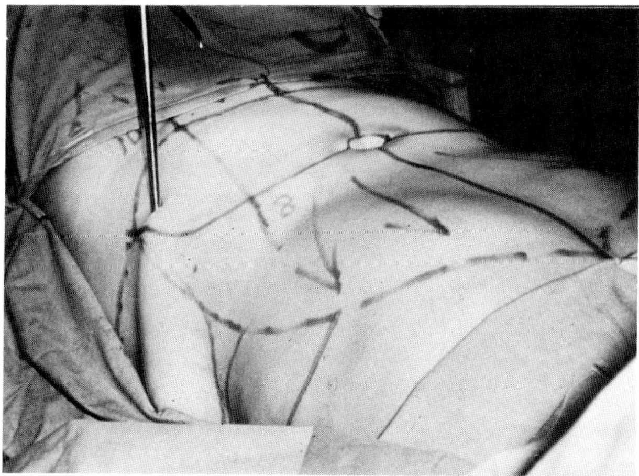

Fig. 29-14. Intraoperative photo showing suction extraction of flank from anterior in case of large excess.

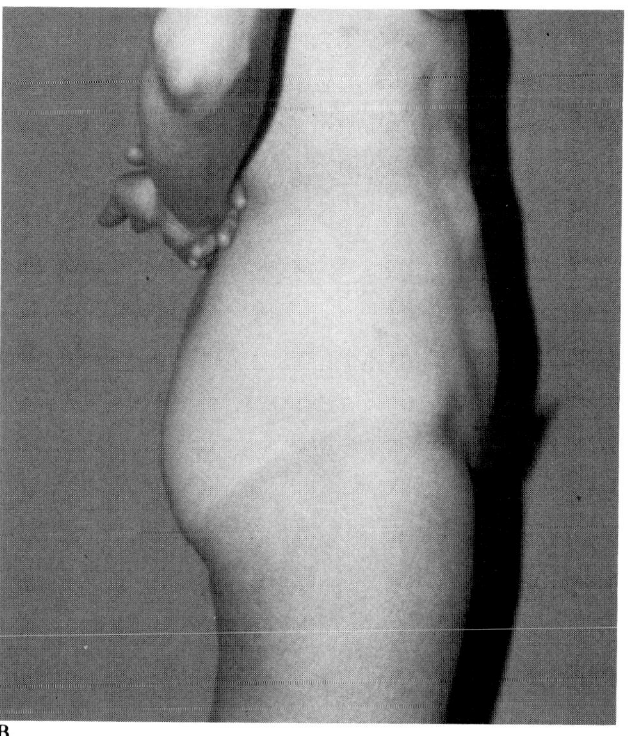

Fig. 29-12.
A. Preoperative view of 33-year-old female with extensive epigastric and flank excess confluent with hypogastric excess. Note matronly appearance.
B. Postoperative view at 18 months following removal of 1600 ml from abdomen and flanks. Note youthful silhouette. (Photographs courtesy of G. Hetter, M.D.)

Usual Case with Mixed Excess of Skin and Fat

This type of deformity is most common in women who are rather plump and who have had one or several pregnancies. In these cases, there is not only obvious skin excess producing a suprapubic transverse roll and relatively large striae, but also a thick adipose panniculus and a diastasis of the recti muscles.

It is undoubtedly the indication for a classical abdominoplasty with musculoaponeurotic plication or reconstruction and a transposition of the umbilicus. But this procedure has no effect on the fat deposits in the superior flap and the flanks. Therefore, the long-term result is often compromised by an unattractive bulge of the superior edge and the persistent lateral roll. *It is now easy to prevent these sequelae by beginning the operation with a suction lipoplasty of the upper part of the abdomen and the flanks* (Fig. 29-14). The advan-

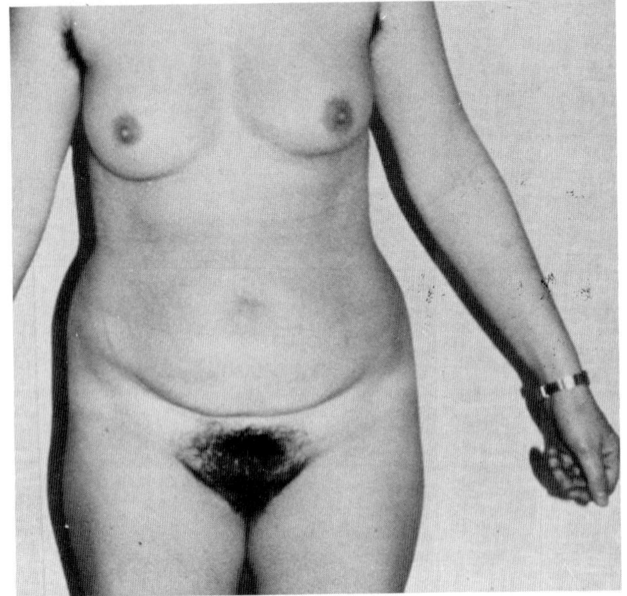

A

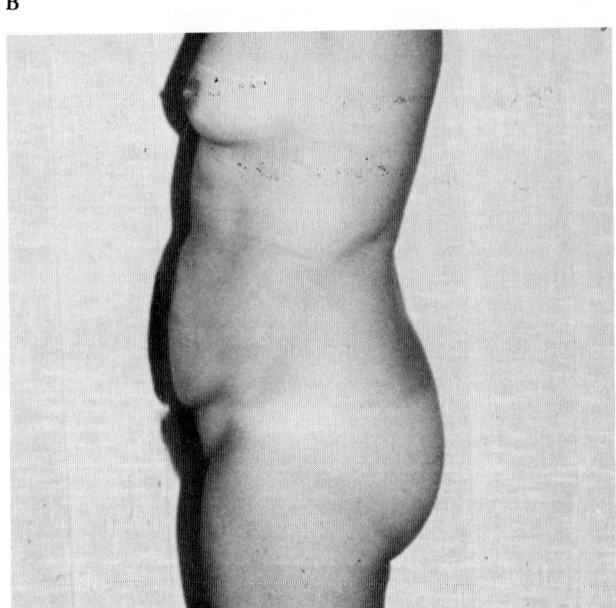

B

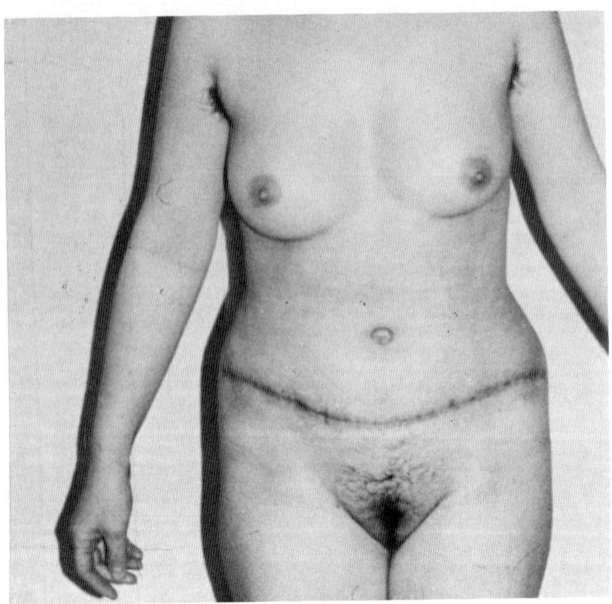

C

D

Fig. 29-15.

A. Preoperative anterior view of young woman with excess of both fat and skin.

B. Preoperative lateral view showing lower abdominal fold.

C. Postoperative 1 month view showing result with scar at upper limit of "bikini line." Note improvement in flanks.

D. One-month postoperative lateral view confirms overall silhouette improvement with absence of dog-ears.

tages are obvious. Suction lipoplasty makes the superior flap thinner, thereby facilitating its mobilization, and reduces the tension at the edges, thus improving the quality of the scar. It reduces the waist and reduces the epigastric and lateral rolls without lengthening the scar. It avoids "dog-ears" at the extremities of the scar.

The disadvantages are negligible. There is no shock phenomenon since the volume of fat removed does not exceed more than a few hundred milliliters. It adds only 10 to 30 minutes to the length of the operation. The small incisions are, of course, situated in the resected skin. The abdominoplasty is completed in the usual manner. Results are particularly satisfying in this group of patients and are permanent (adipocyte theory) (Fig. 29-15).

Abdomen Pendulum

Patients with this deformity are obese people who have undergone one or several slimming diets and who present with important functional complaints such as back pain. There is a major excess of both the skin and the adipose panniculus.

These patients are especially difficult because they may have associated systemic and local disorders (diabetes, high uric acid levels, marked diastasis of the recti muscles, skin infections of the suprapubic fold, etc.). Many of these patients had a high operative risk and were refused classic surgery.

The goal of surgical treatment in these cases is more functional than aesthetic. The technique we propose is safe, quick, and functional. The marking of the dermolipectomy is made with the patient in the standing position. The markings correspond to a large transversal spindle-shaped piece. The lower limit is given by the inferior abdominal fold and the upper limit is obtained by pinching the skin. The marking of the areas to be defatted will guide the operator during the suction part of the procedure. Different vertical guide-marks on each side of the medial line will make the later adjustment of the wound edges easier (Fig. 29-16).

Using several small incisions, we begin with suction of the supraumbilical region, flanks, waist, and lumbar area. This is followed by a dermolipectomy in which the umbilical stalk is removed in the monoblock, *avoiding any undermining* other than what may occur with the suction lipoplasty. Any opening thus created in the aponeurosis is carefully closed with two or three permanent sutures. Of course, any associated hernia will require appropriate procedures (overcoat suture or mesh prosthesis). In the case of a diastasis of the recti, the undermining is limited to the extent necessary to effect the musculoaponeurotic repair. The suture of the wound edges is without tension. Suction drainage is maintained for 48 hours.

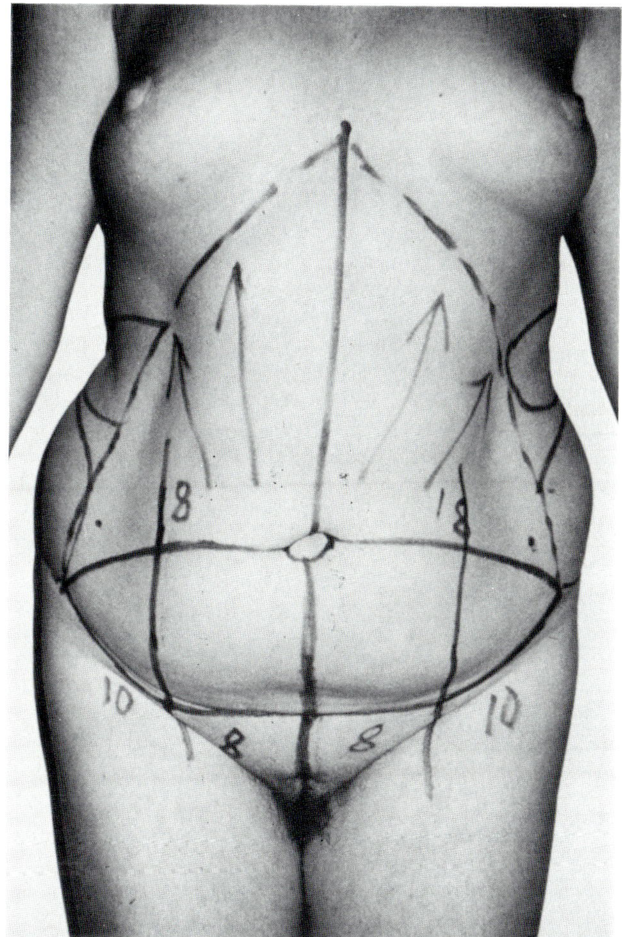

Fig. 29-16. Preoperative markings for an "abdomen pendulum" showing guide marks for reapproximation. Note lower fusiform monoblock resection marked out. Arrows indicate defatting by suction, which allows expansion of superior flap.

To complete the procedure, a neoumbilicoplasty is performed. In the case of obese patients with a short and broad abdomen, the umbilicus is generally situated rather inferiorly near the line joining the anterosuperior iliac spines, and its axis is not longitudinal but transverse. The choice of the site of the neoumbilicus is important, since patients complain more of poor location than poor appearance. The original umbilicus is usually so deformed by obesity that its preoperative appearance will not be missed by the patient and improvement is the rule.

The technique of neoumbilicoplasty that we have used is quite simple and has given us satisfactory results in most cases. Of course, the results in obese patients cannot be judged according to the usual standards for aesthetic abdominoplasty. This kind of surgery is more functional than aesthetic and has a number of advantages.

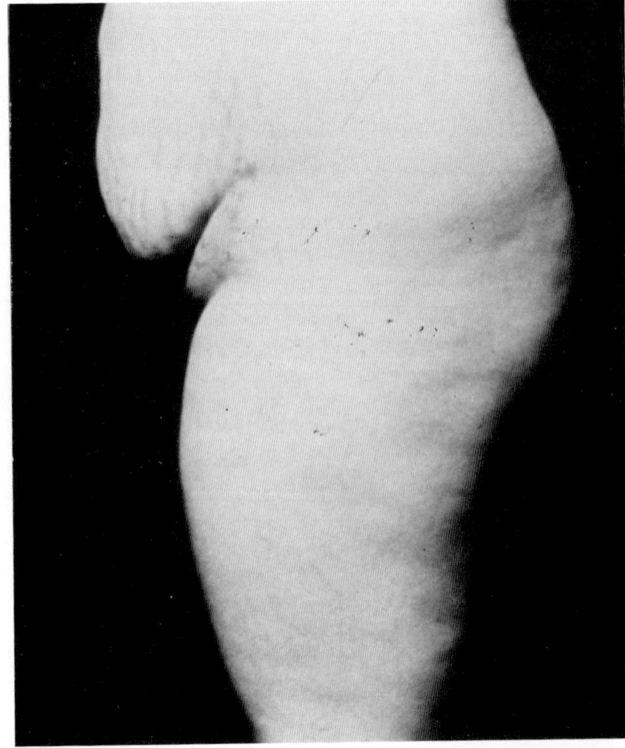

A

B

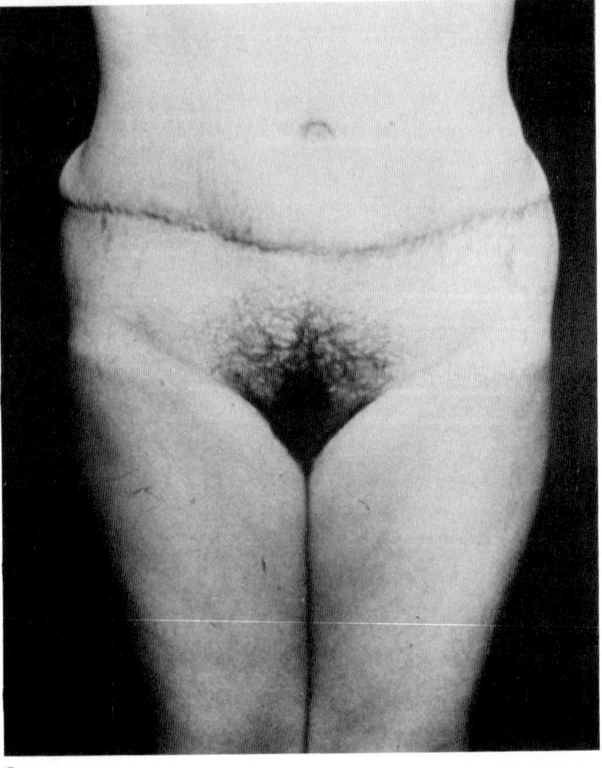

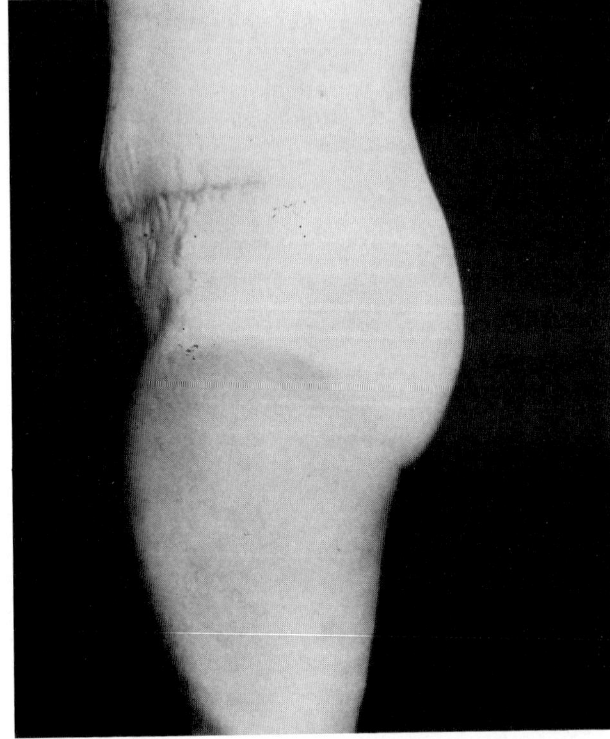

C

D

Fig. 29-17.

A. Preoperative "abdomen pendulum" with poor skin tone, excessive lateral skin, transverse umbilicus, and heavy epigastrium.

B. Lateral preoperative view.

C. Postoperative view at 6 months following suction, der-molipectomy, and neoumbilicoplasty. New umbilicus is an improvement.

D. Postoperative lateral view. The combined technique raises a salvage procedure to a higher level of patient acceptability.

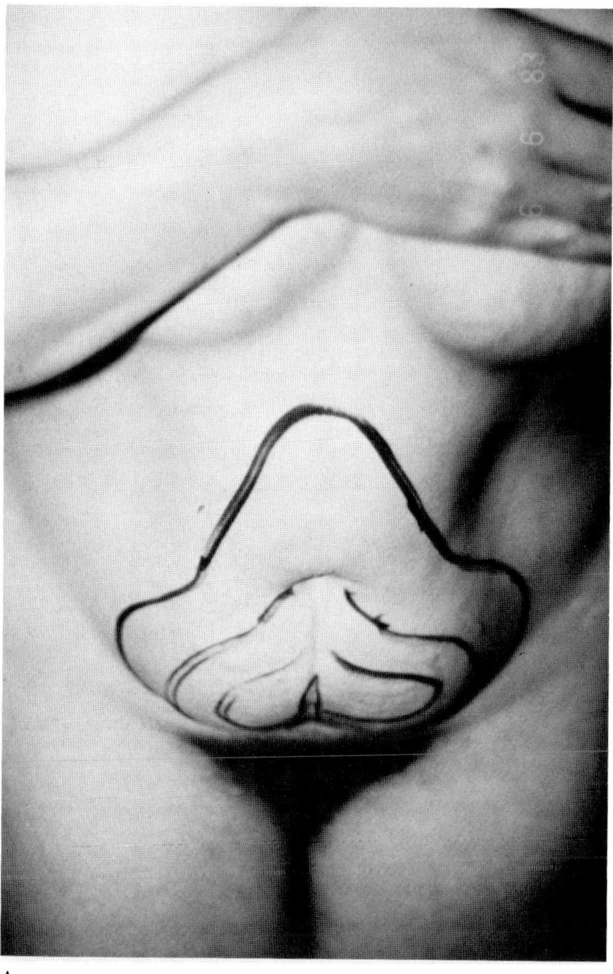

A

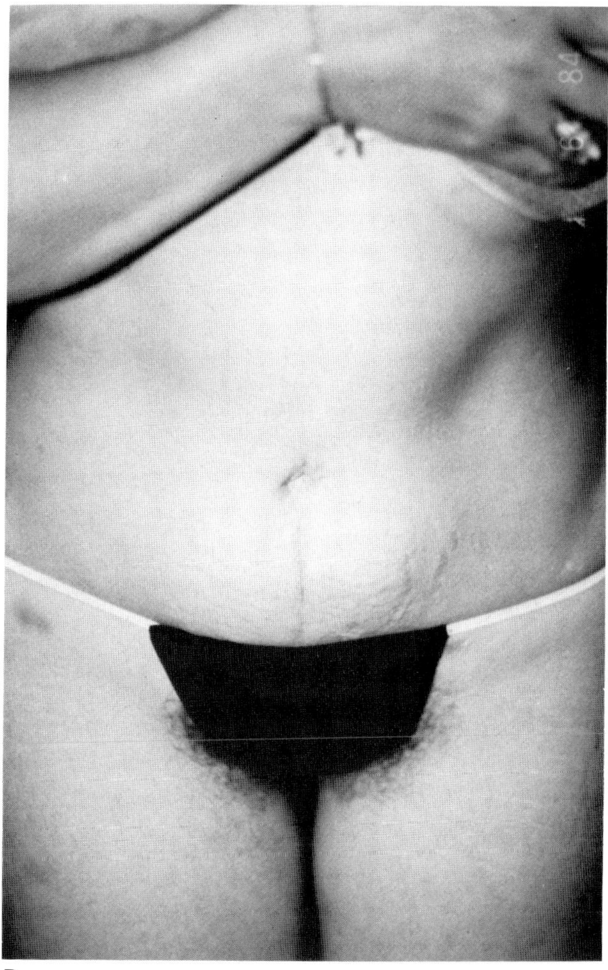

B

Fig. 29-18.
A. Preoperative view of 34-year-old female with midline scar and loose hanging abdomen seen in close-up with flexed pelvis.
B. Postoperative view at one year following scar revision, both horizontal and vertical, and suction lipoplasty. (Photographs courtesy of G. Hetter, M.D.)

The operating time is short (less than one and one-half hours) and hence safer. The dermolipectomy is limited to the anterior part of the abdomen. Immobilization of the patient postoperatively is avoided. The usual large undermining is avoided. There is little or no tension on the wound edges. The reconstruction of the umbilicus is simple and quick.

Even if the aesthetic results and the scar are not perfect, such patients benefit greatly from this operation (Fig. 29-17). They lose between 10 and 20 pounds and their abdominal profile is improved. In addition, their emotional state is usually improved and they are grateful.

Scarred Abdomen

Any abdominal scarring may be poorly accepted by the patient. Obviously, if there is a major skin excess, and if the location of the scar allows for it (for instance, a medial infraumbilical scar), it is possible to do a classic transverse abdominoplasty with or without suction lipoplasty. However, the skin excess is often moderate, and it is the hypertrophy of the pericicatricial adipose tissue that worsens the appearance of the scar.

Here once again, it may be very helpful to do suction lipoplasty before the typical scar revision in order to have a better looking scar and to improve the general aspect of the abdomen (Figs. 29-18 and 29-19). As a rule, the incision necessary for the introduction of the lipoextractor (cannula) will be located in the scar to be resected. However, we are always on the alert for an associated incisional hernia.

Wrinkled Abdomen with Stretch Marks

We choose among a transverse, longitudinal, or mixed

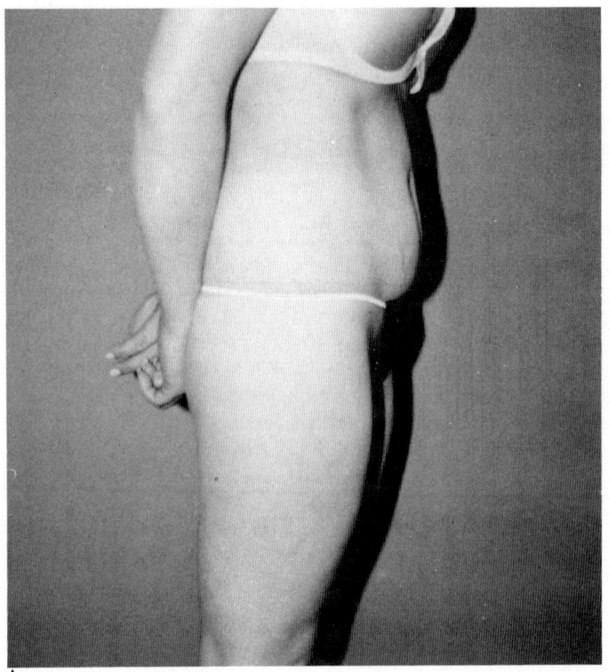

A

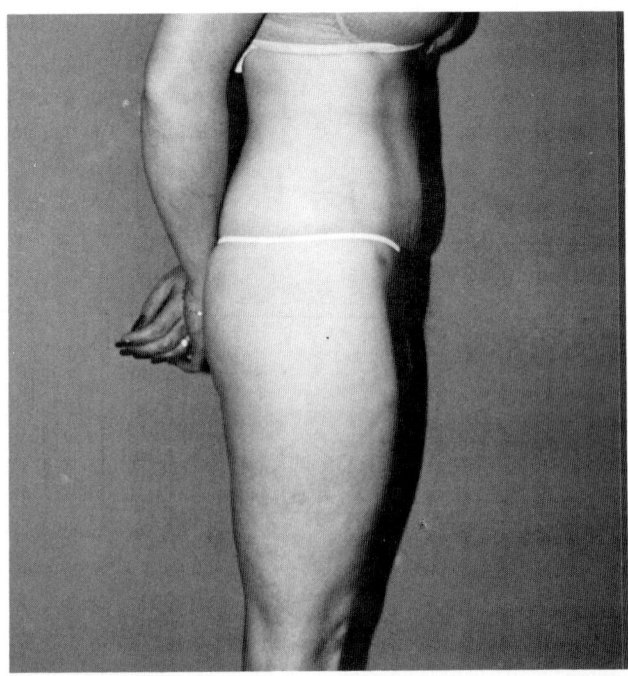

B

Fig. 29-19.
A. Preoperative right lateral view showing protuberant abdomen (same patient as Fig. 29-18).
B. Right lateral view one year postoperatively.

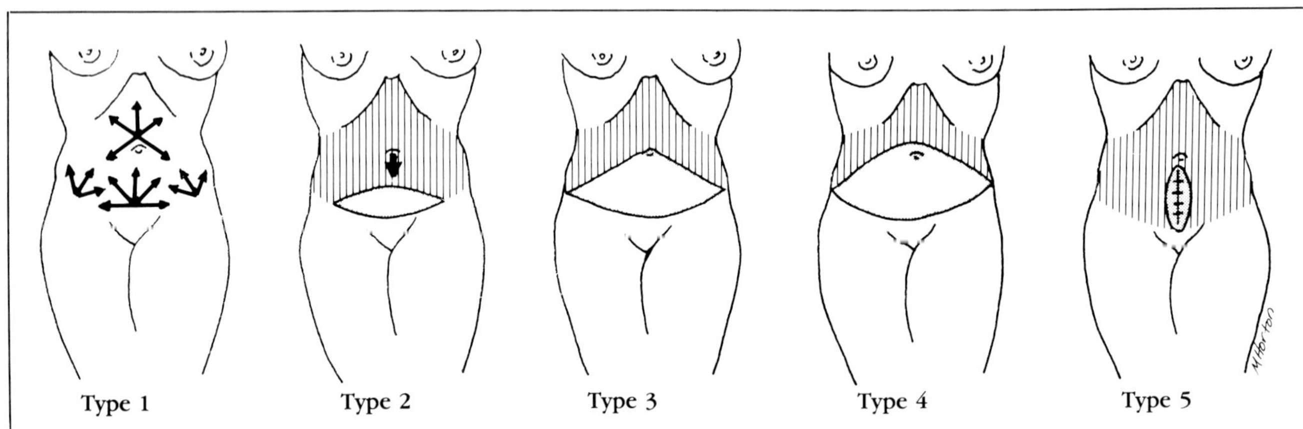

Fig. 29-20. Diagram of the five types of procedures utilizing suction lipoplasty to improve abdominal appearance. 1. Suction alone. 2. Suction combined with localized dermolipectomy with or without disinsertion-reposition of the umbilicus. 3. Suction of the upper flap, flanks, and hips, followed by classic transverse abdominoplasty with transposition of the umbilicus. 4. Suction of the upper flap: dermolipectomy including amputation of the umbilical stem and neoumbilicoplasty. 5. Suction followed by scar revision.

dermolipectomy depending on the topography of the lesions and the type of abdomen—short and broad or long and slim. We do not believe that the transverse abdominoplasty should be routinely applied in every case. By making a low transverse incision, we risk resecting good-looking infraumbilical skin and leaving instead a superior flap damaged by numerous striae. Moreover, if the transverse scar is kept very low we must make sure that there is no exaggerated traction on its edges, which can cause distortion of the mons pubis, and is so commonly seen in published photographs [14].

In summary, the abdominoplasty that leaves the minimum of sequelae should always be chosen. These operations are illustrated in Figure 29-20.

Conclusion

The contribution of suction lipoplasty to aesthetic surgery of the abdomen is of the greatest importance [15]. It can be used as the sole procedure in previously inoperable cases and enables us to obtain truly excellent results with a negligible scar. Results from surgeons all over the world who were trained by Illouz attest to this fact.

When skin damage is too great, suction lipoplasty can be combined with a classic dermolipectomy to improve the results without aggravating the operation.

Finally, suction lipoplasty, as with all plastic surgery, must be carefully planned and performed to avoid complications or unaesthetic results. Unfavorable results are not inherent to the technique but are due to careless examination, inadequate diagnosis, superficial understanding of the technique, or its maladroit application.

References

1. Elbaz, J. S., and Flageul, G. *Plastic Surgery of the Abdomen.* Paris: Masson, 1977.
2. Faivre, J., and Loffredo, V. *Aesthetic Surgery 1978, The Abdomen.* Paris: Maloine, 1978.
3. Illouz, Y. G. A new technique for localized lipodystrophies. *Rev. Chir. Esth. Franc.* 19(6), April, 1980.
4. Illouz, Y. G. A new technique for localized lipodystrophies: Selective lipectomy or lipolysis. *J. Chir. Esth.* Montreuil, November 9–11, 1981. Published in Chirurgie Esthetique, 1981–1982. Pp. 79–92. Paris: Maloine, 1982.
5. Illouz, Y. G. Body contouring by lipolysis: A 5-year experience with over 3000 cases. *Plast. Reconst. Surg.* 72:5591–97, 1983.
6. Fournier, P., and Otteni, F. Treatment of localized lipodystrophies by aspiration. *J. Chir. Esth.* Montreuil, November 9–11, 1981. Published in Chirurgie Esthetique, 1981–1982. Pp. 59–78. Paris: Maloine, 1982.
7. Fournier, P., and Otteni, F. Lipodissection in body sculpturing: The dry procedure. *Plast. Reconstr. Surg.* 72:598–609, 1983.
8. Gonzalez-Ulloa, M. Circular lipectomy with transposition of the umbilicus and aponeurolytic technique. *Chirurgie.* 27:394–409, 1959.
9. Gonzalez-Ulloa, M. Belt lipectomy. *Br. J. Plast. Surg.* 13:179–186, 1960.
10. Juri, J., Juri, C., and Raiden, G. Reconstruction of the umbilicus in abdominoplasty. *Plast. Reconstr. Surg.* 63:580, 1979.
11. Personal communication with Clyde Litton, M.D., who attributed this to Mario Gonzalez-Ulloa.
12. Spadatora, A. *Cirurgia de Obesidad Flaccidez Cutanea Envegecimento: Dermolipectomias y Operationes Conexas.* Buenos Aires: San Marco Lopez Libreros, 1974.
13. Fevrer J. *Chirugie Esthetique del Abdomen.* Paris: Maloine, 1978.
14. Grazer, F., and Klingbeil, J. Body image—a surgical perspective. St. Louis: Mosby, 1980.
15. Otteni, F., and Fournier, P. Surgery of the silhouette: From classical surgery to collapsing surgery. *Rev. Chir. Esth. Franc.* 32(8):13–18, 1983.

CHAPTER 30

Lipolysis of the Flank

Paul L. Schnur

Indications

Excess fatty deposits in the flank area of the male are a sex-related trait, probably mediated by a male hormone. This deformity is frequently seen in men with normal body weight and habitus who have excess fatty deposits in the flanks, with or without excess fat in the lower abdomen. This deformity is as unique to men as the "saddlebag" deformity is to women. Because of the "love handles" or "spare tire," the patient comes to the surgeon with the request for removal. Before the widespread use of suction-assisted lipectomy, the results of the procedure for correction of this problem were not satisfactory. Incisions made to remove the fat in the flank area left unsightly scars that were not accepted by most patients, even when they could be hidden with underwear or a bathing suit.

Preoperative Preparation

Patients present requesting removal of the fat in the flank, either as an isolated deformity or in conjunction with removal of lower abdominal fat. The patients selected for suction-assisted lipectomy of the flanks and abdomen should ideally be men who are at or near ideal body weight. The attempt to remove large amounts of fat in overweight men results in disappointed patients. Even though large amounts of fat can easily be removed in the obese, the final result certainly is not one of improvement in body image. As in other forms of suction lipectomy, there is usually some waviness or irregularity of the skin, but this appears to be less obvious in men than in women. Perhaps this is due to thicker skin and increased body hair in the male.

Anesthesia, in most cases, should be general since it is difficult to establish adequate local anesthesia in the flank and abdominal area. If only removal of fatty tissue from the flank is required, the patient might tolerate this procedure under local anesthesia. If one begins surgery under local anesthesia and finds that the patient tolerates the procedure poorly, the surgeon may compromise the final result by terminating the operation before an adequate removal of fat.

Most procedures can be done on an outpatient basis because large amounts of fat are not removed. Patients are prepared for surgery by a thorough discussion of anticipated accomplishments in relation to expectations. The patient is instructed to purchase an elastic garment such as a supporter with a very wide elastic band. One of the commercially available elastic garments can also be used; however, the ideal line of garments has not yet been developed. The patient is required to wear this support for a period of 6 weeks after surgery. Demerol tablets are prescribed for postoperative pain since milder narcotics are usually not sufficient. Before surgery, the patient is marked in a standing position before a full-length mirror and asked to approve the areas where fat is to be removed. This procedure allows the patient to take an active part in choosing the areas involved in the fat removal. Preoperative photographs are taken before and after the markings have been drawn. The latter is done so that it is possible to later determine exactly what agreement had been reached about what to remove.

Technique

The anesthesiologist hydrates the patient while administering 2 L of Ringer's lactate during and immediately after surgery. The patient is then asked to consume a liter or two of an oral electrolyte solution such as Gatorade during the next 12 hours. The patient is anesthetized in the supine position. The preparation and draping extends into the posterior aspect of the torso because many of the flank deformities extend well onto the back. Rather than turning the patient, he or she can simply be rolled from side to side by the assistant. Before beginning the procedure, the areas that have been previously marked are infiltrated with 0.25% Marcaine with adrenaline. This accomplishes a twofold purpose: long-term local anesthesia for less painful recovery and hemostasis during the procedure.

When fat is removed from the abdomen in conjunction with the flank, it is possible to remove it through a single stab wound incision in the superior pubic hair area. This removal can be done only if the flank deformity does not extend too far posteriorly. If the flank is done as an isolated procedure or if the fat extends well into the posterior trunk, it is necessary to make a stab wound incision laterally. I make an incision at the midaxillary line in the area that would be covered by a brief bathing suit or jockey shorts. These stab wound incisions ultimately become unnoticeable.

I generally start with an 8-mm cannula of appropriate length and curvature. If the fat is extensive, I change to a 10-mm cannula and find that this cannula facilitates rapid removal of large volumes of fat. The length and curvature of the cannula is simply a matter of personal preference. The final smoothing and feathering at the edges is done by reintroduction of the 8-mm cannula.

Generally, only 100 to 400 ml of fat is removed from either flank area. The consistency of the fat in the flank is different than in the thigh, buttocks, or abdomen. It feels as if there are more septa between the skin and the fascia, making fat removal from the flank area more difficult. Sometimes it appears that it is not possible to remove as much fat as is desired, but if one uses the larger cannula and simply continues repeated passage, an adequate amount of fat can be removed.

I find the upper abdomen is similar to the flank in difficulty of fat removal. It is necessary to remove enough fat to produce a slight depression so the final result is adequate. As in any area of suction, it is better to remove too little than too much. Undercorrection is easier to remedy than overcorrection. In any event, it is necessary to work harder and longer to remove fat from the flanks than from other areas.

Once suction lipectomy is completed and it is determined that an adequate amount of fat has been removed, the wounds are closed with interrupted subcuticular Dexon sutures. A small dressing is applied and the patient is placed in the elastic garment.

Postoperative Management

The patient is allowed to resume normal activity the day after surgery but must refrain from strenuous activity for a period of 3 weeks. In the early phase of discoloration, swelling, and weight gain, the patient often has doubts about the final result and must be reassured that the ultimate result will be satisfactory. It is repeatedly stressed to the patient that it is impossible to make a judgment on the adequacy of the final result until 6 to 9 months after surgery. At that time, if necessary, a touchup procedure can be performed.

Patients have generally been very happy with the final results. When fat is removed from the flank area, patients report that they do not change pant size but the fit is much better. In a few patients, secondary procedures must be performed to obtain maximal results. The surgeon should not hesitate to do this. These procedures are usually done under local anesthesia in the office.

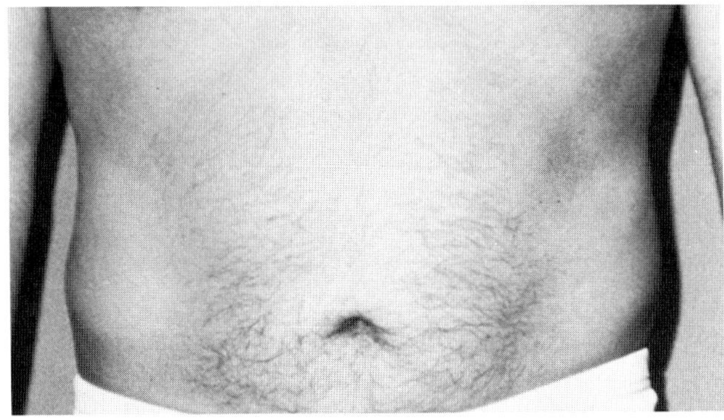

Fig. 30-1. Preoperative photograph of a 48-year-old man complaining of abdominal and flank fullness.

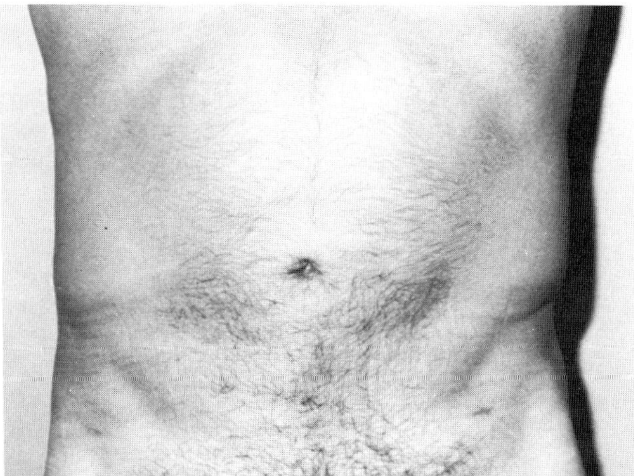

Fig. 30-2. Photograph 6 months after suction lipectomy of the abdomen and flanks.

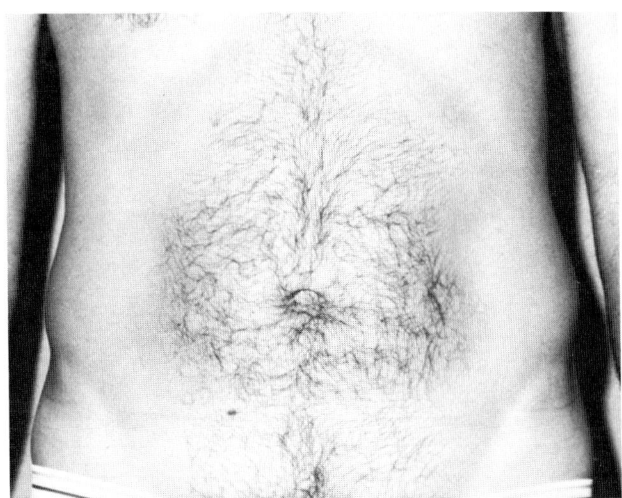

Fig. 30-3. Preoperative photograph of a 38-year-old man complaining of flank and abdominal fat.

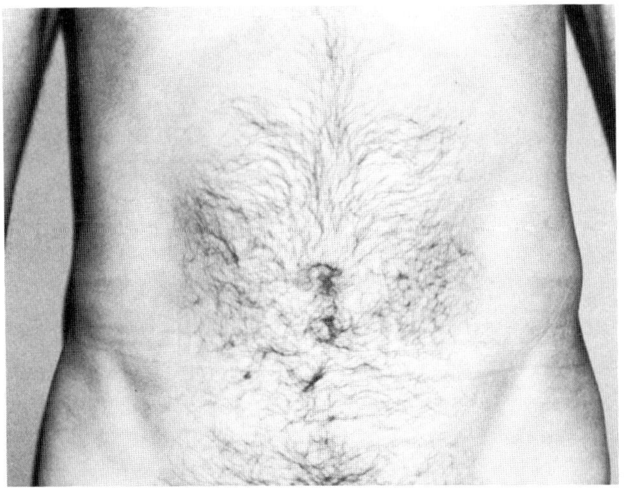

Fig. 30-4. Photograph 4 months after suction lipectomy of the abdomen and flanks with removal of 700 ml.

Case Studies

Case 1: Suction lipectomy of the abdomen and flanks. Figure 30-1 is a preoperative photograph of a 48-year-old contractor who was concerned about the fullness of his abdomen and flanks. His weight was within normal limits for his height. He underwent suction-assisted lipectomy of the abdomen and flanks. Figure 30-2 is his postoperative photograph taken 6 months later. The flank procedure was performed through stab wounds in each groin. Notice that the result on the right side is excellent. On the left side, the result is not as satisfactory. The patient has been offered a second procedure to remove additional fat but has declined because he is satisfied with the results.

Case 2: Suction lipectomy of the abdomen and flanks. Figure 30-3 is a preoperative photograph of a 38-year-old man with minimal amounts of flank and abdominal fat. His weight was within normal limits for his height. A suction-assisted lipectomy was performed through a single midline stab wound just within the pubic hair. Approximately 700 ml of material was removed from the flanks and abdomen. Figure 30-4 is a photograph taken 4 months later with very satisfactory results.

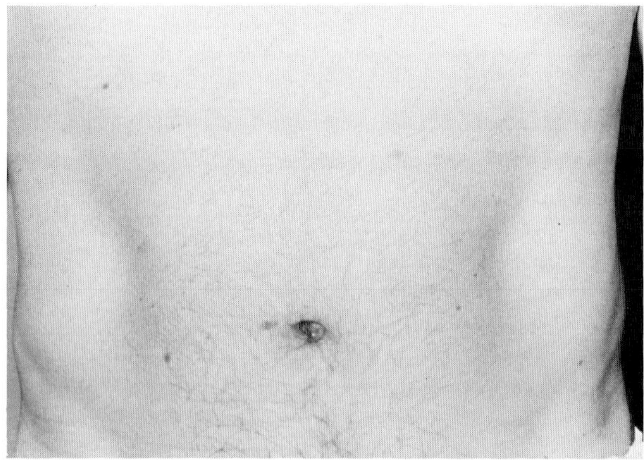

Fig. 30-5. Preoperative photograph of a 41-year-old patient complaining of abdominal and flank excess. (Courtesy of B. Burkhardt, M.D.)

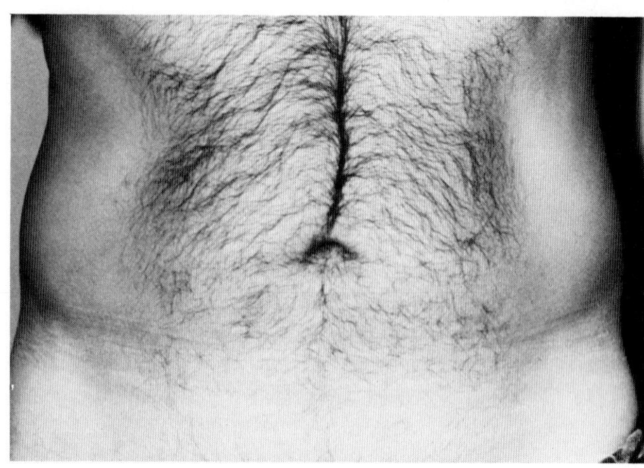

Fig. 30-7. Preoperative photograph of a 36-year-old patient complaining of flank excess alone. (Courtesy of Dr. B. Burkhardt.)

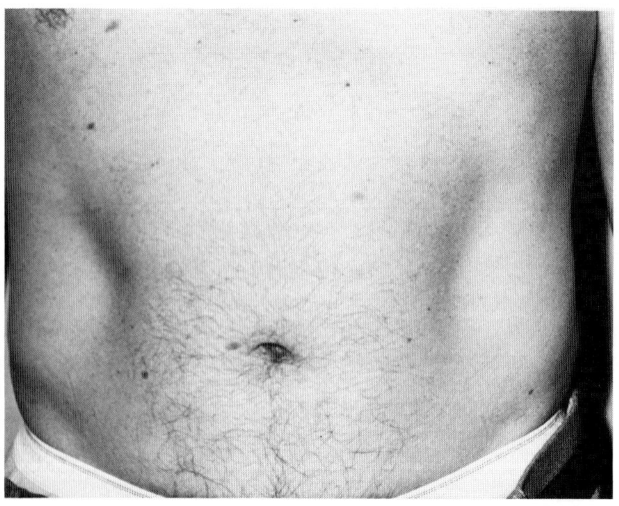

Fig. 30-6. Photograph 1 year after suction lipectomy of the abdomen and flanks with 300 ml removal. (Courtesy of B. Burkhardt, M.D.)

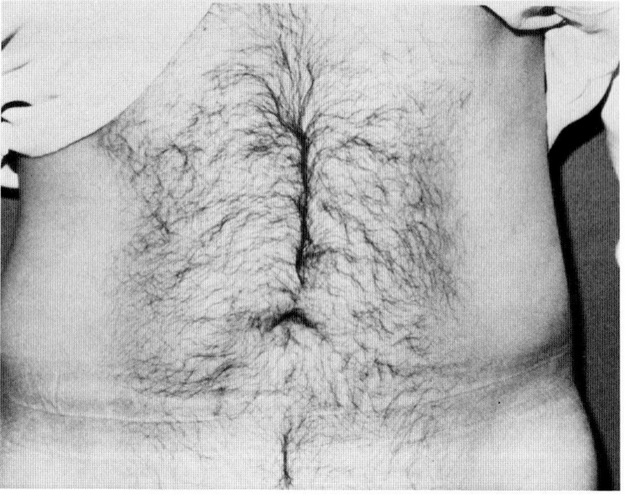

Fig. 30-8. Photograph 6 months after suction lipectomy of the flanks with 500 ml removal. (Courtesy of B. Burkhardt, M.D.)

Case 3: Suction lipectomy of the abdomen and flanks. Figure 30-5 shows the preoperative film of a 41-year-old man who requested removal of fat from the abdomen and flanks. Again, his weight was within normal limits for his height. Approximately 300 ml of material was removed. Figure 30-6 is the follow-up photograph taken 1 year later showing improvement in the flank area. The patient was satisfied with the results.

Case 4: Suction lipectomy of the flanks. Figure 30-7 is a preoperative photograph of a 36-year-old man who had lost a significant amount of weight before consultation. His weight was normal for his height. He requested removal of the fat from the flank area alone. This was done through two lateral stab wound incisions. A total of 500 ml was removed. Figure 30-8, taken 6 months later, shows the patient much improved. He states that before suction lipectomy, flank fat hung over his belt line, but this has been corrected by the procedure.

CHAPTER 31

Lipolysis of the Iliac Crest

Gregory P. Hetter

The iliac crest is the most forgiving area regarding lipolysis. Yet it is one of the areas for which surgeons had no generally accepted procedure to reduce its excess fat. Many abdominoplasties, while satisfactory insofar as the abdomen was concerned, were ultimately not satisfactory because of the fatty extensions laterally around the iliac crest. Scars placed in this area were difficult to conceal, tended to widen, and always marred even a good contour.

I do not remember a case where I have extracted only iliac crest fat. Reduction has always been in association with fatty excess of the abdomen or lateral femoral area.

Examination

The iliac crest fat should always be examined when the patient presents complaining of other areas. This area must be differentiated from flank fat seen often in the male (Fig. 31-1). The pinch test should be performed after the visual examination. The pinch test is applied to the areas confluent with this typical female fat pad. If the thickness is more than twice the surrounding fat thickness, the surgeon should consider treating the area.

Evaluation of the width of the bony pelvis is important to prevent overlooking this uncorrectable bulge. Visual examination often shows an obvious need to reduce this area to bring the whole silhouette into harmony. Asymmetries often due to pelvic tilt or to scoliosis must be pointed out to the patient since these conditions are refractory to fat removal (see Fig. 31-6).

Marking and Incisions

The area is marked out topographically along with the other areas planned for surgery. The site of entry is chosen with the patient's foreknowledge and often with regard to whatever bathing attire the patient finds most appropriate. I find the prone position easiest for removing iliac crest fat and usually use an incision in the gluteal depression. This incision is easily hidden, even by a small bikini (Fig. 31-2), and allows access to the lateral femoral area or buttock, if necessary. Lumbar incisions cause more bleeding and are not as easily hidden, for which reasons I have discontinued their use.

Patient Selection

Generally patients are selected on the basis of the decision regarding their primary area, because they usually

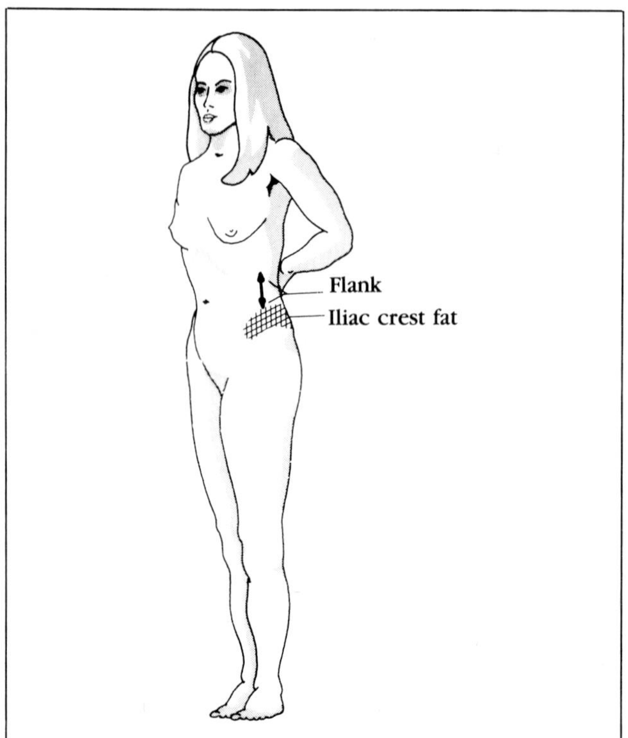

Fig. 31-1. Drawing shows difference between flank between iliac crest and lowest ribs and iliac crest fat *(striped area).*

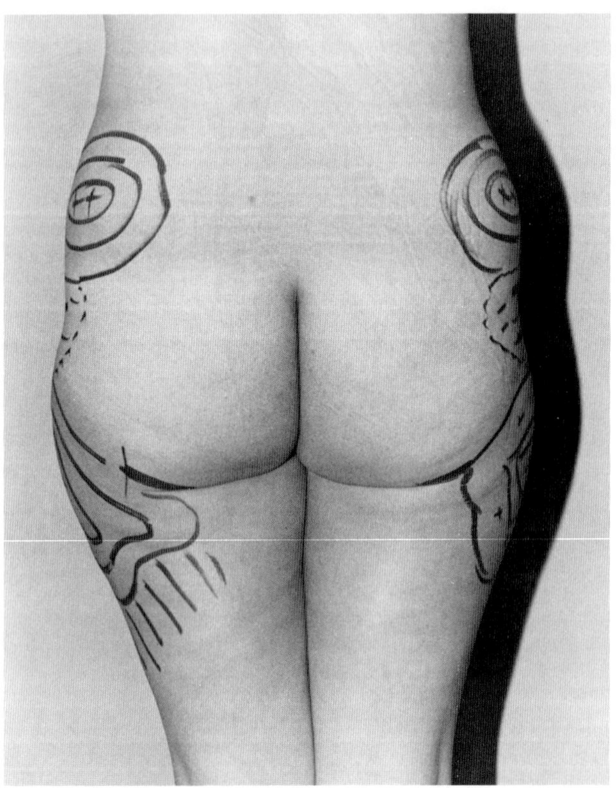

Fig. 31-2. A patient marked for a gluteal depression incision to approach the iliac crest from below.

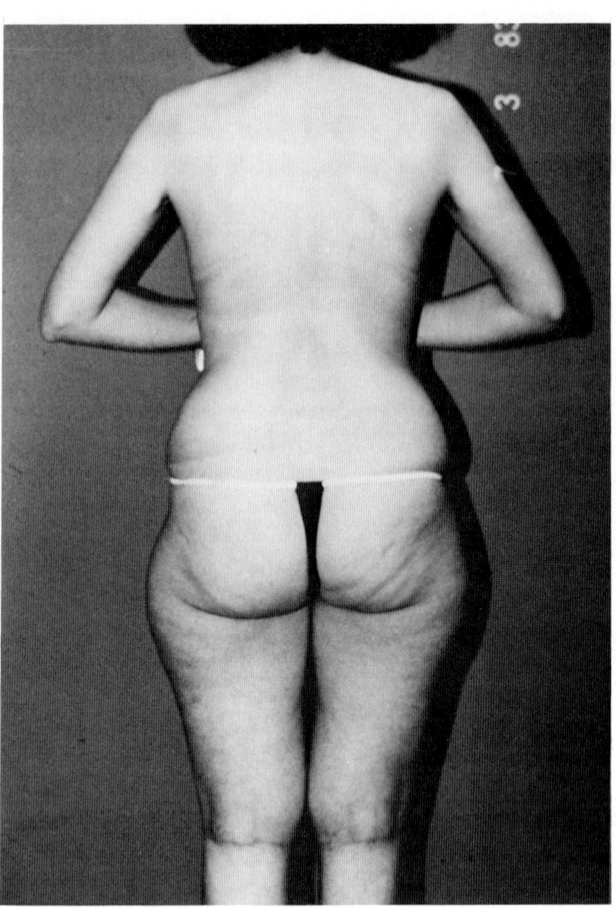

Fig. 31-3. Typical "violin deformity" seen commonly in women of Mediterranean extraction.

have their primary surgery for an area other than the iliac crest.

One of the most common silhouette problems is the "violin deformity" (Fig. 31-3), in which iliac crest fat is combined with lateral thigh excess (see Chap. 32). If the patient is rejected on the basis of unsuitability for the thigh procedure, there is usually no indication to do the iliac crest alone.

Abdominal bulges, especially hypogastric bulges, are probably more often associated with iliac crest bulges than with thigh excess. This hypogastric-iliac crest excess gives a typical pear-shaped silhouette (Fig. 31-4).

The suitability of the patient for this procedure depends on his or her suitability for the primary procedure. When the patient is a candidate for straightforward lipolysis of the abdomen, associated extraction from the iliac crest is common. When the abdomen requires either modified or classical abdominoplasty, the incisions are often shortened and the results improved by defatting laterally in the "dog ear" areas and further into the iliac crest bulges (see Chap. 34).

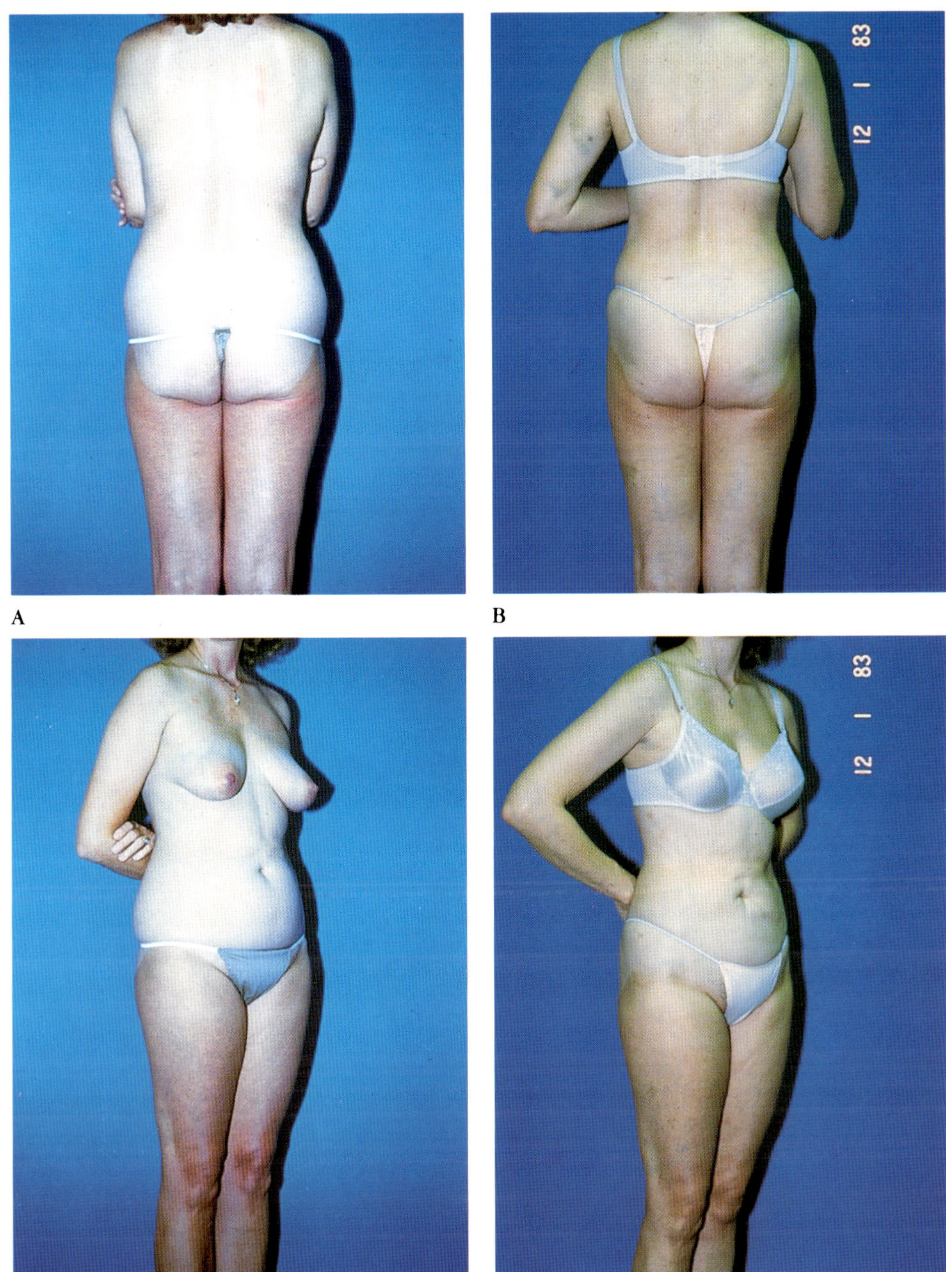

Fig. 31-6.
A. Preoperative posterior view showing irregularity of silhouette due to iliac crest bulges.
B. Three-month postoperative view showing improvement following lipolysis.
C. Preoperative oblique view showing unaesthetic "pear shape" due to confluent iliac crest and hypogastric fat.
D. Three-month postoperative oblique view showing aesthetic improvement from hypogastric and iliac crest defatting.

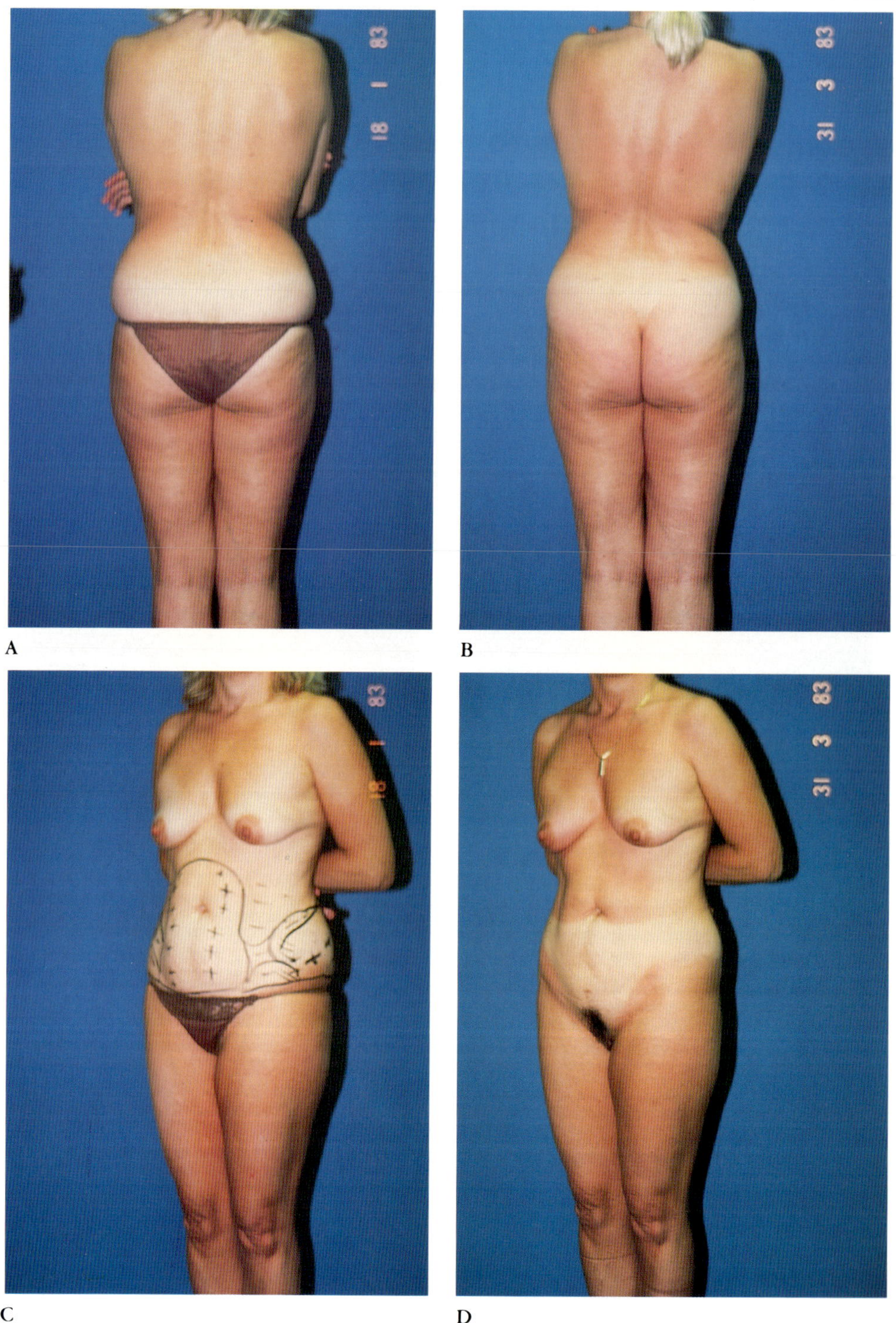

Fig. 31-7.
A. Preoperative posterior view. Note asymmetry due to pelvic tilt.
B. Postoperative view at 2½ months.
C. Preoperative oblique view. Note confluency of fat.
D. Postoperative oblique view showing striking improvement in harmony of form.

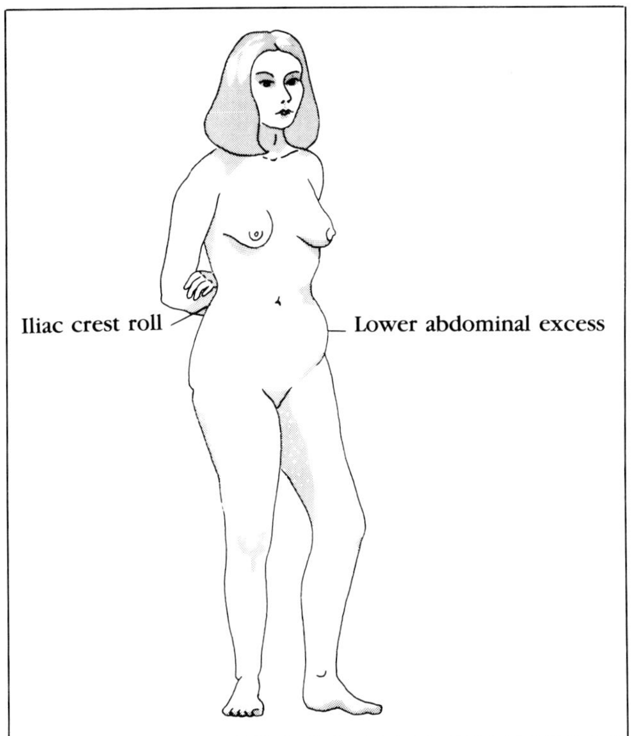

Fig. 31-4. The typical "pear shape" is often seen, even in young patients, and is usually inherited. The "pot belly" is present in the prepubertal years; the iliac crest becomes prominent after puberty.

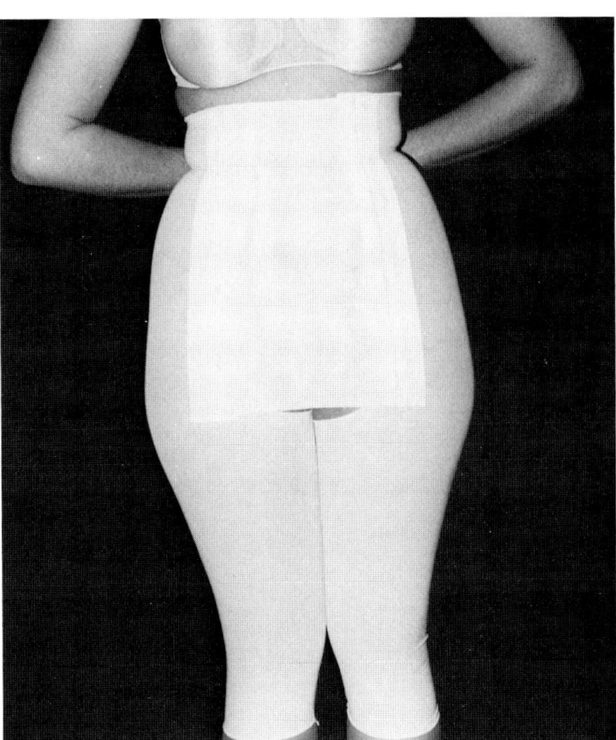

Fig. 31-5. Circumpress garment useful for midtorso procedures including abdomen, flanks, iliac crest, and thigh procedures. (Available from Circumpress, 1625 Godfrey Lane, Virginia Beach, Virginia 23454.)

As yet I have found no upper limit on age for this procedure, as long as the primary procedure is suitable for the patient.

Technique

It is unnecessary to use the criss-cross technique because the iliac crest area is so forgiving. Waves have not been a problem, although rarely an additional removal for asymmetry may be required. The procedure is done under general anesthesia. Pretreatment of this area with low-dose epinephrine solutions is very helpful. This area is higher in vascularity than others and benefits greatly from this pretreatment. To allow for the epinephrine effect, the injections are placed before scrubbing and 10 minutes is allowed to elapse.

For very fatty masses, I use the #10 cannula, with attention to keep the lumen down. A track may be too superficial, yet I have not seen waves subsequent to this problem in the iliac crest area. The #8 Illouz or Padgett is commonly used. Fat should not be extracted as the cannula is removed from the incision site by breaking the vacuum. The pinch test determines when the iliac crest fat has become about as thick as surrounding areas.

Postoperative Care

Any of the girdles commercially available are adequate for compression. The Circumpress girdle with a double row of hooks in front is particularly easy to get on and to open to inspect the abdomen, flanks, and iliac crest areas. The crotch is open for convenience of hygiene (Fig. 31-5). The girdle is worn constantly for 1 week and then worn while awake for the next 2 weeks. Thereafter, I switch the patients to either Sears Cling-A-Long or J. C. Penney Total Support support-type pantyhose for an additional 3 weeks during waking hours.

Results

See Chapter 32 for results associated with thigh procedures and Chapter 34 for results associated with open procedures.

The most striking result is seen in the circumferential hypogastric excess. Examples of this problem are seen in Figures 31-6 and 31-7 in the color plates. This largely hereditary disposition is often seen early in life, even in the prepubertal years. The improvement rendered by lipolysis alone in these fairly young patients is striking.

CHAPTER 32

Lipolysis of the Thigh and Knee

Gregory P. Hetter

There was no procedure before lipolysis that a plastic surgeon, in good conscience, could offer the average woman complaining of "trochanteric lipodystrophy." A misnomer was used to describe this normal, diet-resistant fat deposit, indicating how muddled our view was. The fact that few North American plastic surgeons performed many "classic" thighplasties is a testimonial to the problems associated with this area for most surgeons. Thighplasty was a "long run for a short slide."

Briefly, the problems were as follows: (1) lengthy, often bloody surgery, (2) expensive and unpredictable hospital stays and costs, (3) prolonged and unpredictable recovery time with significant morbidity, (4) destruction of the normal buttock fold, (5) limited improvement of the trochanteric area, (6) frequent recurrence of deformity, and (7) large, unsightly scars. For an intensive look at thighplasty as practiced in North America in the 1970s, the reader is referred to Dr. Frederick Grazer's book, *Body Image* [1].

Most women with small to modest accumulations of fat were rejected for surgery because the "deformity" did not justify any scar, let alone a 15-inch scar. These patients were turned away promptly with little discussion.

Although many complaints about fatty bulges seem frivolous, most plastic surgeons are responsive to a 3-mm hump high on a nasal dorsum because they have a good operation for it. A double fold of the buttock, on the other hand (Fig. 32-1), was greeted with little enthusiasm because surgeons could not reasonably recommend a "buttock lift" for such a small "deformity."

Figures 32-2 to 32-5 illustrate the spectrum of complaints that brought patients in for consultation complaining of "saddlebags." These deposits may occur alone but are often accompanied by a medial superior knee deposit, which gives the knee an ill-defined appearance (Fig. 32-6). Compare this knee with a well-sculptured knee (Fig. 32-7).

When an iliac crest roll accompanies the lateral femoral deposit, the violin deformity results. Often this deformity is accompanied by slim extremities as seen in Figures 32-8 and 32-9. However, it is also seen in more chubby persons (Figs. 32-10 and 32-11).

Large medial and anterior thighs, if accompanied by good skin turgor, are amenable to treatment. This condition may be idiopathic or the result of insulin injection as seen in Figure 32-12. Anterior superior knee accumulations are amenable to treatment and, although not yet common, are occasionally treated.

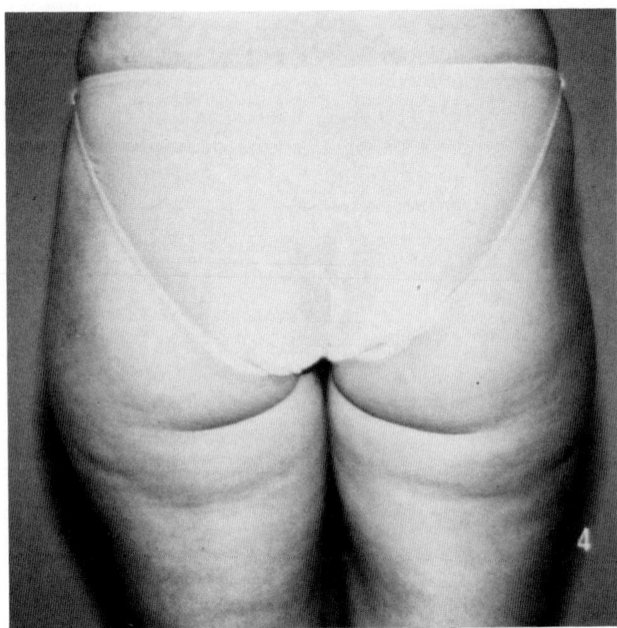

Fig. 32-1. Double fold in buttock of female body builder. Frequent exercise (6 hours per day) could not eliminate this accumulation.

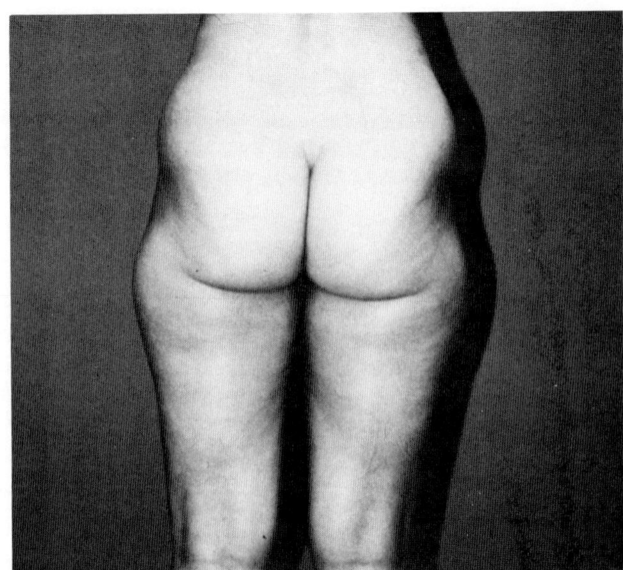

Fig. 32-3. A 28-year-old athletic woman with large lateral thigh deposits accentuated by gluteal depression.

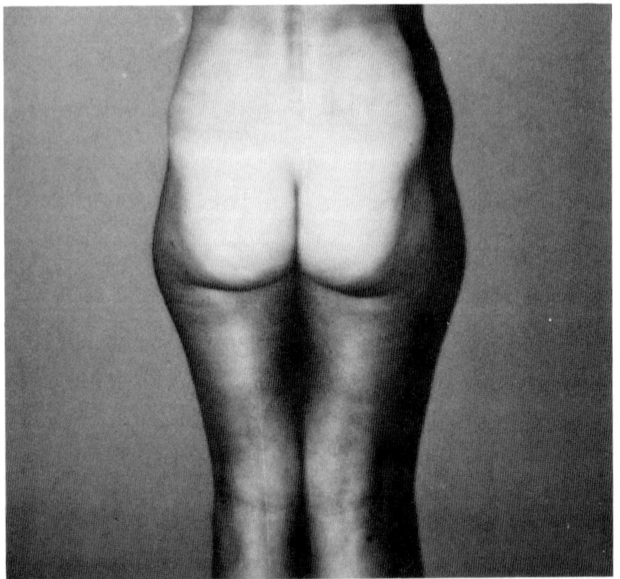

Fig. 32-2. Small 39-year-old trim woman with small lateral thigh deposit not amenable to dietary restriction.

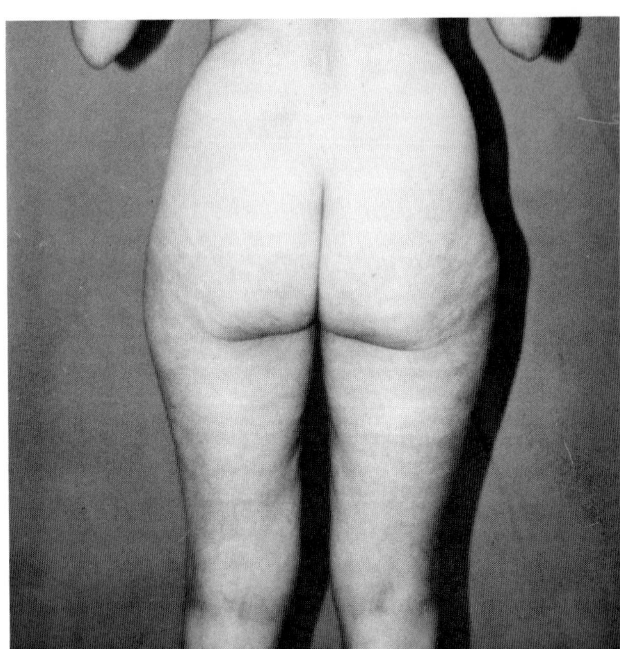

Fig. 32-4. Large-boned 42-year-old woman with fatty accumulations of iliac crest and lateral thighs and knees.

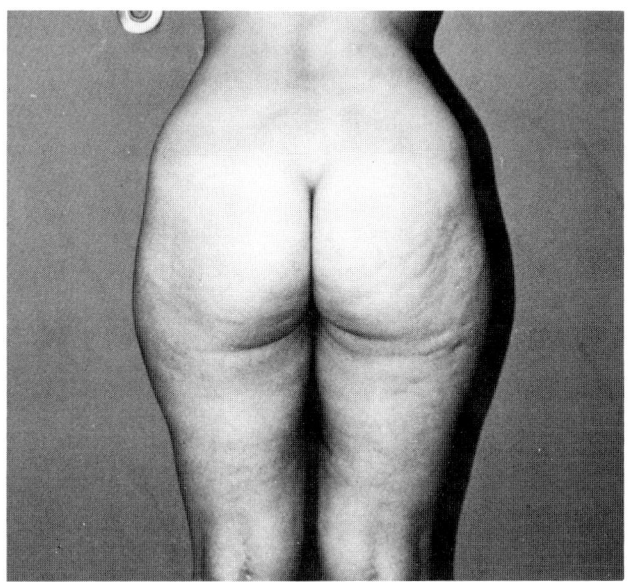

Fig. 32-5. Upper-lower body disproportion in 25-year-old woman with very heavy infragluteal and lateral thigh accumulations.

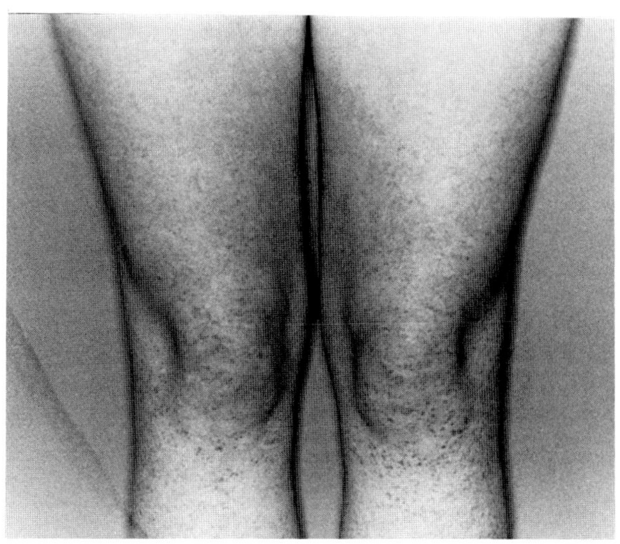

Fig. 32-7. Knees of young slender patient.

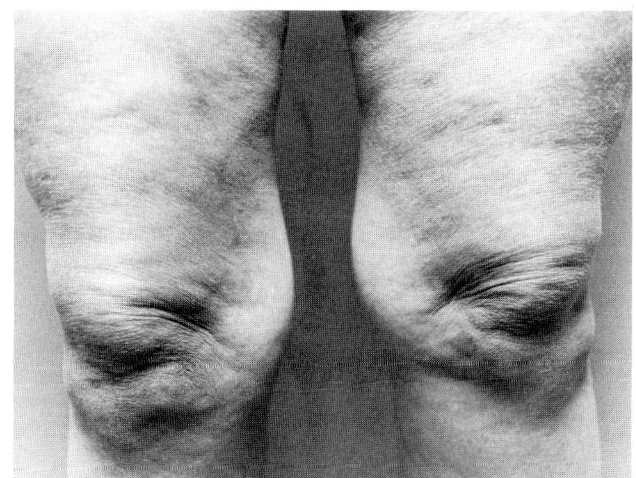

Fig. 32-6. Medial superior knee deposit known as "chubb."

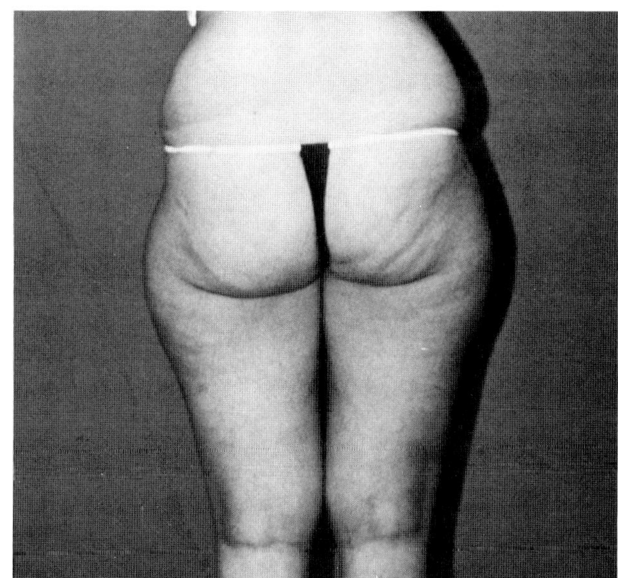

Fig. 32-8. Violin deformity in slender patient.

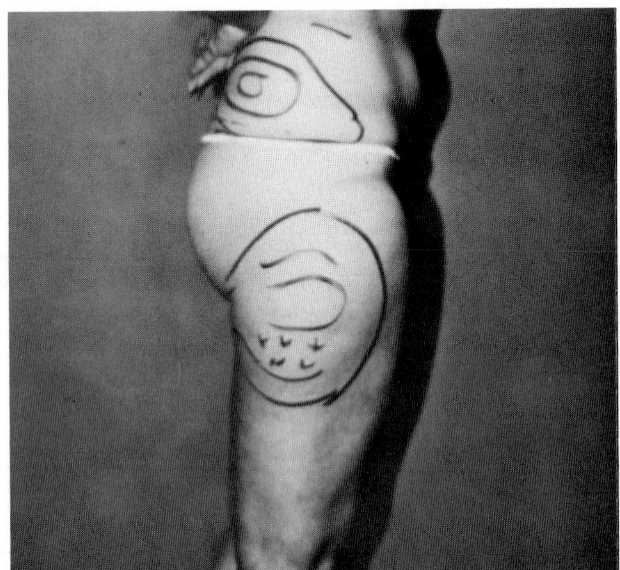

Fig. 32-9. Violin deformity marked for extraction.

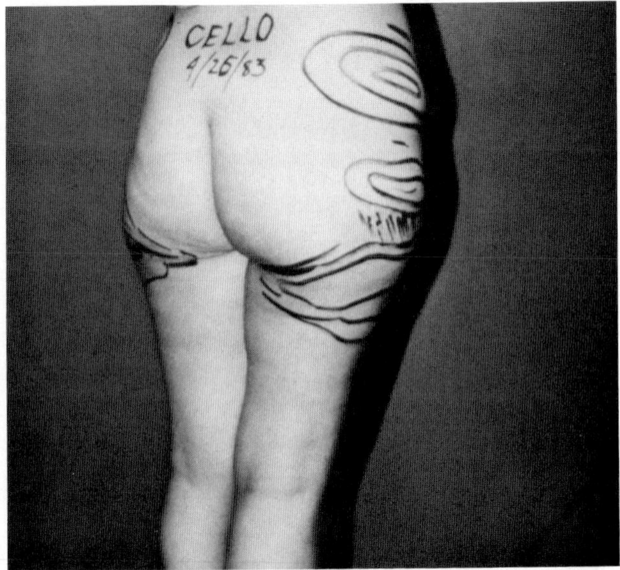

Fig. 32-11. The excess marked for extraction. In this case "cello" seemed more appropriate than "violin."

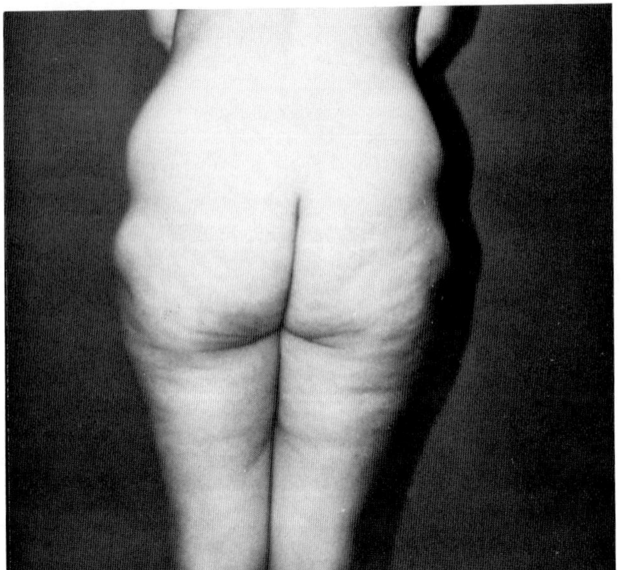

Fig. 32-10. Heavy patient showing violin deformity. Note obliteration of gluteal fold by fat.

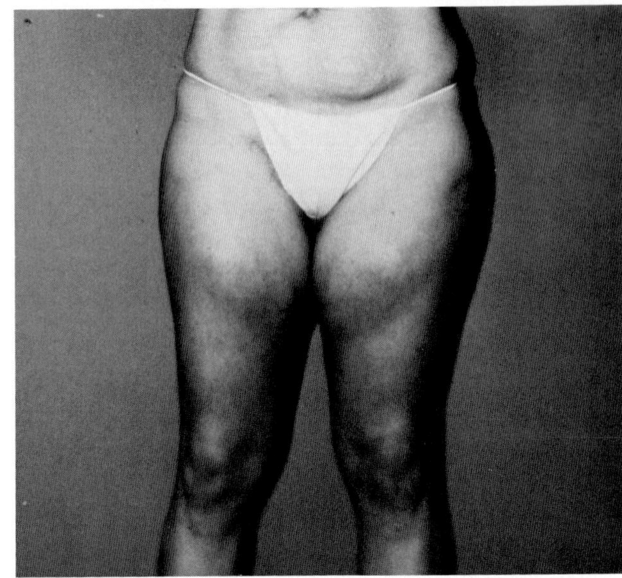

Fig. 32-12. Anterior thigh hypertrophy overlying quadriceps, resulting from insulin injections in an adult "juvenile diabetic."

Evaluation of Skin Contraction

The evaluation of the patient's personality, desires, expectations, and general stability of temperament is performed as described in Chapter 12. If a good psychological candidate, the patient is evaluated from the point of view of the "deformity." The deformity should be significant enough to be recognized by the surgeon and amenable to his or her skills in the procedure. The patient's skin and subcutaneous support should be evaluated by the pinch test, and careful inspection for dermal "lysis" as seen by cross-lighting should be carried out (Fig. 32-13).

"Cascading" skin indicates that skin contraction will not progress well (Fig. 32-14). Firm, taut skin free of stretch marks is a good indicator for the procedure (Fig. 32-15), regardless of the patient's age. Dimpling or a "cottage cheese" appearance (Fig. 32-16) due to fibrous tethers from the dermis to the muscle fascia beneath firm, hard fat is not a contraindication. This dimpling may or may not improve but generally does improve with substantial removals. The patient should not be led to expect *any* improvement in skin appearance and texture but only in contour.

The type of patient who is not a candidate is shown in Figure 32-17. The ideal candidate is shown in Figure 32-18. There is a continuum between these two types of patients. One surgeon's skill and confidence will extend further along that continuum than another's, based on aptitude and experience.

THE PINCH TEST

To evaluate the lateral femoral area, the surgeon should look at the patient from all sides in the nude without any undergarments but, most important, from the front and back. The proportion between upper and lower body, and the relationship of iliac crest fat to lateral femoral fat, should be evaluated. The prominence of the trochanter should be felt and marked; otherwise, a bony prominence may be mistakenly thought to be amenable to treatment. There is usually no more than 2 to 3 cm of fat overlying the trochanter. If this area is the widest part of the saddlebag, no improvement by lipolysis can be expected. The shape of the remainder of the leg, including the knee and calf, should be scrutinized. A patient with only lateral femoral deposits and otherwise slender proportions is the ideal candidate (Fig. 32-18). Such patients are less common than those who have an accompanying medial superior knee deposit (Fig. 32-19), which is the most common combination.

The markings should be done in a skyline view, rotating the patient to see the most prominent areas. A topographical map is drawn as seen in Figure 32-20. Areas of depression are noted with a (−) and avoided during the

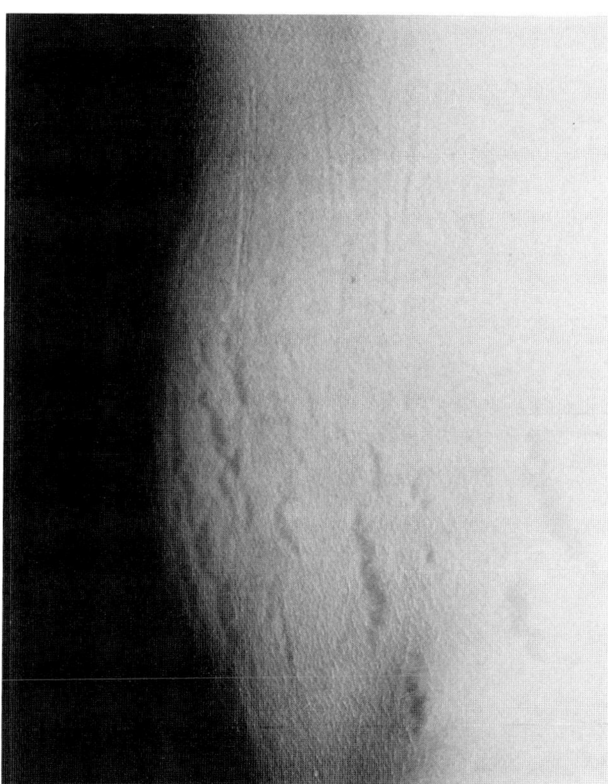

Fig. 32-13. So-called stretch marks or dermal breaks found in many patients.

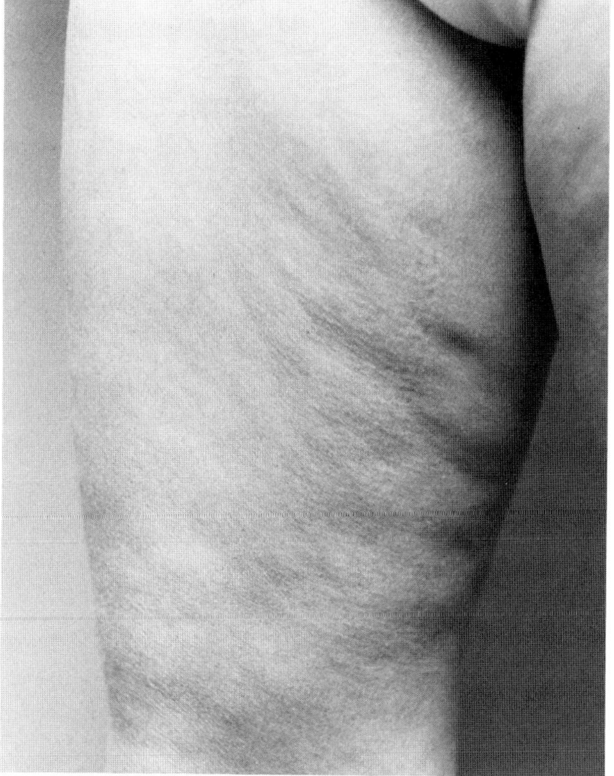

Fig. 32-14. "Cascading" skin seen often in the medial thigh area.

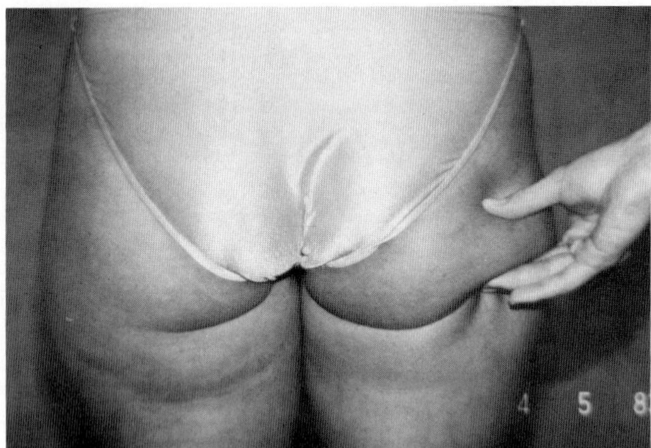

Fig. 32-15. Firm, taut skin (without stretch marks) with firm underlying tissues. Contrast with Fig. 32-16.

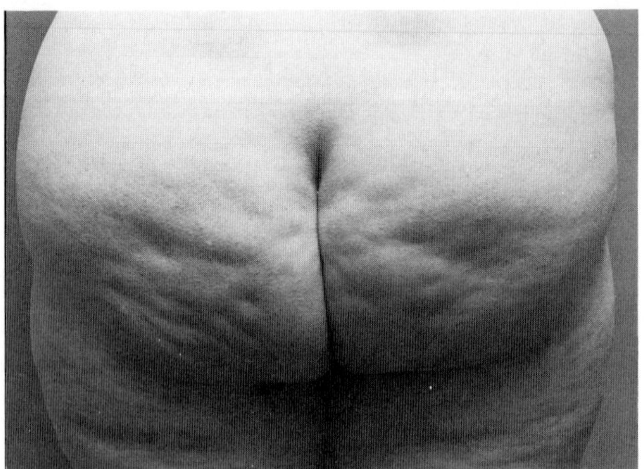

Fig. 32-16. "Cottage cheese" appearance.

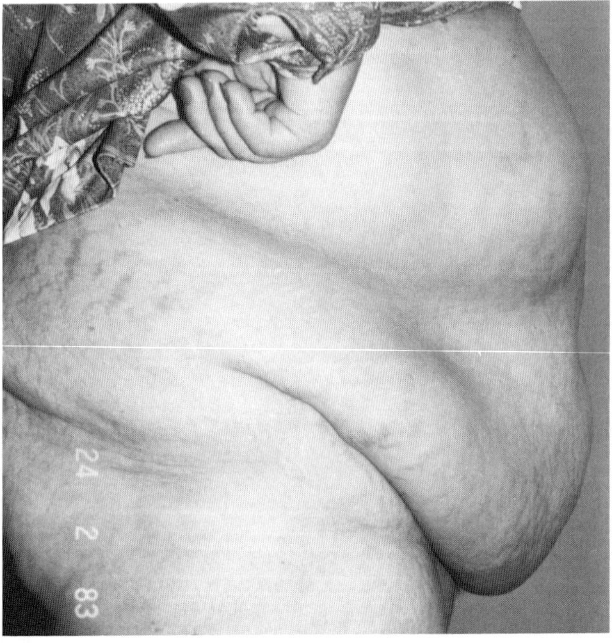

Fig. 32-17. Skin destroyed by gross obesity. This patient would not be a candidate for lipolysis.

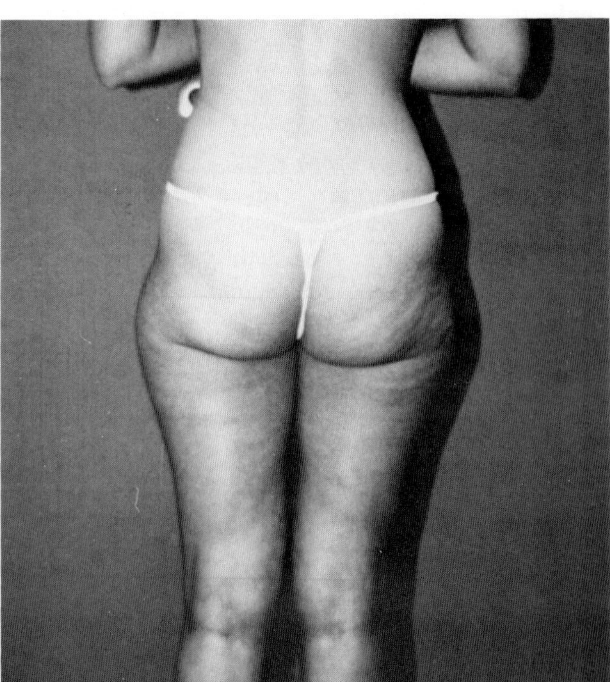

Fig. 32-18. A 27-year-old slender woman with diet-resistant lateral thigh deposits.

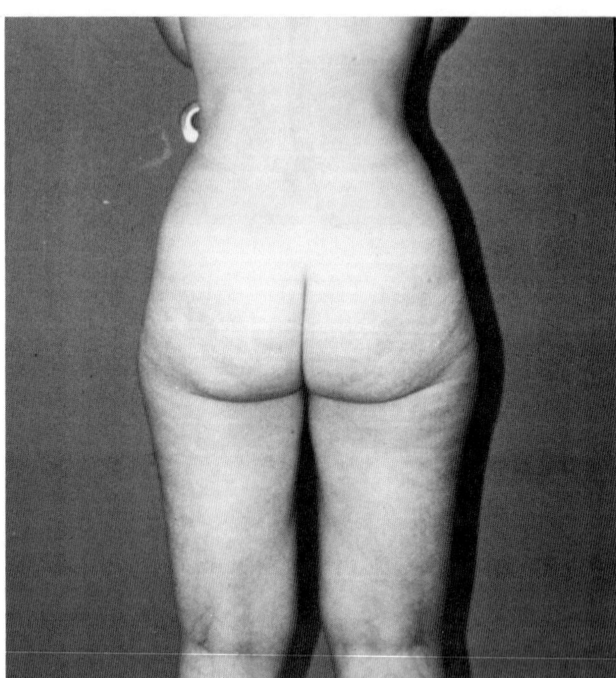

Fig. 32-19. Heavy knee deposits in slender woman with small lateral thigh deposits.

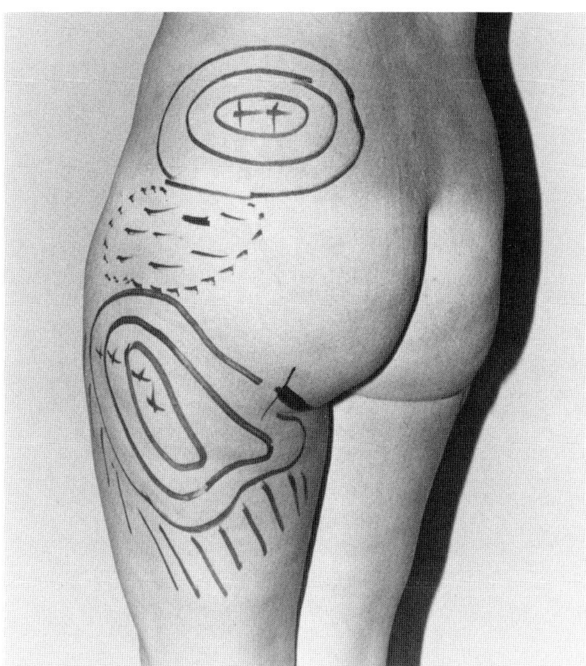

Fig. 32-20. "Surgical map." Areas of depression are noted with (−) signs, areas of greatest excess noted with (+) signs and decreasing circles. New gluteal fold is marked with dark line.

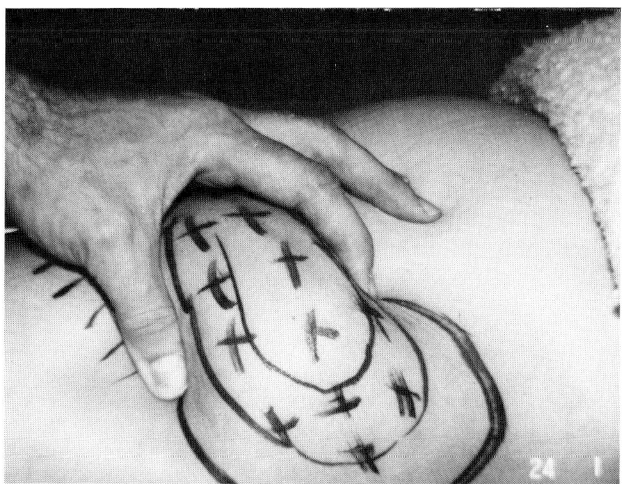

Fig. 32-21. A 10-cm section of lateral thigh fat pinched between thumb and forefinger.

procedure. The most prominent areas by visualization and pinch test are noted with (+) marks. The anticipated end of the gluteal fold is marked out. The surrounding normal areas are pinched and their thickness noted.

An average patient has 3 to 4 cm "pinchable" on the thighs, and the lateral area of concern measures 5 to 10 cm (Fig. 32-21). The goal is to extract enough fat to bring this area into conformity with the surrounding body fat. Obviously wide and prominent trochanteric

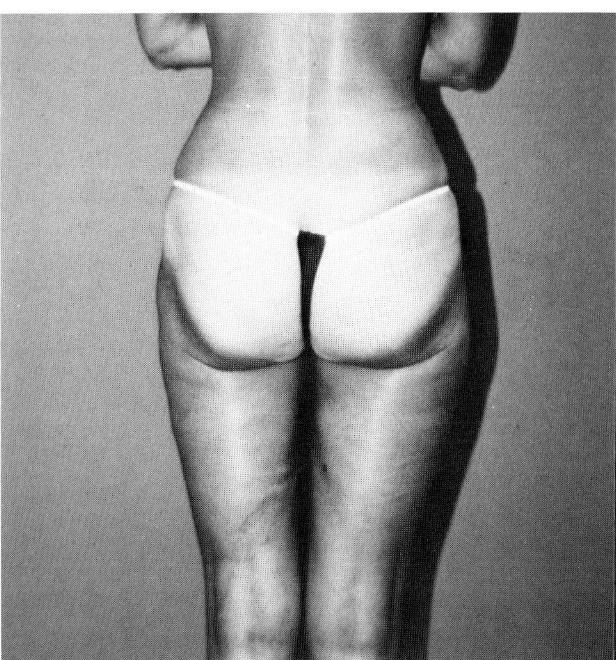

Fig. 32-22. A 45-year-old woman with open curves.

bone prevents the desired silhouette in some cases. It is an error to overextract fat beyond the thickness of neighboring areas. Dimpling, adhesions, and tender bony prominences may result. The atrophy of fat in later years added to the resection could produce an overly cachectic appearance, which should be kept in mind. Remember Fournier's rule: *It is not what you remove, but what you leave behind and where you leave it that is important.*

The desired shape of a beautiful contour is seen in Figure 32-22. It is a subtle series of open curves.

The Gluteal Depression

An absence of fat overlying the gluteal muscle often creates an untreatable depression that may accentuate the lateral femoral bulge (Fig. 32-23). Treatment of the bulge brings the silhouette into better proportion (Fig. 32-24). It is especially important not to pass cannulas through the area of the gluteal depression or this area will be worsened.

The Infragluteal Area and Crease

The infragluteal crease may be present or almost absent as seen in Figure 32-25. It may be square (Fig. 32-26) or appear "sad" by downsloping (Fig. 32-27). The crease may also be a double fold (see Fig. 32-1). A well-defined crease delineates the buttock and is part of a well-turned

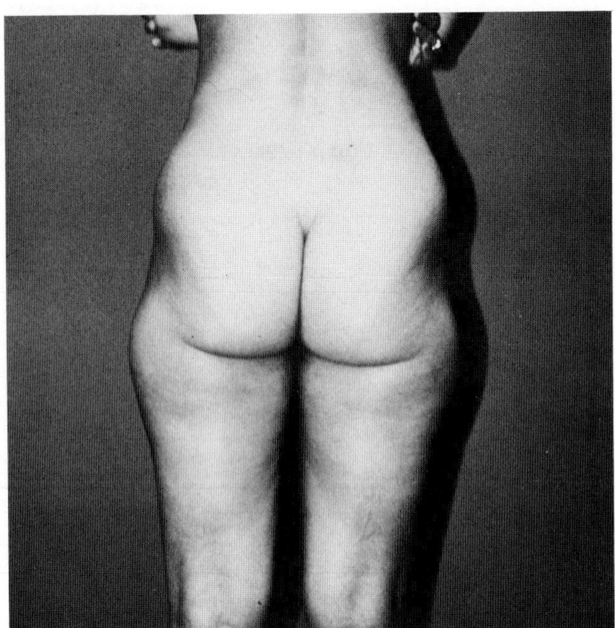

Fig. 32-23. Marked lateral thigh deposits in 27-year-old woman with marked gluteal depression. Exercise and diet have magnified this disproportion.

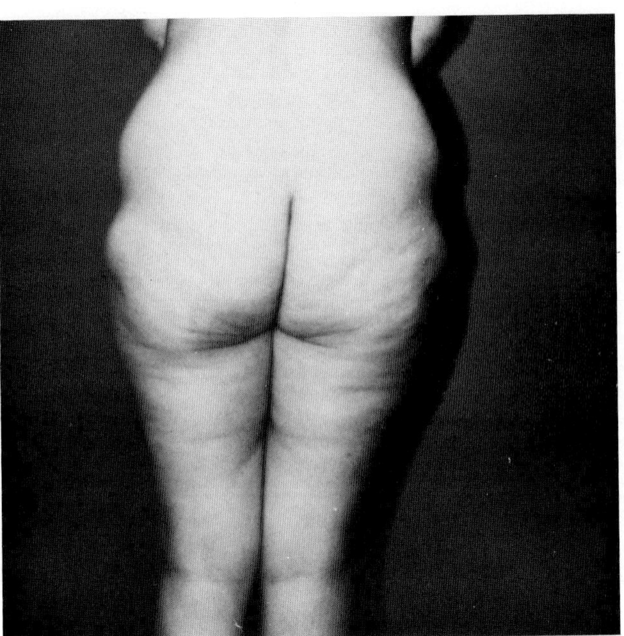

Fig. 32-25. Indistinct gluteal fold caused by fatty accumulations at junction of buttock and posterior thigh.

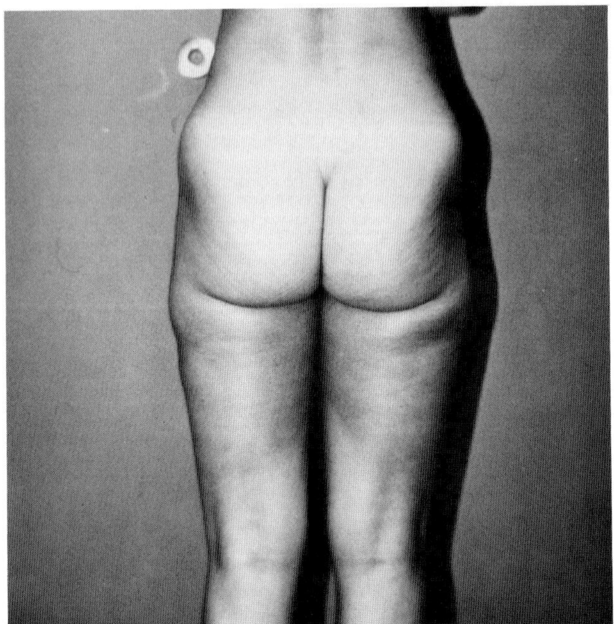

Fig. 32-24. Same patient as in Fig. 32-23 six months after removal of 475 ml total from lateral thighs using gluteal fold approach.

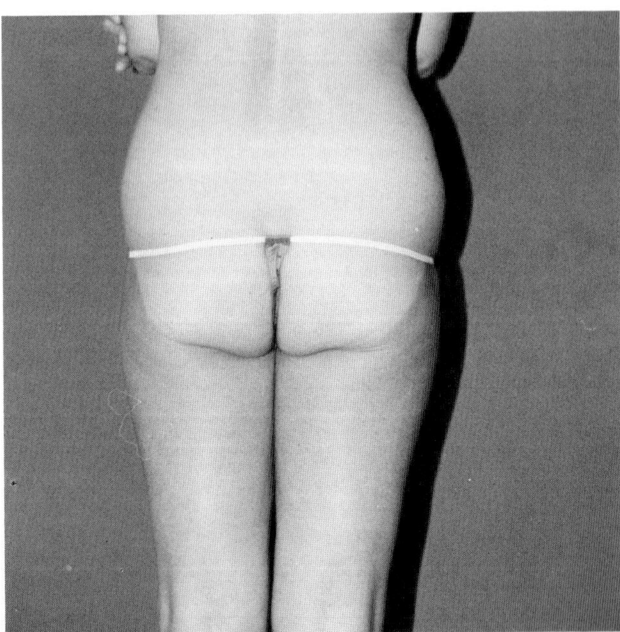

Fig. 32-26. "Square bottom" caused by straight gluteal fold and almost right angle at cleft medially.

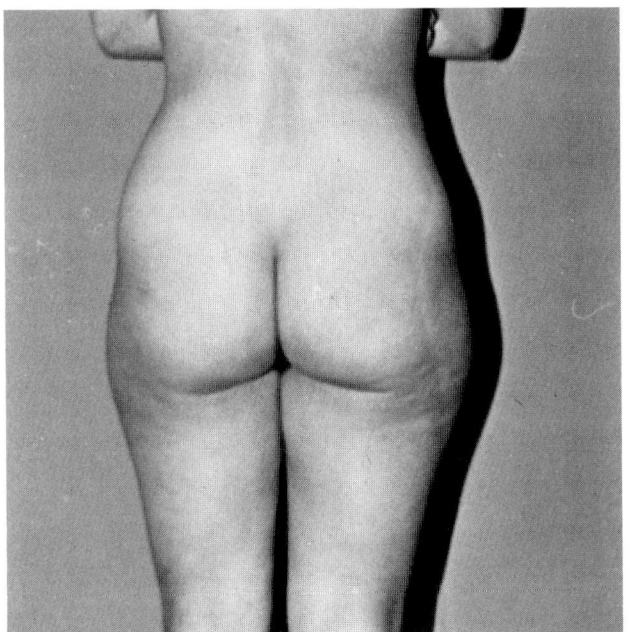

Fig. 32-27. "Sad buttock" caused by downturning gluteal folds.

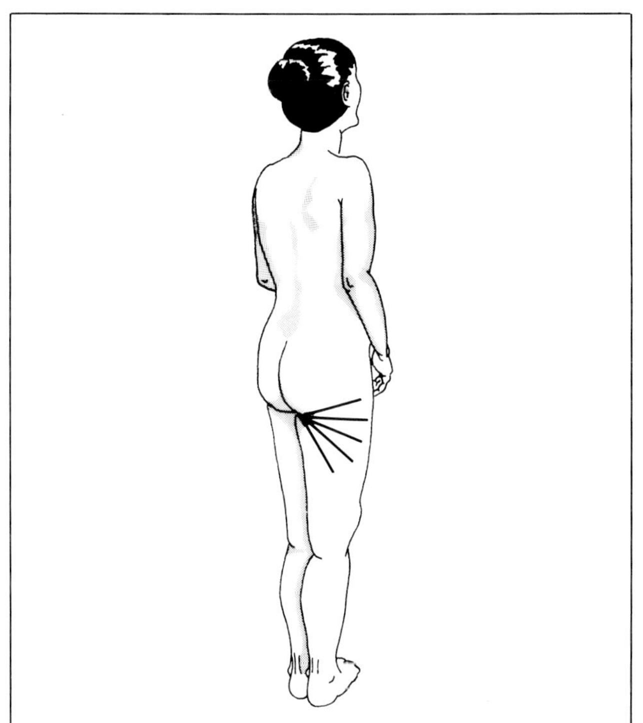

Fig. 32-28. The infragluteal area and most of the lateral thigh can be reached from an incision 3 cm lateral to the ischial tuberosity.

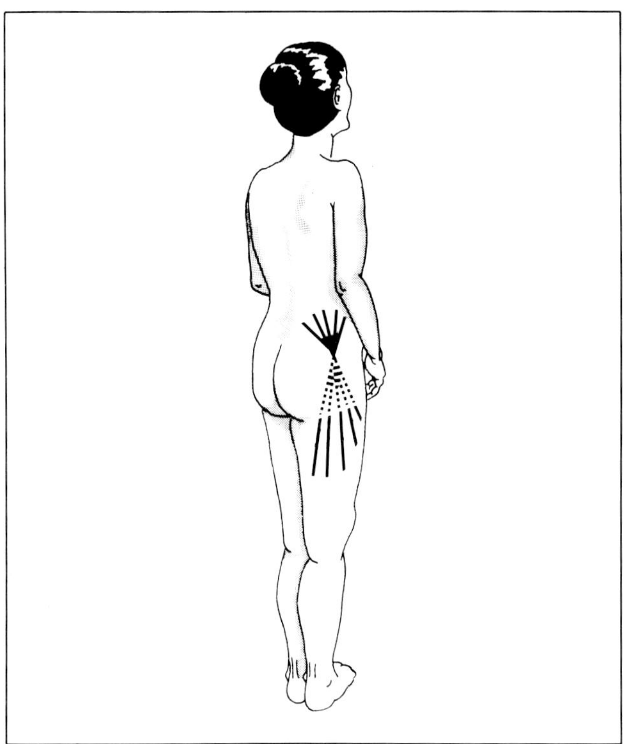

Fig. 32-29. High lateral thigh and more anterior lateral thigh are reached from a gluteal depression incision placed within the bikini shadow. The dotted lines indicate no suctioning in those areas. The iliac crest roll is easily reached with this useful incision, which should not be confused with the highly visible "supratrochanteric" incision.

"derrière." The unaesthetic variants shown in these figures can all be improved by judicious work on the fold by the Illouz technique (see Chap. 17).

The infragluteal area should be carefully marked for excess or noted for paucity of tissue. In the former case, as with a double fold, a medially placed incision in the fold allows parallel strokes beneath the fold with a #6 or #8 cannula (Fig. 32-28). A paucity of tissue and a normal gluteal fold indicate that no incision should be placed in the fold; an incision up in the bikini area of the buttock is a better choice (Fig. 32-29). The iliac crest area can also be reached easily with this incision.

Medial Thigh

If the crural area of the thighs requires some defatting (Fig. 32-30), this should be clearly marked. This area bleeds more, the fat is softer, the skin is finer, and results are less predictable than laterally. Many women are con-

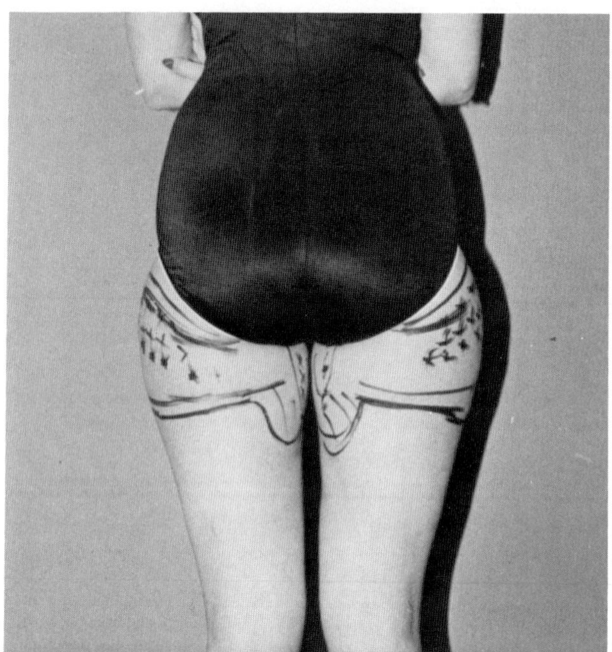

Fig. 32-30. Modest excess of crural area marked for extraction in 39-year-old female with heavy thighs.

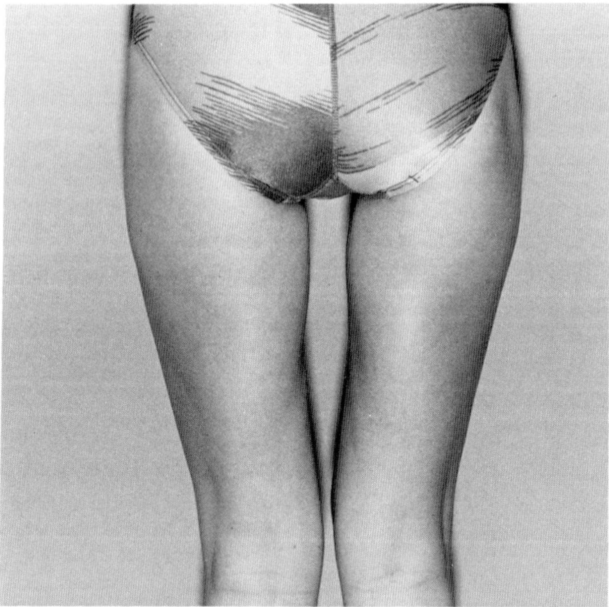

Fig. 32-31. "Slot-like" appearance from lack of normal crural bulge.

cerned with this area because the crural areas touch, and this area is obvious when they wear jeans or other pants. The removal of this fat leaves the thighs apart with a "slot-like" appearance (Fig. 32-31), which is neither normal nor desirable. The surgeon may be pressured to be aggressive in this area and should be very careful.

The crural area is unforgiving. When entering it, use a #6, or at most a #8, cannula and take less fat than you think you should. You can always remove more but can never replace what you have removed.

Planning the Approach

After marking out the areas to be extracted, measure the pinch thickness and record it and the surrounding thickness. The areas to be defatted determine the site of entry.

If medial thigh, infragluteal area, or a gluteal crease is to be altered, a gluteal crease incision is appropriate. From there, all areas including the lateral thigh can be reached. Before placing the incision, place the cannula on the patient to be sure the full extent of the marked deformity can be reached (Fig. 32-32). Some large patients require the infragluteal incision to be made more lateral so the cannula can reach to the edge of the markings for the fatty deposit.

If the lateral thigh deposit is truly lateral with no infragluteal extension and the crease is proper, a gluteal depression incision is better so as not to disturb the fold or extract infragluteal fat (Fig. 32-33). An iliac crest roll and a lateral thigh deposit can both be reached from this same incision. If work is needed on the crease or the medial thigh, this can be added with a separate incision and the "criss-cross technique" used on the lateral thigh (Fig. 32-34).

See Chapter 17 for a description of the actual technique.

The Knee

A common fatty deposit complained of by women is a bulge just at and above the medial condyle (Fig. 32-35). This fatty deposit is very commonly associated with a lateral thigh deposit; however, it may be an isolated finding and carries the colloquial term *chubb.*

The anterior suprapatellar area may ptose over the patella to form another disliked fatty mass. The surrounding integument may be pinched and found to be 2 to 3 cm thick, while the medial knee deposit is 4 to 6 cm. This area is marked carefully including areas to be feathered. The incision is placed superomedially in the

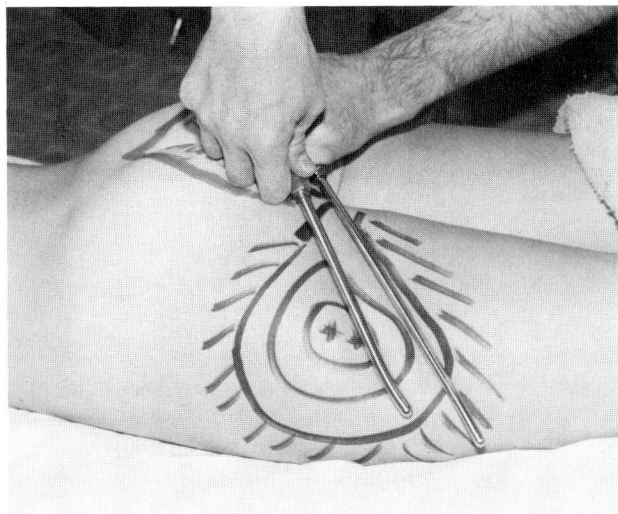

Fig. 32-32. Cannula is placed on area to be defatted to ensure adequate reach from gluteal crease.

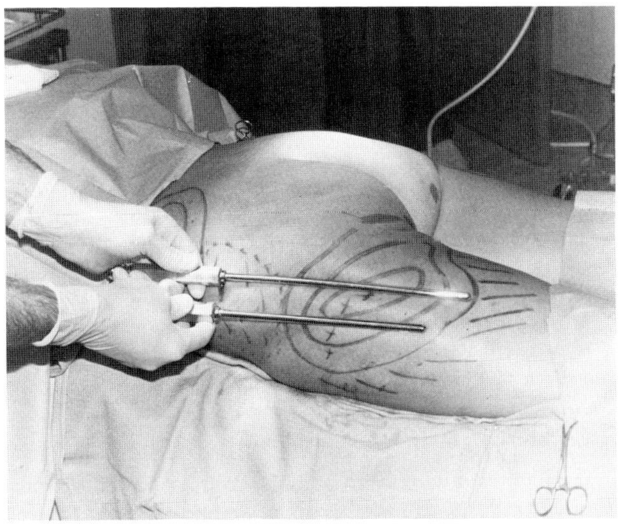

Fig. 32-33. Large cannulas are necessary to reach the edge of the fatty accumulation from a high buttock incision.

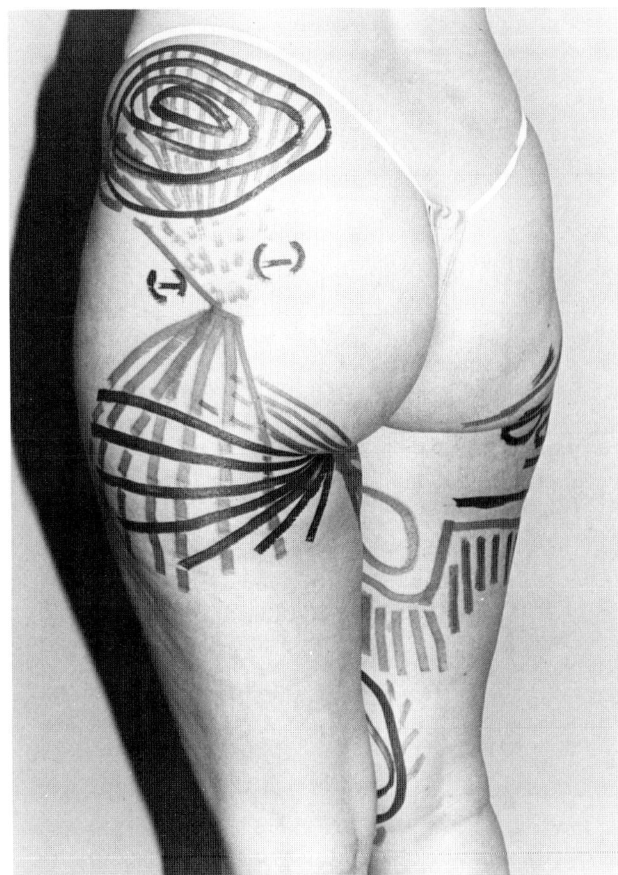

Fig. 32-34. "Criss-cross" technique illustrated on lateral thigh. The iliac crest is reached from the lateral buttock incision.

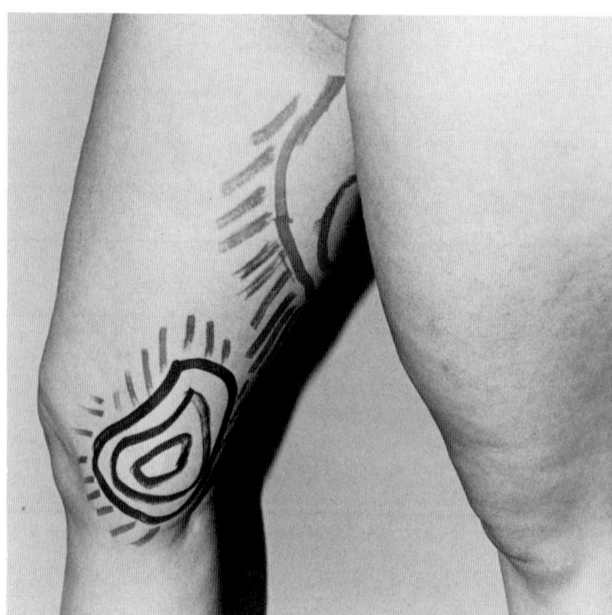

Fig. 32-35. Medial knee deposit and crural area are marked out with contour map for extraction.

popliteal fossa overlying the palpable tendon of the hamstring. The saphenous is far medial to this point. When injecting, however, care should be taken to aspirate the syringe before injecting to prevent a bolus of solution from being injected intravenously.

It is not unusual to enter the greater saphenous vein when injecting the medial knee area. The knee fat comes out easily with a #6 cannula with little force. Be careful not to overtreat below the condyle. Feather the edges and do not "windshield wiper" with the instrument. Keep in tunnels.

The treatment of the knees gives the legs a generally improved shapeliness and is performed in more than half of all patients undergoing thigh lipolysis.

Results of Treatment

A spectrum of patients present for treatment. Most important is to say no to those whom you feel you cannot improve physically or make happy psychologically. *Remember, you make your income from those on whom you operate, and you build your reputation on those on whom you do not operate.*

The following five cases illustrate important points relating to the treatment of these patients and show typical results in my practice of lipolysis.

Case Studies

Case 1: Small, highly localized lateral femoral deposit. Figure 32-36A shows a 37-year-old woman, 115 pounds and 5′4″ tall, who exercised daily and dieted only occasionally. Her highest weight was 118 pounds and lowest was 102 pounds. She considered her ideal weight 110 pounds. Her complaint was excessive, highly localized lateral thigh accumulation ("saddlebags").

Approximately 150 ml of fatty tissue was removed from each lateral thigh with #6 and #8 cannulas under general anesthesia with 1:435,000 epinephrine subcutaneous preparation. Preoperative hematocrit was 40.0% and second postoperative day hematocrit was 39.3%. Postoperative serum iron was low at 31 μg.

Figure 32-36B shows the patient 3 months postoperatively. The patient was pleased but desired more removal because of the gluteal depression, which makes the area beneath appear in excess. No further removal was necessary or appropriate.

Case 2: Large, highly localized lateral femoral deposit with medial knee deposits. Figure 32-37A shows a 33-year-old woman, 120 pounds and 5′5″ tall. Her highest weight was 140 pounds and lowest was 104. The patient dieted constantly. Her concern was the lateral thigh and medial knees.

Approximately 500 ml of almost pure fat was extracted after subcutaneous preparation of the tissue with epinephrine 1:435,000. At the same time a bilateral transaxillary subpectoral augmentation was performed. Preoperative hematocrit was 37.4% and second postoperative day hematocrit was 34.3%. Serum iron was low at 31 μg.

Figure 32-37B shows the patient 6 months postoperatively in a frontal view. The patient had a touchup with removal of 40 ml from small remaining bulges 5 months postoperatively under local anesthesia.

Case 3: Heavier lateral fat accumulation with addition of iliac crest and knees. Figure 32-38A shows the preoperative condition of a 33-year-old woman, 130 pounds and 5′5″ tall, of Mediterranean extraction. Her highest weight was 130 pounds, her lowest 115. Her complaint was inability to lose these accumulations despite 15 years of constant dieting.

About 1000 ml was removed from all three sites. No epinephrine was used in the subcutaneous tissues. The preoperative hematocrit was 40.7% and hematocrit on the second postoperative day was 32.7%. Serum iron was low at 33 μg.

The patient required a "touchup" procedure at 6 months for slight irregularity on each side, at which time 30 ml was removed bilaterally under local anesthesia.

Figure 32-38B shows the result 3 months postoperatively. The patient has better harmony of proportion yet weighs 5 pounds more than preoperatively because she does not diet constantly. Note the incisions near the sacral dimples to access the iliac crest. I use a buttock incision for this now.

Case 4: Very heavy lateral thighs associated with iliac crest, buttock, and knee accumulations. Figure 32-39A shows the preoperative state of a 36-year-old woman who had lovely facial features. The patient weighed 134 pounds. Her highest weight was 148 pounds, her lowest 125, and she was 5′3″ tall. Her complaint was disproportion of her lower body to her thin extremities.

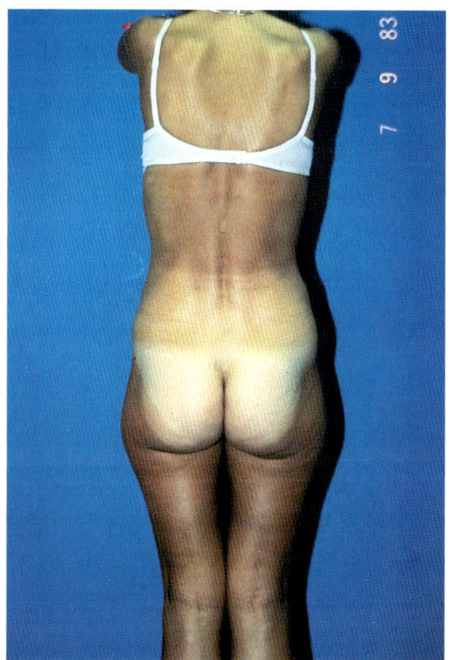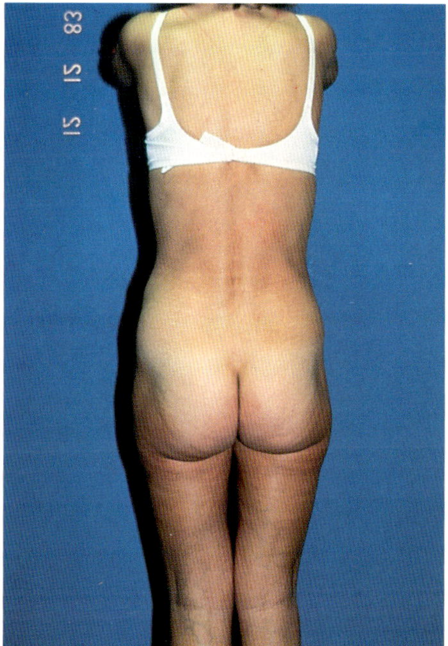

A

B

Fig. 32-36.
A. Preoperative view of 37-year-old, 115-pound woman with "saddlebag" complaint.
B. Postoperative view at 3 months after removal of 150 ml per side.

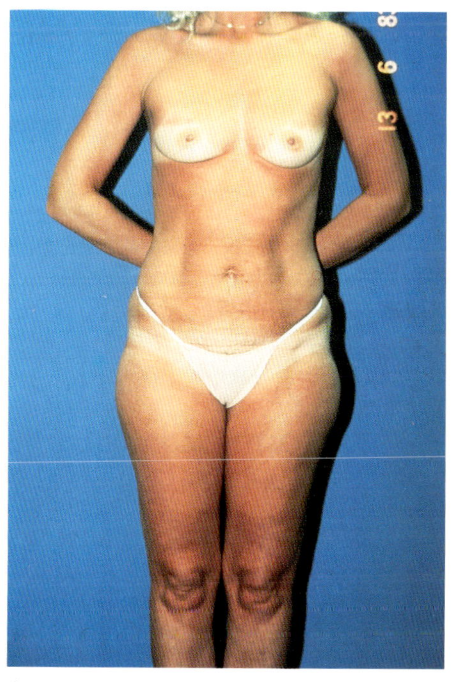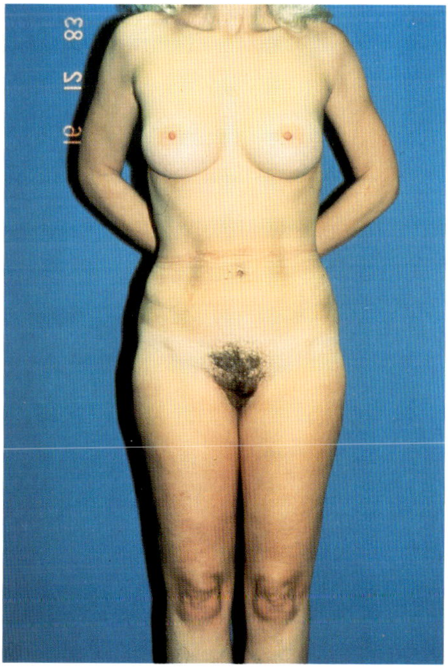

A

B

Fig. 32-37.
A. Preoperative view of a 33-year-old, 120-pound woman with complaint of "saddlebags" and medial knee area.
B. Postoperative view at 6 months after removal of 250 ml per side.

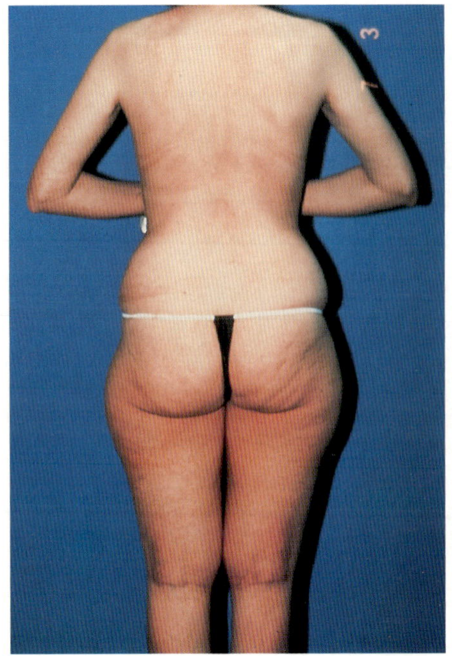 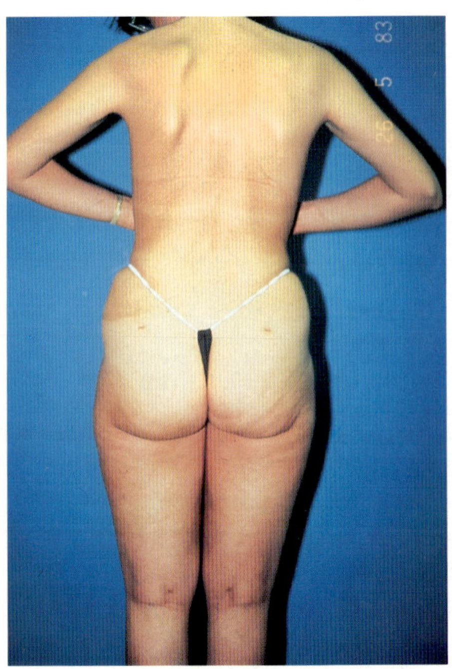

A   B

Fig. 32-38.
A. Preoperative view of 33-year-old, 130-pound woman with complaint of hips, thighs, and knees.
B. Postoperative view at 3 months after removal of 500 ml per side.

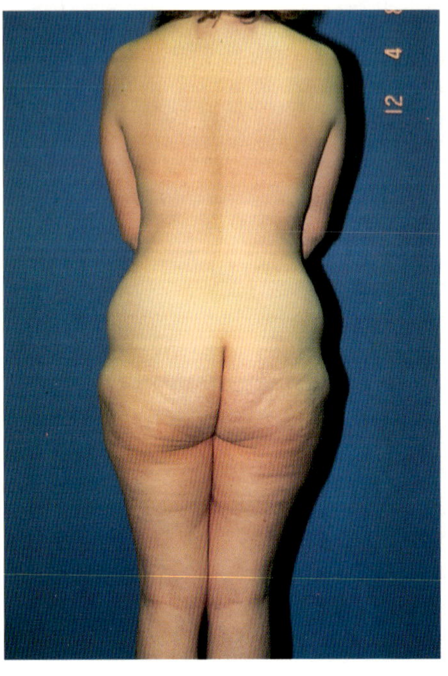 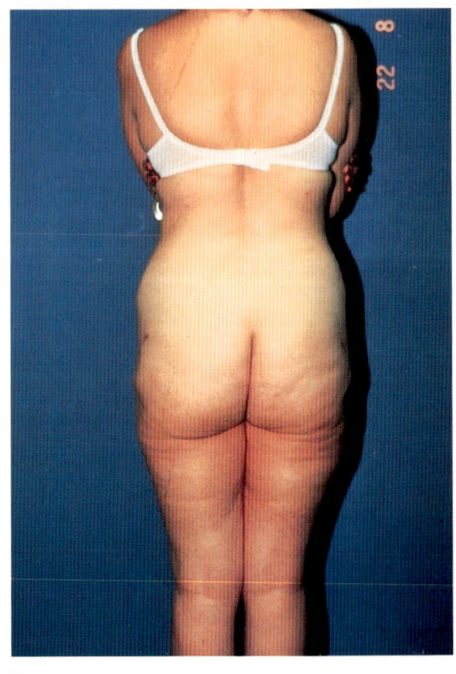

A   B

Fig. 32-39.
A. Preoperative view of 36-year-old, 134-pound woman with complaint of upper-lower body disproportion.
B. Postoperative view at 4½ months after removal of 475 ml per side.

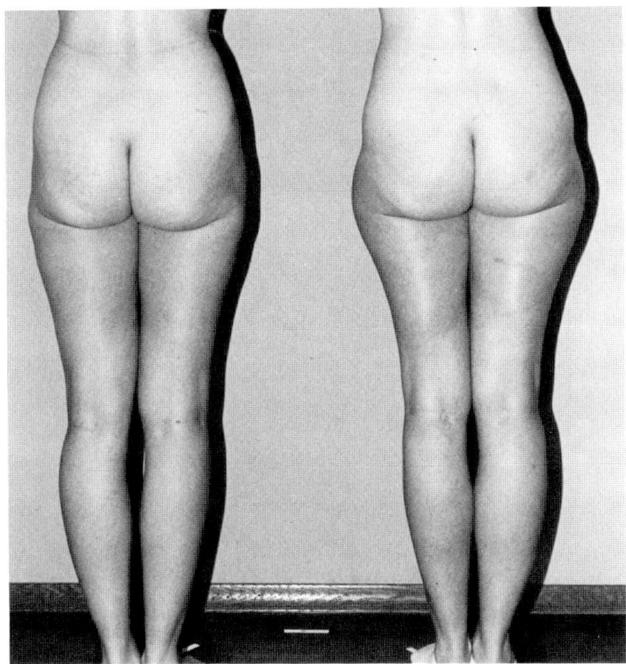

Fig. 32-40. Monozygotic twins; operated patient on left, unoperated twin on right. Operation removed 500 ml total from lateral thighs.

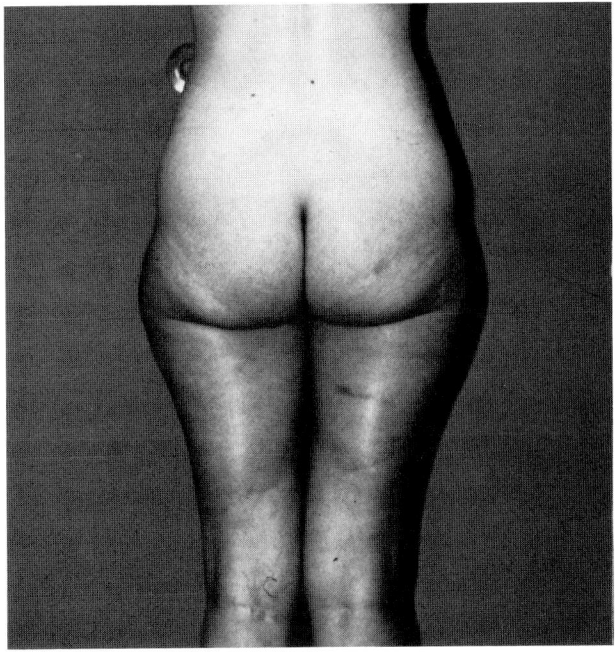

Fig. 32-42. The 29-year-old monozygotic twin to woman in Figure 32-41, preoperative state in early 1984.

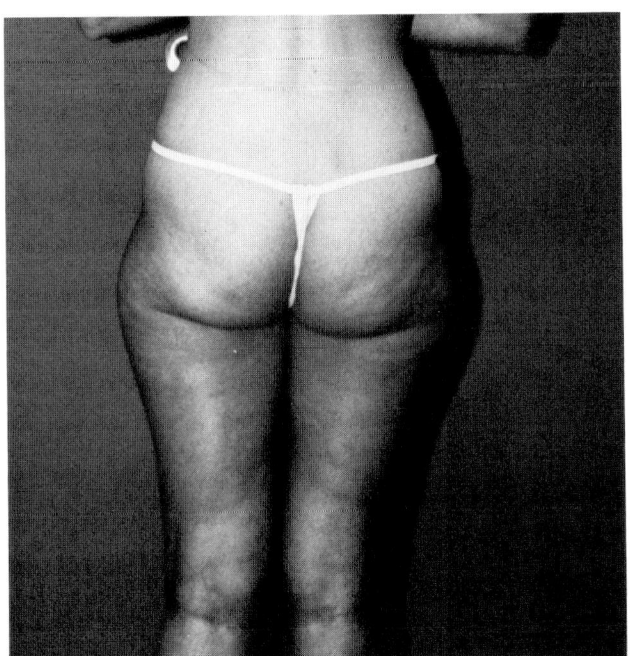

Fig. 32-41. The 28-year-old operated twin at time of preoperative visit in early 1983.

After epinephrine preparation of the subcutaneous tissue, the criss-cross technique was used and 950 ml of almost pure fat was extracted. Preoperative hematocrit was 45% and second day postoperative was 41%, with a modestly low serum iron of 48 μg. Compare these figures with Case 3.

Figure 32-39B shows the results 4½ months postoperatively. There is a better gluteal fold and a more harmonious relationship between the parts. The patient is pleased with her appearance despite remaining heavier than her "ideal" weight.

Case 5: Lateral femoral area diet-resistant fat in monozygotic twins. Figure 32-40 shows a 29-year-old patient 12 months after saddlebag lipolysis, photographed next to her monozygotic twin. In the same photograph the patient's original deformity can be seen in her identical twin. Notice the patient's well-proportioned torso, slender extremities, and lack of excess weight.

This natural laboratory illustrates the hereditary nature of these fatty deposits and their obvious diet resistance. Notice the slight groove on both patients' left midbuttock. This photograph was taken at the time of the unoperated twin's preoperative visit. For a comparison of both twins' preoperative photographs, see Figures 32-41 and 32-42.

Reference

1. Grazer, F. M., and Klingbcil, J. R. *Body Image.* St. Louis: Mosby, 1980.

CHAPTER 33

Lipolysis of the Ankle and Calf

Adrien E. Aiache

Before the introduction of the use of blunt suction lipectomy treatment, fatty ankles were first treated by a procedure described by Schrudde [1]. This procedure consisted of making an incision in the posterior area of the ankle and of using a curette to remove the fat in the area just below the gastrocnemius. The results were interesting; however, the complications were too numerous and the procedure did not gain wide acceptance. The complications consisted mainly of bleeding, infection, and some sloughs.

The advent of blunt suction lipectomy has changed the picture in these cases and, although the results are not always completely spectacular, they have brought improvement to an area that could not be solved in the past.

The usual patient has fatty, heavy lower legs (Fig. 33-1A), especially below the gastrocnemius muscle (Fig. 33-1B shows a normal appearance). The appearance of the leg is deleterious to the aesthetic comportment of these patients. Although in the past these patients have sought improvement surgically, only now can it be offered safely. The problem consists of a fatty deposit interspersed with some fibrous tissue in the whole lower calf area laterally, and especially posteriorly in the lower leg. It is found in certain ethnic groups more often; however, this problem can be found in any ethnic group without distinction.

Technique

MARKING

The patient stands on an elevated stool. The markings are made in that position to assess the exact amount of fat that should be removed. The area most commonly performed in the posterior area of the lower leg is from the lower edge of the gastrocnemius bulge down to the ankle around the Achilles tendon. This area is carefully marked by the pinch test and visual inspection.

The incision is usually made on the lateral side of the Achilles tendon. More anteriorly, some fat deposits may be encountered, although less commonly than posteromedially and posterolaterally. These anterior deposits are usually approached with the same incision although, in exceptional cases, an anterior horizontal foot incision is made to approach the real anterior fat removal. Once the patient has been marked properly in the standing position on tiptoes, the areas to be defatted are marked (Fig. 33-2). The patient then can be taken to surgery.

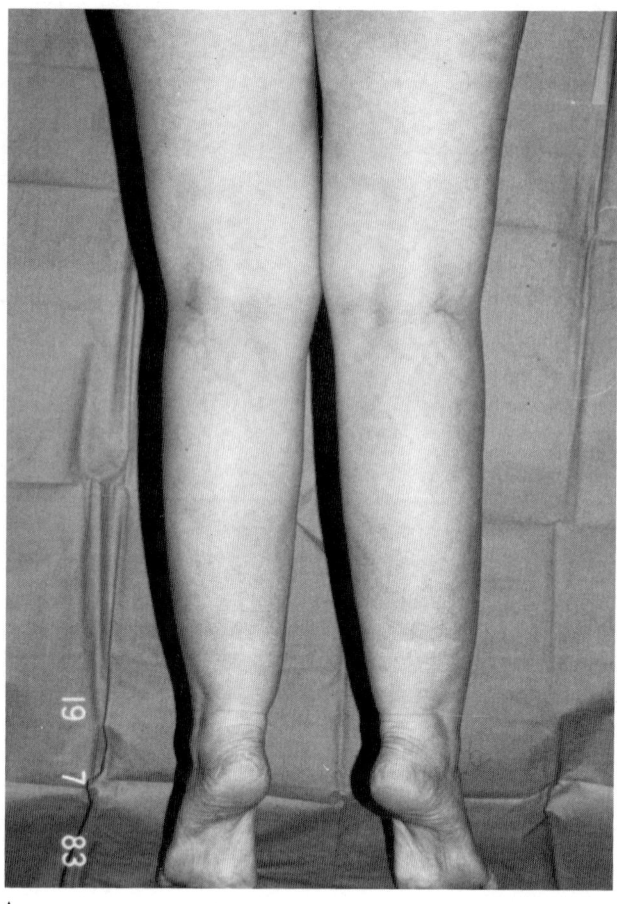

A

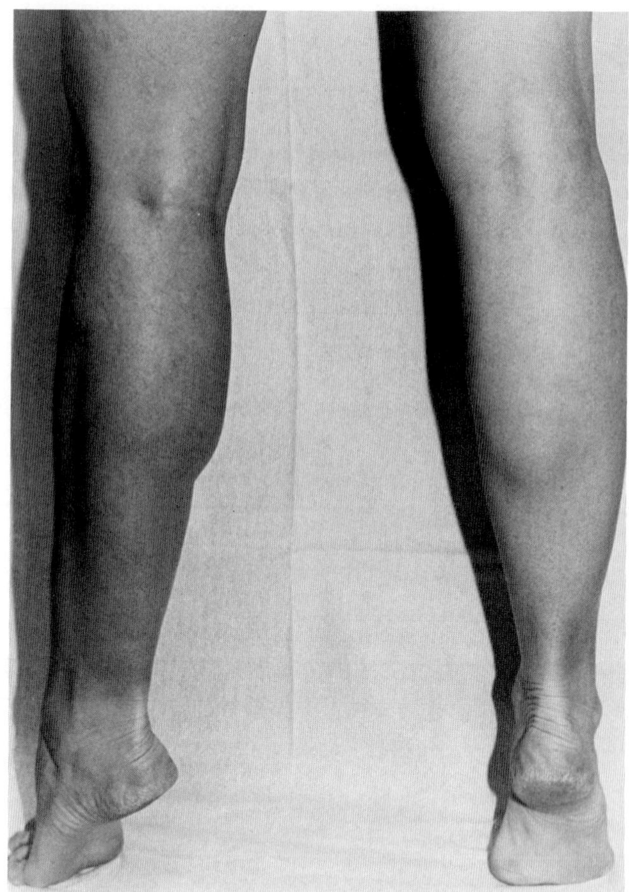

B

Fig. 33-1.
A. A very heavy lower leg with fat obliterating the gastroc outline and ending as a pursestring just above the malleoli.
B. A normal leg with good gastroc relief. (Photographs courtesy of G. Hetter, M.D.)

ANESTHESIA

Anesthesia may be local or general, depending on the extent of the extraction procedure. Local anesthesia is used where the extent of the fat removal is not extensive and where the procedure is performed as a sole procedure. In combined cases, general anesthesia is preferable and usually the prone position is used for adequate removal of all other areas of the leg (Fig. 33-3).

In addition to general anesthesia, infiltration of the area of the lower leg is performed using a solution of Xylocaine 0.25% with epinephrine 1:400,000 (see Chap. 15). In most cases this infiltration is very helpful in reducing the amount of bleeding that occurs with this procedure. In local anesthesia cases, the same anesthetic is used; however, a ring-type of anesthesia is additionally laid down in the upper part of the area to be treated to allow greater anesthesia of the calf below that point.

PROCEDURE

The procedure is performed most often in the prone position, except when the patient needs anterior re-

moval in association with another procedure done anteriorly. The prone position is usually sufficient for the whole area of the ankles and lower calf, including the anterior part.

The incision is made lateral or medial (or both) to the Achilles tendon, and the 4- or 6-mm cannula is introduced (Fig. 33-4). By the usual stroking technique movement, the whole area that needs to be defatted is worked on with the suction (see Chap. 16). The proper progression of the suction technique is checked by palpation and by visual observation, using the pinch and roll test to assess the exact amount of fat that remains (Fig. 33-5). Although the incision in the outer aspect of the Achilles tendon is usually sufficient, in cases where a particular removal is done in the anterior part of the leg, an anterior incision may be made in the lower part of the leg at the junction with the foot. This incision allows defatting of the whole anterior area of the lower leg.

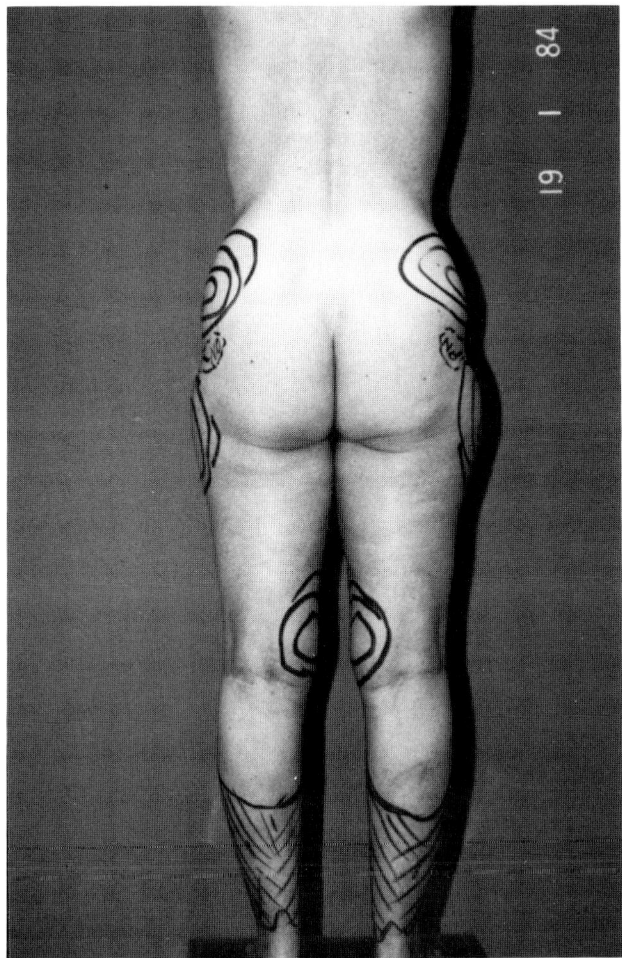

Fig. 33-2. The area to be defatted is marked with the patient standing on her toes to put the gastroc edge in relief. (Courtesy of G. Hetter, M.D.)

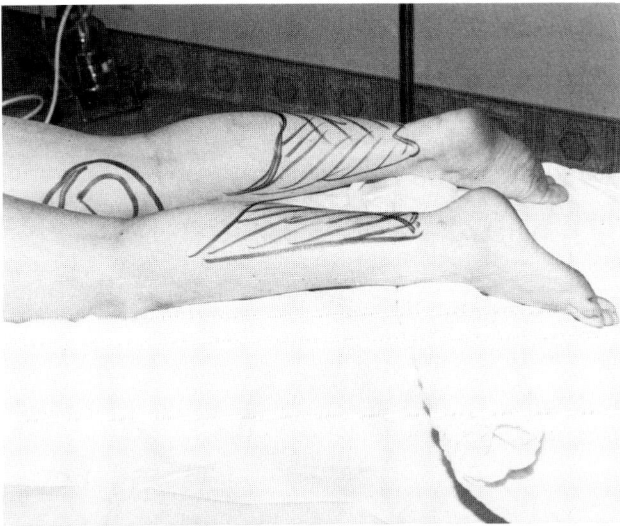

Fig. 33-3. The patient is in the prone position ready for surgery of thighs, knees, and lower calves. (Courtesy of G. Hetter, M.D.)

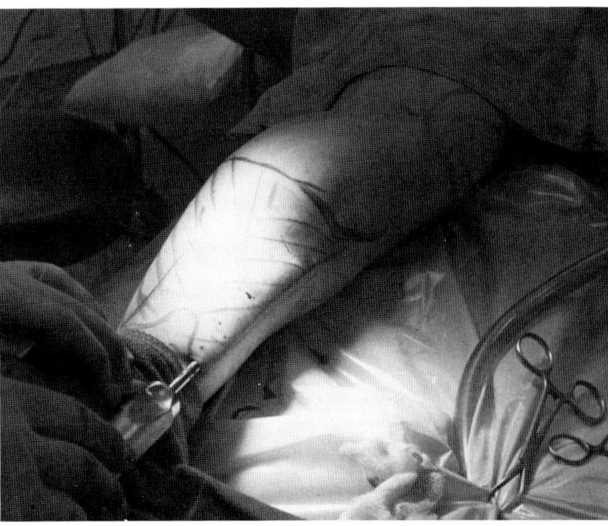

Fig. 33-4. A long #6 Padgett cannula is introduced just medial to the Achilles tendon, defatting the medial posterior calf. (Courtesy of G. Hetter, M.D.)

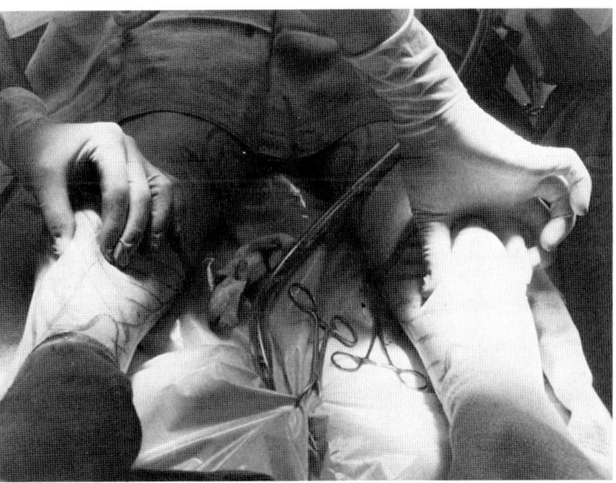

Fig. 33-5. Left calf is defatted, right side is not, illustrating pinch test. (Courtesy of G. Hetter, M.D.)

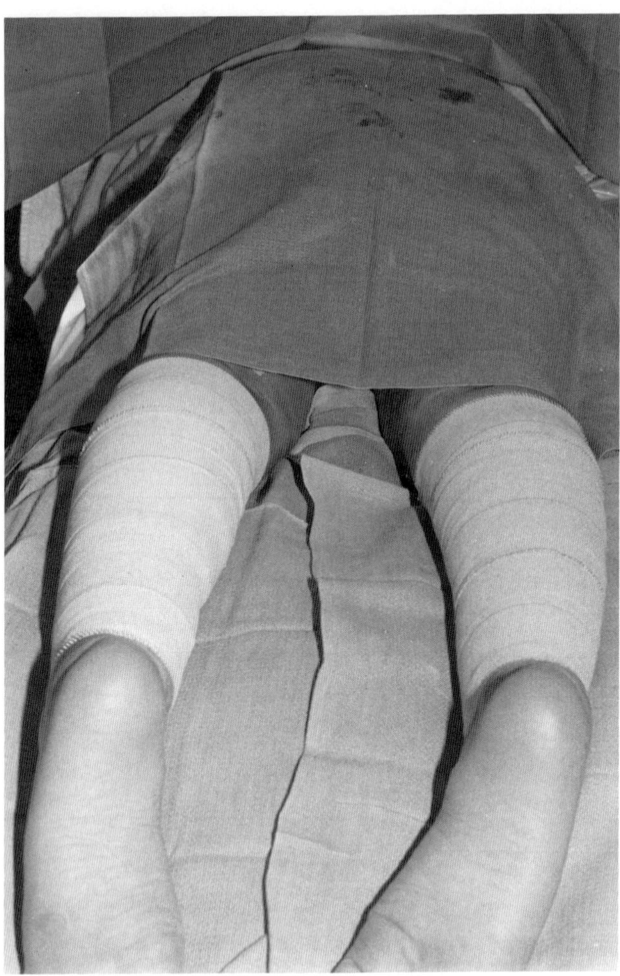

Fig. 33-6. Elastic tape dressing is applied to posterior two-thirds of calf for first week. (Courtesy of G. Hetter, M.D.)

OPERATIVE STEPS

Once defatting is complete and the results checked, the patient is then cleansed and the incision closed using either 5–0 nylon or nonabsorbable suture, reinforced by Steri-Strip. Next, oblique, criss-crossing elastic tape is applied to the leg to afford some compression (Fig. 33-6). Later a support-hose dressing or thromboembolic stocking is applied. The patient is then transferred to recovery and subsequently either discharged home or to a hospital ward, depending on circumstances.

REFINEMENTS IN TECHNIQUE

In cases where large removals are performed in the anterior and posterior area of the lower leg, the refinements are important. They consist of feathering of the junction of the defatted area and the undefatted areas. Feathering consists of defatting in a less aggressive way anteriorly and at the upper junction to avoid a step deformity. Once feathering is completed and the result seems satisfactory to the observer, the area is closed as described.

Postoperative Care

Patients are usually treated with prophylactic antibiotics and pain medication and asked to stay off their feet for a few days, after which they are allowed to ambulate gradually. There is usually a large amount of swelling, pain, and tenderness in the ankle area since the fluid and blood secondary to the surgery cannot be resorbed as easily as in other areas. Massages and exercises are encouraged 10 days after the surgery. Drainage by elevation of the leg is encouraged several times each day. Whirlpool therapy is helpful in improving the general well-being of these patients.

Complications and Sequelae

Noted complications consist of infection and hematoma. Sequelae consist of persistent pain, irregularities, and persisting discoloration in areas where ecchymosis was longstanding. This discoloration is probably a result of the fact that there is no other escape for the blood pigments at this low point in the body. Results are shown in Figures 33-7 and 33-8.

Summary

Blunt suction lipectomy is extremely useful in cases of fatty accumulations of the lower legs in patients who, before this technique, were unable to be improved. It has brought great improvement to these patients and, although the results are not always dramatic, they have been gratifying for the surgeon and patient alike.

Reference

1. Schrudde, J. Lipectomy and lipexeresis in the area of the lower extremities. *Langenbecks Arch. Chir.* 345:127, 1977.

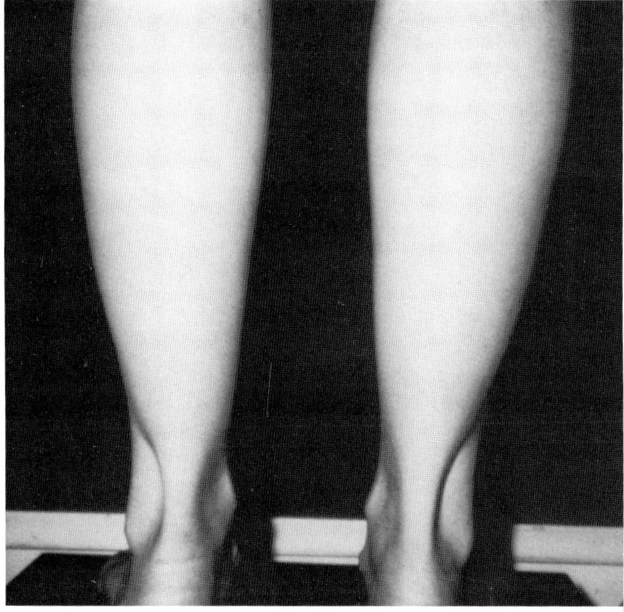

A

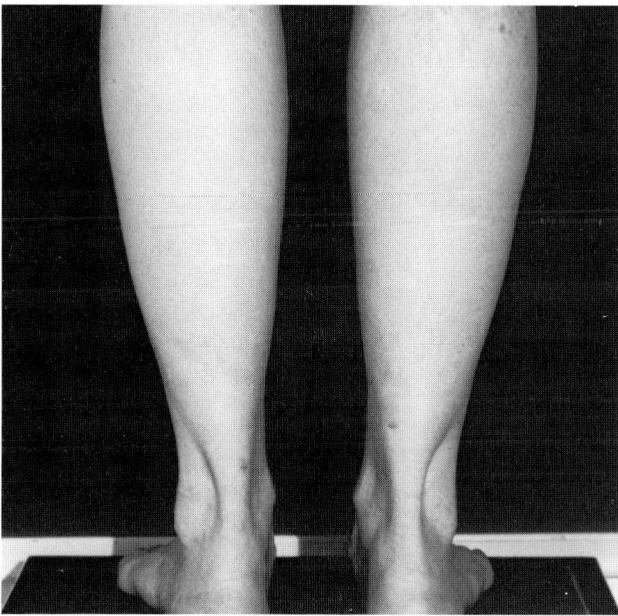

B

Fig. 33-7.
A. Preoperative view of small amount of fat accumulation obscuring the Achilles relief in a 29-year-old woman.
B. Postoperative view showing improvement in the Achilles definition. (Courtesy of C. Lewis, M.D.)

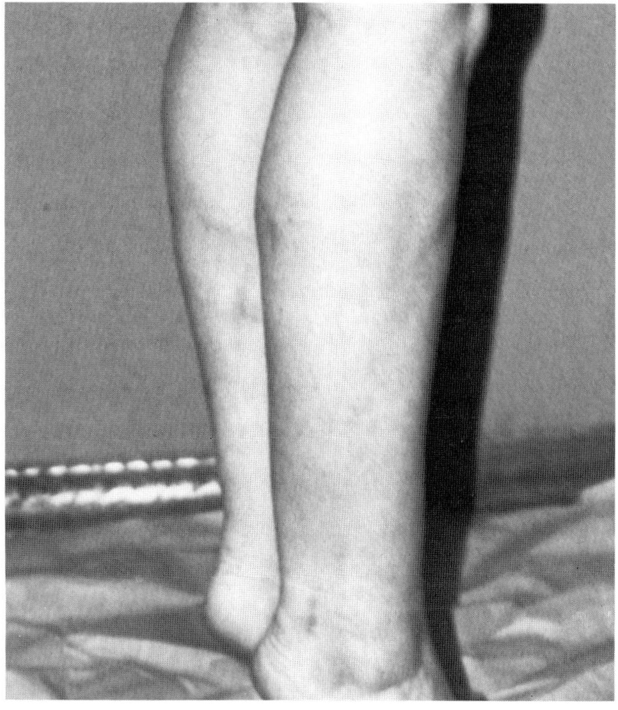

A

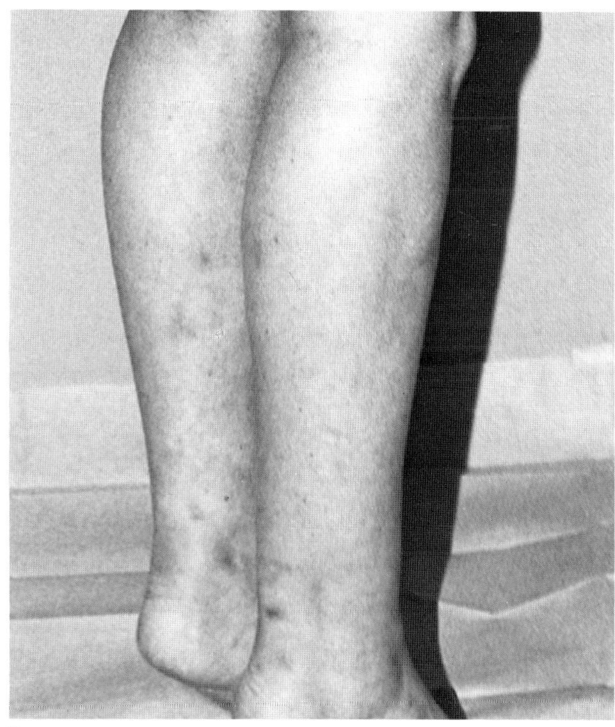

B

Fig. 33-8.
A. Preoperative view of calf with no definition in lower half. The patient is in her fifties.
B. After removal of 150 ml from each calf, there is good improvement in gastroc and Achilles definition. Photos taken 2 months postoperatively. Further improvement continued. (Courtesy of G. Hetter, M.D.)

CHAPTER 34

Lipolysis Combined with Conventional Surgery

Ricardo Baroudi

Ethnic background, weight variations, pregnancies, genetics, hormones, age, and life habits influence the quality of the skin during a lifetime and especially after 40 years of age.

This chapter focuses on the improvement of the body contour, specifically of the abdomen, thighs, and iliac crest, taking into consideration the technical approaches of traditional surgeries combined with blunt suction lipectomy. In the last 20 years, conventional abdominoplasty and thighplasty have been used routinely to improve the body contour in cases of "lipodystrophy,"* skin flaccidity, or both. These surgeries, performed in combined or isolated surgical stages, should always offer an improvement when compared to the preoperative appearance and never equal or worse, whatever the type of residual scar.

In spite of the good quality of scars obtained in most cases, the general public's feeling is still one of criticism of the scarring, regardless of the surgeon's diligence in explaining the impossibility of not leaving scars. There are still some patients who argue with their doctors with the classic question: "Aren't you supposed to perform a plastic suture?" They think this means the scar should not exist.

Traditional abdominoplasty and thighplasty have had a long controversy as to their acceptability by both patients and doctors. The history of these surgeries had three periods. At the beginning, only patients with substantial deformities were submitted to surgery. In the subsequent period, patients with mild problems were accepted for these surgeries. Presently, with the advent of blunt suction lipectomy in the plastic surgery armamentarium, new criteria and refined maneuvers are producing better aesthetic results when compared to previous surgeries.

At the beginning, suction procedures were subject to criticism and restrictions; however, definitive good results have been observed with the Illouz technique. Now, after a period of marked enthusiasm, its indications are becoming clear and allow proper selections. The following is an attempt to present and justify my concepts regarding the use of blunt suction lipectomy in combination with previous techniques of body contour surgery.

Blunt Suction Lipectomy

Blunt suction lipectomy has become an optional surgery for specific problems of localized fatty deposits. Almost

---

* Editor's note: Because of the pervasive use in Portuguese of the term *lipodystrophy* for all heavy, localized fatty deposits, Dr. Baroudi's text has been left unchanged in this regard. See Chapter 9, Nomenclature.

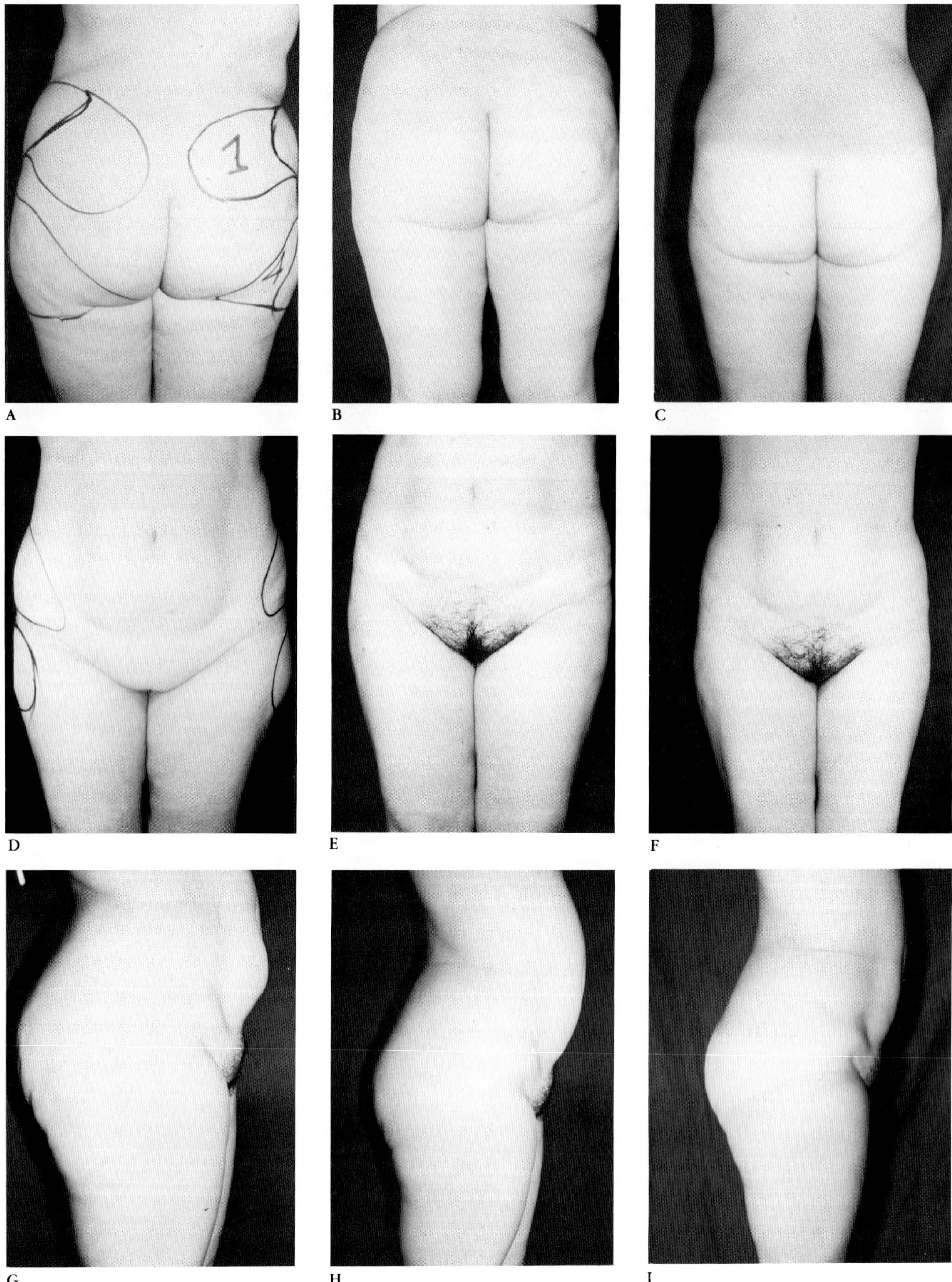

all regions of the body may be suctioned, leaving inconspicuous scars and producing gratifying results. As with any other surgery, it has its advantages and disadvantages.

The advantages of blunt suction lipectomy are (1) minimal scars, (2) minimal risks, (3) modest discomfort, (4) quick recovery, and (5) nonrecurrence of fatty deposits. The disadvantages are (1) it is a blind surgery, where mild to aggressive complications may occur when the basic surgical details are not followed, (2) it cannot be recommended when skin flaccidity is present, and (3) a second and even third suction stage may be necessary when poor results are obtained.

Technical discussions are outside the realm of this chapter. No specific philosophy is presented here; however, some points are important to give a didactic guideline about suction lipectomy.

1. Based on what has been published, selected cases that were previously submitted to conventional surgery are now indicated for suction.
2. The same results can be obtained with blunt suction lipectomy (as with a conventional body contour surgery) with a minimal scar and with all the advantages already described regarding recovery.
3. Suction lipectomy should be indicated after previous loss of weight and when physiotherapy treatment fails.
4. If poor results are obtained, a second and even a third suction stage should be included in the doctor's regimen with the patient's understanding. If the unacceptable result persists, the patient must have already been informed that a conventional body contour surgery is recommended as the final stage of the regimen.
5. Blunt suction lipectomy should be used for specific cases where body contour surgery is also indicated. This combined procedure improves the final result and can be done in the same or in different surgical stages.
6. When the patient does not lose weight and when physiotherapy methods fail, blunt suction lipectomy is recommended. The improvement of the patient's silhouette may motivate them psychologically to lose additional weight and reach their desired appearance faster (Fig. 34-1).

The Present State of Body Contour Surgery

The traditional abdomen, hip, and thighplasties have been described in the literature and have been used in the specialty for more than 20 years in patients with lipodystrophy, skin flaccidity, or both. In spite of the appearance of the large scar, it is still an excellent procedure to improve body contour.

Blunt suction lipectomy and conventional surgery have been combined to improve results. To reach these conclusions, certain details had to be evaluated. Four basic characteristics involve suction lipectomy, traditional body contour surgery, or their combined procedures, specifically on dysmorphism of the abdomen, hips, and thighs. These characteristics are discussed in the following sections.

PURE LIPODYSTROPHY

Patients, mostly in their twenties and thirties, sometimes present with protruding epi- or hypogastriums or both with what has been referred to as localized lipodystrophy. No flaccidity or striae exist (Fig. 34-2). The fat is about 3 cm thick. Others present flat abdomens and a gynecoid fat distribution. The iliac crest is fatty and bulging, the buttocks and the thighs are voluminous. The trochanteric regions are also frequently voluminous and protruded with an indentation between it and the iliac crest. The upper-inner thigh regions are frequently fat and usually rub against each other when the patient walks. No flaccidity exists and the skin is firm (Fig. 34-3).

There are innumerable individual variations apart from this basic type of body shape described. For these patients, blunt suction lipectomy is highly recommended. A final good result is always expected in one or two suction stages. The skin retracts over the new reduced fat volume.

Fig. 34-1.
A. Preoperative posterior view of a typical lipodystrophy in an overweight 25-year-old patient with no flabbiness in whom diet and exercise failed.
B. Eight months after first suction stage, where excess of fat was eliminated according to previous demarcated areas. Iliac crest and trochanteric regions are improved.
C. Four months after a second suction lipectomy was performed on the same lateral torso areas. Effective improvements of the body contour are observed. The patient's behavior changed after the second suction lipectomy, and she lost 8 pounds.
D. Preoperative frontal side view of same patient.
E. Postoperative frontal view 8 months after her first suctioning.
F. Final postoperative frontal view after second suctioning and 8-pound weight loss compared to 34 1E.
G. Preoperative lateral view of same patient.
H. Postoperative lateral view 8 months after first suctioning with good improvement of hypogastrium.
 I. Postoperative lateral view 4 months after second suctioning and 8-pound weight loss. The patient was psychologically motivated at this point to lose weight and to maintain her weight to keep the final result.

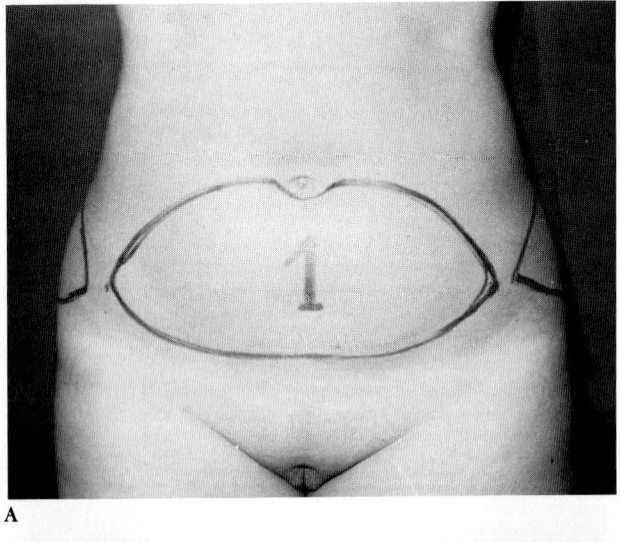

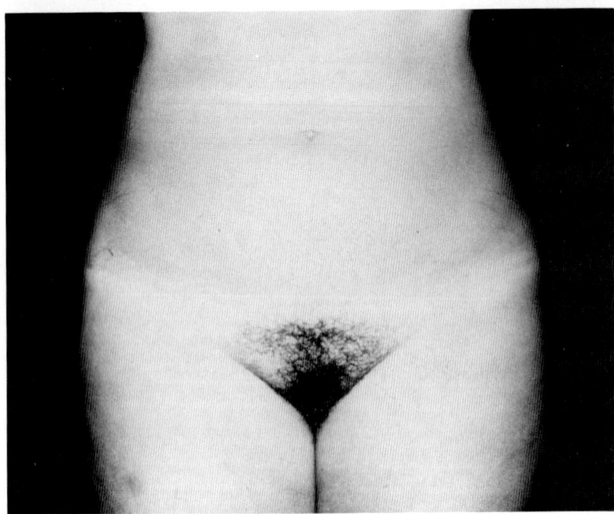

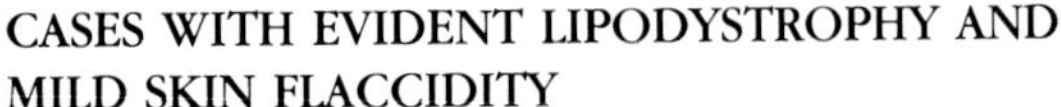

A

B

Fig. 34-2.
A. Typical hypogastric fat deposit of a patient in her twenties. No flabby skin or striae are seen. Frontal preoperative view.
B. Three months after suction lipectomy. The shape of the lower abdomen is improved and no skin waviness is observed.

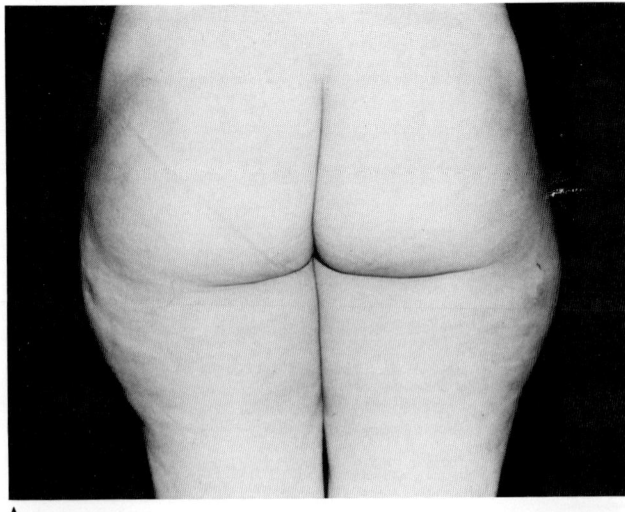

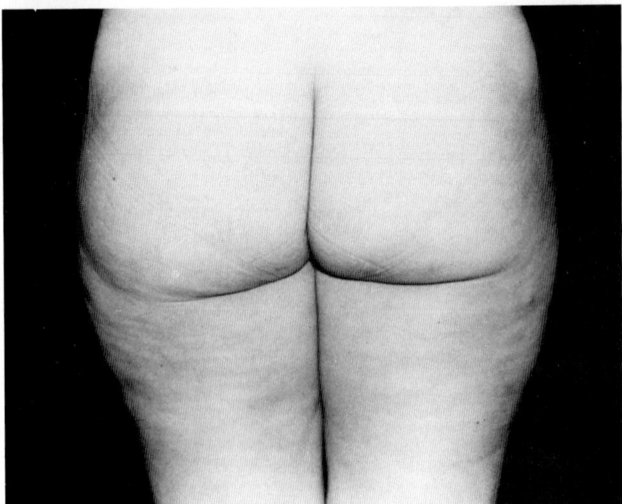

A

B

Fig. 34-3.
A. Preoperative posterior view of a 30-year-old patient with typical trochanteric lipodystrophy with no flabby skin.
B. Postoperative posterior view after routine blunt suction lipectomy, which provided an acceptable final result without any secondary wave problem. The contour is improved.

CASES WITH EVIDENT LIPODYSTROPHY AND MILD SKIN FLACCIDITY

Moderate skin flaccidity is commonly seen in patients with lipodystrophy of the abdominal wall, iliac crest, buttocks, and thighs. All varieties may exist in each specific region. When the patient's skin is pinched between the fingers, it shows a thickness of about 5 cm of fat. These patients are mostly in their thirties and forties.

Blunt suction lipectomy is still highly recommended for patients with this type of problem. Nevertheless, a basic detail should be considered: The volume of suctioned fat should be moderate. In these patients the skin flaccidity provides less retraction capacity. Any suction beyond the limits could bring secondary problems. There is no way to put the fat back in place. Therefore, moderation when removing fat is very important. The exact limit is difficult to tell. The surgeon's experience and judgment should indicate the correct moment to stop the suction before ever reaching the intended limit (Fig. 34-4).

Patients should be informed during the preoperative program that *a second and even a third suction stage may be necessary* around the fifth or sixth month, in

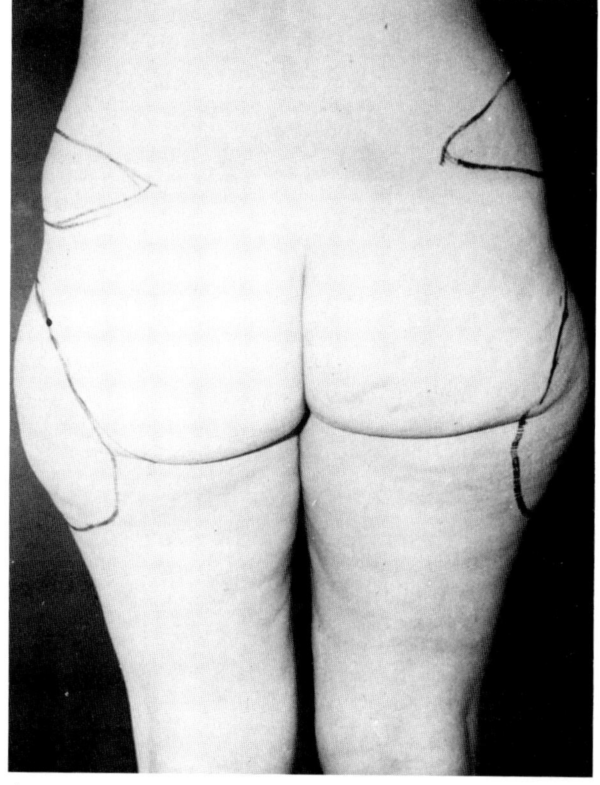

A

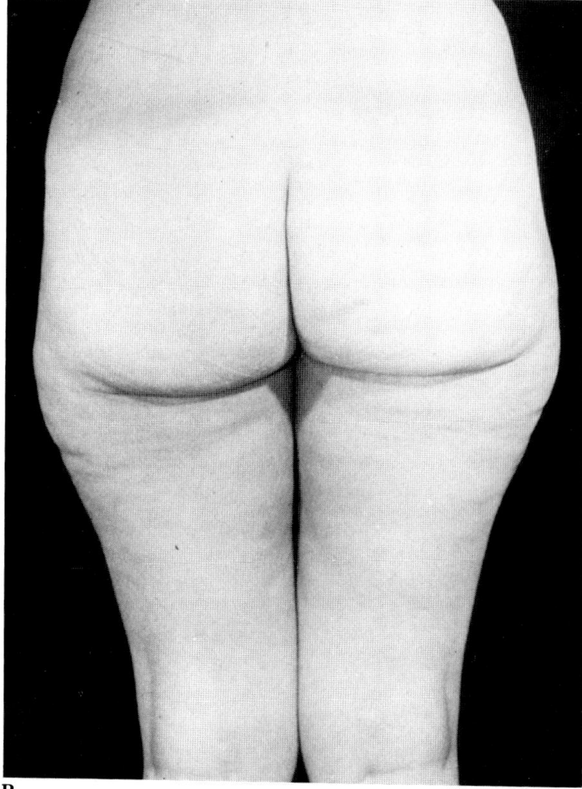

B

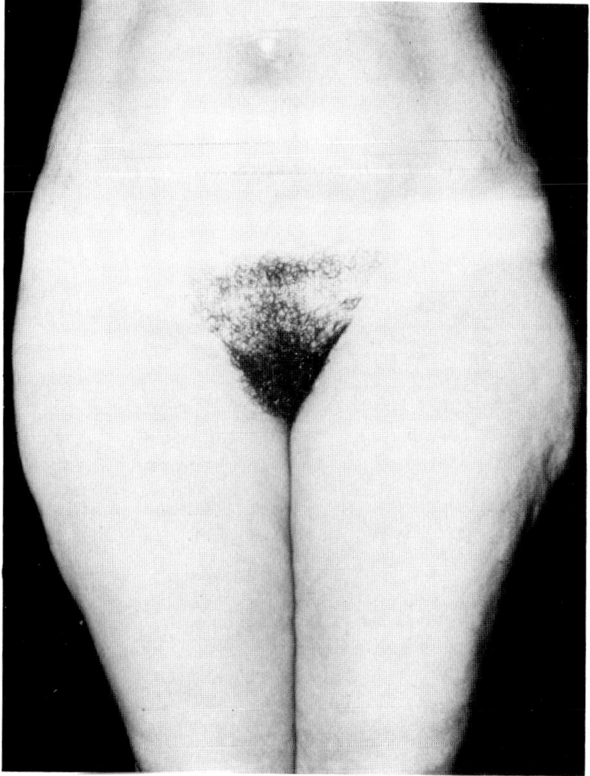

C

D

Fig. 34-4.

A. Preoperative appearance in the posterior view of a 39-year-old patient with iliac crest and trochanteric lipodystrophy. The skin was not firm and some flabbiness was evident by tactile exam.

B. The postoperative result shows the improvement of the contour with some waviness and removal limitation based on the skin flabbiness. Fat suction was interrupted before the ideal limits. Some skin waves can be observed in the trochanteric regions.

C. Preoperative anterior view.

D. Postoperative anterior view.

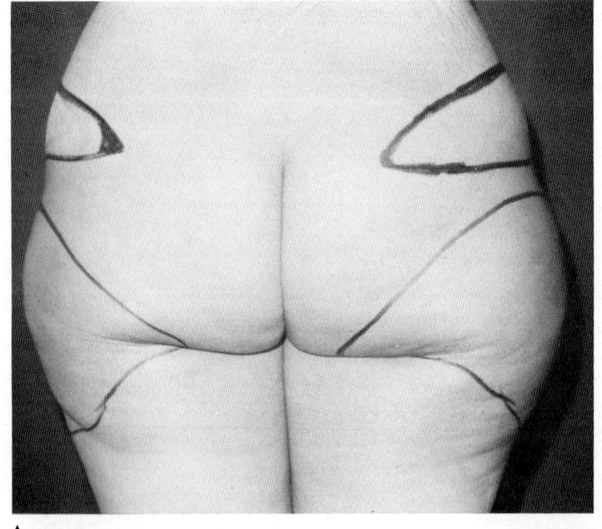

A

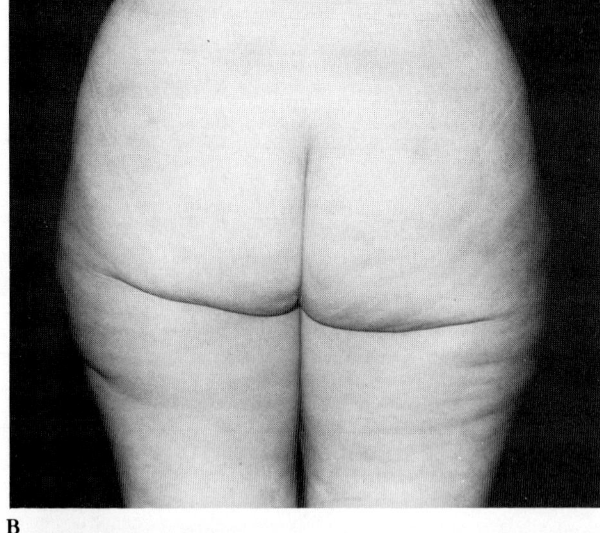

B

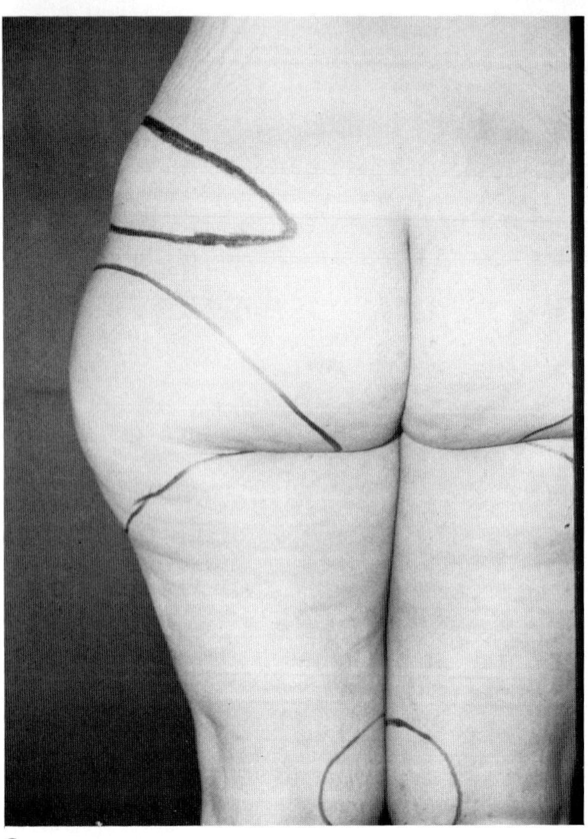

C

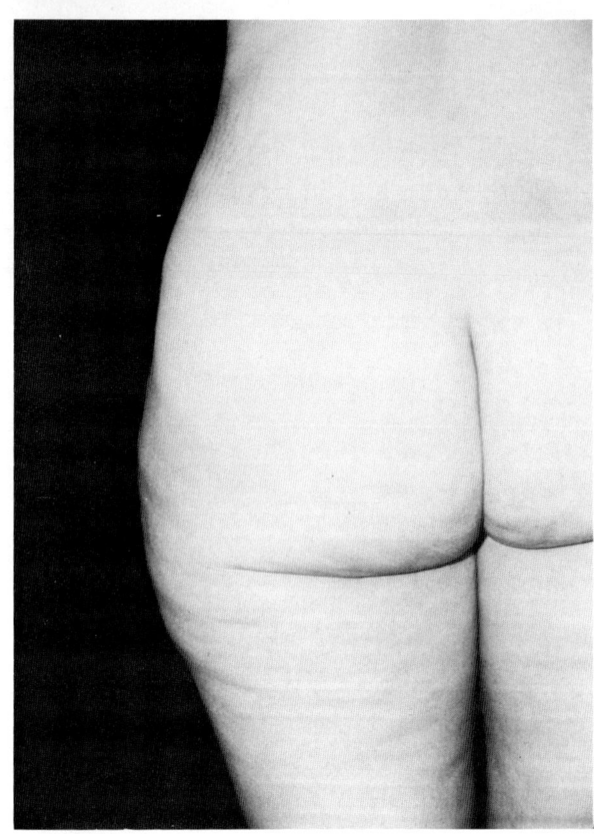

D

Fig. 34-5.

A. Preoperative posterior view of a 45-year-old patient.
B. Postoperative view 4 months after two consecutive suction stages with an 8-month interval. Effective volume reduction of the trochanteric areas and iliac crests is evident, but skin flabbiness remains with some depressions and waves of the skin surface. Such patients should be informed of this possibility previously. Body contour improvement should be sufficient to compensate for this secondary problem.
C. Left side view of the patient preoperatively marked.
D. Postoperatively, the bulging hips have been removed. The contour appears more natural, but flabby skin is evident. This result is more frequent in patients over 40.

accordance with the retraction process of the skin and the aesthetic results obtained. In spite of the extreme care used during the procedures, local skin waves may appear, compromising the final result (Fig. 34-5).

EVIDENT SKIN FLABBINESS AND LIPODYSTROPHY

Evident skin flabbiness with lipodystrophy is the result of the natural aging of the skin and is frequently observed in patients over 40. It may, however, also exist in puberty. Poor skin quality, fat distribution, and marked fluctuation of weight are the main causes in younger patients. Blunt suction lipectomy has two distinct indications. First, if the patient does not accept conventional surgery and does not mind the increased flaccidity, suction may be performed in one or more stages. The basic consideration is the body shape improvement. Many patients want to wear pants, tighter dresses, and bathing suits that reveal the body contour excesses (Fig. 34-6). As a second possibility, a combined procedure is really better to solve these problems, that is, suction along with the traditional body contour surgery. Both procedures can be performed during the same stage or in different stages.

Three specific examples of evident skin flabbiness and lipodystrophy illustrate this problem.

THIGHS, BUTTOCKS, ILIAC CREST, AND TROCHANTERIC LIPODYSTROPHY COMBINED WITH SKIN FLACCIDITY

When thighs, buttocks, and trochanteric lipodystrophy present no flabbiness, blunt suction lipectomy is usually indicated. When flaccidity is evident, classic surgery remains the only really satisfactory solution. Conventional technical procedures have been published, and the scars they leave should be compensated for by a significant aesthetic improvement.

With blunt suction lipectomy, new types of combinations with classic contour surgery now offer better final results. This surgery may be done in the same or in different surgical stages, according to the necessity and to the primary results produced. Selective regional suction is performed to better delineate the region (Figs. 34-7 and 34-8). In the traditional body contour surgeries, a great volume of tissue is undermined and resected. When blunt suction lipectomy is combined in the same surgical stage, it is best to perform it through a different access point than through the surgical cavities created by the dermolipectomy. This discontinuity may reduce possible infection. In general, large areas of dead space increase morbidity.

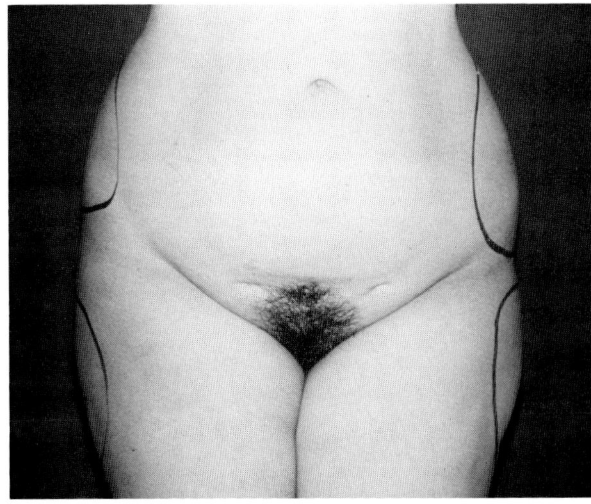

A

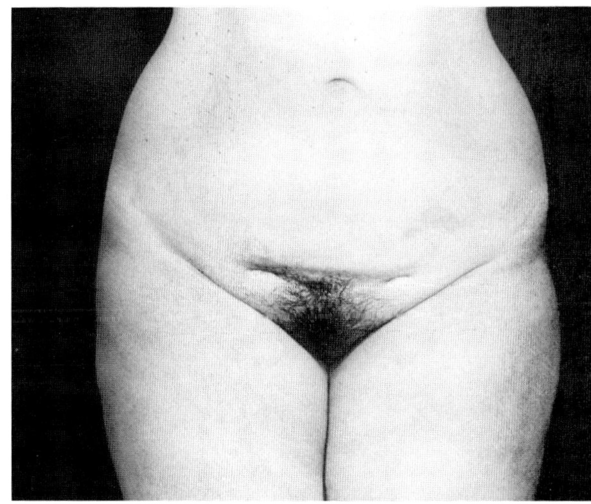

B

Fig. 34-6.
A. Frontal preoperative view of a 32-year-old patient with iliac crest and trochanteric excess and adipose abdomen. The skin in these regions was not firm and the patient was 20 pounds overweight but was accepted for suction lipectomy after unsuccessful weight loss. Conventional abdominoplasty was refused by the patient.
B. Four-month postoperative view after hips and abdomen were suctioned. Poor results are observed. The skin did not retract sufficiently and the body contour still remains quite similar to the preoperative appearance. Mild improvement of the abdomen. Suction volume was approximately 800 ml (less than normal) in an attempt to avoid skin waves.

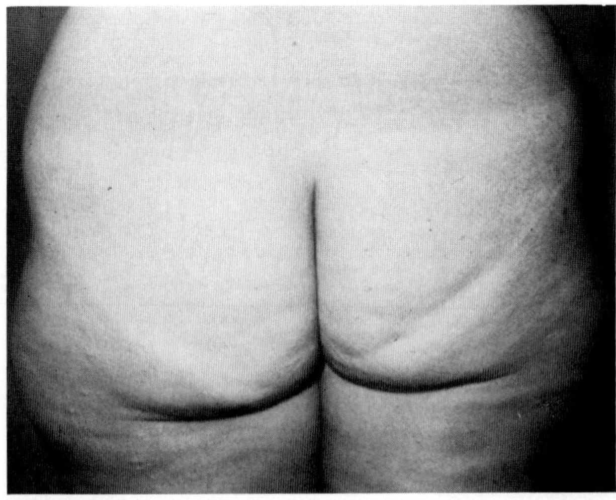

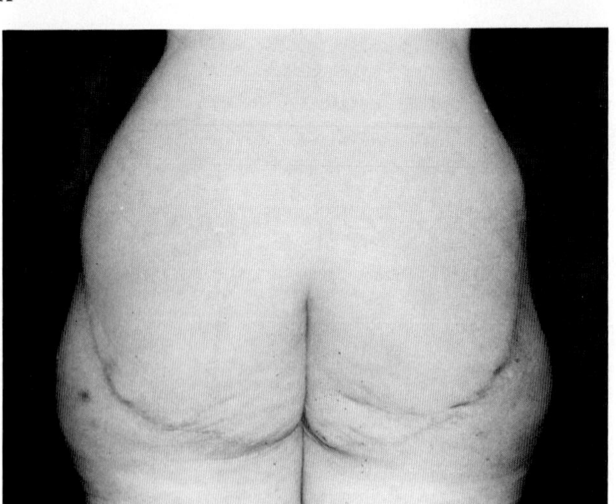

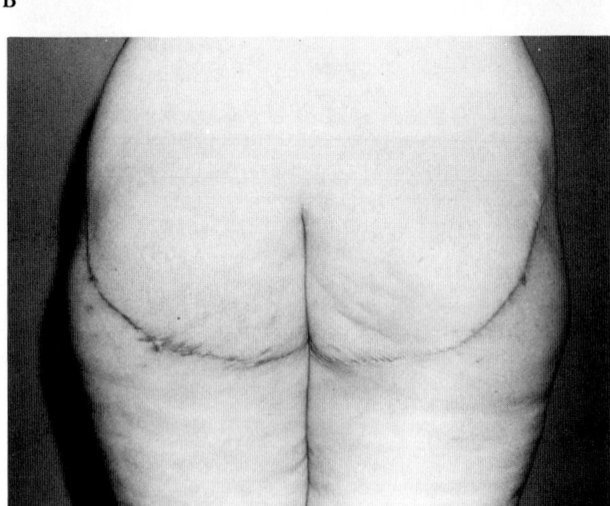

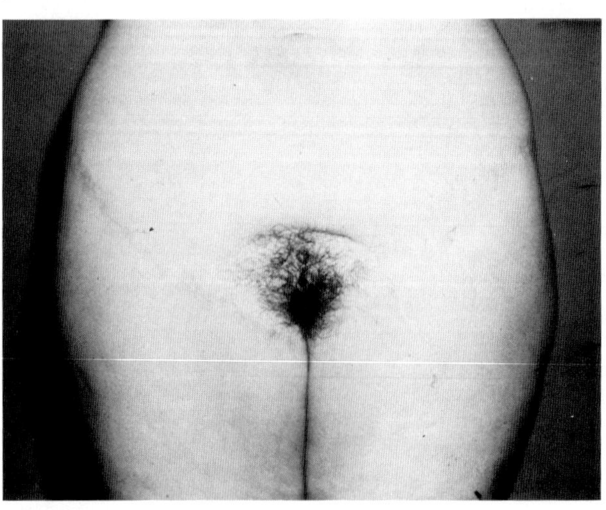

Fig. 34-7.
A. Frontal view of a 27-year-old woman when first admitted for consultation in 1975.
B. Posterior view of same patient showing the signs of previous buttock and thigh reduction operated on elsewhere after consultation in 1975. The patient complained about the residual volume on hips and skin flaccidity.
C. After two surgeries for thigh reduction, secondary deformity still persisted. At this stage, patient submitted to dermal suspension and suction lipectomy of the iliac crest and trochanteric regions.
D. Posterior view after third postoperative appearance. The contour shows a better shape. The final scars are still recent.
E. Final anterior view 4 months after three surgeries for circular thigh reduction, performed over 9 years. Evident body contour improvement is noted. Compare to 34-7A.

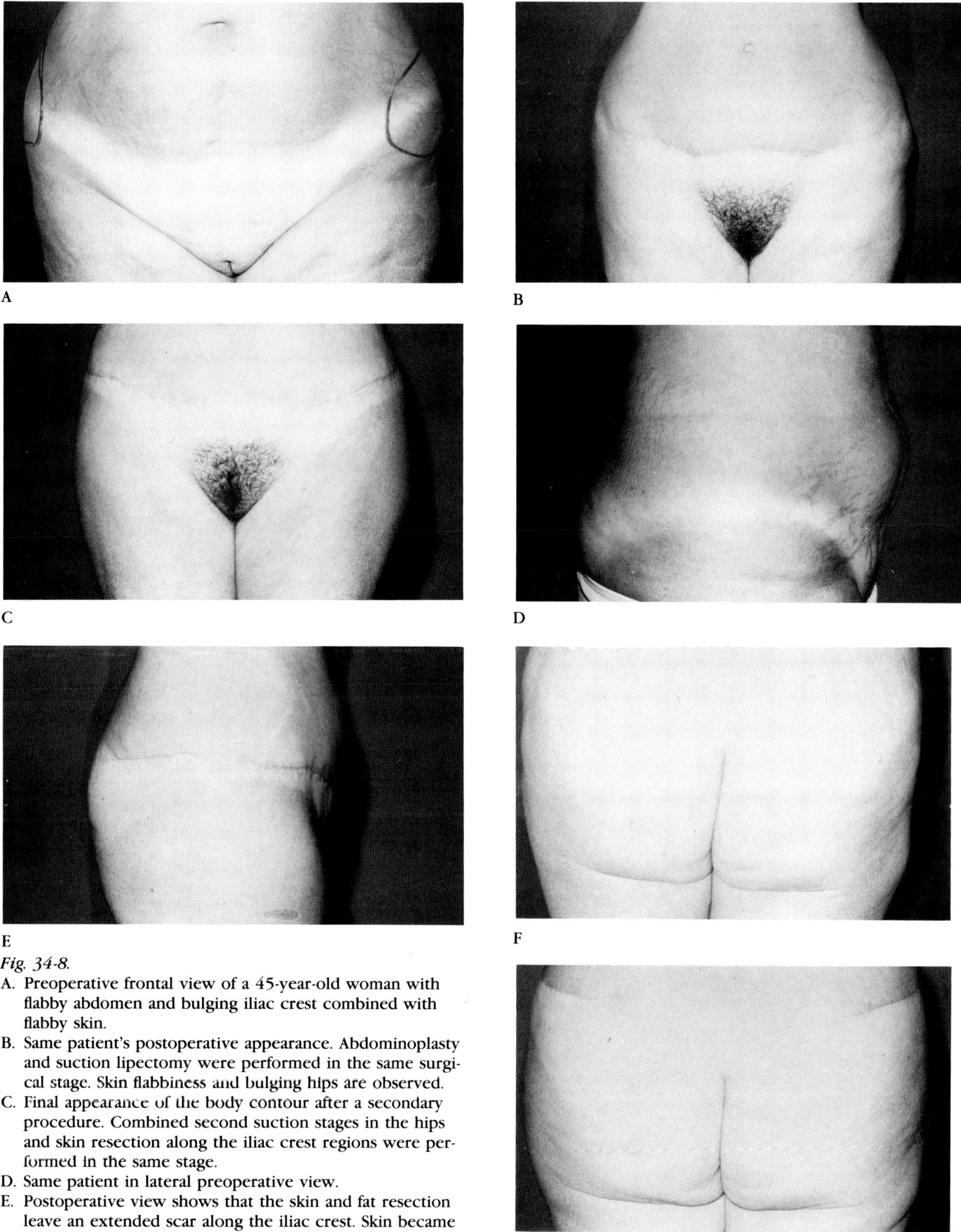

Fig. 34-8.
A. Preoperative frontal view of a 45-year-old woman with flabby abdomen and bulging iliac crest combined with flabby skin.
B. Same patient's postoperative appearance. Abdominoplasty and suction lipectomy were performed in the same surgical stage. Skin flabbiness and bulging hips are observed.
C. Final appearance of the body contour after a secondary procedure. Combined second suction stages in the hips and skin resection along the iliac crest regions were performed in the same stage.
D. Same patient in lateral preoperative view.
E. Postoperative view shows that the skin and fat resection leave an extended scar along the iliac crest. Skin became firm, and the contour improved.
F. Preoperative posterior view.
G. Acceptable final results support the good quality of the method in spite of the extended scar.

ABDOMINOPLASTY WITH BULGING EPIGASTRIC LIPODYSTROPHY

Conventional abdominoplasty has as its highlights removal of the excess of skin and fat from the lower abdomen, and improvement of the aesthetic characteristics of the waistline and navel. Some patients complain of a protruding epigastrium after the surgery, which they did not notice before. This secondary problem occurs when the epigastric fat is already thick, combined or not with projecting or flared lower ribs. The fat layer in this region is about 5 cm thick (Fig. 34-9).

Two possibilities may be used in such cases. First, blunt suction lipectomy of the epigastric region may be carried out immediately before the traditional abdominoplasty. The thickness of epigastric fat is reduced, and the skin flap undermining is performed in a routine manner.

Second, a surgical resection of this fat may also be done. After the resection of the lower portion of the flap excess, a sharp resection of the fat to the level of the superficial fascia is performed to reduce its thickness by one-half. The fat resection must be limited within a triangular area to avoid the lateral vascular supply (Fig. 34-10).

ABDOMINOPLASTY WITH ILIAC CREST LIPODYSTROPHY

One of the most common secondary problems after abdominoplasty can be observed at the iliac crest. The abdominal wall becomes flat while the iliac crest becomes more prominent because of localized lipodystrophy. Patients often complain about this problem.

Two solutions may be used in such cases (Fig. 34-11). First, suction lipectomy along the iliac crest may be performed at the time of the abdominoplasty. The same procedure can also be performed several months after the abdominoplasty if no fat in that area was appreciated at the time of the abdominoplasty (Fig. 34-12). If suction is performed together with the abdominoplasty, the entry site is through the abdominal incision laterally. Another possibility, with a questionably better margin of safety, is to use a separate site of entry for the cannula. Infection may be reduced.

A second surgical procedure for the removal of the iliac crest prominence is indicated for patients with excessive flaccidity of the skin in the area. In this case, blunt suction lipectomy is restricted (Fig. 34-13). One of the most common regional deformities observed in a feminine body contour is the indentation between the iliac crest and the trochanteric region (so-called gluteal depression, see Chap. 9, Nomenclature). The bulging aspect in these two regions leaves a supratrochanteric depression that compromises a harmonious body con-

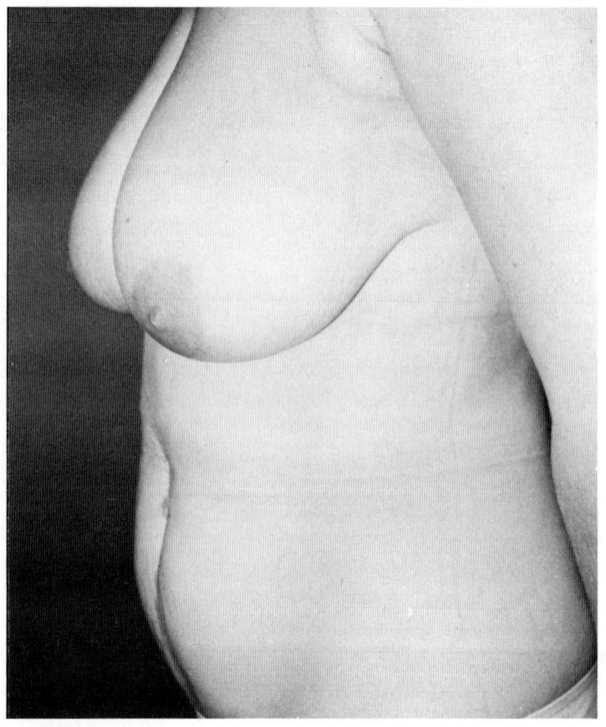

A

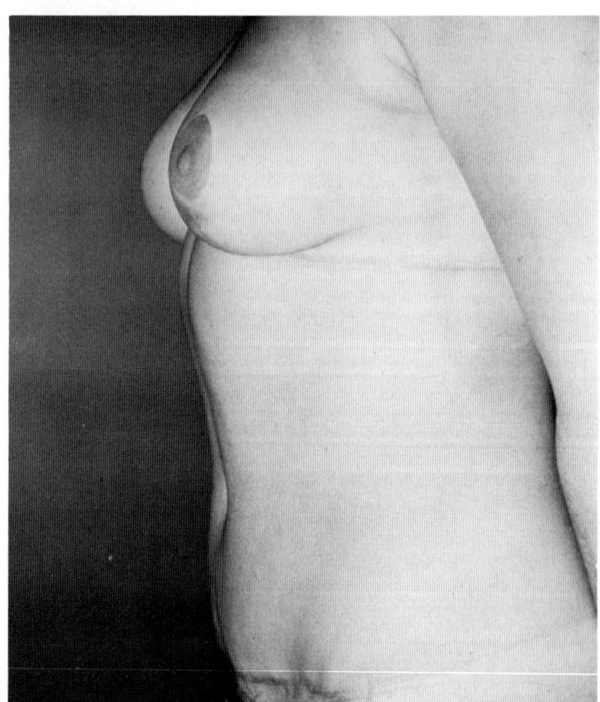

B

Fig. 34-9.
A. The epigastrium is partially hidden by the breast and voluminous hypogastrium.
B. Postoperative view after a breast reduction combined with an abdominoplasty in one stage. The epigastrium seems to protrude because of the existence of the thick fatty tissue in the subxiphoid area. Patients commonly complain about this occurrence.

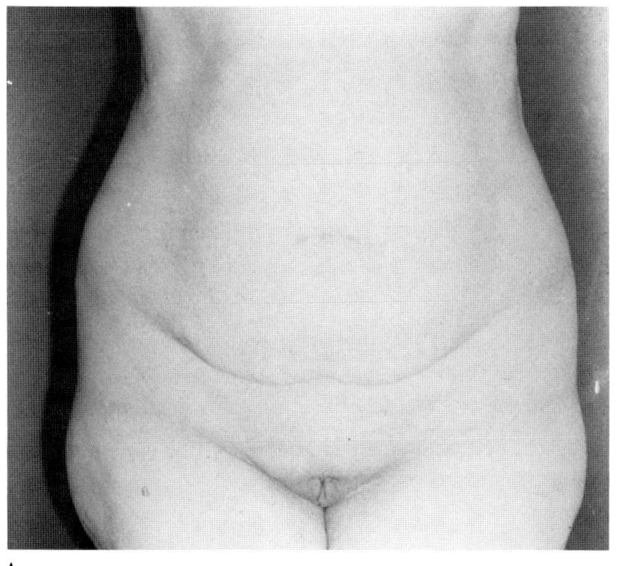

A

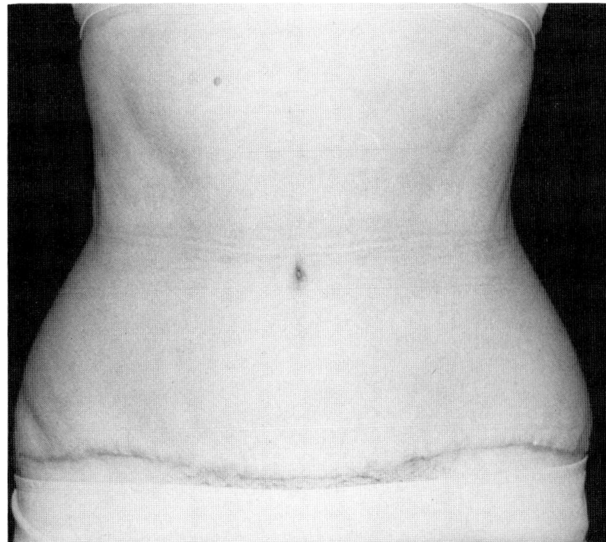

B

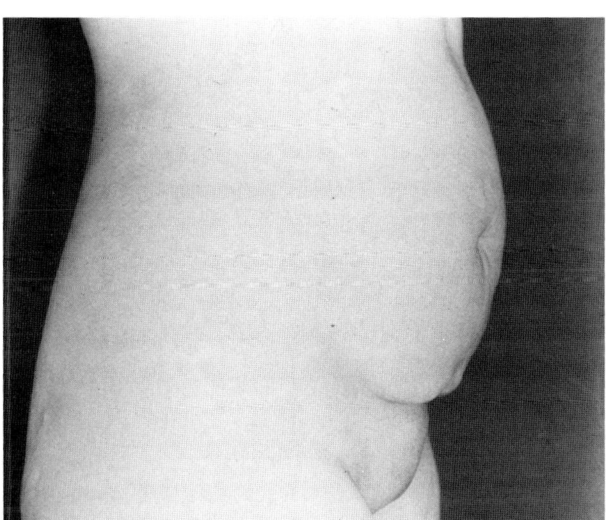

C

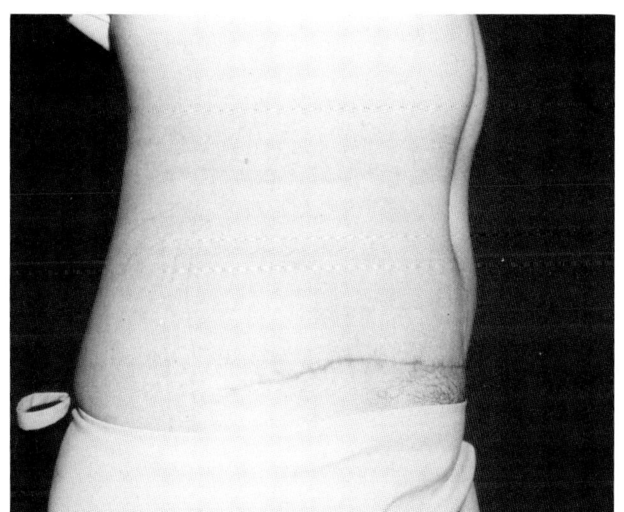

D

Fig. 34-10.
A. Preoperative frontal view of a 42-year-old patient with a flaccid and fatty abdomen.
B. Final result after a conventional abdominoplasty.
C. Preoperative lateral view.
D. Postoperative lateral view showing the body contour improvement.
E. After the excess flap resection, the upper portion of the flap is defatted to the level of the superficial fascia. The fat excess resection should not go laterally on the skin flap to avoid blood supply problems.

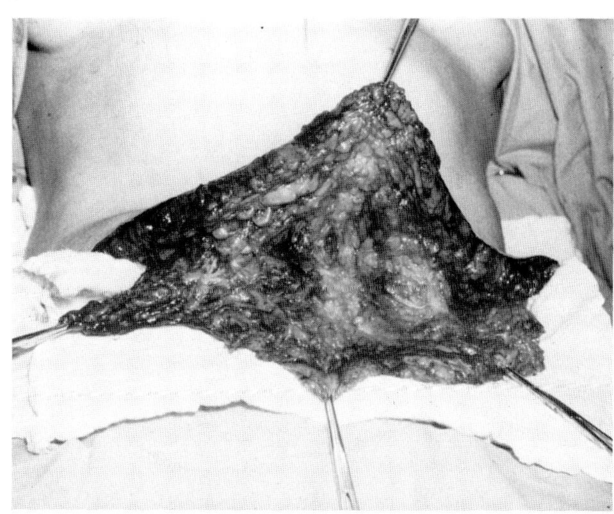

E

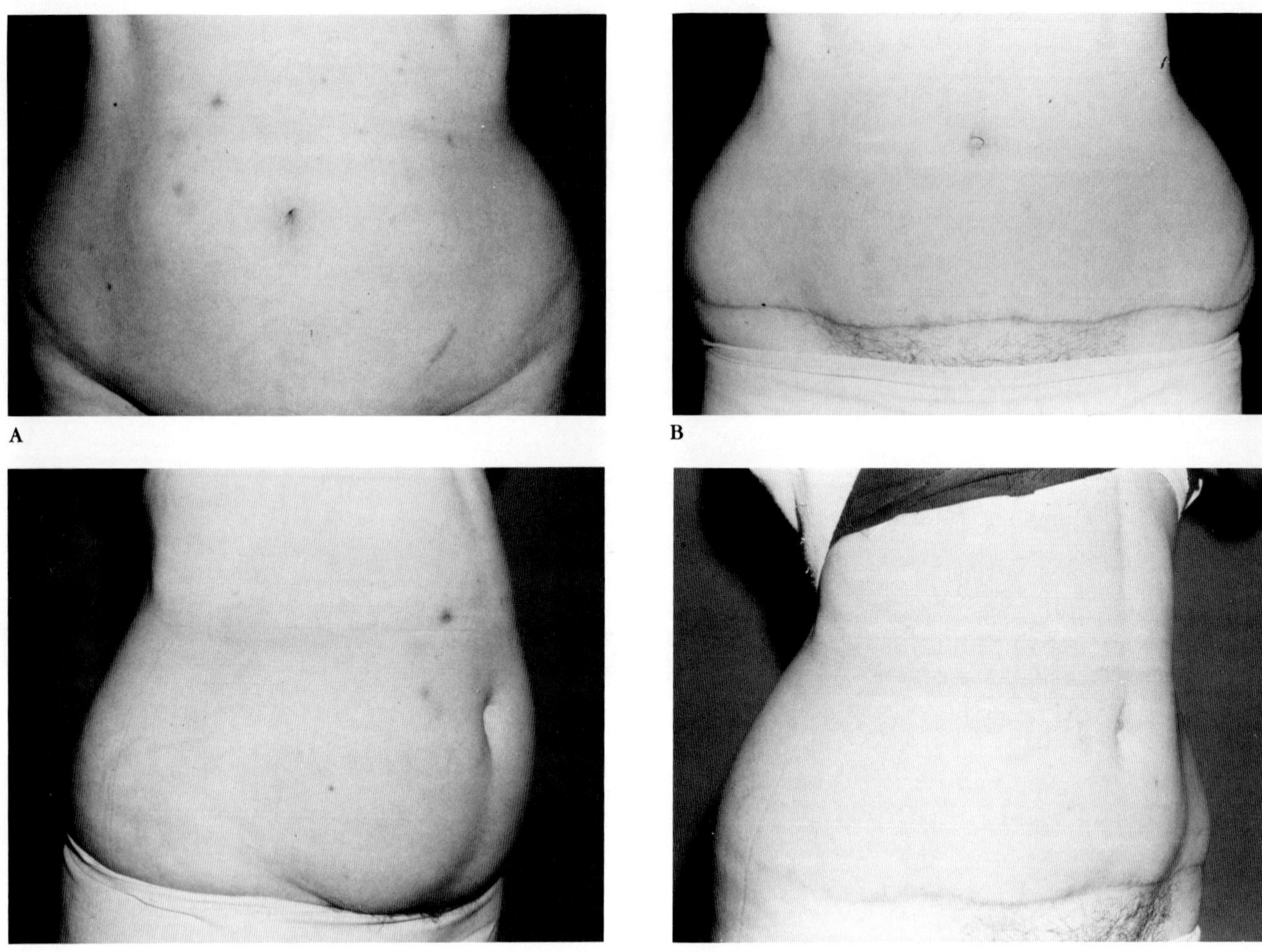

Fig. 34-11.
A. Preoperative appearance of a globular abdomen in a fat patient with adipose hips.
B. After abdominoplasty the abdomen became flat but the unpleasant iliac crest fat excess remains.
C. Preoperative right oblique view.
D. Postoperative photograph shows secondary deformity of the hip region.

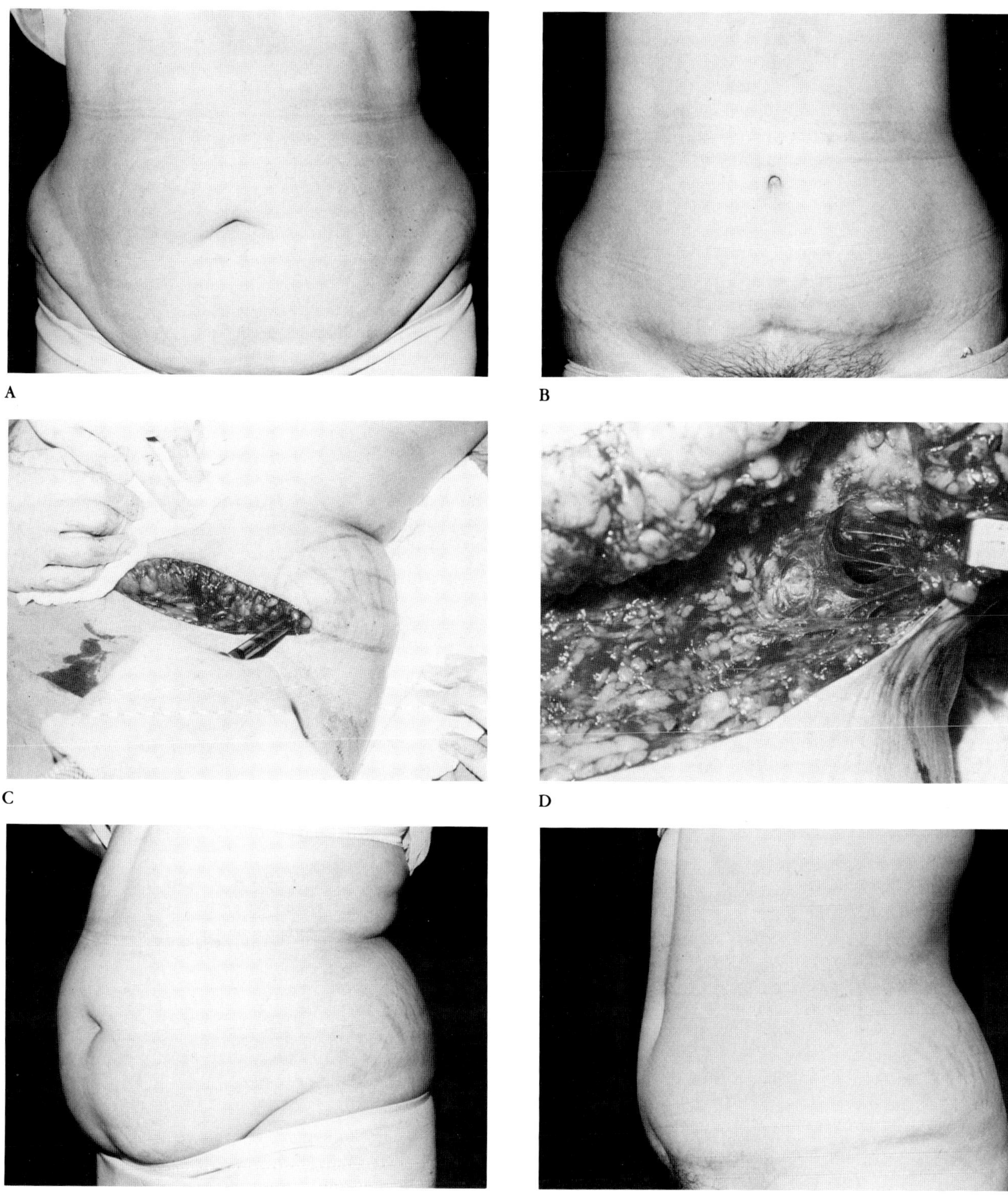

Fig. 34-12.

A. Preoperative frontal view of a 48-year-old woman with a pendulous, fat abdomen who presented for an abdominoplasty.

B. Frontal view 2 years postoperatively. Patient lost 8 pounds after the surgery. Combined surgery with suction lipectomy of the iliac crest was performed in the same surgical stage.

C. Site of entry for suction was through the incision for the abdominoplasty.

D. Close-up of suctioned area. Tunnels through the fat tissue and vascular network can be observed.

E. Left oblique preoperative view.

F. Postoperative appearance can be compared. The body contour improvement is evident using the combined method as well as patient's general weight loss.

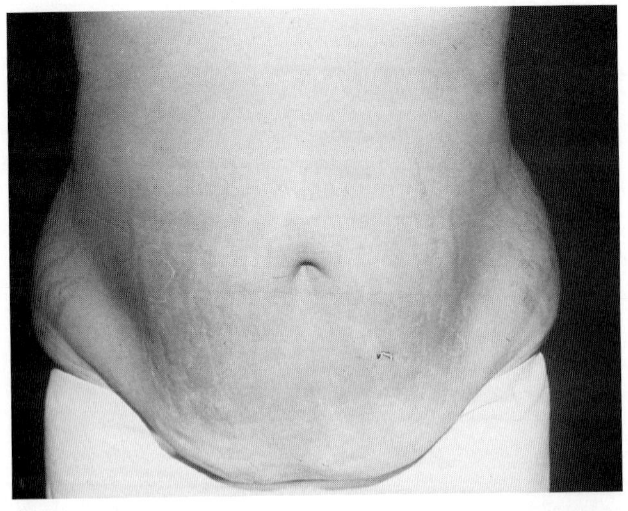

A

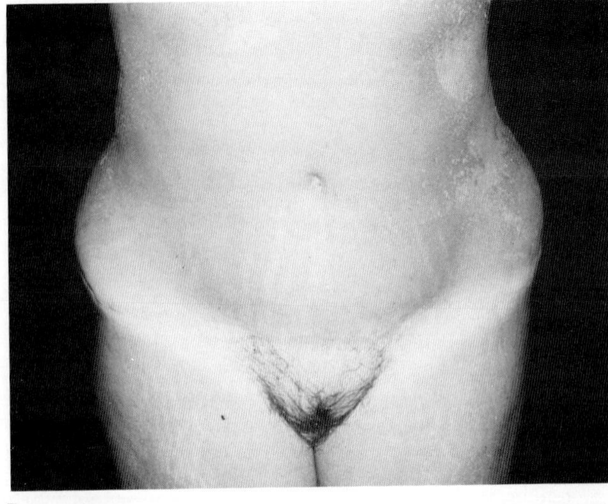

B

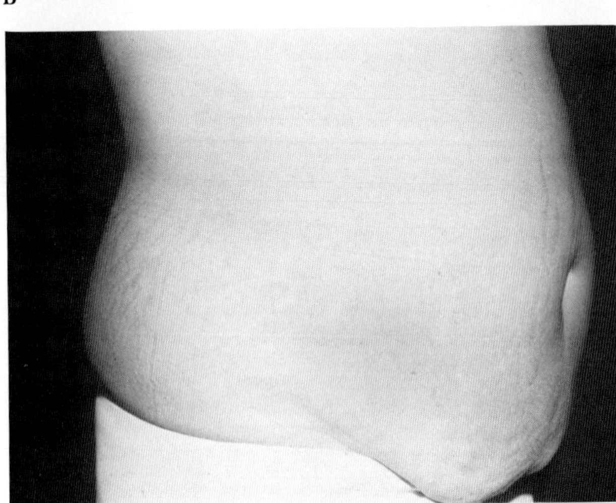

D

C

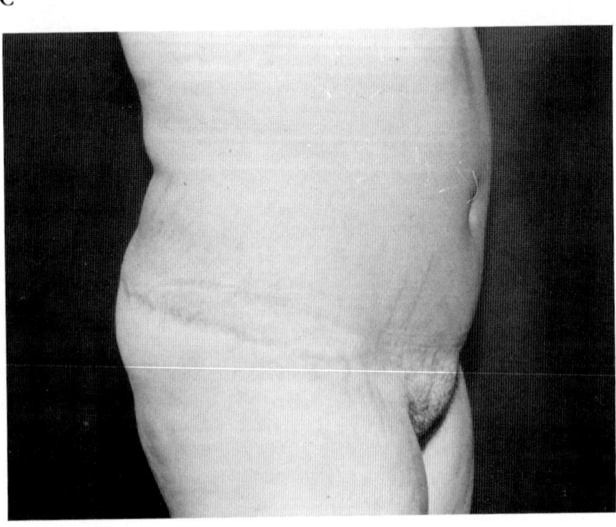

E

Fig. 34-13.
A. Preoperative frontal view of a 45-year-old woman with pendulous abdomen, thick fat skin, and bulging iliac crest.
B. Frontal view 2 years postoperatively showing improvement of the abdominal wall but persisting bulging iliac crest following conventional surgery.
C. A surgical revision for excess tissue of the crest was performed as a combined procedure with suction lipectomy in the same area. Body contour became effectively better in spite of the final scar.
D. Same patient in lateral position before the abdominoplasty.
E. Postoperative lateral view showing the final scar going around the iliac crest region, through the elongation for the residual abdominoplasty scar.

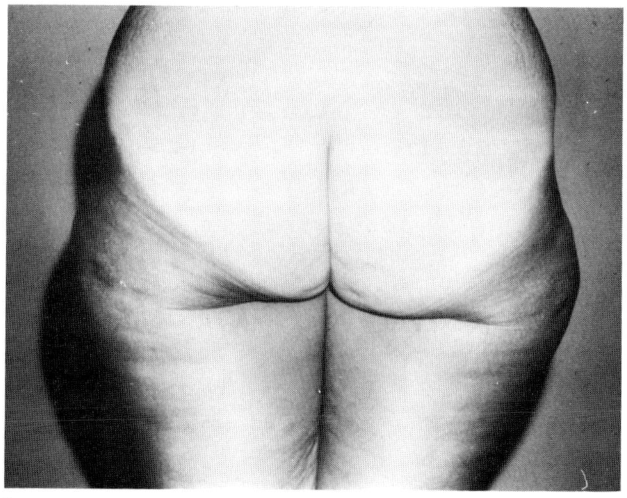
A

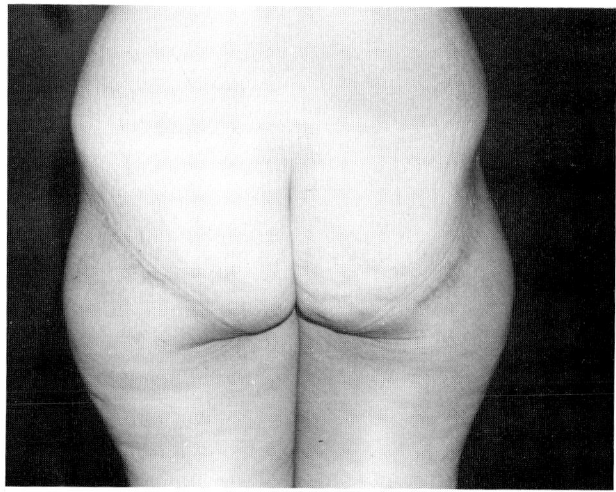
B

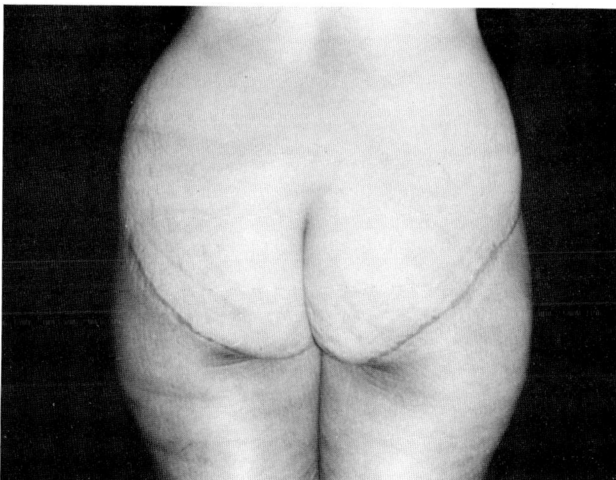
C

Fig. 34-14.

A. Preoperative posterior view of a 48-year-old woman with trochanteric lipodystrophy and flabby skin of the buttock and flank regions. Patient underwent circular thigh reduction.

B. Three-year postoperative view shows a secondary deformity with indentation in the body contour.

C. Surgical revision was performed. Recent final result can be observed. Dermal suspension of the trochanteric region was performed to correct the indentation, combined with suction lipectomy in the trochanteric and iliac crest regions.

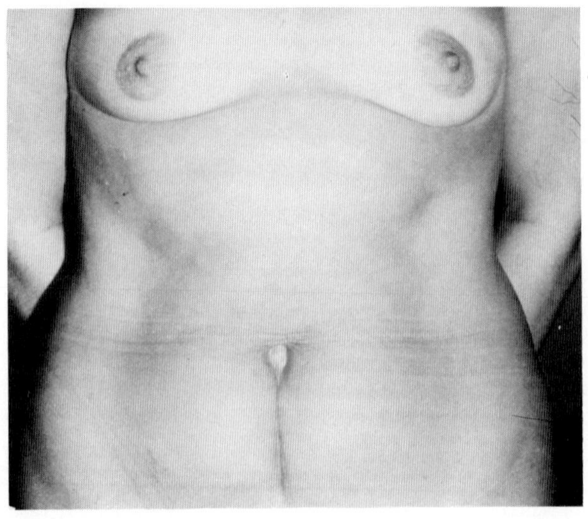

A

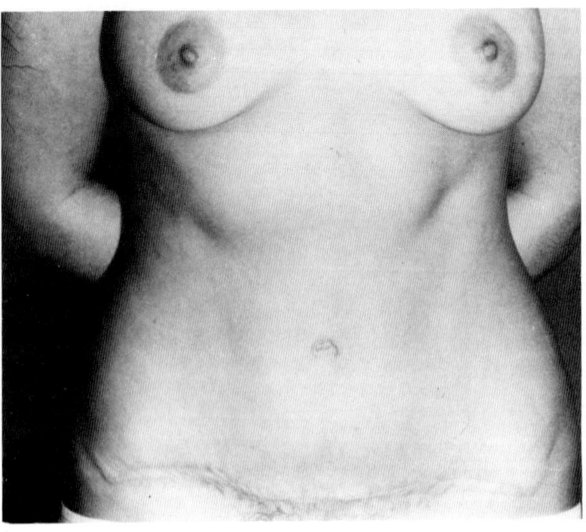

B

Fig. 34-15.
A. Preoperative case of vertical infraumbilical scar and mild fat deposits. Suction lipectomy was not indicated because the patient would not accept the vertical scar.
B. Two-year postoperative view. The result justifies the scar.

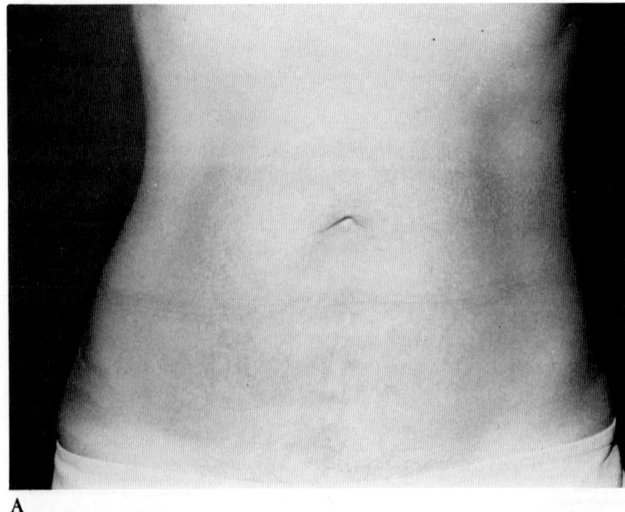

A

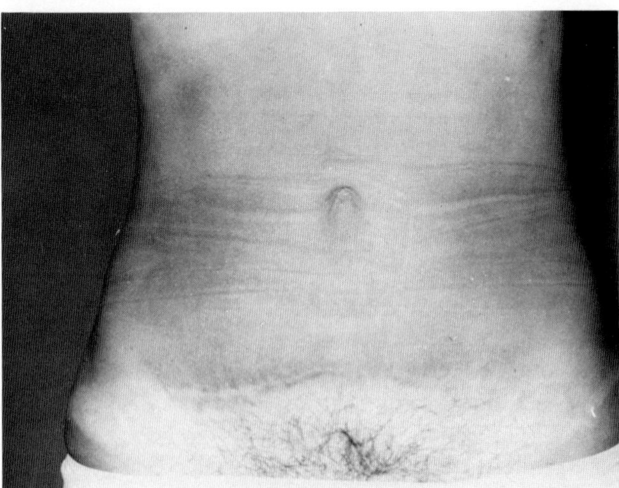

B

Fig. 34-16.
A. Case of an abdomen with no fatty tissue but with flabby skin with a vertical infraumbilical scar. Suction lipectomy was not indicated.
B. Conventional abdominoplasty was performed for the scar and skin excess. Final result justifies the scar.

tour. The suction or surgical procedures or both are performed with the aim of directly removing these bulging regions in an attempt to give a better contour (Fig. 34-14).

SKIN FLACCIDITY WITH NO LOCALIZED LIPODYSTROPHY

Basically, patients with skin flaccidity with no localized lipodystrophy present with flat but crepey abdominal skin with or without scars after previous celiotomy. Striae are very common. These patients usually have a slim figure with no voluminous hips or epigastrium (Figs. 34-15 and 34-16). No suction lipectomy is indicated for these patients. Classic surgery is the only option. Final results should always be better than the previous appearance, in spite of the resulting scar.

Discussion

Blunt suction lipectomy, when combined with conventional body contour surgery, offers better final results in selected patients. Added mechanisms of refinement make the surgery more gratifying for both the surgeon and the patient. The conventional surgeries will, of course, continue. For the patient's benefit and information, it is important to have a treatment regimen outlined in accordance with his or her specific problem: (1) Any overweight distortions possible to solve with diet and exercise should be so treated. (2) If these treatments fail, blunt suction lipectomy should be the elective treatment in one or more suction stages, depending on the patient's skin condition. (3) Finally, if the suction presents poor results, the door should always have been left open for conventional surgery with all of its repercussions.

In cases where blunt suction lipectomy is not indicated, surgery should be chosen. With the new firm skin obtained, any fat residual not appreciated initially may be suctioned just as in a planned combined procedure.

In conclusion, the new approach has avoided a large number of traditional surgeries with their scar dissatisfactions. The results obtained by classic body contour procedures have also been improved by combining it with blunt suction lipectomy.

Bibliography

Agris, J. Use of dermal fat suspension flaps for thigh and buttock lifts. *Plast. Reconstr. Surg.* 59:817, 1977.

Andrews, J. M. Nova técnica de lipectomia abdominal e onfaloneoplastia. In *Transactions of the Third Latin American Congress of Plastic Surgery,* 1956.

Baroudi, R. The present and future aspect of the sculpturing surgery. In *Transactions of the Eighth International Congress of Plastic Surgery.* Montreal, 1983.

Baroudi, R. Umbilicaplasty. *Clin. Plast. Surg.* 2:431, 1975.

Baroudi, R., Keppke, E. M., and Tozzi Neto, F. Abdominoplasty. *Plast. Reconstr. Surg.* 54:161, 1974.

Carvalho, C. G. S., Baroudi, R., and Keppke, E. M. Anatomical and technical refinements for abdominoplasty. *Aesth. Plast. Surg.* 1:217, 1977.

Courtiss, E. H. (Ed.) Aesthetic Surgery: Trouble—How to Avoid It and How to Treat It. St. Louis: Mosby, 1978.

Delerm, A., and Cirotteau, Y. Plastie cruro-fémoro-fessière ou circum fessière. *Ann. Chir. Plast.* 18:31, 1973.

Ducourtioux, J. L. Technique and indications for crural dermolipectomies. *Ann. Chir. Plas.* 17:204, 1972.

Elbaz, J. S., and Fanguel, G. Chirurgie Plastique de L'abdomen. Paris: Masson & Cie, 1977.

Fournier, P. F., and Otteni, F. M. Lipodissection in body sculpturing: The dry procedure. *Plast. Reconstr. Surg.* 72:598, 1983.

Franco, T., and Rebello, C. *Chirurgia Estetica.* Rio de Janeiro: Livraria Ateneu, 1977.

Goldwyn, R. M. The Unfavorable Result in Plastic Surgery (2nd ed.). Boston: Little, Brown, 1984.

Gonzalez-Ulloa, M. Belt lipectomy. *Br. J. Plast. Surg.* 13:179, 1960.

Grazer, F. M., and Klingbeil, J. R. Body Image: A Surgical Perspective. St. Louis: Mosby, 1980.

Guerrero-Santos, J. Lipectomies: arms, abdomen and thighs. Study session, Section I. Annual Meeting of the Educational Foundation of the American Society of Plastic and Reconstructive Surgeons. Houston, October, 1981.

Hetter, G. P., Herhahn, F. T., and Aiache, A. E. Experience with the Illouz technique of suction assisted lipectomy (lipolysis). In Transactions of the Eighth International Congress of Plastic Surgery. Montreal, 1983, p. 566.

Illouz, Y. G. Body contouring by lipolysis: a 5-year experience with over 3000 cases. *Plast. Reconstr. Surg.* 72:591, 1983.

Juri, J., Juri, C., and Raiden, G. Reconstruction of the umbilicus in abdominoplasty. *Plast. Reconstr. Surg.* 63:580, 1979.

Kesselring, U. K. Regional fat aspiration for body contouring. *Plast. Reconstr. Surg.* 72:610, 1983.

Lewis, J. R. *Atlas of Aesthetic Plastic Surgery.* Boston: Little, Brown, 1973.

Pitanguy, I. Surgical reduction of the abdomen, thighs and buttocks. *Surg. Clin. North Am.* 51:479, 1971.

Planas, J. The "vest over pants" abdominoplasty. *Plast. Reconstr. Surg.* 61:694, 1978.

Psillakis, J. M. Abdominoplasty: Some ideas to improve results. *Aesth. Plast. Surg.* 2:205, 1978.

Regnault, P. Abdominoplasty by the W technique *Plast. Reconstr. Surg.* 55:265, 1975.

Schrudde, J. Lipectomy and lipexeresis in the area of the lower extremities. *Langenbecks Arch. Chir.* 345:127, 1977.

Vilain, R., Dardour, J. C., and Straub, S. Extra fat surgery with and without a scar: A new approach. In Transactions of the Eighth International Congress of Plastic Surgery. Montreal, 1983.

CHAPTER 35

Lipolysis in Blacks, Including Treatment of Steatopygia

Pierre F. Fournier
Francis M. Otteni

During the past few years, the number of operations performed on black women has increased considerably, while the number remains low for black men and does not appear to be increasing. This desire of black women for an improved appearance is rarely associated with a desire to modify themselves to identify with the indigenous population, but rather a wish, as in other ethnic groups who have turned to aesthetic surgery, to remedy natural dysmorphias (e.g., steatopygia) or acquired ones (age, obesity, postpartum defects). The desire is to perfect a normal morphology and to refine their appearance. The closed techniques of lipoplasty influence this desire for contour improvement because blacks are often the ideal candidates for such operations.

Classically, black skin is said to react badly to the scalpel. A surgeon hesitates to propose an aesthetic operation for a minor or moderate dystrophy without a functional component. Because of the tiny incisions necessary for suction extraction of fat, these fears, which I feel were exaggerated, are disappearing. There is no disputing, however, that the proportion of poor-quality scarring (hypertrophies and keloids) in blacks is greater than that observed in whites; however, this need not be a deterrent.

My clinical impression from working with blacks in Africa and the West Indies is that the classic belief that blacks have three times as much scarring as whites is hardly justified. I believe black patients have only approximately twice as much problem scarring as whites. Therefore, the indications for operations for dystrophies should be approached with more optimism than was previously thought.

Finally, for women in many black ethnic groups, localized or associated general adiposities are much more common than for white women. Steatopygia, of course, is not really dysmorphic but a racial characteristic often combined with an exaggerated lordosis.

Study of Black Morphology

It is a current belief that many black ethnic groups have a morphology identical to whites. The adipose layer, however, is thinner on the torso of blacks. The localized adiposities that are usually treated in such cases are identical in distribution and location to those of whites.

In other ethnic groups, especially in Africans, certain dysmorphias are worth noting:

1. Classic steatopygia, pure or associated with peripelvic adiposity, is well documented. It is accentuated by the hyperlordosis that is seen in many black populations, their pelvis being more forwardly inclined. The treatment of such dysmorphias should be inspired

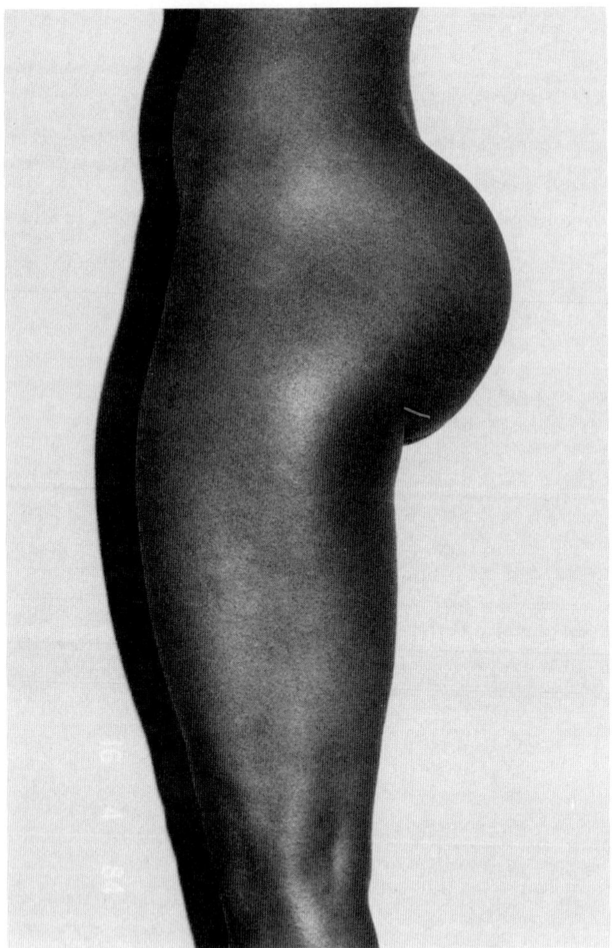

Fig. 35-1. Lateral view shows classic steatopygia in a young, slender black woman with fine classic black racial proportion. Patient nicknamed "bubble butt" in college. (Courtesy of G. Hetter, M.D.)

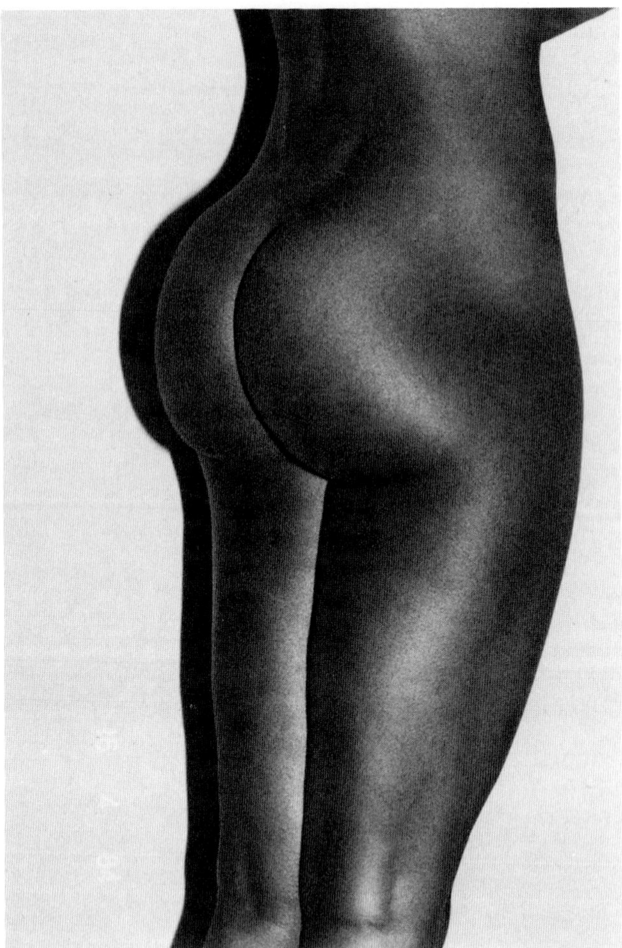

Fig. 35-2. Posterior right oblique view shows hyperlordosis, which accentuates the steatopygia. Strobe highlight shows the excess of lateral buttock confluent with high trochanteric excess. (Courtesy of G. Hetter, M.D.)

by their normal morphology and should not be overcorrected; neither should a natural hyperlordosis be confused with a steatopygia (Figs. 35-1 and 35-2).

2. Localized trochanteric adiposities are often greater (more accentuated and angular) than in whites, less diffused, and should be treated with certain precautions (Fig. 35-3).

3. Certain extremity adiposities are rhizomelic, regular, very defined yet with an almost normal distal extremity. Very developed thighs may be observed, necessitating a circular lipoplasty. One may see upper arms and thighs that contrast with the normal morphology of the forearm or of the calf (Fig. 35-4). The separation between the two segments of the extremity is very clear. The segmentary extremity adiposity may be regular, isolated, or associated with localized, trochanteric, intercondylion, or internal thigh adiposities. It is important to accurately inform the patient about what is

achievable as well as the limitations of the treatment of *localized* adiposities to avoid misunderstandings. We have only just begun to perform circular lipoplasties of the extremities. They are much more difficult to perform than localized lipoplasty.

4. Angular lumbosacral dysmorphia is frequent and is specific to certain West African races. Isolated treatment is always requested while the treatment of other associated peripelvic adiposity is not. Lipoplasty is not a treatment for this skeletal form.

5. Posterior and lateral thoracic and anterior axillary adiposities are present more often than in whites.

6. Distal adiposities of the limbs are seen more rarely than in whites. These adiposities seem much less frequent in blacks.

7. Cervicofacial adiposities, on the other hand, are

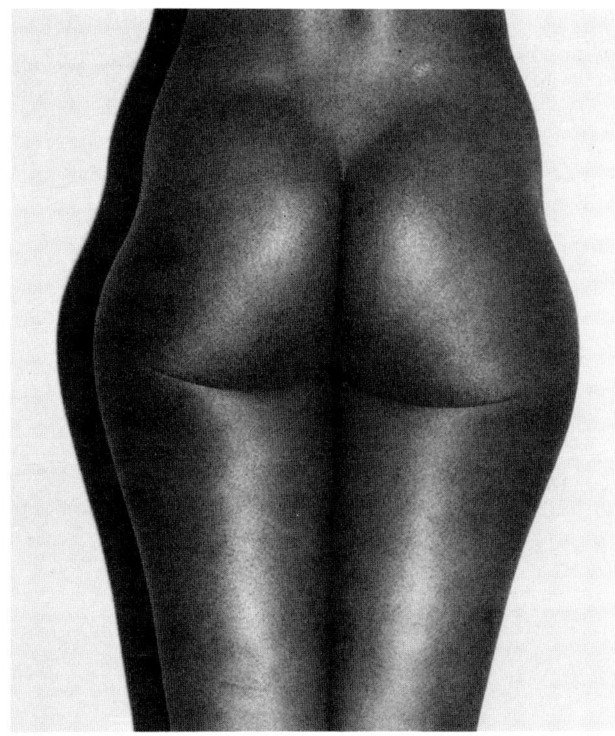

A

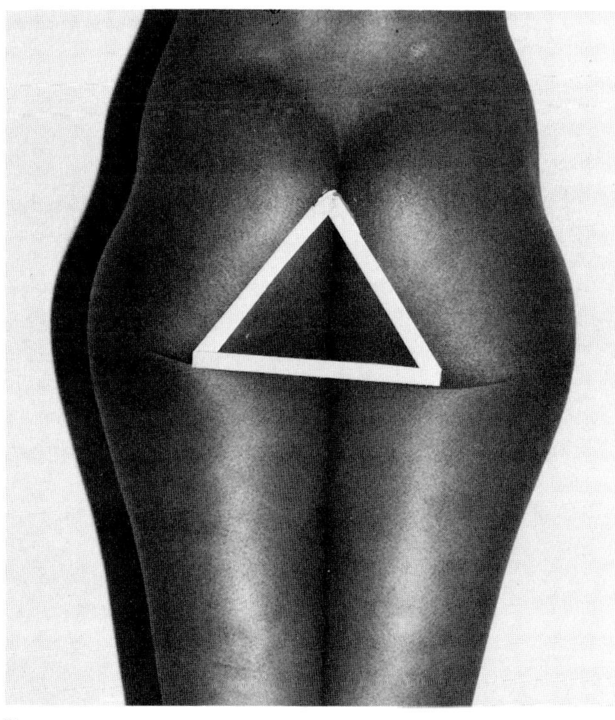

B

Fig. 35-3.
A. Posterior view shows high trochanteric position of excess. Strobe highlight perfectly outlines Illouz "Bermuda Triangle."
B. Bermuda Triangle outlined. Concurrent treatment of buttock and trochanteric area lateral to these markings is necessary for improvement of either. Solitary treatment is contraindicated. (Courtesy of G. Hetter, M.D.)

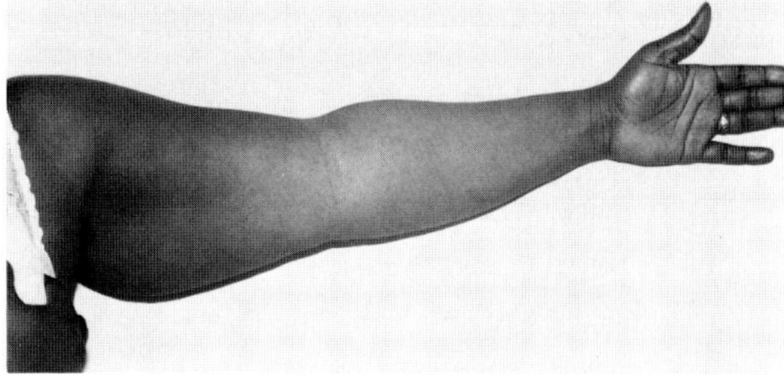

Fig. 35-4. Upper and lower arm segmental fatty disproportion is evident. (Courtesy of G. Hetter, M.D.)

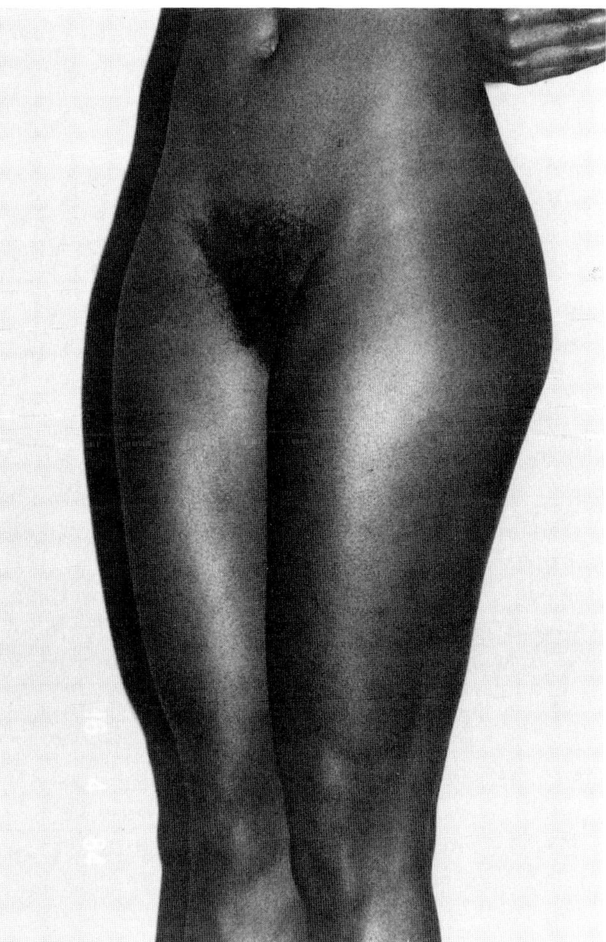

Fig. 35-5. Anterior left oblique view shows the confluency of the high trochanteric adiposity with the steatopygia. Note the circular thighs yet bony knees and flat abdomen without much hypogastric fat. (Courtesy of G. Hetter, M.D.)

treated as often as in whites (e.g., nasolabial folds, jowls, submental, and submandibular areas). However, they are only treated if exaggerated. Associated facial ptosis appears to be rarer in blacks than whites. I believe this is due to the excellent quality of the black skin and the abundance of fatty facial tissue, in contrast with the thinness of the adipose layer of the body in normal black subjects.

8. When treating trochanteric adiposities, one should be aware that the deformity is increased by the weight of the buttocks. The surgeon should not remove too much from the outer thigh, and a lipoplasty of the buttock should always be considered if it is not a pure trochanteric adiposity (without increase of the volume of the buttock) (Fig. 35-5).

Histology of Black Skin and Black Adipose Tissue

The practice of combined procedures (the open technique combined with the closed technique) necessitates a brief review of the microscopic anatomy of the skin of blacks pertinent to the surgeon.

The epidermal corneal layer is much thicker in blacks than in whites and explains the skin's resistance to the scalpel and to needles. Likewise, the connective tissue is more abundant as are the vessels of the dermal and subdermal plexi. I believe the prevalence of elastic muscular fibers explains in part the exaggerated scarring reactions.

Melanin, which is very abundant, is either present freely or contained in the melanocytes throughout the thickness of the epidermis. As in whites, it is absent from the granular layer and from the corneal layer.

Keloids appear to be related to the skin's degree of pigmentation, at least partially. Depending on the ethnic group, the darker the skin color, the more it is to be feared. Keloids are not observed on the palms of the hands or on the soles of the feet, which normally contain no pigment.

The adipose tissue contains more retinacula cutis, fibrous ligaments tethering the skin to the deep fascia, and is more vascularized. Clinically, this makes the adipose tissue seem firmer at the time of the pinching maneuver of the superficial tissue. The adipose layer is more abundant in the face than in Caucasians yet is thinner over the rest of the body in normal subjects.

Operative Impressions

The firmness of superficial tissue is due to skin elasticity and to the abundance of the connective tissue in the adipose layer.

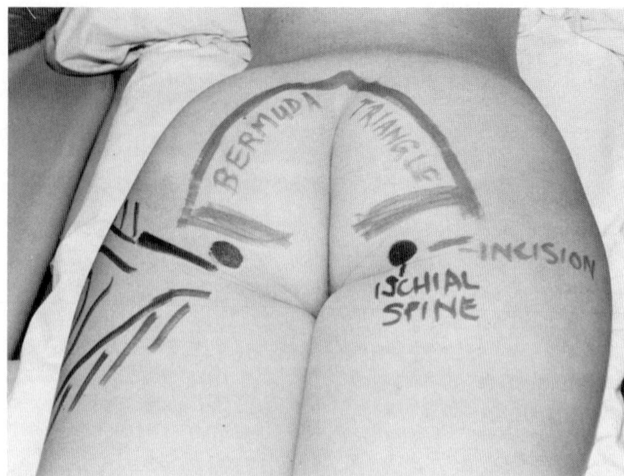

Fig. 35-6. Posterior view shows buttock landmarks on a model.

Operative experience has shown that (1) more force is necessary to pass the lipodissectors (cannulas) in blacks than in whites; this is due to the more abundant connective tissue, and that (2) bleeding appears more common due to the richer vascularization.

Useful Techniques

1. Small-caliber cannulas (#4 or #5) with three openings facilitate the fat extraction and I believe cause less operative bleeding.
2. Decreasing the force of the suction to about 0.7 atm at sea level seems to decrease the bleeding but prolongs the operative time.
3. The use of a low-dose epinephrine solution is useful as recommended by Dr. Hetter, or refrigeration anesthesia may be considered.
4. In combined procedures, a lesser degree of cutaneous pigmentation (all degrees of pigmentation are seen in the black races), or the presence of stretch marks makes poor-quality scars less likely.
5. Vigorous peripheral mesh undermining is necessary despite the excellent skin elasticity due to the high number of retinacula cutis, which prevent the repositioning of the skin over the underlying tissue.
6. The use of an awl instead of a blade to allow penetration of the lipodissector (cannula) through the skin is recommended.

Operative Indications

The indications for an operation are identical to those in Caucasians. However, one must be aware that the size of the adiposities often dictates multiple stages, even if tissue ptosis is never observed due to the excellent skin quality. Combined procedures are particularly frequent

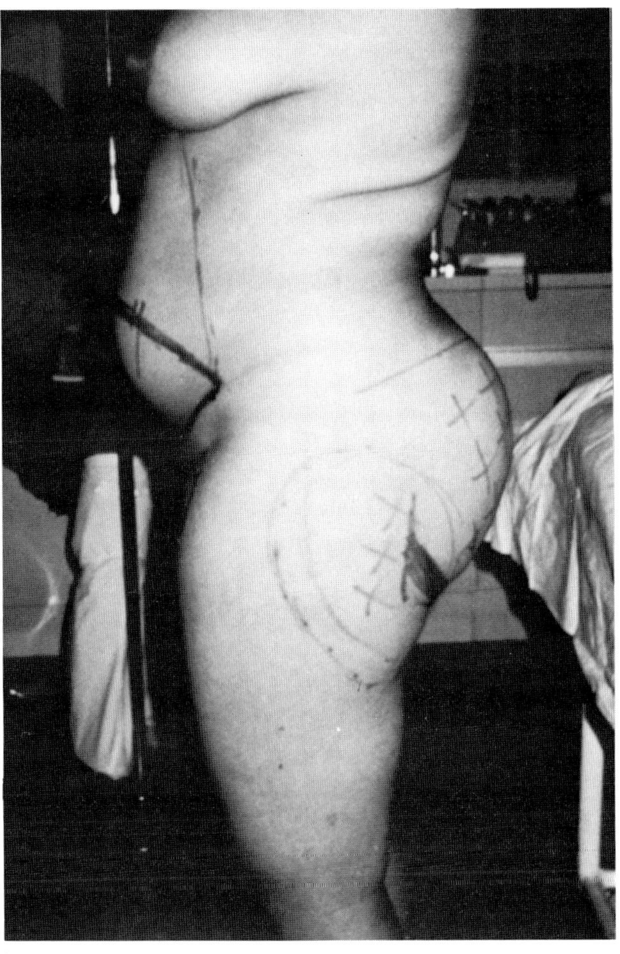

A

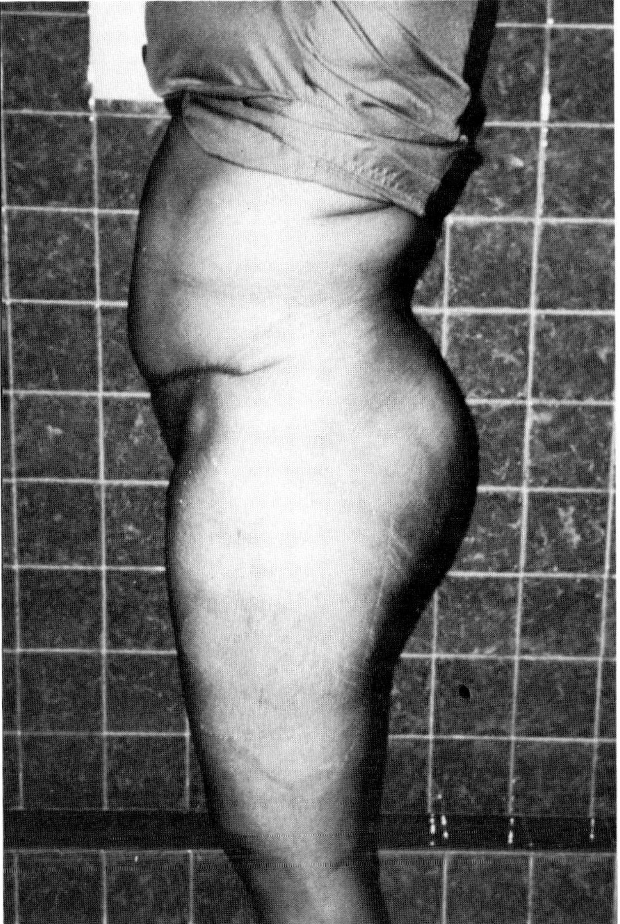

B

Fig. 35-7.
A. Preoperative lateral view of 37-year-old black female with buttock and abdominal excess.
B. Postoperative lateral view at 6 months showing reduction of excess combined with abdominal lipoplasty.

for more general torso obesity or for too many or too early pregnancies. (See Chap. 34). Circular lipoplasties frequently are indicated much more than in whites. Skeletal dysmorphias must be clearly separated from fatty dysmorphias to avoid failure.

Complications

SURGICAL COMPLICATIONS

1. Bleeding is more frequent and more abundant in blacks than in whites.
2. Hematomas have not been observed, but they are more likely in blacks than in whites.
3. The postoperative course is otherwise not different from whites.

AESTHETIC COMPLICATIONS

1. Ptosis has not been observed, even in the case of a block lipectomy leading to a false bursa.
2. Surface irregularities are to be feared less due to the excellent skin elasticity, if associated with a wide peripheral mesh undermining.
3. Poor quality of the scar is the most common aesthetic complication. Scarring in the combined procedures does not differ in the least from scarring of other similar procedures. However, the lessening of the tension on the skin flaps from the defatting seems to be very favorable.

Lipoplasty of the Buttock

The buttock may have considerable amounts of fat, and extractions range from 500 to 3000 ml. The fat is easily removed, especially with small lipodissectors (cannulas).

EVALUATION

Evaluation consists of a visual examination, photographs, and pinch test. The surgeon must appreciate skeletal limitations of silhouette improvement and communicate these limitations to the patient. If the buttock excess is confluent with the trochanteric excess, both should be treated at the same time. Large removals should be staged and the patient forewarned of this necessity.

INCISION

The gluteal depression incision is the most common from which both buttock and trochanteric areas can easily be reached. An infragluteal incision may also be used for criss-cross purposes but alone is much less versatile.

TECHNIQUE

The patient is marked in the standing position. The "Bermuda Triangle" of Illouz is spared (Fig. 35-6). An infragluteal incision is placed at least 3 cm lateral to the ischial spine to avoid unnecessary postoperative pain when sitting. With small cannulas, the gluteal depression incision may be placed wherever swimwear and scant underclothes will cover the tiny scar, and more than one may be placed to allow criss-crossing.

POSTOPERATIVE CARE

Taping with Elastikon or other pressure tape is very useful to splint the buttock, especially if the trochanteric areas are also treated. A compression-type garment or girdle, if properly fitting, is also useful. These garments need to be fitted before the procedure to ensure good fit. The care otherwise is similar to other procedures.

Reduction in buttock mass allows more standard clothing styles to be worn. Figure 35-7 shows the typical improvement obtained by the removal of 1200 ml fat.

Summary

Simple or combined lipoplasty is frequent in blacks. The morphology in certain cases can differ from that of Caucasians, and the differences noted in the operating room can be explained by the histological appearance of the integument.

Aesthetic complications are less common than in Caucasians due to the excellent skin elasticity and its resistance to waviness, ptosis, and aging.

CHAPTER 36

Contour Deformities of the Upper Thigh

Norman Martin

Contour deformities of the upper thigh represent the largest single area of patient and physician dissatisfaction after suction extraction procedures to that region. The upper thigh is also the location of the greatest number of secondary revisions. The anticipation or avoidance of a contour deformity is of paramount importance if success with this technique is to be achieved.

As the initial postoperative bruising and swelling subsides, the physician and patient begin to note the emergence of residual bulges, apparently new folds, or, occasionally, depressed areas in the skin and subcutaneous fat. Some of these manifestations are temporary and resolve in time. Most of these conditions present for 3 months or more are permanent. The large majority could have been anticipated or avoided.

Based on an analysis of 800 consecutive lipolysis procedures on the upper thighs over a 3-year period, a classification of contour deformities has been developed.

An ongoing periodic review of the pre- and postoperative photographs of most of these patients was performed. An analysis of the specific surgical techniques used during the initial procedures, as well as an analysis of the surgical techniques used in secondary procedures, was made. This experience has led to a method of anticipating, minimizing, or avoiding many of the contour deformities listed in Table 36-1.

Preexisting Contour Deformities

Protruding localized bulges of fat obviously are the reasons that the patient has presented himself or herself. However, certain types of body configurations and skin textures lend themselves less well to suction lipectomy and are predestined to result in a contour deformity no matter how carefully and extensively the fat extraction has been performed (Figs. 36-1, and 36-2). Certain other contour deformities noted postoperatively can actually be seen, but are not readily recognized in the preoperative photographs (Figs. 36-3 and 36-4). These incipient contour deformities become noticeable because they become *smaller* after surgery. Recognition during surgery is extremely difficult since the gravitational pull on the prone patient is anteroposterior, as opposed to superoinferior in the erect patient. Therefore, it is extremely important to recognize the incipient problem before surgery, so that additional fat can be removed in that area. A useful maneuver to judge the adequacy of fat removal to the upper outer thigh during surgery is described in Figure 36-5.

Developmental concavities located at the lateral buttock area (gluteal depression) just below the iliac crest and above the upper lateral thigh have very little fat, and

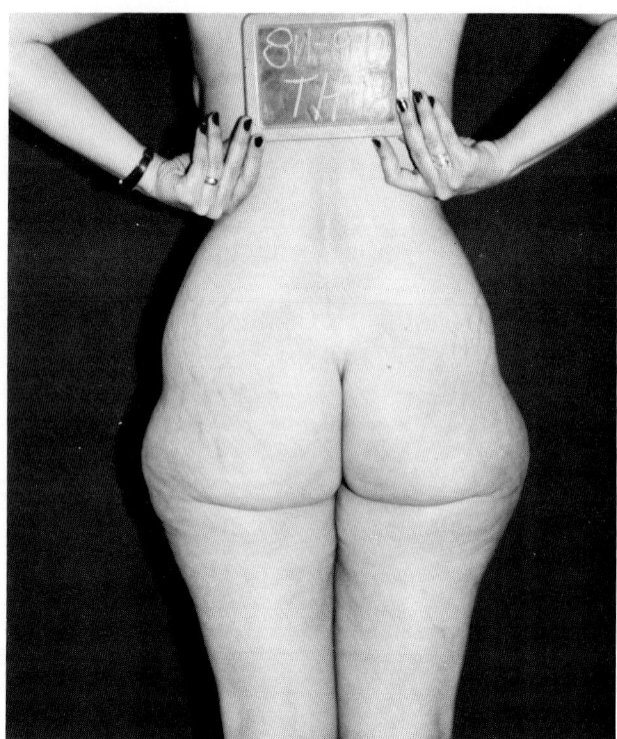

Fig. 36-1. Photograph of patient before suction lipectomy. Note severe striae.

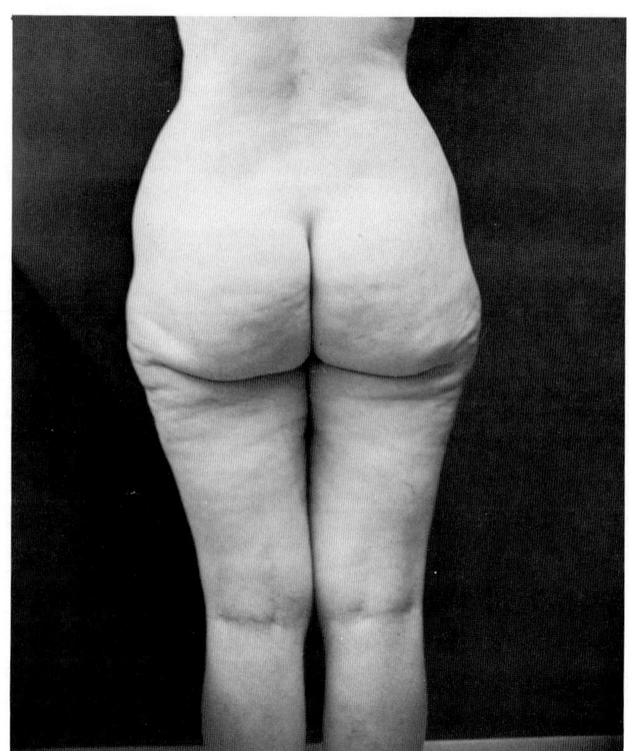

Fig. 36-2. Same patient as in Fig. 36-1 21 months after surgery. Contour deformities are due to an inability of skin to contract further.

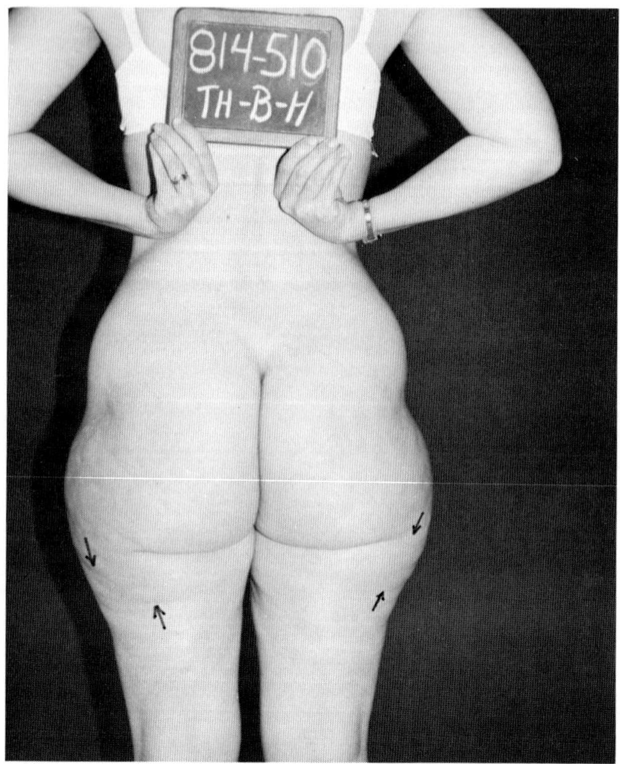

Fig. 36-3. Preexisting incipient contour deformity *(arrows)*.

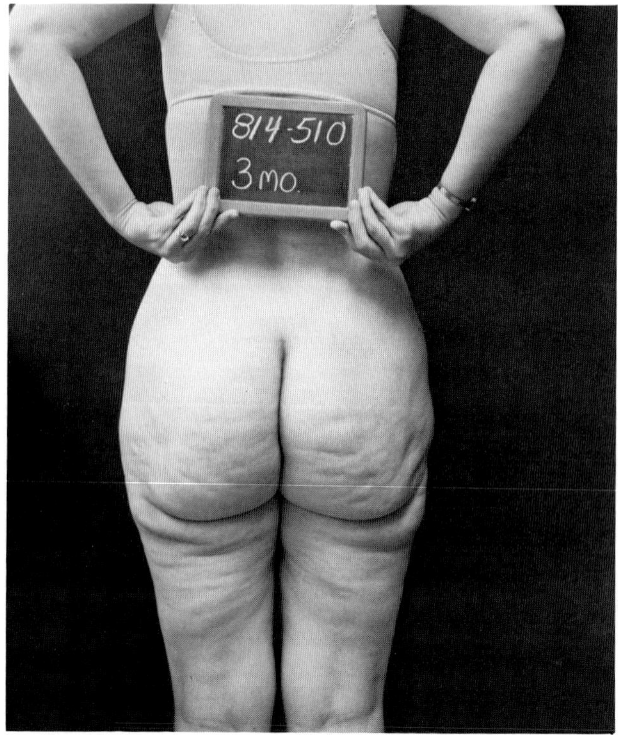

Fig. 36-4. Banana-type contour deformities 10 months after the operation.

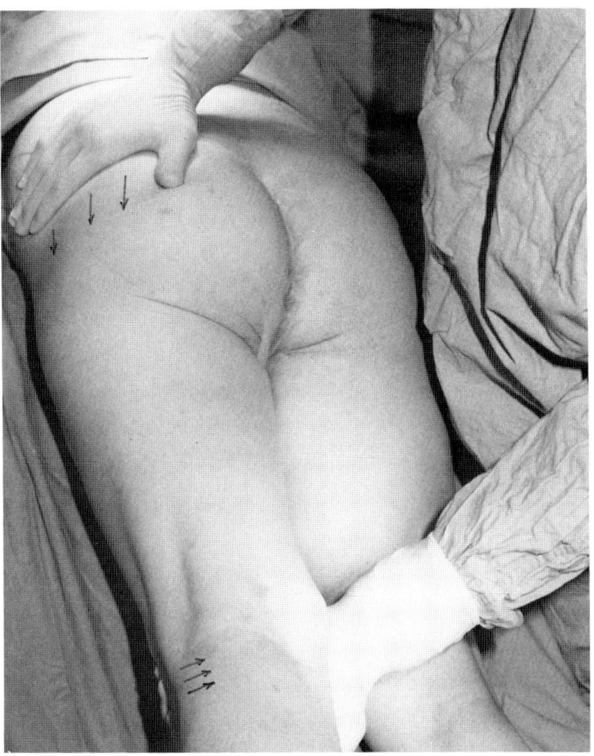

Fig. 36-5. Gravitational forces on the upper lateral thigh can be simulated in the prone patient by elevating the extended knee while at the same time making downward pressure on the upper buttock area (Martin Maneuver).

Table 36-1. Classification of contour deformities of the upper thigh

I. Preexisting deformity
  A. Protruding
    1. Apparent
    2. Inapparent
  B. Receding
    1. Large concavities
      a. Developmental
      b. Traumatic
      c. Postoperative
    2. Dimpling
      a. Localized
      b. Diffuse
    3. Waviness
  C. Asymmetry
II. Postoperative deformity
  A. Temporary
  B. Permanent
    1. Waviness
    2. Asymmetry due to structural differences
    3. Deformity due to loss of elasticity
  C. Avoidable
    1. Lateral thighs
    2. Posterior thighs
III. Iatrogenic deformity
  A. Dents and depressions
  B. Waviness
  C. Asymmetric fat removal
  D. Fat removal from areas that should be avoided
  E. Drooping buttocks
  F. The gluteal fold

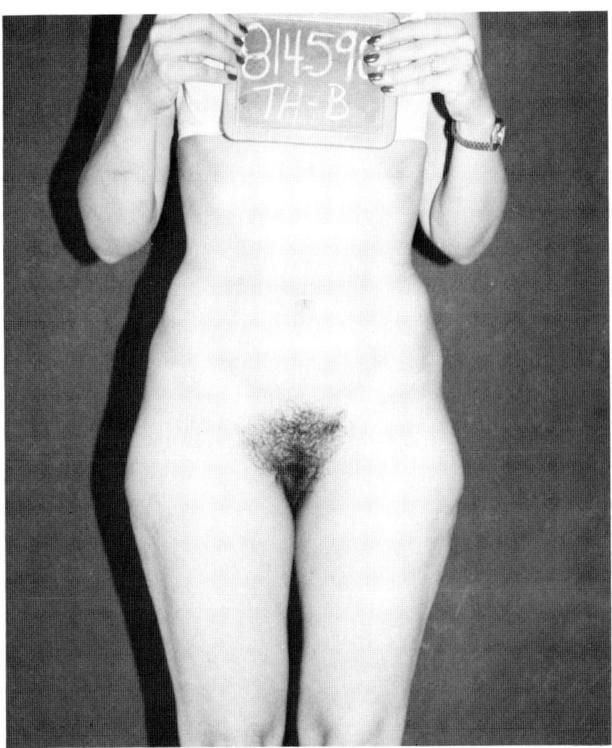

Fig. 36-6. Lateral thigh concavities in preoperative photos.

therefore no suction is indicated in this hollow. A relative contour deformity can result in such patients when lateral thigh fat is removed and no iliac crest fat is extracted.

A shallow anatomical concavity over the tensor fascia lata is present in many women (Fig. 36-6), particularly in those with excellent muscle tone. Suction must be extremely judicious in this area to avoid producing a localized depression in the mid- and lower-lateral thigh (Fig. 36-7). This anatomical concavity is best visualized with the patient in the standing position. The change from concavity to bulge in the contour of the lateral thigh can sometimes be abrupt, and delicate "feathering" is required to achieve a smooth postoperative contour.

Traumatic and surgical concavities and contour deformities are relatively common (Fig. 36-8). Careful evaluation of the surrounding fat is important to avoid enlarging the defect. Secondary fatty deformities of the lateral thighs, resulting from previous surgery for "epitrochanteric" fat deposits, readily respond to the lipolysis technique.

Localized dents and dimples usually involve the skin and subcutaneous fat and therefore usually remain after the lipolysis procedure. It is extremely important to document and point out these isolated contour deformities to the patient *preoperatively.* Diffuse dimpling (the "cottage cheese" look) implies poor skin elasticity

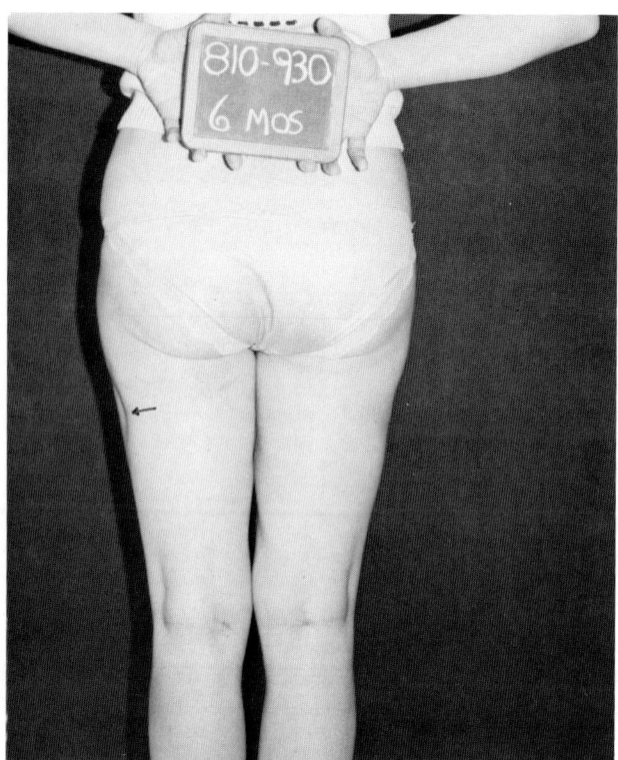

Fig. 36-7. Surgically induced localized concavity *(arrow)*.

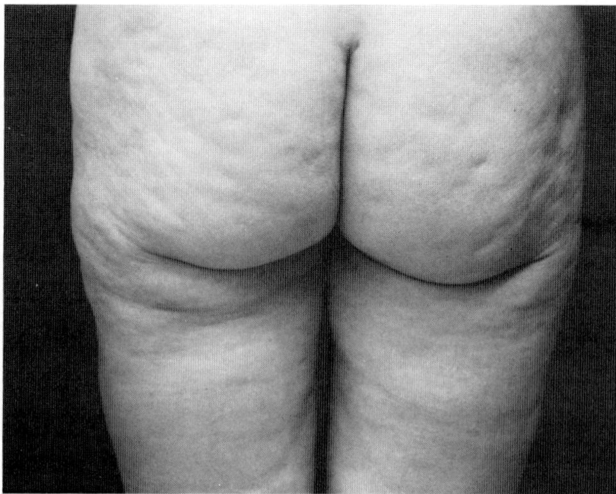

Fig. 36-9. Diffuse dimpling.

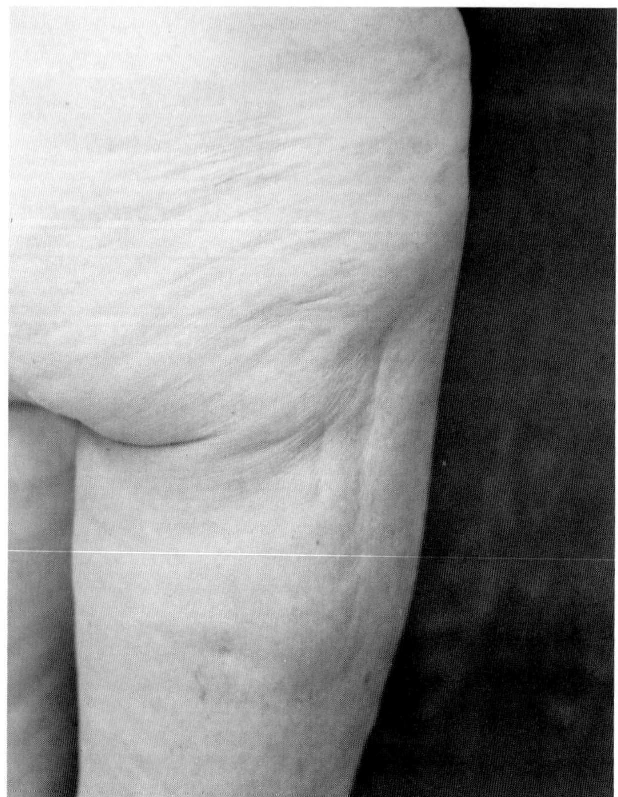

Fig. 36-8. Preexisting, surgical, and traumatic contour deformities of the lateral and posterior thigh.

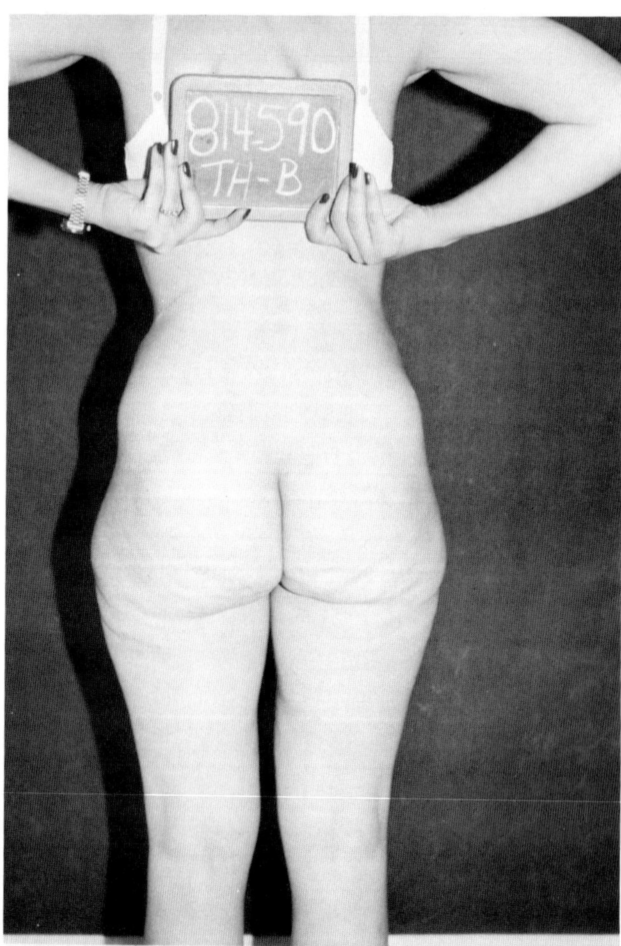

Fig. 36-10. Preexisting waviness.

and almost certain postoperative contour deformities of both the segmental and depression variety (Fig. 36-9).

Preexisting waviness is often found in older patients, particularly those who have had repeated significant weight changes or multiple pregnancies (Fig. 36-10).

Asymmetry of the lateral thigh area is frequently the result of slight skeletal abnormalities such as scoliosis or leg length inequality. Such asymmetry should be carefully searched for preoperatively and documented photographically. It is important to begin lipolysis on the "larger" side.

Postoperative Contour Deformities

Temporary irregularities for up to 3 months are expected sequelae to the procedure and vary with the operator and the extent of the surgical procedure, as modified by the patient's own tissue response, age, and physical condition.

Extensive lipolysis procedures on the posterolateral thigh performed on patients with decreased skin elasticity either due to age, weight fluctuation, or excessive solar exposure inevitably lead to waviness or segmental contour deformity focused at the lateral aspect of the gluteal fold (Figs. 36-11 and 36-12). This waviness or deformity can be prevented, or at least minimized, by avoiding aspiration of the posterior thigh and by "planing" off the bulge at the inferolateral aspect of the buttock-lateral thigh area while at the same time staying extra deep to the skin with the cannulization.

Severe structural abnormalities, either bony or muscular, may produce asymmetries of fatty tissues that cannot be equalized with the lipolysis technique. When dealing with a severe asymmetry, always suction the *larger* side first.

The technique and method of cannulization used on the lateral thigh area can determine the extent of contour deformity present after surgery. In general, the suction cannulization should be carried out first in the deepest portion of the fatty bulge, with gradual feathering motions circumferentially. At all times it is paramount to avoid creating a large cavity or undermining of the area, because this will always result in an undesirable contour deformity both above and below the previous bulge. Cannula thrusts should be varied as to their plane within the fat, particularly in the 1 to 3 inches immediately lateral to the incision to avoid creating a waviness. The general rule on lateral thighs is the deeper into the fat the cannulization, the less chance for a contour deformity.

Fat extraction in the posterior thighs should be approached with caution, particularly in patients over 40 years of age and in obese patients without excellent skin

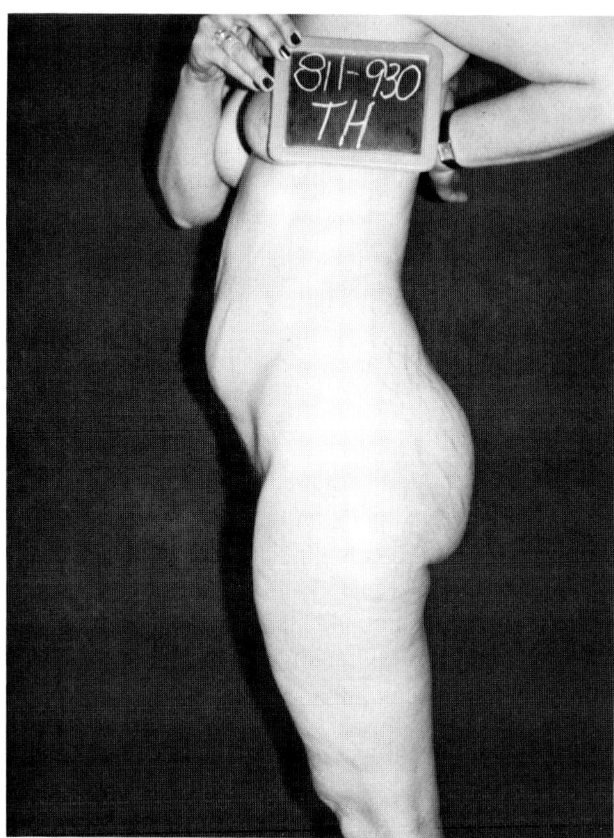

Fig. 36-11. Preoperative view showing incipient buttock ptosis.

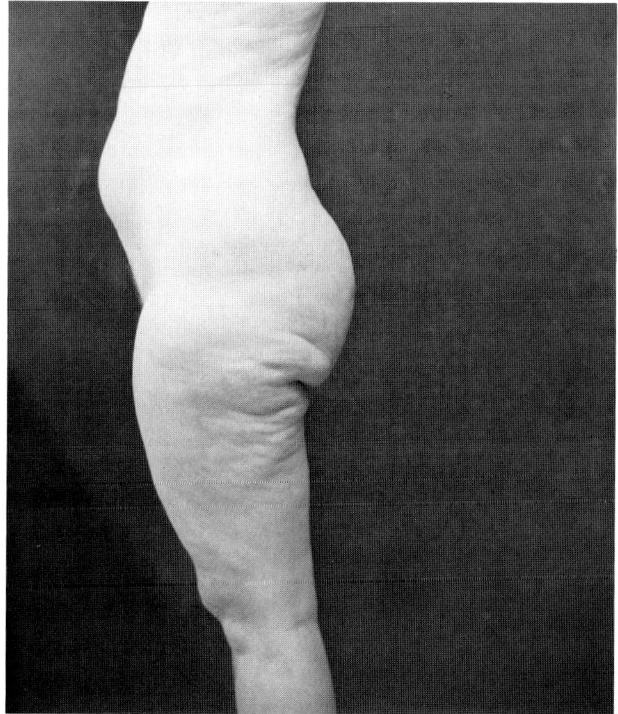

Fig. 36-12. Waviness and segmental contour deformities 21 months after extensive lipolysis of the posterior and lateral thighs with aggravation of buttock ptosis.

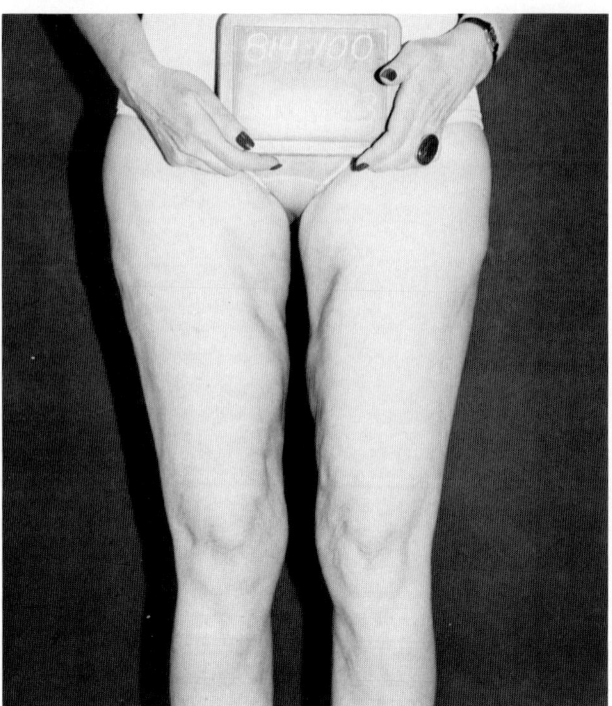

Fig. 36-13. Medial thigh contour deformity due to extensive fat removal in patient with poor tissue elasticity.

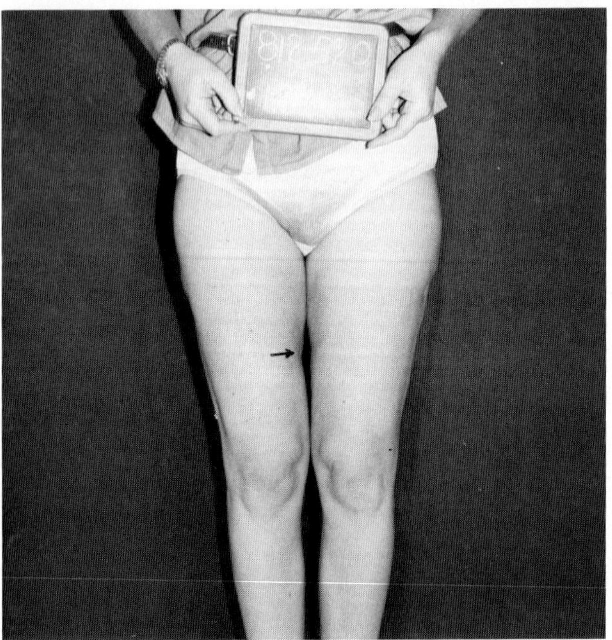

Fig. 36-14. Suction in the midmedial thigh area *(arrow)* should be avoided, otherwise a bow-legged appearance will result.

elasticity. There appears to be a buttressing effect by the posterior thigh fat on the lower buttocks and injudicious fat removal in this area produces an apparent drop of the buttocks (Figs. 36-11 and 36-12).

Iatrogenic Contour Deformities

Dents and depressions (see Figs. 36-7 and 36-13) on the lateral and medial thighs represent the largest and most disconcerting group of contour deformities. *Most are not correctable by secondary procedures.* The obvious cause of such depressions is the loss of fat from the superficial layer, thereby causing a lack of support for the cutaneous tissues. Several factors can account for the inadvertent superficial cannulization:

1. The cannula is inserted too superficially.
2. Suction is applied while the cannula opening is facing the undersurface of the skin.
3. The cannula is twisted by a too-rigid suction tubing without the operator realizing it.
4. Angulated cannulas seem to tent-up the tissues on the lateral thigh and suck in superficial fat at the distal tip.

Waviness to a greater or lesser degree appears to be a function of the technique. It is related to the patient's age, skin condition, and amount of fat removed (provided the procedure is carried out properly and at the proper levels).

Asymmetric fat removal is the easiest contour deformity to correct. Secondary procedures involving small areas can be readily carried out under local anesthesia. Small-caliber cannulas (6 mm) allow for adequate vacuum, easy feathering motions, and minimal pain and discomfort for the patient.

Avoided areas include the medial thigh area midway between the knee and inguinal area (Fig. 36-14). Suction of the *anterior* thigh fat results in a washboard appearance of the skin surface. As mentioned previously, suctioning in developmental concavities of the lateral buttock and mid- and lower-lateral thighs should be approached judiciously. Suction around the natal cleft is to be avoided since a flattened buttock will result. Removal of the inferior buttock bulge in all but the lateral aspect results in a more accentuated drooping (see Figs. 36-11 and 36-12).

The attempt to create a gluteal fold where little or none existed previously carries several risks: (1) a double fold may result (Fig. 36-15), (2) removal of posterior thigh fat can result in a slight drooping appearance of the buttocks on side view (Figs. 36-16, 36-17 and 36-18), and (3) fold length may be unequal and necessitate a second procedure for correction.

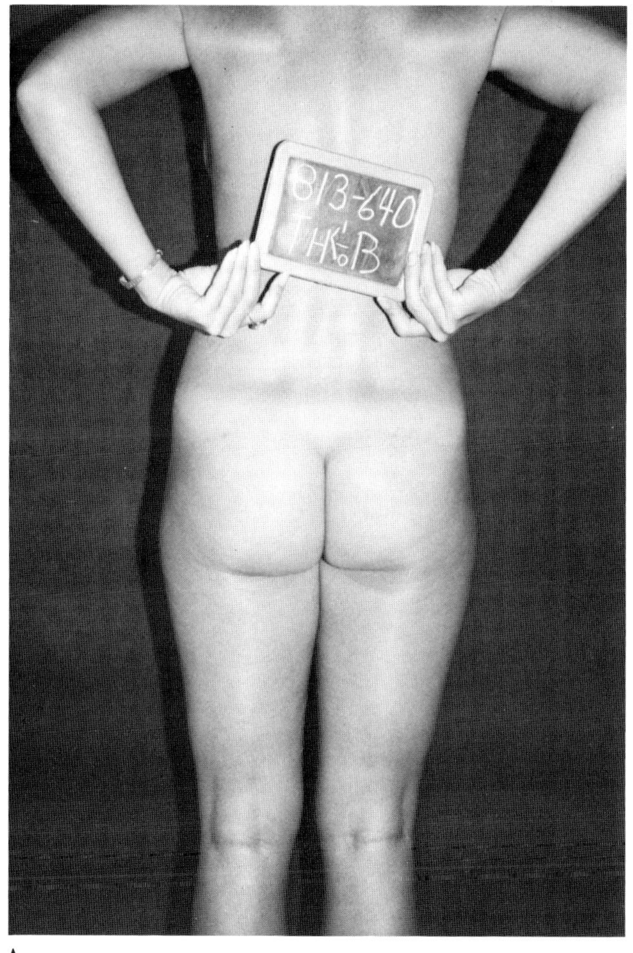
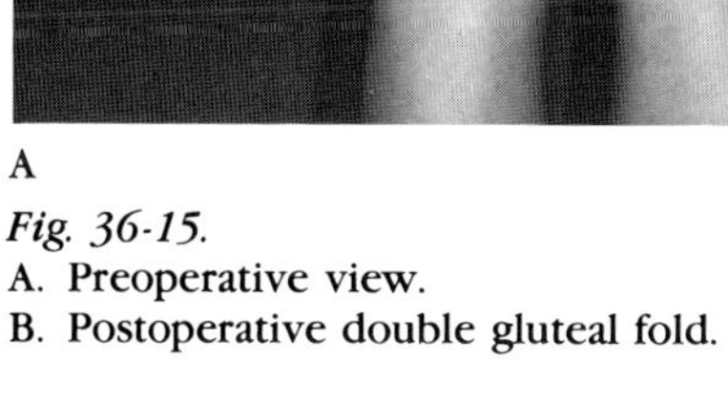

A

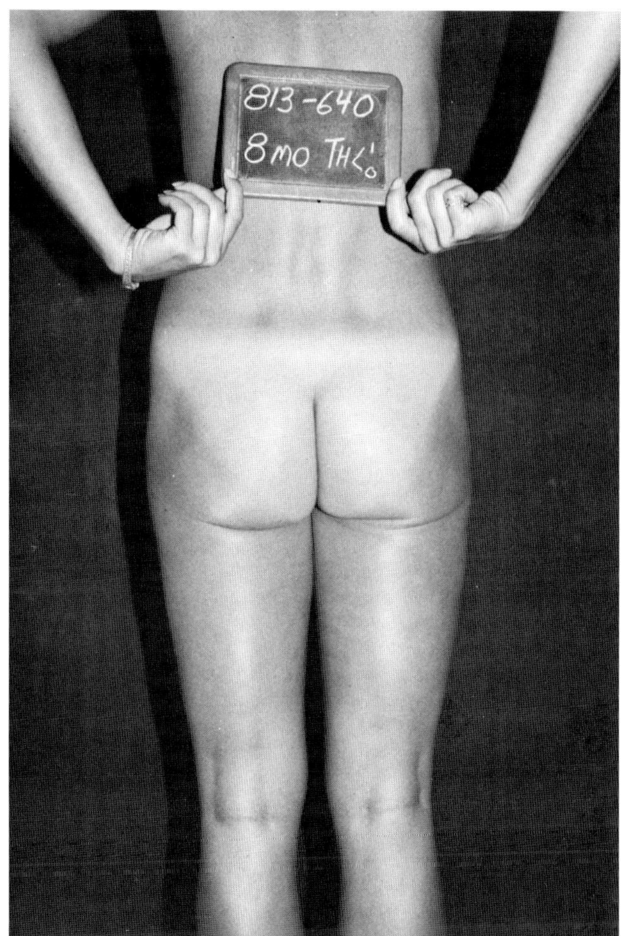

B

Fig. 36-15.
A. Preoperative view.
B. Postoperative double gluteal fold.

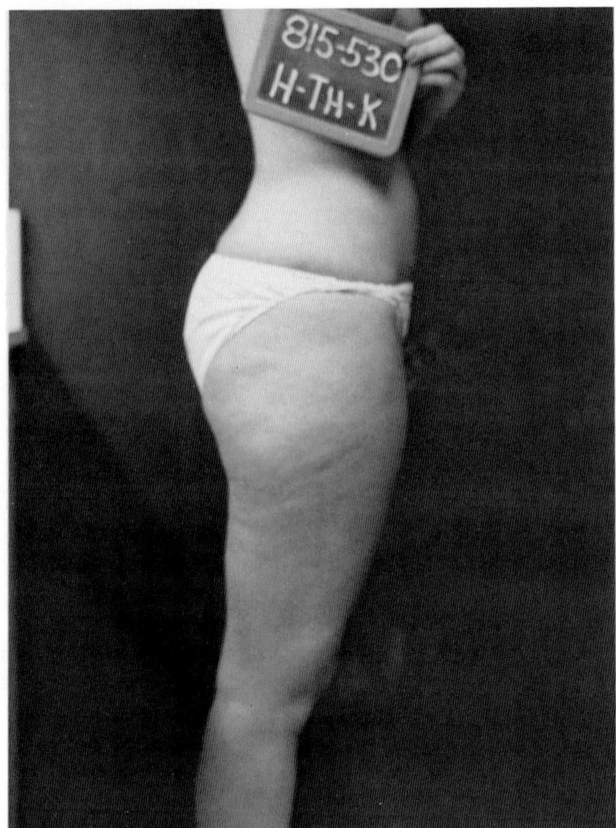

Fig. 36-16. Preoperative gluteal fold and posterior thigh fat removal.

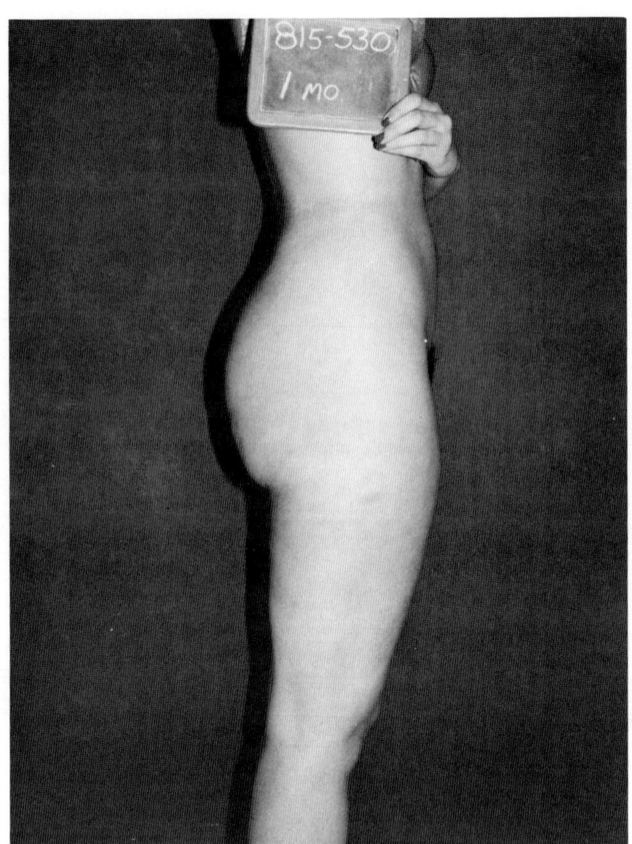

Fig. 36-17. Same patient as in Fig. 36-16 one month later.

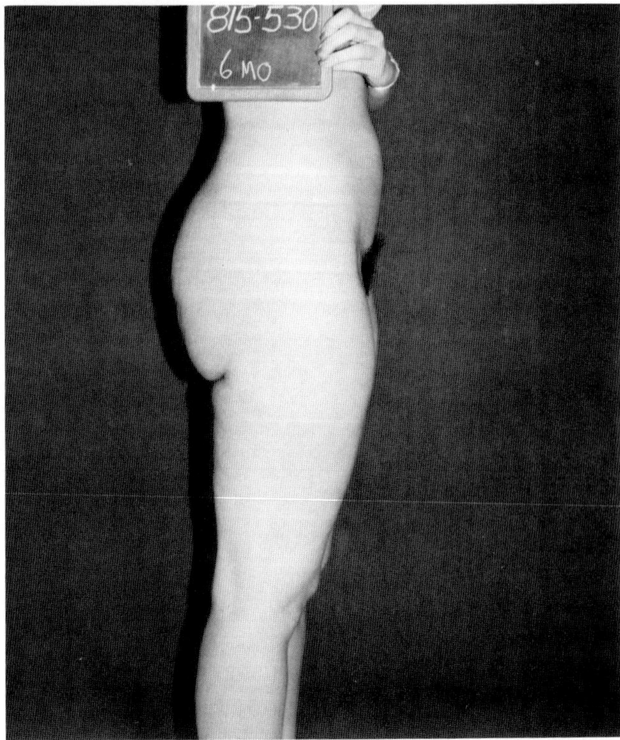

Fig. 36-18. Same patient as in Fig. 36-16 six months after the operation. Note buttocks droop.

CHAPTER 37

The Defatting of Flaps by Lipolysis

James O. Stallings

Lipolysis by the Illouz blunt cannula technique represents a major new weapon system in the treatment arsenal of the reconstructive plastic surgeon. The mind-set of the patient is critical. The reconstructive patient is generally satisfied with only an improvement; however, the aesthetic patient frequently expects and often demands a miracle. Proceeding on the premise that the body is nothing more than a series of complex flaps, this chapter presents 11 case studies that exemplify the uses of lipolysis in reconstructive plastic surgery.

Case Studies

Case 1. J.C. is a 33-year-old woman who sustained a gunshot wound to her mandible (Fig. 37-1). She lost her mandible from angle to angle, with a loss of overlying soft tissue and a considerable loss from the floor of the mouth. Figure 37-1B shows her in front view after a one-stage mandibular reconstruction from angle to angle, using a microvascular free flap of iliac crest based on the deep circumflex iliac artery and vein. Additional soft tissue in the form of a tensor fascia lata microvascular free flap based on the lateral circumflex femoral artery and veins was also used. All microvascular anastomoses were done end-to-side to the external carotid artery and internal jugular vein.

Figure 37-1C shows an intermediate stage of the reconstruction after extensive lipolysis and standard flap revision using some of the extra tissue to reconstruct the floor of the mouth. Lipolysis at no time ever compromised the vascularity of the flap. Further stages of surgery are planned to get the optimal reconstruction for this patient.

Case 2. S.S. is a 23-year-old man who sustained an industrial-related injury to his right hand. All the skin distal to the wrist on both the flexor and extensor aspects of the hand was avulsed as seen in Figure 37-2A. He had stumps of index and middle fingers left intact; after several debridement procedures, a large microvascular free flap of tensor fascia lata as a myocutaneous flap was transferred (17 cm wide, 45 cm long).

Anastomosis of the lateral circumflex femoral artery was done end-to-side to the ulnar artery. One lateral circumflex femoral vein was anastomosed end-to-side to the basilic vein and the other end-to-side to one of the ulnar vena comitantes. Figure 37-2C shows the early bulky flap. Figure 37-2E shows an intermediate result after three episodes of lipolysis and standard flap revision, including an iliac bone graft to give length to the index and middle finger stumps. S.S. has MP flexion and extension, so that he has a mobile post. His thumb was not significantly injured. At no time did lipolysis compromise the vascularity of the flap. This patient has returned to work. Further revision is planned to obtain the optimal result.

Case 3. V.A. is a 45-year-old right-handed man who sustained industrial trauma, including burns to his right hand with expo-

The author acknowledges the assistance of the following surgeons, who are members of the Mercy Hospital Medical Center Department of Plastic and Reconstructive Surgery, Microvascular, and Microsurgical Team, in the management of these patients: Justin Ban, N. K. Pandeya, Lee Abramsohn, Ronald S. Bergman, and Carlene Dam.

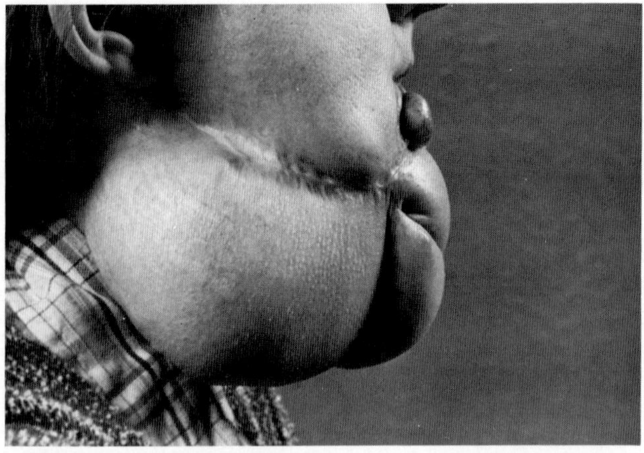

A

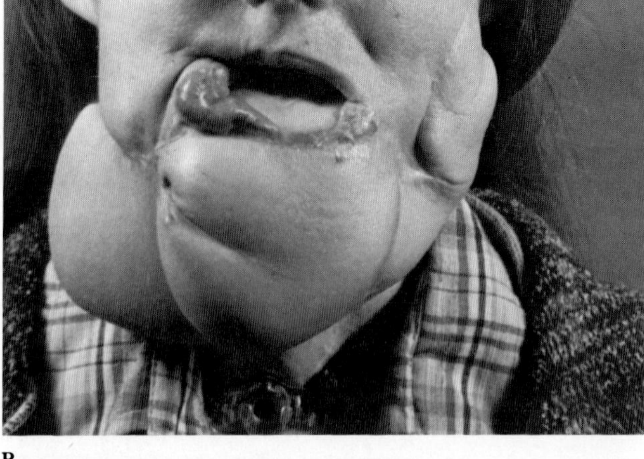

B

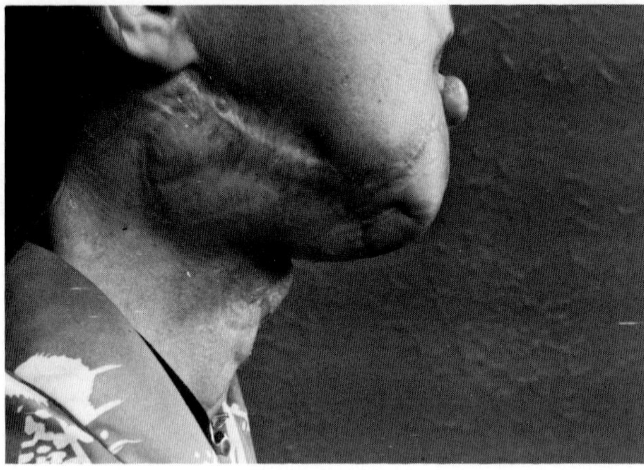

C

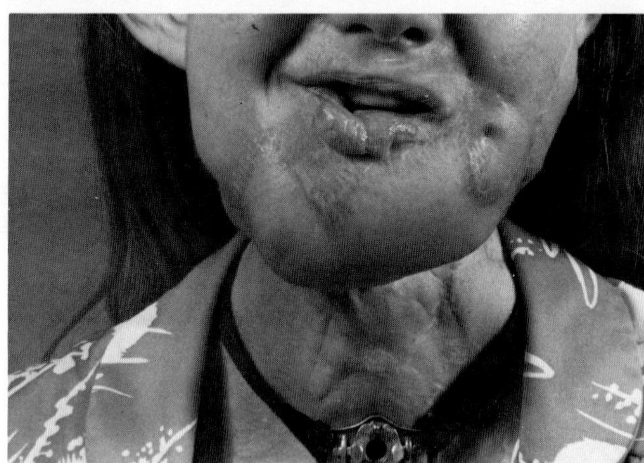

D

Fig. 37-1.
A. Right lateral view after microvascular free flap transfer of iliac crest and associated tensor fascia lata as a myocutaneous flap to reconstruct mandible and floor of mouth from angle to angle.
B. Front view of the same procedure.
C. Right lateral view after lipolysis and standard flap revision.
D. Front view after the same procedure.

Fig. 37-2.
A. Volar view of avulsion injury to right hand.
B. Dorsal view of avulsion injury to right hand. The thumb was not seriously injured.
C. Dorsal view of bulky microvascular tensor fascia lata myocutaneous free flap.
D. Radial view of the same flap.
E. Dorsal view after extensive lipolysis and standard flap revision and iliac bone grafting to the index and middle finger stumps.
F. Volar view after extensive lipolysis and standard flap revision and iliac bone grafting to the index and middle finger stumps and skin grafting to the palm to give a better gripping surface. The tensor fascia lata flap formerly on the palm was elevated and advanced distally to make room for the iliac bone graft on the index and middle fingers; then the palm was skin grafted.

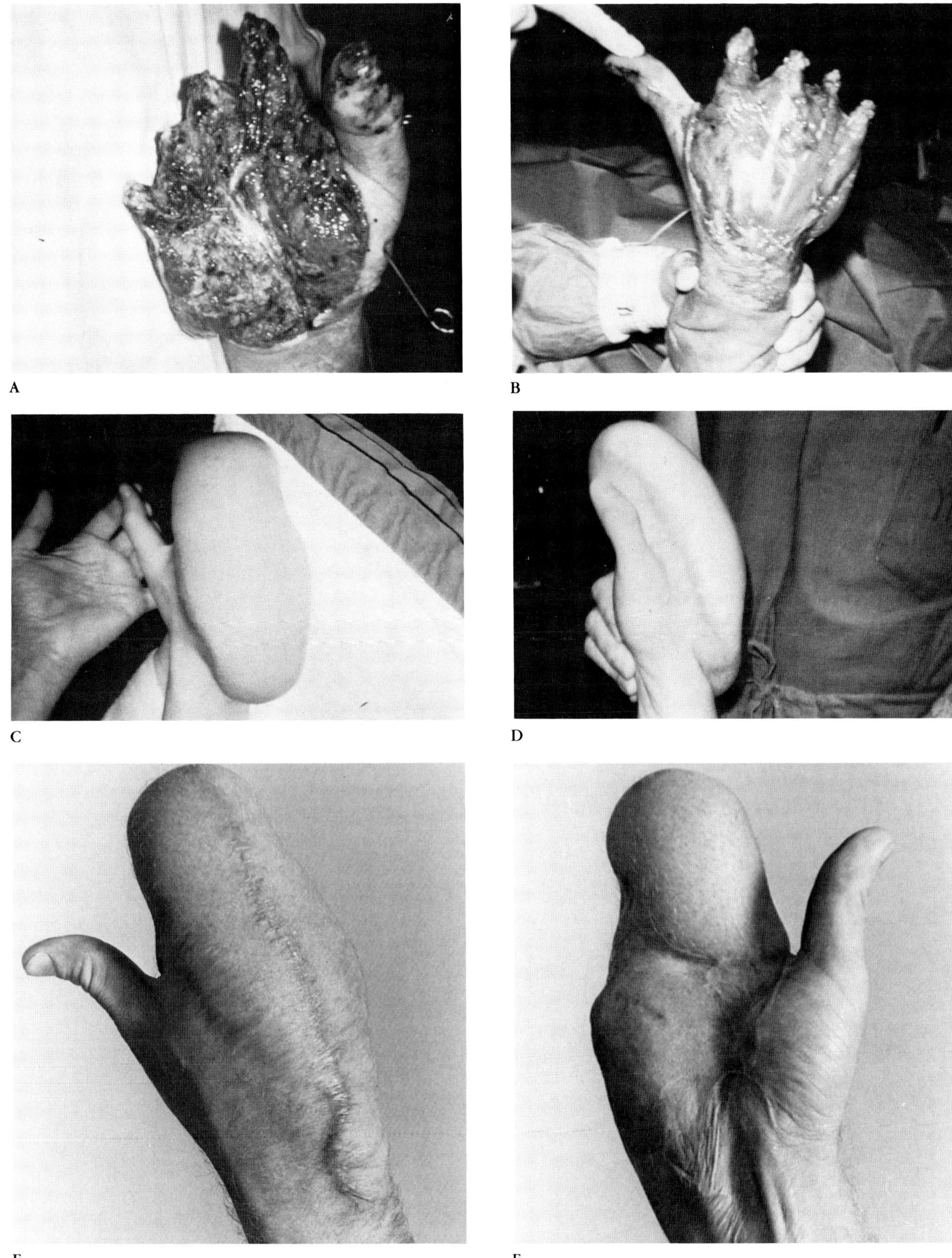

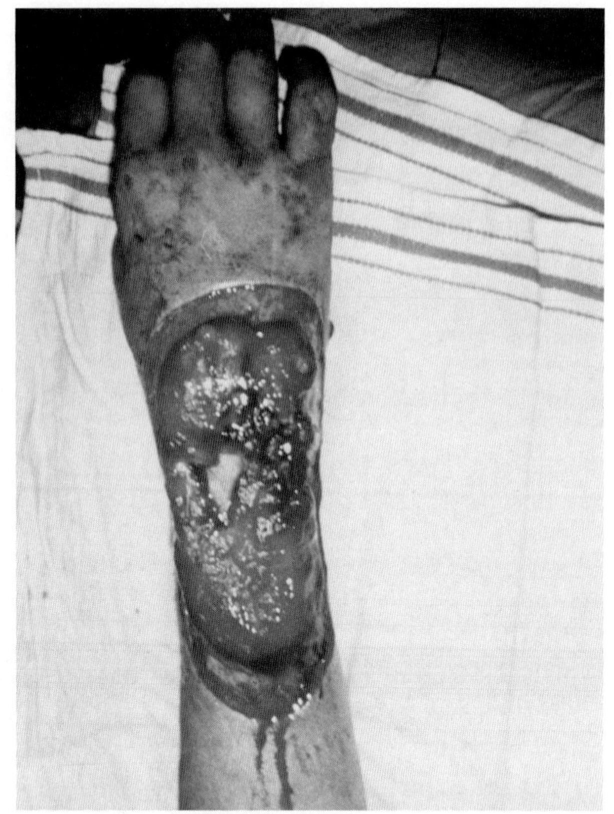

A

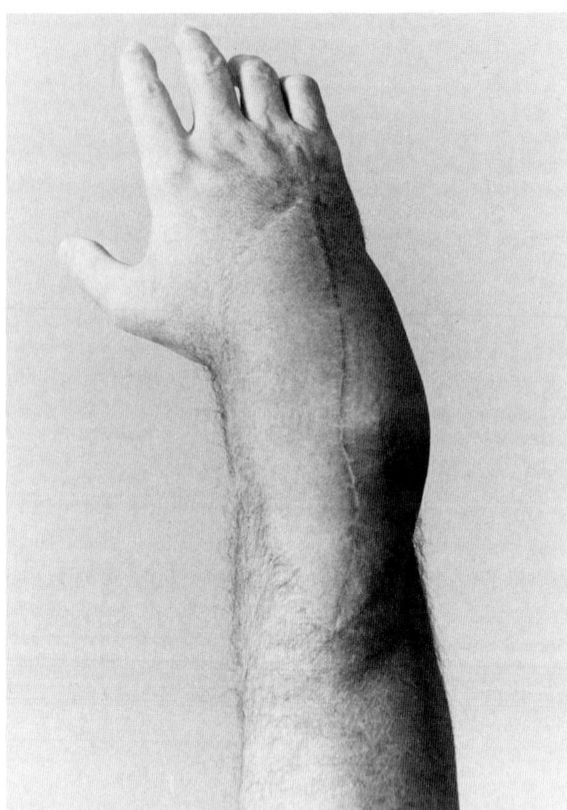

C

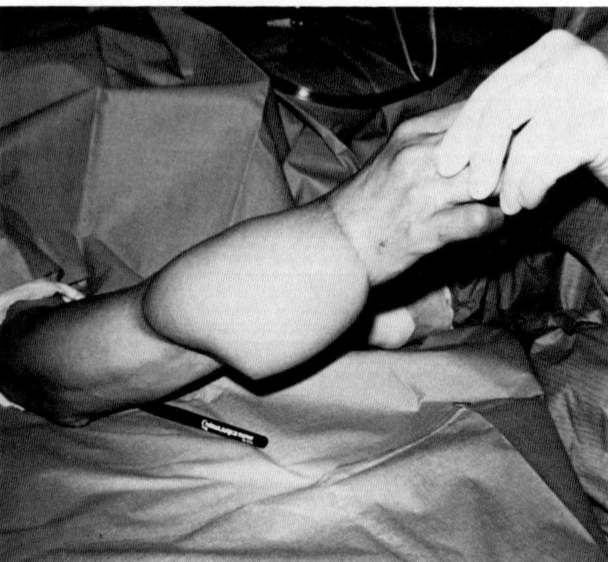

B

Fig. 37-3.
A. Avulsion injury of right forearm with exposed radius and ulna.
B. Bulky microvascular latissimus dorsi myocutaneous free flap.
C, D. Intermediate stage of reconstruction after extensive lipolysis, standard flap revision, and multiple tendon transfers to restore extension to the wrist and fingers.

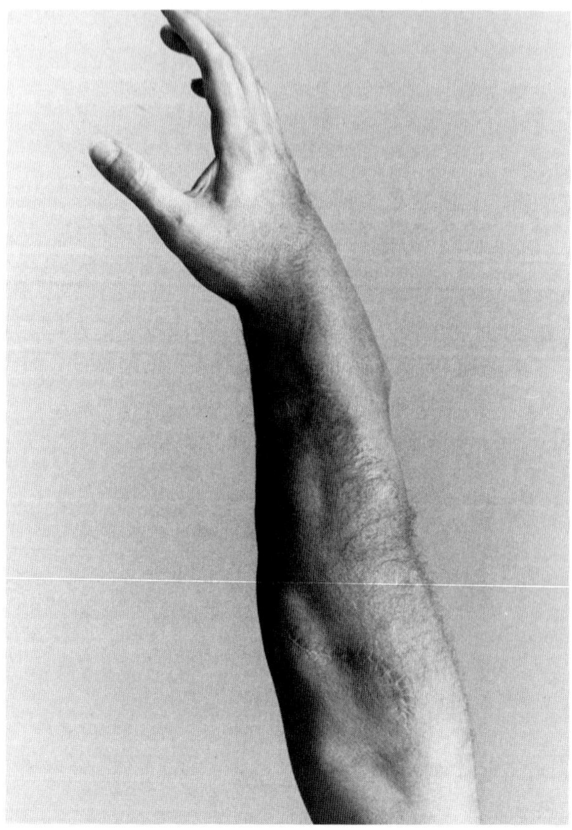

D

sure of the radius and ulna and avulsion of all the extensors of the hand and wrist, except the extensor pollicus brevis. He had multiple burns of his body, so a local trunk flap was not deemed suitable. Accordingly, a large latissimus dorsi microvascular myocutaneous free flap (measuring 16 cm wide by 22 cm long) was transferred to his right forearm as the first stage of reconstruction. The thoracodorsal artery was anastomosed end-to-side to the radial artery, and the thoracodorsal vein was anastomosed end-to-end to the radial vena comitantes.

Figure 37-3A shows the wound, and Figure 37-3B shows the successfully transplanted latissimus dorsi myocutaneous microvascular free flap. Figure 37-3C shows an intermediate stage of reconstruction after standard flap revision, including lipolysis and reconstruction of wrist and finger extension using pronator teres and flexor carpi ulnaris tendon transfers extended by tensor fascia lata grafts. At no time did lipolysis interfere with the vascularity of the flap. Further work is planned.

Case 4. J.W. is a 36-year-old woman who had a basal cell carcinoma on the dorsum of her nose that was treated with Mohs' chemosurgery by one of our local dermatologists, Dr. Roger Ceilley. The defect was through-and-through, and she requested that no additional scars of the cheeks and lower face be caused by the reconstruction, so we mutually agreed on the scalping flap technique of Converse as the procedure of choice.

Figure 37-4A shows the original defect. Figure 37-4B shows the scalping flap in place according to the technique of Converse. Figure 37-4C shows the excessive tissue after the return of the scalping flap and after skin grafting of the forehead. Figure 37-4D shows an intermediate result after extensive lipolysis and standard flap revision. At no time did lipolysis cause vascular embarrassment to the flap. The patient is very content with the result and currently desires no further surgery, although more improvement is possible.

Case 5. E.W. is a 55-year-old woman who had a right radical mastectomy and a left simple mastectomy. The right radical mastectomy was followed by postoperative irradiation, and she developed lymphedema of the right arm. She underwent right latissimus dorsi myocutaneous flap to the right chest, along with left simple mastectomy as the first stage. Figure 37-5A shows the preoperative situation.

The patient wished to keep the donor site on her back to a minimum, so she asked that I not completely resurface her right chest, which detracts from the final result, but I acceded to her request. Figure 37-5B shows the right latissimus dorsi myocutaneous flap in position along with the left simple mastectomy. Figure 37-5C shows a later stage of bilateral breast reconstruction. Figure 37-5D shows our latest result after lipolysis of the reconstructed right breast, along with judicious lipolysis of the posterior aspect of the lymphedematous upper extremity. Standard flap revision was also done on the reconstructed right breast. At no time did lipolysis cause any vascular embarrassment to either flap.

E.W. reports that the judicious lipolysis of the lymphedematous right upper extremity has relieved quite a bit of the tenseness and discomfort caused by the tightness of the arm. She continues to wear a supportive elastic stocking on the right arm and has lost 2 cm in circumference, measuring preoperatively at 34 cm and postoperatively at 32 cm. The patient is delighted with her surgery, although the irradiated upper anterior chest skin does detract from the final result.

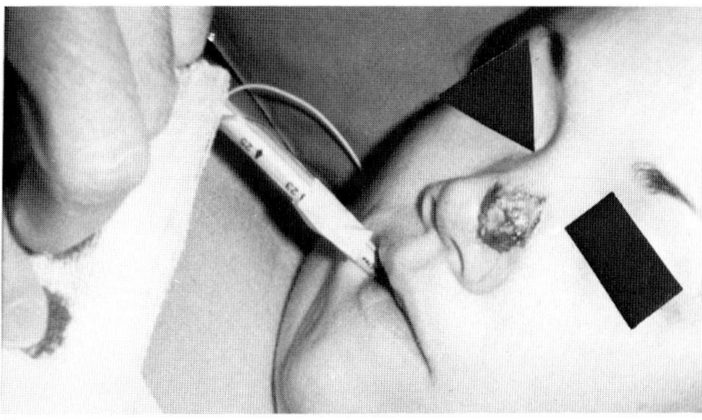

A

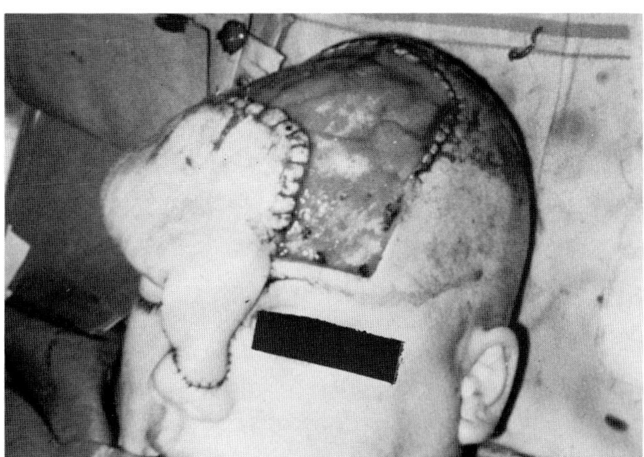

B

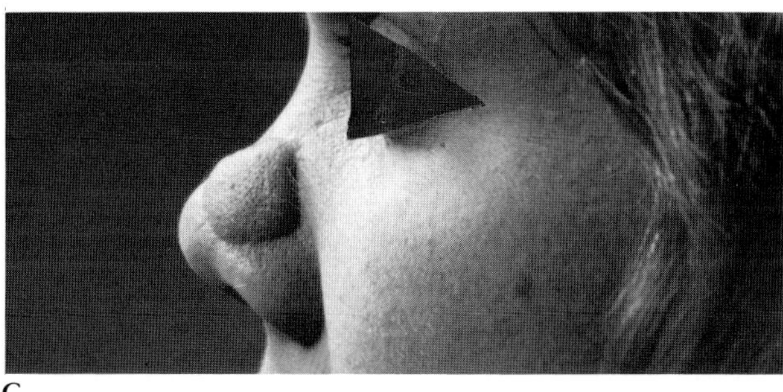

C

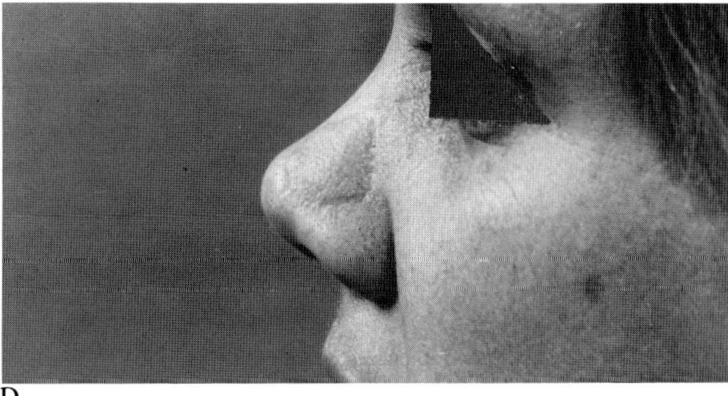

D

Fig. 37-4.
A. Large through-and-through defect of the nose following Mohs' chemosurgery for basal cell carcinoma.
B. Scalping flap in place according to the technique of Converse.
C. Bulky forehead flap on the nose.
D. Intermediate result after extensive lipolysis and standard flap revision.

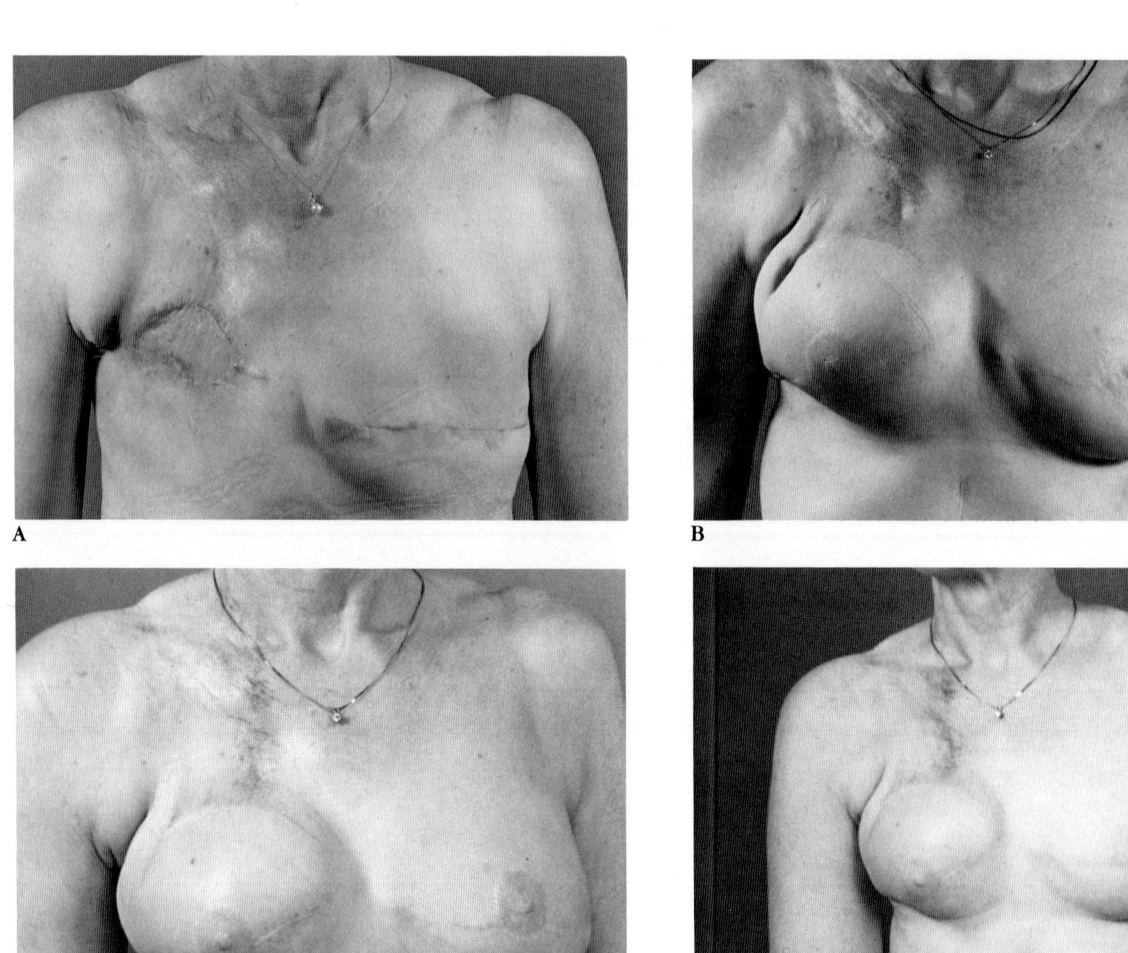

Fig. 37-5.
A. Front view of right radical mastectomy. Note the severely irradiated tissue over her upper chest.
B. Front view of right latissimus dorsi myocutaneous flap in position along with the left simple mastectomy (reconstructed).
C. Intermediate stage of bilateral breast reconstruction after lipolysis and standard flap revision.
D. Most recent result after extensive lipolysis of the reconstructed right breast along with standard flap revision, and also after judicious lipolysis of the posterior aspect of the lymphedematous right upper extremity.

Case 6. L.R. is a 16-year-old girl who sustained severe burns of her right upper extremity. She received excellent treatment at one of the Shriner's Hospitals, including skin grafting and a pedicled groin flap to her right wrist and forearm. Figure 37-6A shows the way she originally presented to me with multiple scars and a bulky groin flap to her right wrist and forearm. Figure 37-6C shows an intermediate result after two flap revisions, including lipolysis and standard flap revision. Lipolysis was done not only at the bulky groin flap, but also to help blend in the area around the ulnar aspect of her elbow. At no time did lipolysis compromise the vascularity of the flap. Further work is planned to obtain the best result. She is pleased with her progress.

Case 7. C.L. is a 19-year-old woman who had a Clark level 3 malignant melanoma that was widely excised from her left shoulder and upper arm with skin grafting by a general surgeon. Figure 37-7A shows the way she presented to me with the large defect of her left shoulder and upper arm. Figure 37-7C shows an intermediate stage after several serial excisions, including lipolysis, to more harmoniously blend in the depressed skin graft area with the surrounding tissues. At no time did lipolysis compromise the vascularity of the flap. Further work is planned.

Case 8. L.Q. is a 27-year-old left-handed man who sustained an industrial burn to his left wrist, causing severe impairment of motion. This problem could have been treated with a trunk flap, but the patient preferred a microvascular free flap of tensor fascia lata as a myocutaneous free flap (34 cm long and 15 cm wide). Anastomoses were done end-to-side to the radial artery, cephalic vein, and radial venae comitantes. Figure 37-8A shows the bulky tensor fascia lata myocutaneous microvascular free flap. Figure 37-8C shows an intermediate stage using lipolysis with a #3 cannula. Figure 37-8E shows the most recent result after lipolysis and standard flap revision. Further work is planned. At no time did lipolysis cause any vascular compromise of the flap.

Case 9. O.C. is a 43-year-old woman who had a longstanding, painful ulcer on her left foot. Arteriograms showed impaired arterial circulation beginning near the junction of the upper calf and middle calf areas. She and her family physician asked me to try to save the foot through microsurgery, and our microvascular team did just this. We transferred a large latissimus dorsi myocutaneous microvascular free flap measuring 14 cm wide by 30 cm long. Anastomosis of the thoracodorsal vein was done end-to-side to the posterior tibial vein, and anastomosis of the thoracodorsal artery was done end-to-side to the posterior tibial artery. Figure 37-9A shows the ulceration on the sole of her left foot. Figure 37-9B shows the large microvascular flap of latissimus dorsi as a myocutaneous free flap. Figure 37-9D shows the most recent result after two flap revisions including lipolysis. At no time did lipolysis compromise the vascularity of the flap. She is now able to walk and get around just fine. Further work is planned.

Case 10. R.B. is a 30-year-old right-handed man, who approximately 10 years ago severed his brachial artery and ulnar nerve. He was primarily repaired in another city by another surgeon. His complaints when he came to see me were not only the obvious deformity shown in Figure 37-10A, but also severe cold intolerance in his hand and absolutely no padding on the ulnar aspect of his hand.

The first stage of his reconstruction was to reconstruct his ulnar artery, which was completely occluded. The technique

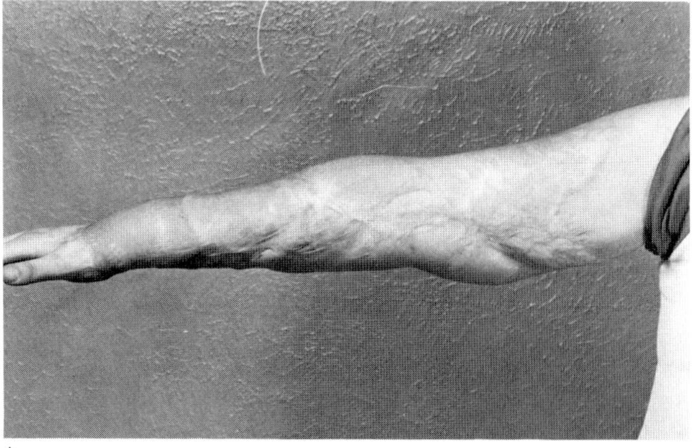

A

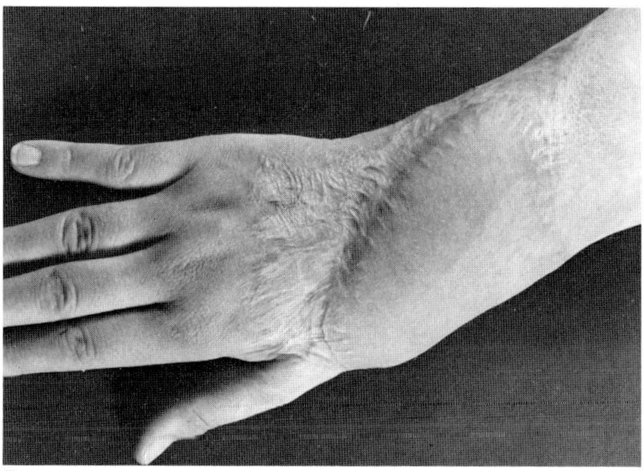

B

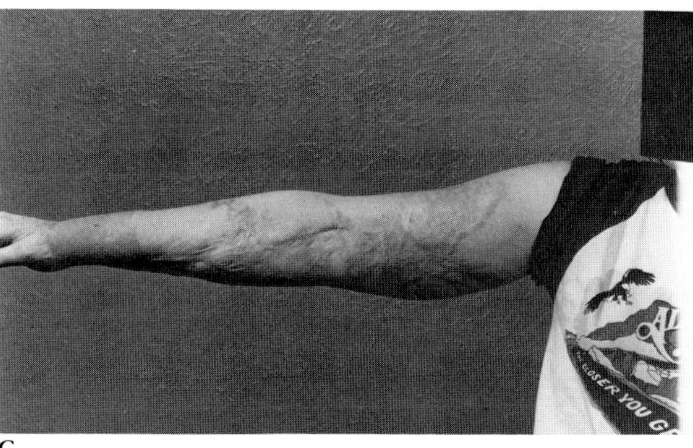

C

Fig. 37-6.
A. Multiple scars of right wrist, forearm, and upper arm with a bulky groin flap when first seen by me.
B. Close-up of bulky pedicled groin flap to right wrist, hand, and forearm.
C. Intermediate result after extensive lipolysis of bulky groin flap and judicious lipolysis of upper arm along with standard flap and scar revision.

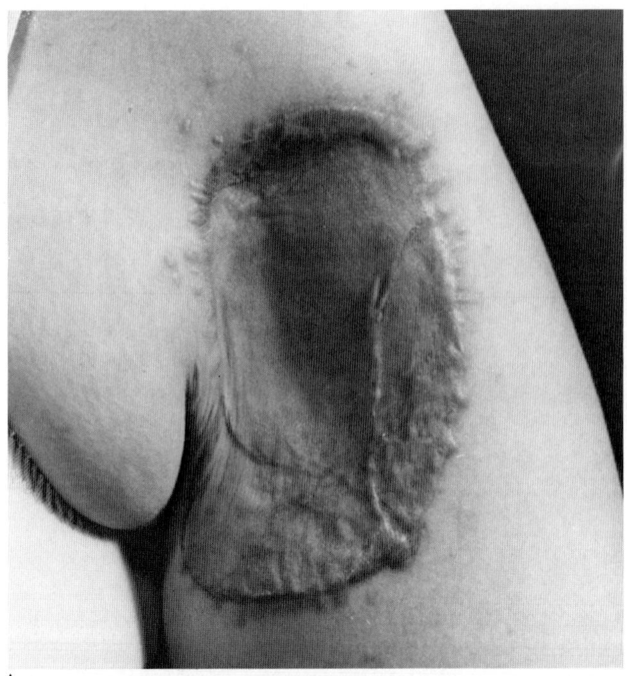

A

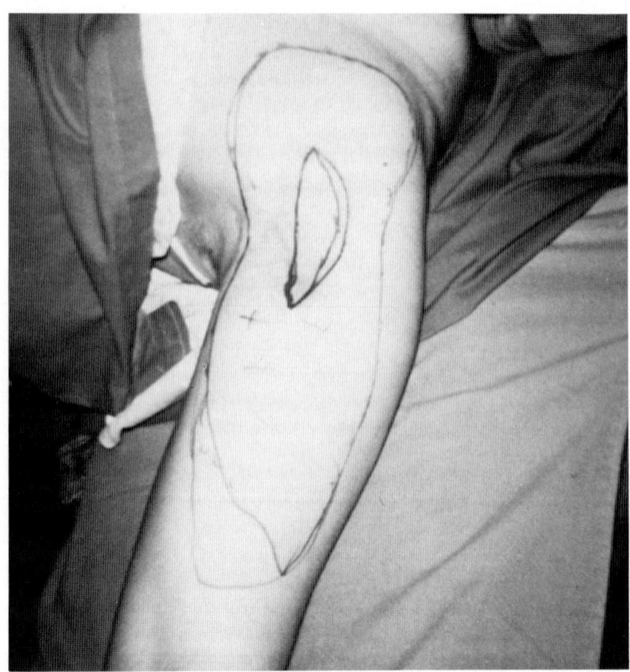

B

Fig. 37-7.
A. Status after excision of malignant melanoma from the left shoulder and upper arm, with skin grafting.
B. Intraoperative photograph depicting area of serial excision and extent of lipolysis of the anterior axillary fold and shoulder and upper arm areas.
C. Intermediate stage after several serial excisions, including extensive lipolysis.

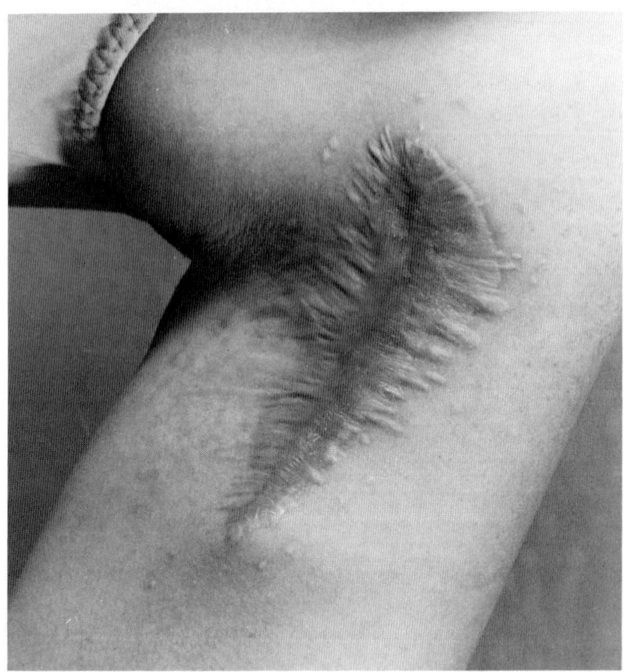

C

Fig. 37-8. ▶
A. Volar view of bulky microvascular tensor fascia lata myocutaneous free flap to right hand, wrist, and forearm.
B. Dorsal view of the bulky tensor fascia lata free flap.
C. Intermediate stage intraoperative photograph showing lipolysis of the flap using a #3 cannula.
D. Fat is seen in the cannular tubing.
E, F. Most recent result after extensive lipolysis and standard flap revision in two views.

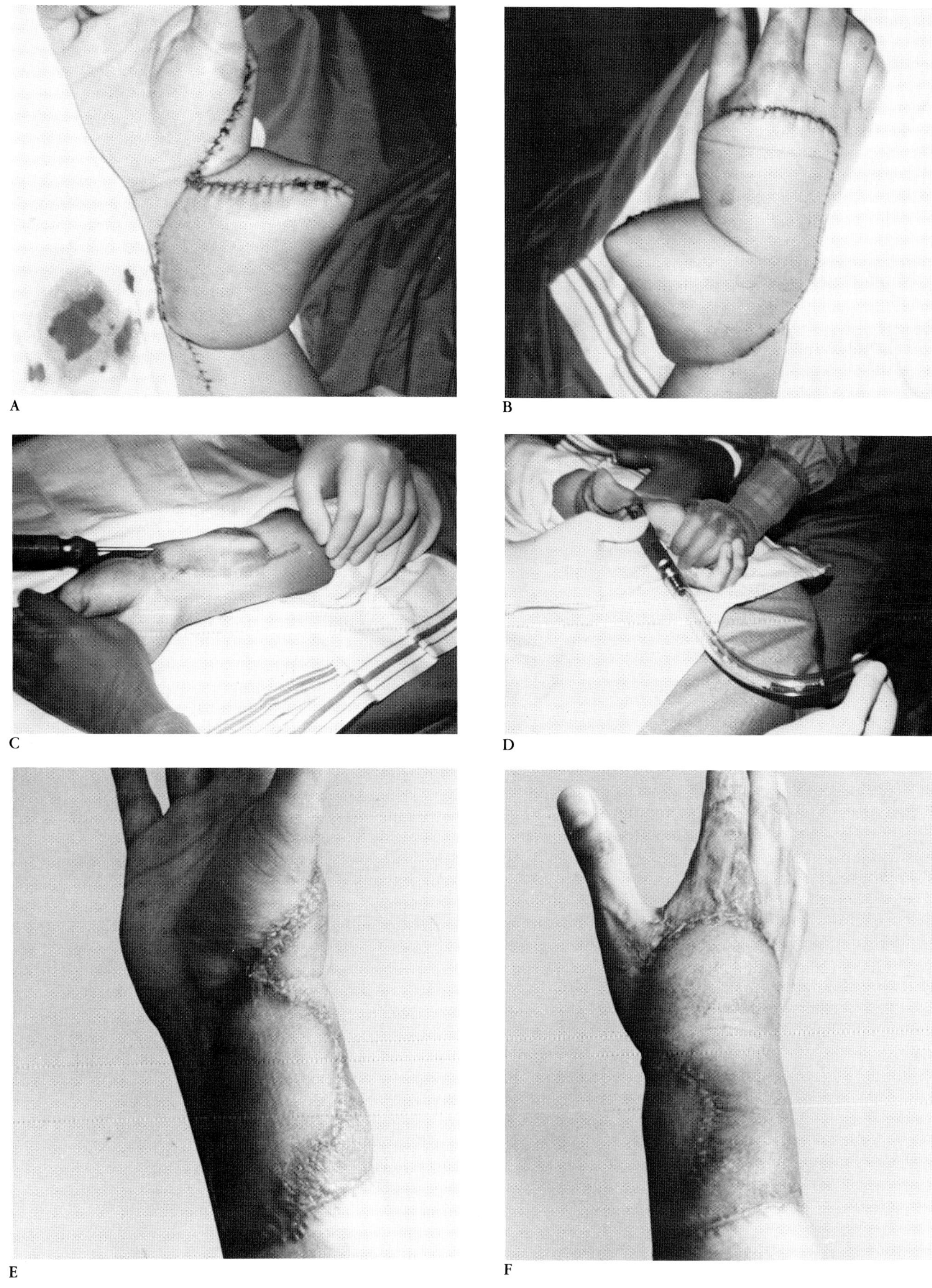

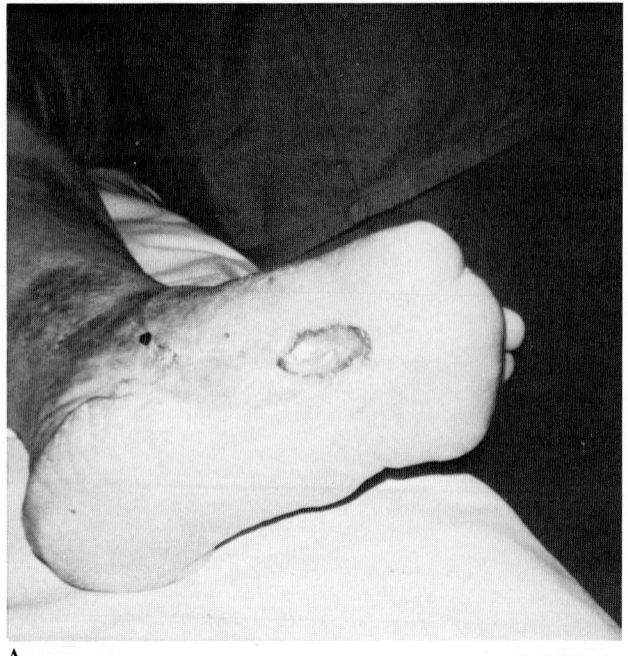

A

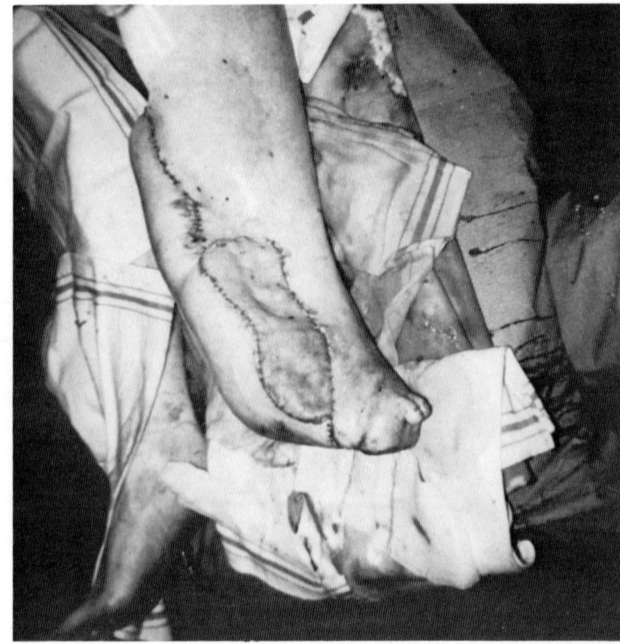

B

C

Fig. 37-9.

A. Longstanding ulceration on the bottom of the left foot, along with poor-quality skin more proximal in the ankle area.

B. Intraoperative view of large, bulky latissimus dorsi myocutaneous microvascular free flap to left leg and foot.

C. Intraoperative photo of standard flap revision. The areas outside the ink underwent extensive lipolysis.

D. Most recent result after extensive lipolysis and standard flap revision.

D

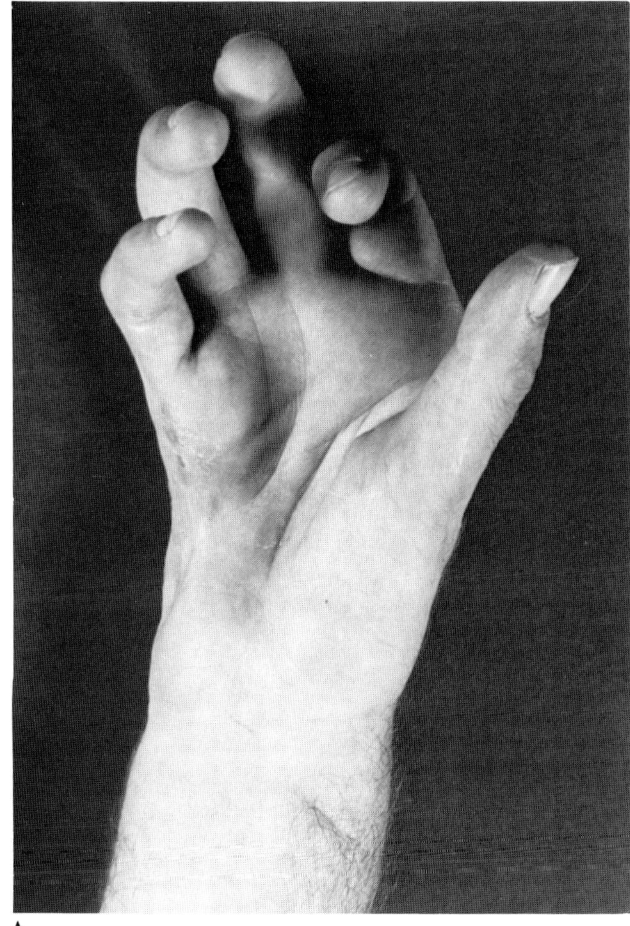

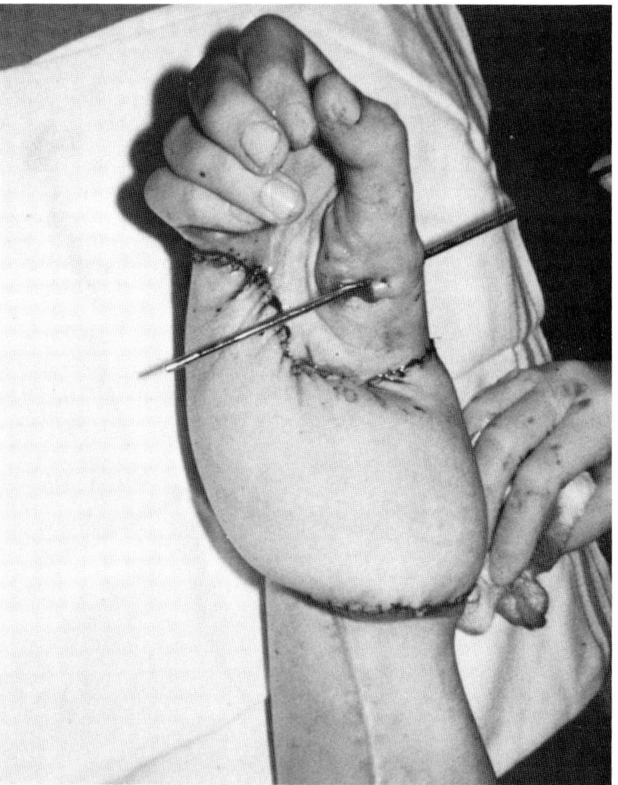

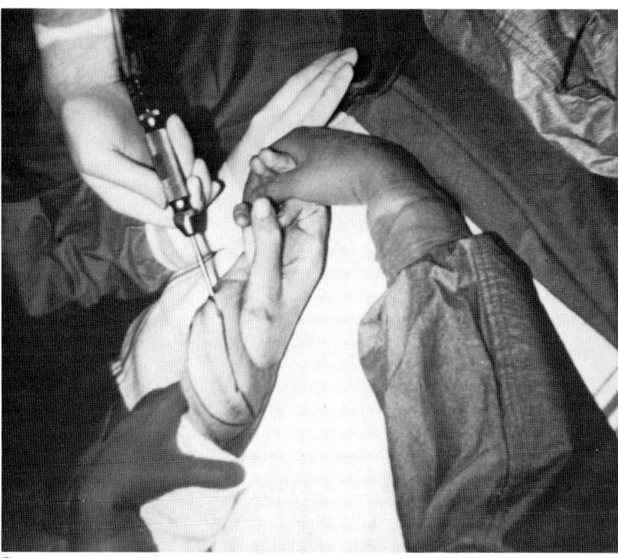

Fig. 37-10.

A. Volar view of right hand. Note the lack of padding on the ulnar aspect and the claw deformity, as well as the trophic changes on the ulnar aspect of the hand.

B. A large tensor fascia lata microvascular myocutaneous free flap was transferred to the right hand, wrist, and forearm. A Steinmann pin has been placed through the thumb metacarpal to aid in postoperative elevation of the right hand and arm.

C. Intraoperative photograph showing lipolysis with a #3 cannula outside the inked area, which will be excised.

D. Intermediate stage after extensive lipolysis and standard flap revision.

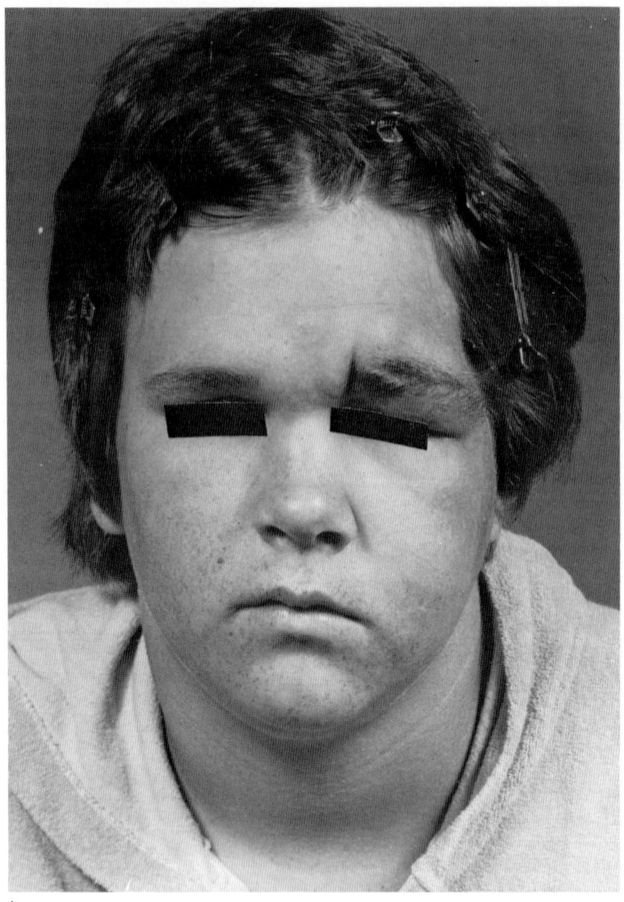

A

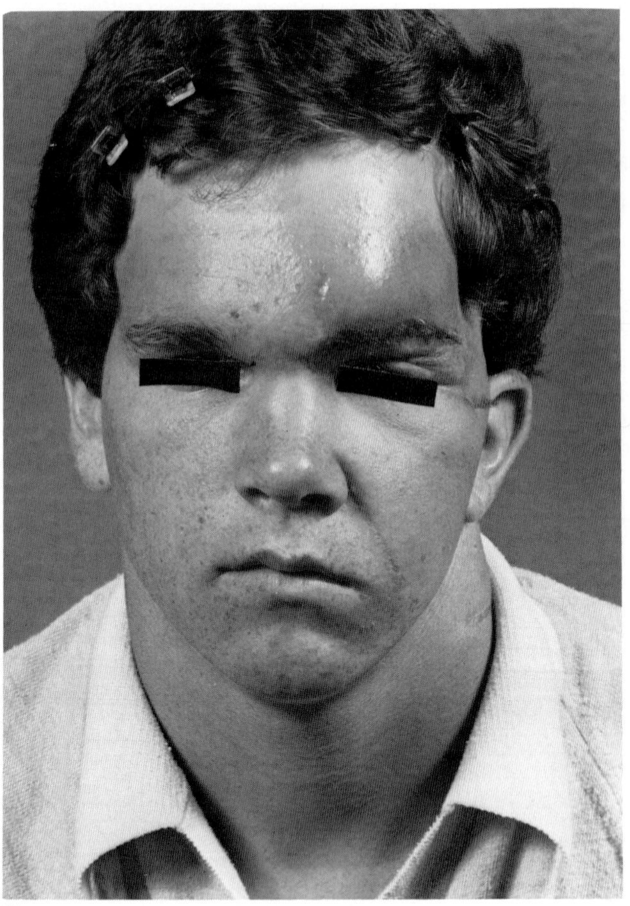

B

Fig. 37-11.
A. A young man born with extensive neurofibroma of the left face and neck. He has already had considerable plastic surgery at another institution by another surgeon.
B. Patient's appearance just before extensive lipolysis of the entire left face and entire neck. Fat only was removed and not neurofibroma. His mandibular and frontal branches of the facial nerve have been nonfunctional from the time I first saw him. Postoperatively, he has no weakness of the remaining branches of his facial nerve.

used was reversed saphenous vein graft end-to-side from his brachial artery hooked side-to-side to three different locations along his ulnar artery. Later, a tensor fascia lata microvascular free flap as a myocutaneous unit was transferred to his right hand and wrist (15 cm wide by 30 cm long).

Anastomoses were end-to-side to the radial artery, cephalic vein, and radial venae comitantes. The purpose of this procedure was to give padding to the ulnar aspect of his hand and to use the excess tissue as shown in Figure 37-10B for further reconstruction. Figure 37-10C shows an intermediate stage of lipolysis plus standard flap revision. At no time did lipolysis interfere with the vascular integrity of the flap. His cold intolerance is now completely gone, and he has padding on the ulnar aspect of his right hand. Further work is planned.

Case 11. J.B. is an 18-year-old man who was born with extensive neurofibroma of the left face and neck. Figure 37-11A shows the way he presented to me several years ago, after already having had a great deal of reconstructive plastic surgery at another hospital by another surgeon.

Figure 37-11B shows the way he looked just before his last surgery, which included extensive lipolysis of the entire left face and neck. His facial nerve branches to the frontal and mandibular areas were nonfunctional or absent by the time I first saw him. At this time, I did extensive lipolysis of the entire left side of the face and the entire neck. There was absolutely no damage to the remaining branches of the facial nerve, nor was there any vascular impairment to the flap. To clarify, I

removed *only* fat and *not* neurofibroma. I wanted to get a better contour for him. Also, I took a palmaris longus graft and looped it around the left side of his mouth.

At a second stage, I will take a plantaris tendon and do a static suspension of the drooping left corner of the mouth. Alternatively, I have discussed with him a microvascular free muscle transfer, such as extensor digitorum brevis with cross-facial nerve juncture across the upper lip to one of the opposite normal buccal branches with microvascular anastomosis end-to-side to the external carotid artery and internal jugular vein. He has yet to decide about the microsurgery.

This last case is recent (January 1984), so there is no long-term follow-up as yet. The main lesson to be learned from this case is that as long as you know precisely where the facial nerve is located, you will not damage it when using lipolysis with a #3 or #4 cannula by the Illouz blunt cannula technique.

Discussion

My beginnings in lipolysis were prudently modest and highly selective after I spent some time with Dr. Illouz in Paris. I operated initially only on the reconstructive patients. Gradually, I began aesthetic lipolysis, but only on patients on whom I had either operated before or were members of a family on whom I had operated. Iowa is a very conservative state, and I wanted to be suitably conservative about introducing this procedure to Iowa. So far, thankfully, all of our patients, both in the reconstructive and the aesthetic categories, have been very pleased. There have been no complications.

Initially, I was quite concerned about causing vascular embarrassment to the flap through lipolysis; however, if the principles set down by Illouz using his blunt cannula technique are followed, the flap will not be devascularized. A caveat, however, is that anything can be overdone. It takes skill, experience, judgment, and artistry to achieve the best result.

It is highly recommended that plastic surgeons be very cautious in their early attempts at lipolysis until they fully understand and are proficient in the technique. One suggestion is to have the plastic surgeon begin lipolysis on the lower abdomen of the abdominoplasty patient where the tissue will be discarded anyway. In this procedure, learning is maximal, no harm is done, and the surgeon can get the feel of the instruments.

Regarding the aesthetic patient, I initially operated only on those patients on whom I had performed other aesthetic or reconstructive surgery, or on their family members, or friends of a former patient. These patients are predisposed to be happy, because they, or their family member or a friend, have been happy with whatever surgery I performed for them. In the early stages it is best not to operate on strangers.

On the upper and lower extremity, I always use a pneumatic tourniquet without any thought of injection. Dr. Greg Hetter kindly suggested a form of injection for aesthetic lipolysis that I have used with great success. Whenever I am unable to use a tourniquet in the reconstructive aspects of lipolysis, I always use the Hetter injection. Also, since I almost always combine lipolysis of flaps with standard excisional revision techniques, I rarely ask the patient to wear any type of support dressing, as I always do in aesthetic lipolysis surgery. On microvascular free flaps to the lower extremity, however, I have the patient continue to wear supportive stockings after any type of revision of the flap, even before the days of lipolysis. This was my standard routine, and I have continued using it with lipolysis. So many of our lower-extremity, free-flap patients have such severe arterial or venous disease that long-term wearing of the pressure stocking just seems prudent.

Summary

Our series of patients in the reconstructive plastic surgery category on whom we have used lipolysis numbers 32. Eleven of these cases have been presented in some detail to exemplify the uses of lipolysis by the Illouz blunt cannula technique.

There has been no vascular impairment of any flap and, furthermore, there have been no complications to any of these flaps. I would like to repeat what I stated at the beginning of this chapter: lipolysis by the Illouz blunt cannula technique represents a major new weapon system in the treatment arsenal of the reconstructive plastic surgeon. If this technique is used wisely and prudently on carefully selected patients in both the reconstructive and aesthetic categories, my sincere belief is that it represents the most major advance in plastic surgery within the past 5 years. Depending on the size of the flap, I generally use the following sizes of cannulas: 3, 4, 6, and occasionally 8. Also, it appears that lipolysis can be prudently and wisely used in any area of the body frequented by the plastic surgeon.

CHAPTER 38

The Use of Lipolysis for Unusual Diseases

Conditions other than aesthetic refinement have been shown to benefit from suction lipoplasty. The three case histories that follow illustrate these applications.

Treatment of Insulin Induced Fat Hypertrophy
Gregory P. Hetter

A 25-year-old diabetic white female presented with irregular hypertrophy of the hypogastric fat and both anterior thighs. The patient had been diabetic since the age of 7. She took 15 units of regular and 15 units of NPH insulin per day. She had successfully borne two children.

The patient had used the anterior thighs for her insulin injections until five years before consultation. She then began using the abdomen, the upper buttocks, and the upper outer arms.

Several months before consultation she noted rapid onset swelling of the anterior thighs and could no longer wear her pants. This swelling was regular and even, as shown in Figure 38-1. The hypogastric area, scarred from previous surgeries, showed irregular areas of hypertrophy because of the scarring, as shown in Figures 38-2 and 38-3.

First, a biopsy was obtained under local anesthetic to verify the apparent normal histologic appearance of the tissue. Later standard Illouz-type lipolysis was carried out through one of the abdominal scars with good improvement (Fig. 38-4) and through a direct approach over each anterior thigh bulge (Fig. 38-5). A #6 Illouz cannula was used. There were no problems extracting the hypertrophic fat using a low-dose epinephrine (1:435,000) injection into operative areas on an outpatient basis under short general anesthesia. Histologic examination was unremarkable.

The patient's insurance company reimbursed her for 84% of the total charges related to this procedure, accepting the disease-based etiology of the patient's problem.

Treatment of Large Lipoma of the Back
Carson M. Lewis

Over a 5-year period a 71-year-old male noted growth of a soft tissue tumor on the mid-scapular area of the back. As the mass became larger, it became progressively symptomatic, and it became difficult for the patient to lie on the area.

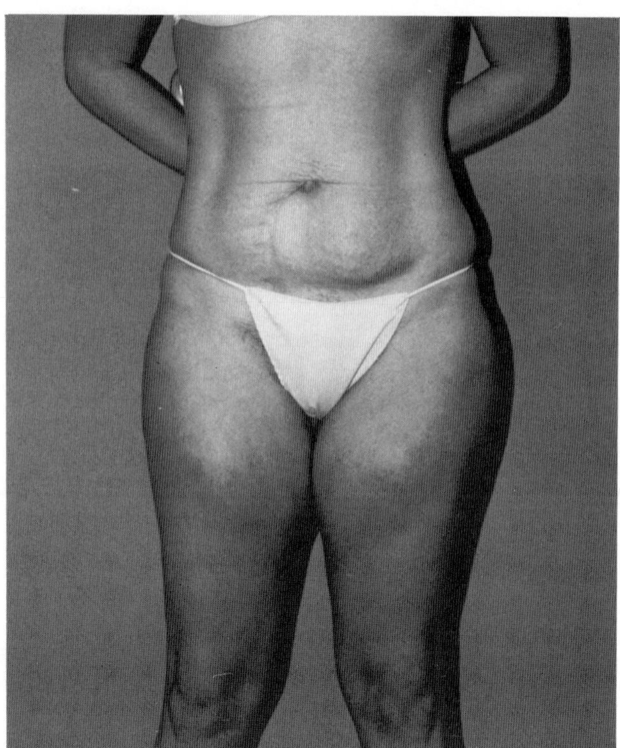

Fig. 38-1. Preoperative anterior view of patient showing hypertrophic bulges of anterior thighs.

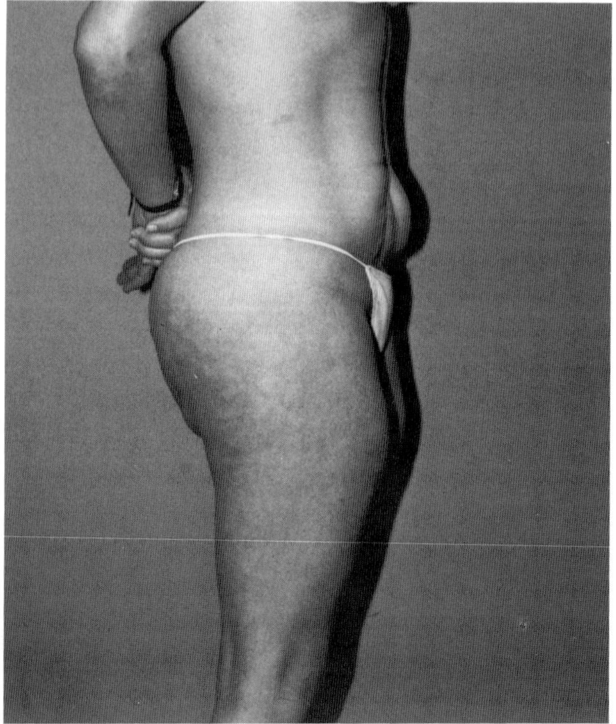

Fig. 38-2. Preoperative lateral view showing the abdomen.

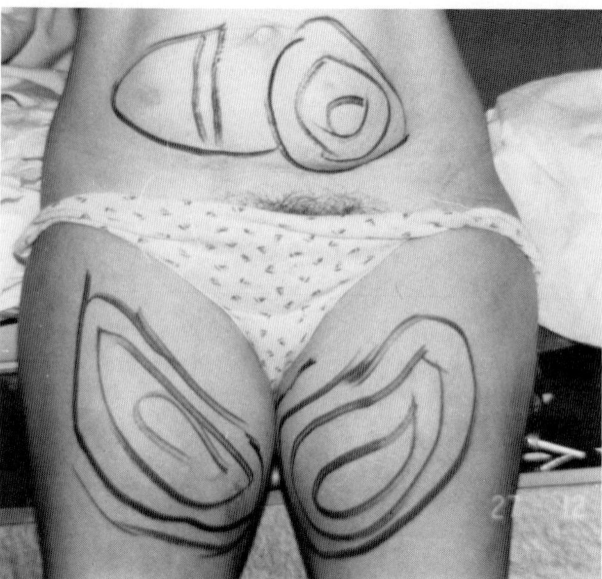

Fig. 38-3. Preoperative marking of thighs and abdomen showing vertical scar that tethered hypertrophic bulging.

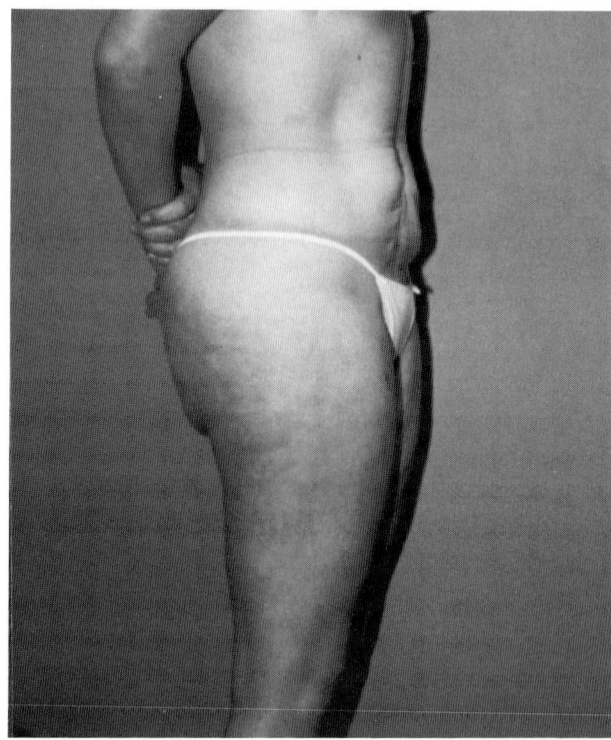

Fig. 38-4. Lateral view 3 months postoperatively.

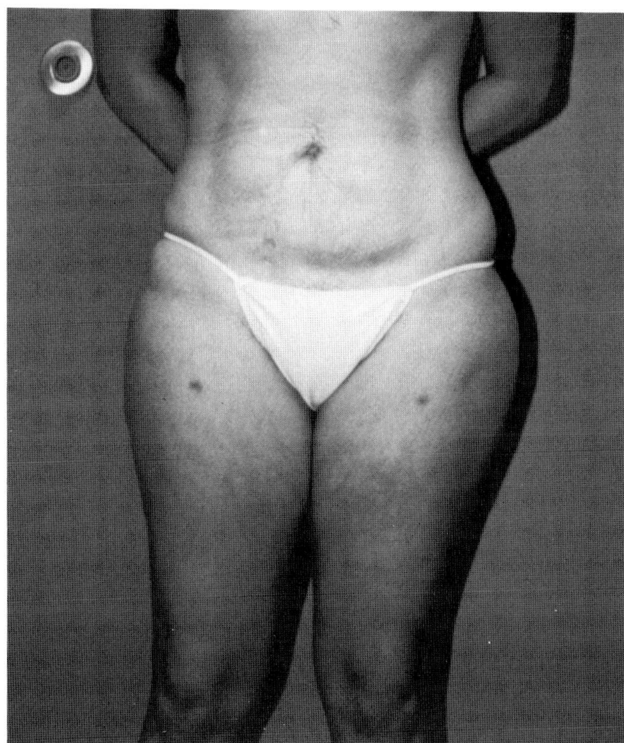

Fig. 38-5. Anterior view of patient 3 months postoperatively. Note small scars at bulge sites on thighs.

PROCEDURE

The 15 × 12 cm area was measured and marked (Figs. 38-6, 38-7, 38-8), the patient placed in the prone position, and an intravenous solution of Valium and Sublimaze started. The patient was infiltrated with less than 100 ml of 0.25% Xylocaine containing 1:400,000 epinephrine. The area was prepped routinely with Betadine, and a small transverse incision was made beneath the mass. Using #8 and #6 blunt cannulas fatty tissue was removed. The fat was superficial and more fibrous than in other areas of the body. Removal was similar to fat removal in the upper abdomen. The total amount removed by lipolysis was 175 ml, and the removal appeared to be complete. The peripheral area was feathered. The specimen was sent for a permanent histologic examination. The area was palpated, and there was an attempt to express any fluid. None was obtained. Subcuticular closure with Vicral sutures was used; Steri-Strips and elastic dressings in a figure-of-8 were placed over the defect. Estimated blood loss was less than 25 ml. The postoperative course was uneventful. The tape was removed at 7 days. The patient's activities were not limited. At 6 months there was no evidence of recurrence or residual tumor (Figs. 38-9, 38-10).

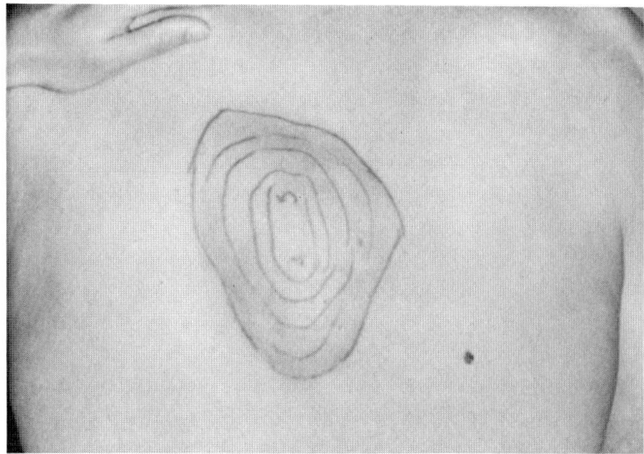

Fig. 38-6. Preoperative posterior view of a 71-year-old man with large lipoma of the intrascapular area.

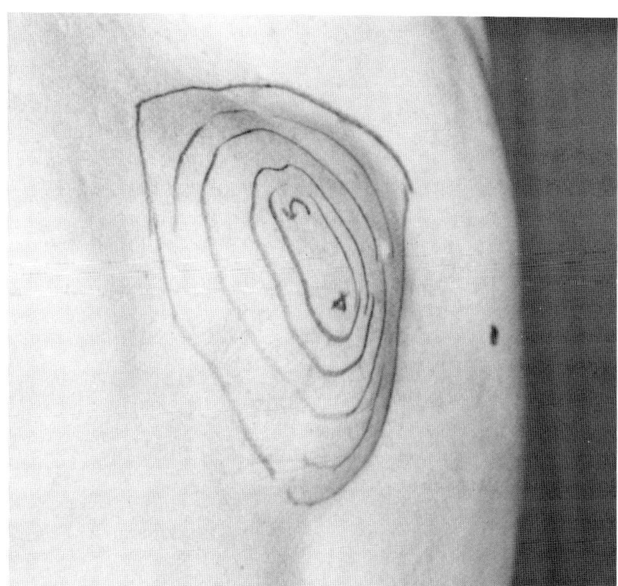

Fig. 38-7. Close-up view of area.

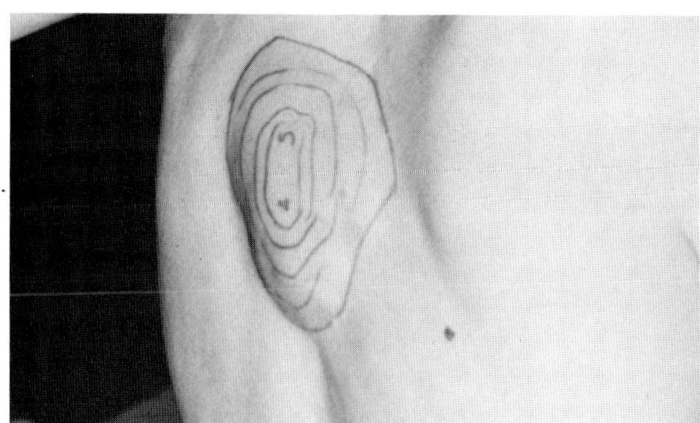

Fig. 38-8. Preoperative right oblique view.

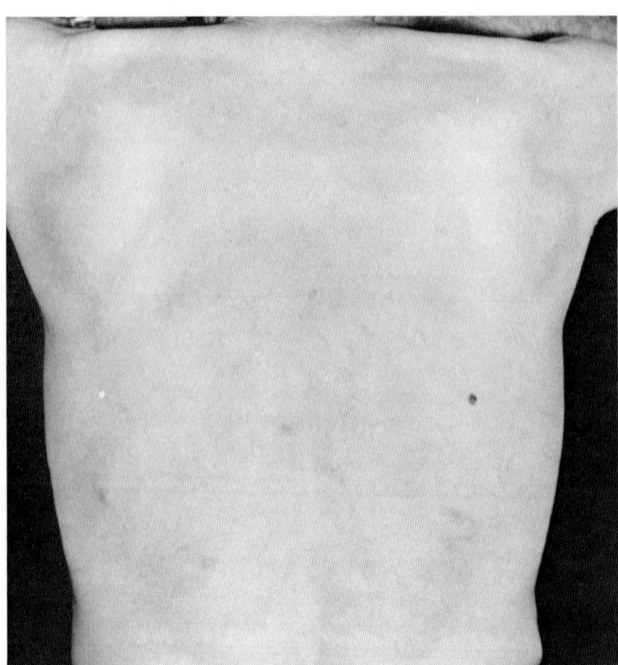

Fig. 38-9. Postoperative view 6 months following removal. There is no hint of recurrence.

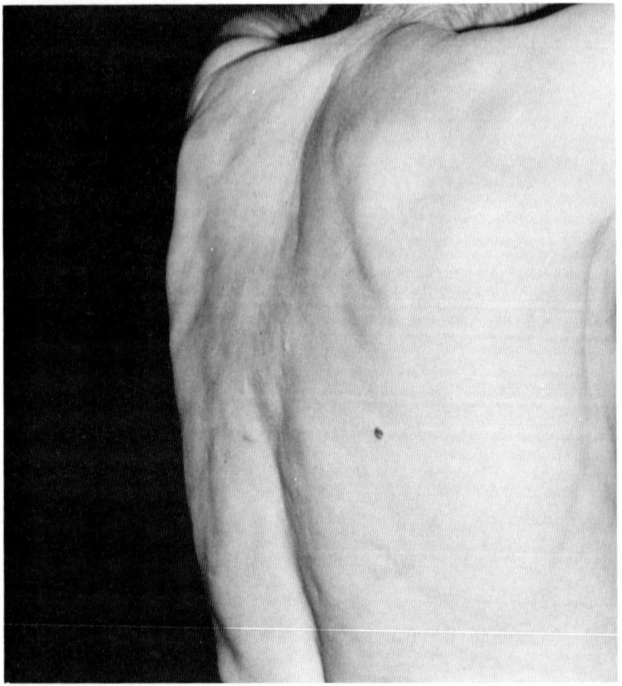

Fig. 38-10. Postoperative right oblique view at 6 months.

Treatment of Congenital Lymphedema of the Lower Extremity
Robert B. Winslow

Despite well-reasoned attempts to improve the surgical treatment of congenital lymphedema of the lower extremity [1,2,3,4,5], no technique has evolved that approaches the ideal operation—one that is simple, safe, reliable, reproducible, and improves physiology of the treated area. Only the techniques of Homans [7,8] and Thompson [9] have survived to take their place in the armamentarium of the modern surgeon.

Homans described staged subcutaneous excision beneath flaps, a procedure that is fraught with danger because it destroys all connections between overlying skin and underlying fascia. This destruction inevitably includes all vertical septa, which may include arterial supply to the skin, venous drainage from the skin, and any rudimentary or residual lymphatic connections. Usually the superficial saphenous system is destroyed or at least damaged. It is this trauma that may be self-defeating when using this approach; the benefit of reduced bulk of the extremity and removal of abnormal tissue may be counterbalanced by ischemia of the overlying skin and/or increased venous and lymphatic stasis in the dependent extremity.

The Thompson procedure attempts to address some of these problems by providing a buried dermis flap as a conduit between the superficial and deep lymphatic drainage systems, systems between which there is usually no connection [10,11]. Even in experienced hands, however, it is a difficult and complex procedure, and results are not expected to be as reliable as those reported by Thompson [12], Larson [13], and others [14,15].

The removal of abnormal subcutaneous fat from the lower extremity by avulsion, while at the same time preserving the vascular and lymphatic connections that presumably reside to a greater or lesser extent in the vertical septa between the skin and underlying tissue, are goals that might be accomplished by suction-assisted lipo extraction, and, furthermore, would overcome the objections of previous techniques. The healing process that follows suction-assisted lipo extraction includes a phase of neovascularization and usually results in close coaptation of overlying skin to underlying fascia. Such an outcome might provide a wide area of improved circulation of the lower extremity.

A 29-year-old white male with Prader-Willi syndrome and massive obesity has been treated for congenital lymphedema with suction-assisted lipo extraction. Prader-Willi syndrome is congenital rounded face, almond-shaped eyes, strabismus, low forehead, hypogonadism, and mental retardation. The patient is 5'5" tall and, at one time, weighed as much as 300 pounds

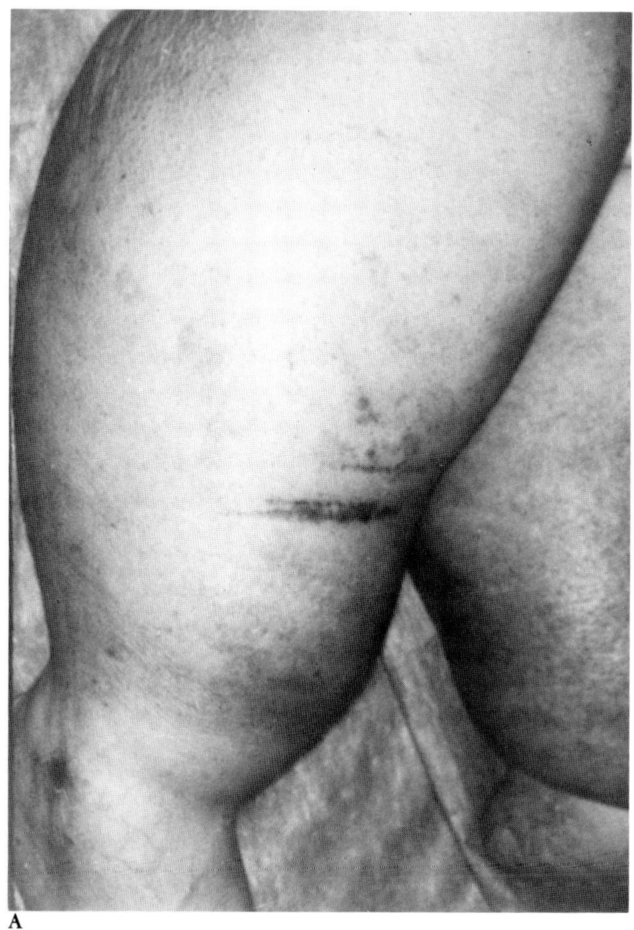

A

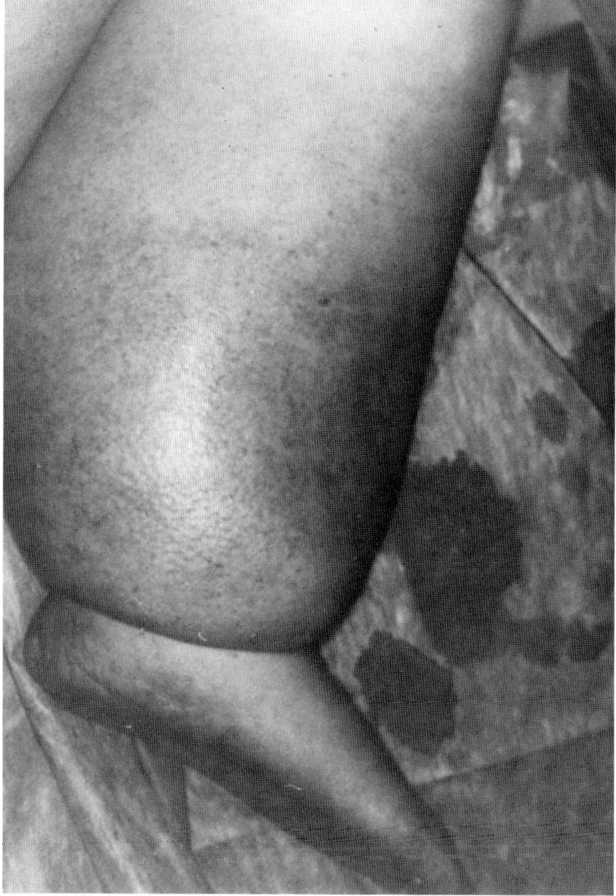

B

Fig. 38-11. Right lateral (A) and left medial (B) lower legs. Patient is unable to stand. There is thickened hyperkeratotic skin and massive enlargement with overhanging of the left medial maleolus. The maleolus is completely obscured even though the patient is recumbent. Bruised area on the anterior aspect of the right leg is result of prehospitalization trauma.

but lost 136 pounds before surgery. The patient had massive enlargement of his legs, typical of congenital lymphedema (i.e., nonpitting enlargement and thickened hyperkeratotic skin) (Fig. 38-11).

The planned surgical approach was staged subcutaneous excision beneath flaps: the Homans operation. The first operation involved excision of redundant skin and all subcutaneous fat under anterior and posterior flaps on the lateral aspect of the right leg and the medial aspect of the left leg. No suctioning was used. Considerable dense fibro-fatty tissue of the type associated with chronic lymphedema was excised. The operation proceeded well but the long saphenous system on the left medial leg was destroyed. Satisfactory healing ensued except for small areas of skin slough around the suture line on the lateral aspect of the right leg indicating a certain degree of vascular compromise (Fig. 38-12).

One month later, the patient returned to the operating room for the second stage. Disenchanted by the destruction of the saphenous system and the skin slough associated with the first operation, we elected to treat the medial aspect of the right leg and lateral aspect of the left leg by suction technique. By a combination of suction followed by skin resection, 660 ml of tissue was removed from the right medial leg and 605 ml of tissue was removed from the left lateral leg (Fig. 38-13). The tissues were very difficult to penetrate. At the time of the skin resection, no undermining of the flaps was necessary. It was easy to visualize (1) the empty spaces or tunnels from which fat had been removed by suction, (2) intact vertical fibro-septa between the skin and fascia, and (3) an intact saphenous system on the right. No bleeding was noted, and closure was by a single layer of staples. This operation took less time than the first stage. Rapid healing ensued without any evidence of vascular compromise to the wound margins. The pathology report revealed slightly dilated lymphatic or vascular channels. Results were satisfactory. When seen 5 months postoperatively, the patient was sitting and standing without the use of compressive garments and

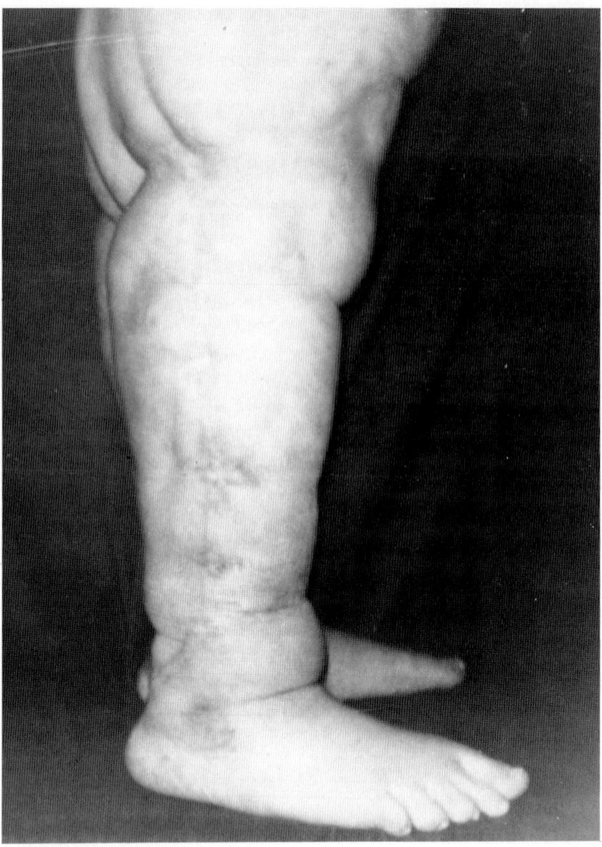

A

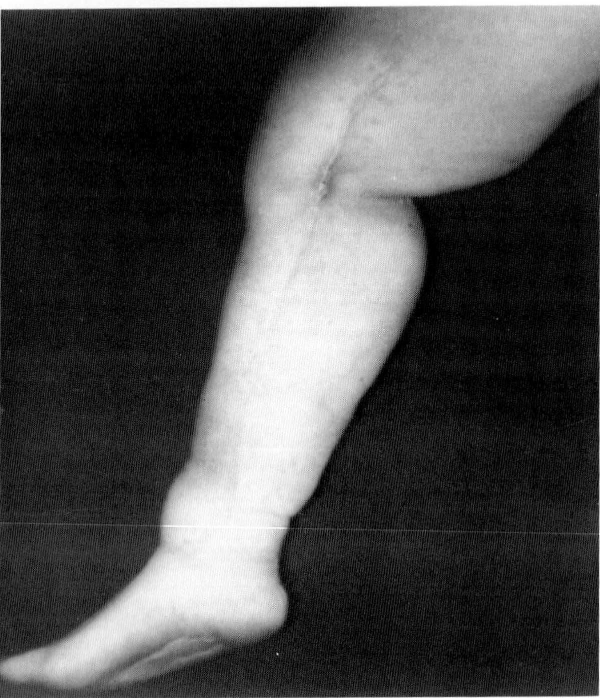

B

Fig. 38-12. Right lateral (A) and left medial (B) legs after surgery. Three small skin grafts are visible on the lateral aspect of the right leg.

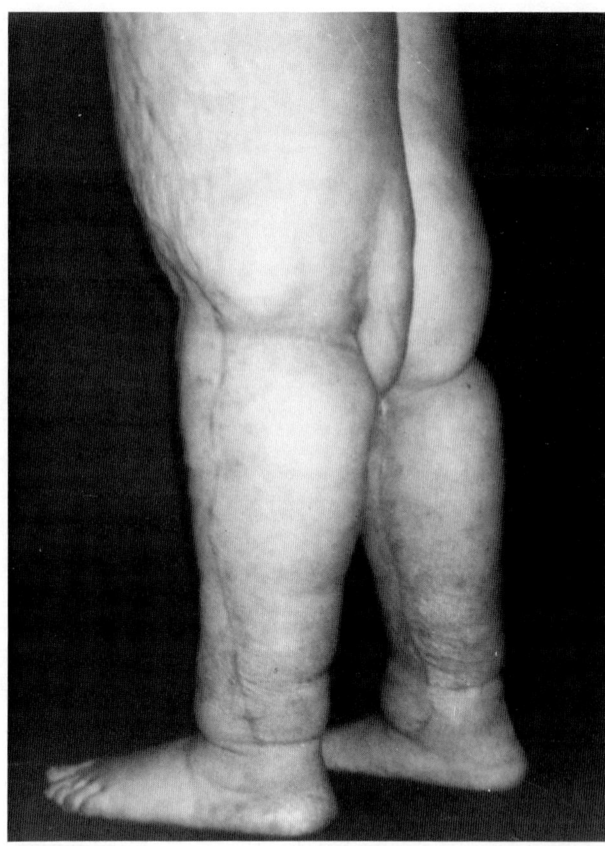

Fig. 38-13. The right medial and left lateral sides after treatment bysuction-assisted lipo extraction and resection of redundant skin.

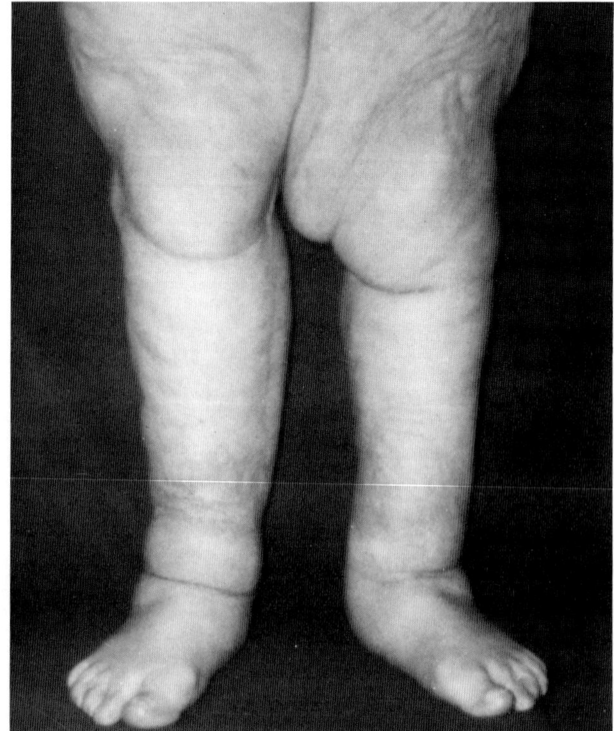

Fig. 38-14. Five months after surgery with no use of support garments.

without any evidence of recurrence of his edema (Fig. 38-14).

A tentative conclusion based on this experience is that congenital lymphedema can be treated by suction-assisted lipoextraction combined with resection of redundant overlying skin. At least four questions are raised: (1) Is this experience reproducible? (2) Was this really congenital lymphedema or rather lipodystrophy of the lower leg (a rare anomaly called lipedema)? (3) Using this technique, is it necessary to stage the procedure? (4) Does the adhesive bond that forms between the skin and the underlying fascia after full recovery carry more or less vascular/lymphatic connections than before? None of the answers is available yet but based on this one experience, it may well be that suction-assisted lipo extraction offers a means to treat congenital lymphedema that may be treated more reliably and safely than previous means. If so, the concept of an ideal surgical treatment for this condition in which we combine ablation of abnormal tissue with improvement of physiology in the treated area may be emerging.

References

1. Handley, W. S. Lymphangioplasty: A new method for the relief of the brawn arm of breast cancer and for similar conditions of lymphatic edema: Preliminary note. *Lancet* 1:783, 1908.
2. Silver, D., and Puckett, C. Lymphangioplasty: A ten-year evaluation. *Surgery* 80:748, 1976.
3. Kondoleon, E. Die operative Behandlung der elephantiastischen Oedeme. *Zentralbl. Chir.* 39:1022, 1912.
4. Goldsmith, H. S., and de los Santos, R. Omental transposition in primary lymphedema. *Surg. Gynecol. Obstet.* 125:607, 1967.
5. Goldsmith, H. S., de los Santos R., and Beattie, E. J. Relief of chronic lymphedema by omental transposition. *Ann. Surg.* 166:572, 1967.
6. Charles, R. H. *A System of Treatment* (vol. 3). London: Churchill, 1912.
7. Sistrunk, W. E. Further experiences with the Kondoleon operation for elephantiasis. *J.A.M.A.* 71:800, 1918.
8. Homans, J. The treatment of elephantiasis of the legs: A preliminary report. *N. Engl. J. Med.* 215:1099, 1936.
9. Thompson, N. Surgical treatment of chronic lymphedema of the lower limb. *Br. Med. J.* 5319:1567, 1962.
10. Malek, P., Belan, A., and Kocandrle, V. L. The superficial and deep lymphatic system of the lower extremities and their mutual relationship under physiological and pathological conditions. *J. Cardiovasc. Surg.* 5:686, 1964.
11. Thompson, N. The surgical treatment of chronic lymphedema of the extremities. *Surg. Clin. North Am.* 47:445, 1967.
12. Thompson, N. Buried dermal flap operation for chronic lymphedema of the extremities. Ten-year survey of results in 79 cases. *Plast. Reconstr. Surg.* 45:541, 1970.
13. Larson, D. L., Coers, C. R., Doyle, J. E., Rappaport, A. S., Kloehn, R., and Lewis, S. R. Lymphedema of the lower extremity. *Plast. Reconstr. Surg.* 38:293, 1966.
14. Edwards, J. M., Negus, D., and Kinmonth, J. B. A review of operations from lymphedema. *J. Cardiovasc. Surg.* 10:110, 1969.
15. Fontaine, R., and Fontaine, J. L. Die operative Therapie des Lymphodems. *Arch. Chir.* 325:89, 1969.

Index

Index

Abdomen
  dressings, 164
  nomenclature, 68
  perforation, 153
  preoperative markings, 139
  subcutaneous fat, 46–47
Abdominal binder, 237
Abdominal dermolipectomy. *See* Abdominoplasty
Abdominal lipolysis
  cannulas, 129, 130
  with iliac crest extraction, 253–255
  incisions, 156, 157
  including flanks, 251–252
  markings, 138, 243
  operative approach selection, 148, 238
  regional anesthesia, 111
Abdominoplasty
  in combined procedures, 28–29, 237–238
  history of, 277
  indications
    fat with skin excess, 238, 241
    fat without skin excess, 238–241
    mixed excess of skin and fat, 241–243
    pendulous abdomen, 243–245
    scar revision, 245
    for wrinkles and stretch marks, 245, 247
  markings, 138, 243
  navel depression and, 25
  preoperative considerations, 235–237
  sequelae, 19, 233
    epigastric lipodystrophy, 286, 287
    iliac crest lipodystrophy, 286, 288–291, 293
  types, 233–235
    classic transverse, 246
    quadruple V, 235
  umbilicus disinsertion, 234
  umbilicus transposition, 234
Acetone, for tape removal, 164
Adenosine monophosphate, cyclic, (cAMP), 44
Adenosine triphosphate (ATP), 44
Adenylate cyclase, 43–44
Adipose tissue
  brown, 41
  catecholamine sensitivity, 43
  cell number, 25
  differences by diet, 46
  function and development, 41–42
  insulin sensitivity, 44
  metabolism, 43–47
  physiological role(s), 41, 46, 47
Adiposuction, 75
Adolescent(s), dissatisfaction with body size, 49–50
Adrenaline, 195, 250, 255
Air pressure
  reference pressure, 119, 120

Air pressure—*Continued*
  relationship to altitude, 120–121
  units of measurement, 119–120
Airway
  maintenance, 107–108
  postoperative obstruction, 112
Albolene, 177
Albumin
  adipose tissue metabolism and, 41, 42
  intravenous administration, 110
  and serum changes following lipolysis, 169–171
Alcohol withdrawal, 112
Alcoholism, bulimia and, 52
Alkaline phosphate, 170
Alpha-adrenergic activity, lipolysis and, 44
Alpha-glycerol phosphate, 41–42
Altitude, effect on air pressure, 120–121
American Society of Plastic and Reconstructive Surgeons (ASPRS), 35
Amidate (etomidate), 107
Anaphylaxis, from local anesthetics, 111
Android fat distribution, 46, 65, 67
Anesthesia. *See also specific procedure(s)*
  and airway maintenance, 107–108
  delayed emergence from, 112
  induction, 107
    sedation and, 105–106
  informed consent, 103–104
  lipodissection, dry procedure, 34
  in lipolysis
    of abdomen, 233
    of arms, 211
    of breast, 228
    of calves and ankles, 272
    of face, 187
    of flank, 249, 250
    with glandular resection, 220
    of thighs, 257
  maintenance, 108–110
  and patient positioning, 141, 142
    prone, 141
    supine, 155, 157
    supine lateral decubitus, 157–159
  preoperative visit and, 105
  for rhytidectomy, 202
  subarachnoid, 111–112
Ankle
  dressings, 164
  lipolysis, 271
    cannula(s), 132
    dressings, 274
    incisions, 272
    indications, 271
    procedure, 272–274
    results, 274, 275
    skin marking, 271, 273
    technique, 271
  measurements, 61
  terminology, 72
Anorexia nervosa, 51

Antacids, preoperative, 106
Anthropometry, 61–63
Antibiotics, prophylactic, 152
Anticholinergic drugs, 106, 107
Anticholinesterases, 105, 108
Anticoagulant drugs, 105
Anticonvulsant drugs, 105
Antihypertensive drugs, 105
Antiinflammatory drugs, 105
Anxiety, patient selection and, 92, 93
Aphrodite, 56
Arm(s)
    dressings, 164
    lipolysis
        cannulas, 132, 133
        case study, 212–215
        with dermatolipectomy, 216
        incision, 155, 156
        indications, 211
        technique, 211–213
Art, feminine figure in, 3–12
Arteriosclerosis, 46
Ascorbic acid, 174
Aspiration, gastric, 106
Aspiration procedures. *See also specific
    procedures*
    curette techniques, 20–21
    surgical perspective, 16–17
ASPRS (American Society of Plastic and
    Reconstructive Surgeons), 35
Ativan (lorazepam), 106
Atracurium (Tracrium), 108
Atropine
    bradycardia and, 108, 113
    induction, 107
    side effects, 106, 112

Background, photographic, 78–79
Banana deformity. *See* Buttocks, folds
Bandage phase, 180
Bandaging techniques, postoperative,
    29
Barbiturates, 106, 107
Beauty, feminine
    in art, 62–63
    in Egyptian civilization, 3, 4
    modern concept of, 3
    parameters, 62
Beauty industry, effect on female shape,
    15–16
Benzodiazepines, 106
Bermuda triangle, 28, 297, 300
Beta blockers, 105, 113
Betadine, 141
Bikini resection, 234, 238, 242
Billing disputes, 88–89
Birth control pills, 105
Blacks
    histology of skin and adipose tissue,
        298
    morphology, 295–298
    operative impressions and indica-
        tions, 298
    steatopygia, 295–297
    surgical complications, 299

Bleeding
    intraoperative, 26, 150, 152
    postoperative, 115–116, 221, 225,
        299
Blepharoplasty, 72, 73, 193
Blood chemistry, changes after lipolysis,
    169–171
Blood count, complete, (CBC), 169, 170
Blood gases, arterial, 169, 171
Blood pressure, postoperative, 112
Blood transfusion, autologous, 110
Blunt suction lipectomy (Illouz tech-
    nique). *See also* Lipolysis;
    specific sites
    advantages, 279
    cannulas
        for ankles and calves, 132, 133
        for arms, 132, 212
        for epigastric and hypogastric area,
            129, 130
        facial, 133, 186
        for thighs, 129, 266
        types, 122–127
    combined with conventional surgery,
        277, 279, 293
    dressings, 164, 165
    hematocrit in, 115–116
    historical perspective, 17, 20–22
    indications
        ankles, 271
        arms, 211, 217
        breast, 227
        of epigastric region, 238, 286
        face, 184
        flank, 249
        gynecomastia, 225
        iliac crest, 253
        knee, 266
        lipodystrophy with skin flaccidity,
            280–285
        as surgical complement, 230–231
        thigh, 261
    physical exhaustion of surgeon, 160
    postoperative care, 88
    preoperative evaluation, 87, 88
    pretreatment with epinephrine, 115,
        144
    pretunneling, 159–161
    risk management, 87–89
    suction pressure, 122, 123
    technique, 137
        dissemination of, 34–35
        dry technique, 21
        Illouz technique, 21, 26
    terminology, 75, 76
    and unrealistic patient expectations, 86
    vacuum pump, 132, 134–135
Body contour surgery. *See* specific sur-
    gical procedures
    comparison of closed techniques,
        21–23
    present state, 279
Body image disturbances
    background factors, 49–51
    eating disturbances and, 51–53

Body weight and measurement, 61–63
Botticelli, portrayal of the female, 3, 5
Brachial adiposity, 99
Bradycardia, 108, 112, 113
Breast. *See also* Gynecomastia
    dressings, 164
    lipolysis
        positioning and incision, 228
        preoperative preparation, 227–228
        surgical technique, 229–230
    psychological outcome of surgery, 53
    reconstruction, 313, 314
Brevital, 106, 107
Bruising, postoperative, 29–30
Buccal fat lipolysis, 200, 206–207
Bulimia, 50–53
Bupivacaine (Marcaine), 111, 187, 250
Buret settlement, depiction of female
    figure in, 11
Bust measurement, and figure propor-
    tion, 61
Buttocks. *See also* Infragluteal area
    folds
        double, 68, 69, 258
        location, 68, 69
        raising or accentuating, 150, 151
        secondary, 306–308
    lift, 257
    lipodystrophy with skin flaccidity,
        283–285
    lipoplasty, in blacks, 299–300
    reduction, 27–28
    sad, 150, 151, 263, 265
    smiling, 151
    square, 65, 66, 263, 264
    steatopygia, 295–297
    terminology, 68

Calcium, 169, 170, 171
Calcium channel blocker(s), 113
Calf
    lipolysis
        anesthesia, 272
        cannulas, 132, 133
        incisions, 159
        marking, 271, 273
        procedure, 272–274
        results, 274, 275
    measurements, 61
    posterior fat, 70, 72
Cameras
    focus and f-stop, 82
    height adjustment, 82, 85
    standard for surgical offices, 77
Candidates, ideal surgical, 95–97
Cannulas
    blunt, 32–34
    Brazilian, with air leak channel, 124
    design, 27
    facial, 185–187
    Fournier modification, 34
    general considerations, 128, 133
    Grazer-Grams modification, 124, 127
    Hetter-Padgett modification, 124,
        128, 130

Cannulas—*Continued*
  Illouz design, 127, 133
  Illouz technique, 122, 123
  modifications related to techniques, 124–127
  resistance related to diameter, 128–129
  shark mouth, 150, 151
  size
    criss-cross technique and, 148
    drain usage and, 150
    related to deformity, 138, 139
  for specific areas, 129–132
  suction, 75, 237
  techniques, 144–145
    closed, 21–23
    dry, 21
    Illouz, 21–23
    improvements, 25–26
    postoperative contour deformity and, 305
Carotid triangle area, anterior, 72, 73
Catecholamine, 43–44, 47
CBC (complete blood count), 169, 170
Cellulite, 61
Cellusuctiotome, 20, 33, 34
Central neural block, 111–112
Cephalosporin, 152
Cervicomental angle, 73, 192
Chajcher technique, 122
Chart documentation, 88
Cheeks
  lipolysis cannulas, 129
  terminology, 72, 73
Chin
  augmentation with facial lipolysis, 192
  double, 35
  implant, 155, 156
    clinical results, 193, 194
  lipolysis cannulas, 129
Cholesterol, serum changes following lipolysis, 170
Chubb, 70, 71, 259
Cimetidine (Tagamet), 106
Clotting time, 107
Cocaine, 110
Collapsing surgery, 20
Colloid fluid therapy, 110
Complaint duration, patient selection and, 92
Complication(s). *See also specific operation*
  aesthetic, 152, 301–308
  cardiovascular, 113
  hematocrit drop, 115, 116
  inclusion in consent form, 103
  respiratory, 112
Compression garments
  for abdominal lipoplasties, 237
  design and disadvantages, 166–168
  for gluteal fold surgery, 150
  for midtorso procedures, 255
Consent. *See* Informed consent
Consent form, 38

Contour deformities. *See also specific deformity*
  degree of, compared to anxiety level, 92
  iatrogenic, 306–308
  postoperative, 305–306
  preoperative, 305–306
Convalescence, phases of, 180–181
Counseling, patient, 53, 105
Courtiss procedure, 122
Creatinine, serum, 106
Creatinine phosphokinase (CPK), 108
Criss-cross technique, 266, 267
Crows feet, 189
Crural area
  complications of, 306
  location of fat, 68, 70
  marking for lipolysis, 265–266
Crush-type injury, 163
Crystalloid fluid therapy, 110
Culotte de cheval. *See* Riding breeches deformity
Curare, 107
Curettes
  techniques
    compared to cannula techniques, 21–23
    consequences, 22
    seroma rate, 20
    suction, 20–21
    uterine, 20
  types, 124, 125
Cushing's disease, 46

Dantrolene sodium (Dantrium), 108
Delirium, postoperative, 112
Depressed patients, as surgical candidates, 92–93
Dermal lysis, 261
Dermolipectomy
  abdominal, 233–235
  arm, 212, 216, 217
  combined procedures, 277
  comparison of techniques, 21–23
  historical perspective, 19
  with suction lipoplasty, 246
Diabetes
  effect of on lipolysis, 44
  fat hypertrophy secondary to insulin, 260, 323
  insulin resistance and, 45–46
Diazepam (Valium)
  for induction, 107
  ketamine and, 109
  premedication, 106, 111
Diet, postoperative, 182
Dieting, 50, 61
Dilantin (diphenylhydantoin), 112
Dimpling, diffuse, and skin elasticity, 303, 304
Diphenylhydantoin (Dilantin), 112
Disappointment phase, 181
Disinsertion-reposition, of umbilicus, 234, 235
Dissatisfaction, surgical, 92, 93
Diuretics, 105

Dopram (doxapram), 112
Dorsal thoracic folds, 74, 75
Doxapram (Dopram), 112
Drains, 150, 152
Draping, heat loss during surgery and, 141, 143, 144
Dressings
  abdominal, 167, 237
  axillary breast, 164
  chest wall, 164
  gluteal crease, 150, 152
  iliac crest roll, 164, 165
  knee, 167
  thigh, 165, 167
  types, 163
    combination of tape and compression garments, 168
    compression garments, 166–168
    elastic tape, 163–166
Droperidol (Inapsine), 106, 112–113
Drug abuse, 50, 52
Drug withdrawal, 112
Duranest, 187
Dürer, Albrecht, 3, 5, 57–59

Eating disorders, 50–53
Ectomorph, 62
Edema, postoperative, 110, 180
Edrophonium (Tensilon), 108, 113
Education, patient, 93, 102
Effleurage, 176, 177
Endomorph, 62
Enflurane (Ethrane), 108, 109
Enzyme studies, serum, 170
Epidural anesthesia, 111–112
Epigastrium. *See* Abdomen
Epinephrine
  blood chemistry changes and, 170
  drain usage and, 150
  effect on blood loss and hematocrit, 38, 116–117
  general anesthetics and, 109
  local anesthetics and, 107, 111, 228
  toxic dose limit, 109–110
  and Wydase, 220
Esterification process, 41–42
Ethanol, 105, 110
Ether, for tape removal, 164
Ethrane (enflurane), 108, 109
Etomidate (Amidate), 107
European Paleolithic Age, 6, 7
Eutonyl (pargylin), 105
Exercise
  ineffective for localized fat loss, 15
  postoperative, 181, 182
Expectations, patient, 88, 93

Face. *See also* Facial lipolysis
  dressings, 164
  and nerve palsy, 194–195
  nomenclature, 72, 73
  photographic technique, 80, 81
  proportions of, Fibonacci series in, 58, 60
  psychological outcome of surgery, 53

Face-lift. *See* Rhytidectomy
Facial lipolysis
 areas, 186
 cannulas, 185–187
 clinical results, 196, 197
 combined with other procedures, 192
 complications, 192, 194
 for neurofibroma, 320
 and patient interview, 194–195
 postoperative care, 195, 197
 preoperative planning, 195
 with rhytidectomy, 200–202
 technique, 187–189, 195
Fashion
 female shape and, 13–16
 surgical consideration of, 60
Fasting, and adipose tissue metabolism, 44, 47
Fat embolism, 110
Fat tissue
 catecholamine sensitivity, 43
 determination of excess, 61
 distribution, 19, 65, 67
 insulin sensitivity, 44
 metabolism, 46
 removal, judgment of adequacy, 301, 303
 reserves, historical origins of, 12
Fatigue phase, in convalescence, 180
Fear, patient selection and, 93
Feathering technique, 220, 274
Females, fat distribution in, 65, 67
Femoral area
 aesthetic complications, 152, 306
 dressings, 165, 167
 lateral, dressings for, 164, 165
 lateral fat, treatment of, 263, 264
 lipolysis, 269
 markings, 137, 261, 263, 266, 268
 nomenclature, 70
 subcutaneous fat, 46–47
 technique, 144, 257
Fentanyl (Sublimaze), 108–109, 112
Fetus, adipose tissue development in, 42
Fibonacci series, 57–59
Film, photographic, 78, 82, 85
Fischer technique. *See* Lipectomy, Fischer technique
Flank
 defined, 68
 lipolysis, 249–252
  cannula, 129, 130
  case studies, 251–252
  with lipoplasty, 240, 241
  postoperative management, 250
  preoperative preparation, 249–250
  technique, 250
 location, 68
 preoperative markings, 140
Flap revision
 for breast reconstruction, 313, 314
 for forearm, hand, and wrist reconstruction, 309, 312, 313

Flap revision—*Continued*
 for hand injury, 309, 310–311
 in mandibular reconstruction, 309, 310
 for nose, 313
Fluid replacement therapy, 38, 110, 115
Follow-up, after lipolysis, 181–182
Foodstuffs, in nutritional support of surgical recovery, 174
Forane (Isoflurane), 108, 109, 116
Forearm reconstruction, 309, 312, 313
Form, female
 perceptions of, 60–61
 standards
  artistic, 55–57
  mathematical, 57–60
Fournier's rule, 263
FRC (functional residual capacity), 113
Free fatty acids (FFA)
 high levels, 46
 storage, 41–42
 turnover rate, 42
Friction, in massage, 176, 177
Frog position, 157
Functional residual capacity (FRC), 113

Gallamine, 108
Gastrointestinal bypass surgery, 53
Genetics, hip structure and, 12, 13
Gigantomastia, 229
Girdles. *See* Compression garments
Globulin, 170
Glucose, blood, 44–46, 106
Gluteal depression, 263, 264
 contour harmony and, 286, 301, 303
 nomenclature, 68, 70
Gluteal folds. *See* Buttocks, folds
Gluteus, 68
Glycopyrrolate (Robinul)
 bradycardia and, 108, 112
 premedication, 106, 107, 113
Golf bag deformity, 145, 147
Greece, feminine figure in art of, 3, 4, 55, 57
Gynecoid fat distribution, 46, 65, 67
Gynecomastia
 case history, 222
 historical treatment methods for, 219, 221
 lipolysis
  with glandular excision, 219, 222–225
  patient positioning, 155–158
 treatment techniques, 21, 22

Halothane, 108
Hand, avulsion injury, 309, 310–311
Heat loss, draping and, 141, 143, 144
Height-weight proportion, ideal, 61–63
Hematocrit
 decrease
  effect of epinephrine, 116–117
  following lipolysis, 115, 169, 170
 preoperative screening, 106–107

Hematomas
 postoperative, 115, 221
  cannula technique, 22, 115
  curette technique, 22, 115
 racial differences, 299
Hemoglobin
 changes following lipolysis, 169, 170
 preoperative screening, 106–107
Hemorrhage. *See* Bleeding
Hernia, 238
Hetastarch (Hespan), 110
Hetter formula, 144
Hetter-Padgett modified cannula, 124, 128, 130
Hibitane tincture, 141
High-pressure suction machines, 122, 124
Hips
 anatomical terminology, 65, 68
 evolution in female, 12–13
 measurements, 61
History, feminine figure in, 6–12
Hormones, effect on adipose tissue, 43–47
Humeral area, posterior, defined, 73, 74
Hyaluronidase, 21
Hyperlordosis, 295, 296
Hyperpigmentation
 in blacks, 298
 minimizing, 153–154
 postoperative, 29, 153–154
Hypertension, postoperative, 112, 113
Hyperthermia, malignant, 108, 109
Hyperthyroidism, 44
Hypertriglyceridemia, 46, 47
Hypogastrium
 lipolysis results, 239–242, 278, 280
 location, 68
 surgical approaches, 148, 149
Hypotension, postoperative, 111–113
Hypotonic solutions, 16
Hypoventilation, postoperative, 112
Hypovolemia, 153

Iliac crest
 cannulas, 129, 131
 combined surgical procedures, 283–287
 dressings, 164, 165
 lipolysis, 150, 253–255
 roll, 68, 69
Ilio-femoro-rotulian line, 3
Ilium, defined, 68
Illouz technique. *See* Blunt suction lipectomy (Illouz technique)
Inapsine (droperidol), 106, 112–113
Incisions. *See specific incisions*
Inderal (propranolol), 113
Informed consent
 and patient education, 93
 risk management and, 87–88
 specific topics in form, 103–104
Infragluteal area. *See also* Buttocks; Thigh
 cannulas, 132
 lipolysis, 263–265

Insulin
    effect on adipose tissue, 43, 44–46
    and induced fat hypertrophy, 323–
        325
Intravenous fluids, anesthesia and, 110
Iron supplementation, 174, 180
Isocarbozid (Marplan), 105
Isoflurane (Forane), 108, 109, 116
Isoniazid, 105

Jowls. *See also* Nasolabial folds, upper;
        Preantral area
    lipolysis
        cannula, 129
        with rhytidectomy, 200–202, 205
        technique, 189
    location, 72, 73, 185, 186
Juri's procedure, 234

Karman cannula, 34
Keflex, 152
Keloids, 298
Kesselring procedure
    complications of, 145, 147
    curette, 124, 126
    first publication, 16–17, 20
    suction pressure, 122
Ketamine, 106–109, 112
Knee(s)
    comparison of appearance, 257, 259
    dressings, 164
    lipolysis, 266
        case studies, 268–269
        positioning and incisions, 157
    location of fat deposits, 70, 71
    operations, 28

Laboratory determinations, changes fol-
        lowing lipolysis, 169–171
Lactic acid dehydrogenase (LDH), 169,
        170
Laugh lines, 189
Lenses, photographic
    for body work, 82–83
    for facial work, 77–78
    focal length, 80–82
Levodopa, 105
Lidocaine
    contraindication, 108
    with epinephrine, 109–111, 170
Lifestyle, postoperative changes, 182
Lighting, photographic, 79–80
Lipase, 44, 45
Lipectomy. *See also* Blunt suction lipec-
        tomy; Lipoextraction; Lipolysis;
        Lipoplasty
    with abdominoplasty, 28–29
    closed techniques, 20
    compared to lipolysis, 195
    Fischer technique, 33–34
        improvements, 25–26, 29–30
        terminology, 75
    Fournier technique, 34
    historical development, 17, 20–22
    Illouz technique, 26–30

Lipectomy—*Continued*
    Kesselring technique, 20
    open techniques, 19
    Schrudde technique, 20
    suction-assisted (SAL), 75
    technical modifications, 34
    terminology, 75
Lipexeresis technique, 16
Lipodissection, dry technique, 34
Lipodystrophy. *See also specific site*
    and evident skin flabbiness, 283
    and mild skin flabbiness, 280–283
    pure, 279–280
    trochanteric
        misnomer, 70
        surgical instrumentation, 33
Lipoextraction. *See* Blunt suction lipec-
        tomy; Lipolysis; Lipoplasty
Lipoextractor. *See* Cannulas, suction
Lipolysis. *See also* Lipectomy; Lipoex-
        traction; *specific site*
    advantages compared to lipectomy,
        195
    alternatives, 103
    bulimia and, 52–53
    cannula techniques, 21
    combined with abdominal der-
        molipectomy, 97
    complications, 38, 152
        aesthetic, 153, 301
        delayed sequelae, 153
        immediate, 152–153
        major irregularities, 153, 301
    development of technique, 25–30
    first course in English language, 35
    with flap revision
        of groin flap, 315
        of hand, wrist, and forearm, 315,
            316, 317, 319, 320
        of leg and foot, 315, 318
        of neck and face, 320
        of shoulder and arm, 315, 316
    Fournier's rule, 263
    with glandular excision, 221
    incisions, 144, 145
        for breast lipolysis, 228
        requiring prone position, 145
        requiring supine position, 155–
            157
    introduction in United States, 37–
        38
    lectures and supervision of first cases,
        31–32
    patient selection, 94, 95, 104
    photography of patients, 82, 85
    preoperative screening, 53
    presentation of technique, 30–31
    pretreatment with epinephrine, 144
    pretunneling, 159
    repeat procedures, 89
    surgical privileges, 89
    surgical technique, 144–152
        criss-cross, 148
        mesh undermining, 148
        terminology, 65, 75

Lipolysis—*Continued*
    in treatment of
        congenital lymphedema of lower
            extremity, 326–329
        insulin-induced fat hypertrophy,
            323–325
        lipoma of back, 323, 325, 326
Lipolysis Society of North America, 154
Lipomas
    of back, lipolysis for, 323, 325, 326
    removal, 26
Lipoplasty. *See also* Blunt suction lipec-
        tomy; Lipoextraction; Lipolysis;
        specific sites
    aspirative, 17
    circular, 296, 299
    technical modifications, 34
    terminology, 75–76
Liposuction, 17, 75
Lithium carbonate, 105
Litigation. *See also* Malpractice
    dissatisfaction related to, 93
    magnification of unsatisfactory result
        and, 89
    prevention, 87–89, 91–94, 103–104
Lorazepam (Ativan), 106
Love handles. *See also* Flank
    incision, 157
    location, 65, 68
    suprapubic incision, 156
Lower body
    congenital lymphedema, 326–329
    disproportion of, 69
    dressings, 164
    terminology, 68–72
Low-pressure suction machines, 124
Lumbosacral dysmorphia, angular, 296
Lymphedema, congenital, 326–329

Macromastia, 74, 75
Malar area
    lipolysis
        locations, 185, 186
        with rhytidectomy, 200–201
        technique, 189
    location, 72, 73
Males, fat distribution in, 65, 67, 68
Malpractice. *See also* Litigation
    dissatisfaction related to, 92
    first suit, 20
    lipolysis and, 38
    prevention, 87–89, 91–94, 103–104
Malta, depiction of female form in, 10,
        11
Mammoplasty, reduction
    with blunt suction lipectomy
        postoperative management, 230
        sequelae, 230
        surgical technique, 229–230
    dressings, 164
    historical treatment, 227
    limitations of excision approach, 221
    preoperative preparation, 227–228
    results, 230–231

Mandible
  lipolysis with rhytidectomy, 206
  reconstruction, 309, 310
Marcaine. *See* Bupivacaine
Marplan (isocarbozid), 105
Mask, advantages of anesthesia by, 107,
      155
Massage
  benefits, 175–176
  hemosiderin staining and, 181
  hyperpigmentation and, 153
  regimen, 177
  techniques, 176
Mathematical standards, of human pro-
      portion, 57–60
Measurements, body weight and, 61–63
Melanin, 298
Mesh undermining
  in blacks, 298, 299
  peripheral, 235
  technique, 148
Mesomorph, 62
Mestinon (pyridostigmine), 105, 108
Methohexital (Brevital), 106, 107
Methoxyflurane (Penthrane), 109
Metocurine, 108
Mineral oil, for tape removal, 164
Monoamine oxidase inhibitor(s), 105
Muscle contracture test, 108
Muscle relaxants, 107, 108, 112
Mytelase, 105

Naloxone (Narcan), 112
Narcotic(s)
  in anesthetic maintenance, 108
  in induction, 107
  premedication, 106
  preoperative discontinuance, 105
  reversal, 112
  spinal, pain relief from, 112
Narcotic antagonists, 112
Nardil (phenelzine), 105
Nasolabial folds, *upper,* 200–201. *See
      also* Jowls; Preantral area; Rhy-
      tidectomy
Nasolabial grooves, 189
Nausea, postoperative, 112–113
Neck. *See also* Facial lipolysis
  anatomical terminology, 72, 73
  dressings, 164
  lipolysis, 29, 199, 320
    facial, 192
    during rhytidectomy, 200–202
Neolithic period, 11
Neostigmine (Prostigmin), 105, 108
Neoumbilicoplasty
  indications and steps, 234–235
  in obese patients, 243–245
Nerve blocks, central, 111–112
Neurofibroma, face and neck lipolysis
      for, 320
Neuromuscular blocking drugs. *See*
      Muscle relaxants
Nitroprusside, 108
Nitrous oxide, 108, 109

Nose, reconstruction, 313
Nutritional support, of surgical recov-
      ery, 173–174

Obesity
  adipose tissue development and, 42–
      43
  alteration of lipolysis, 44
  classification, 46, 47
  forms, 43
  insulin and, 45, 46
  subcutaneous fat deposition, 46–47
Office personnel, importance of, 89
Organophosphates, 105
Outcome
  predictors, 53
  surgical, 179–180
  unsatisfactory, 89
Overextraction, 192
Overweight, standards of, 61
Oxygen, supplemental, 113

Pain medications, 88, 112
Paleolithic cultures, depiction of female
      form in, 6–12
Pancuronium, 108
Paranoia, patient selection and, 93
Pargylin (Eutonyl), 105
Patients
  average, 97–99
  ideal candidates, 95–97
  informed, 180
  less than ideal, 97, 100–102
  selection
    importance, 38, 179
    medical aspects of, 105
    physical aspects of, 95–102
    of proper procedure, 95
    psychological aspects, 91–93
    risk management and, 87
Pear-shaped deformity, 68, 69
Pectoral area, lateral extension, 74, 75
Penthrane (methoxyflurane), 109
Pentobarbital, 105
Pentothal (thiopental), 106, 107, 187
Perianesthetic period, 105
Peritrochanteric fat
  as misnomer, 70
  surgical perspective, 16–18
Personality disturbances, bulimia and,
      50, 52
Pétrissage, 176, 177
Phenelzine (Nardil), 105
Phi, in body proportion, 58, 59
Phosphodiesterase, 44, 45
Photographic documentation
  film, 78
  lens, 80
  lighting, 79
  of operative markings, 137–140
  patient position and attire for, 82–85
  photograph quality
    average, 77–78
    good, defined, 77
    ideal, defined, 77

Photographic documentation—*Con-
      tinued*
  preoperative, 102–103, 104
  risk management and, 87
  technical considerations, 77–82
  views, 83, 84
Physician, second opinion, 89
Physics, of pressure, 112–124
Physiotherapy, 16, 175. *See also specific
      therapies*
Physostigmine (Antilirium), 112
Pigmentation. *See* Hyperpigmentation
Pinch and roll technique, 188, 189, 229
Pinch test
  in female breast lipolysis, 228, 229
  for gynecomastia, 220, 221
  for iliac crest fat, 253
  in lateral femoral area, 138, 150, 152,
      261, 263
  preoperative preparation and, 137–
      138
Pitanguy's operation, 19
Plane dissection, 23
Planotomé, 33
Polydrug abuse, 50, 52
Positioning of patient
  for face and neck, 155
  prone, 141
  supine, 155–157
  supine lateral decubitus, 157–159
  for ultrasound and massage, 177
Postoperative period
  and care after rhytidectomy, 202
  convalescence, 179–182
  delayed sequelae, 153
  dressings, 163–168
  follow-up, 154
  hospitalization costs and epinephrine
      usage, 115–117
  hypovolemia, 110, 115, 153, 171
  limitations and informed consent, 104
  nutrition in, 173–174
  physical therapy, 175–178
  recovery room complications, 112–
      113
  risk management and, 88
  touch-up procedures, 89, 153, 182
Prader-Willi syndrome, 326
Preantral area. *See also* Jowls; Nasola-
      bial folds, upper
  cannula, 129
  defined, 72, 73
  fat extraction, 190
  lipolysis
    location, 185, 186
    technique, 188, 189
Preauricular fat lipolysis, 200–201
Prehyoid adiposity, clinical results, 196
Premature ventricular contractions
      (PVCs), 110
Premedications, 105–106
Preoperative period
  evaluation
    interview and examination, 102–
      103, 194–195

Preoperative period, evaluation—*Continued*
limiting physical factors, 102
limiting psychological factors, 91–93
risk management and, 88
SAFE, 93, 94
informed consent, 103, 104
patient positioning, 141
photographic records, 77–85, 87
prepping, 141
records, 89
screening tests, 106–107
skin marking, 137–140
Preparotid fat
extraction, 191
lipolysis, 185, 189
with rhytidectomy, 206–208
Pressure, physics of, 112–124
Pressure garments. *See* Compression garments
Pretreatment, with subcutaneous injections, 144
Pretunneling. *See* Tunnel creation
Proportion
classic, 55–57
Golden, 58, 59
perceptions of, 60–61
Vitruvian diagram, 55, 57
Propranolol (Inderal), 113
Prostigmin (neostigmine), 105, 108
Protein
nutritional requirements, 173–174
serum changes following lipolysis, 169, 170
Pseudocholinesterase, 107–108
Psychological aspects
patient selection, 91–94
postoperative sequelae, 52–53
Psychotic patients, as unsatisfactory surgical candidates, 92–93
Pursestring appearance, of ankle, 70, 72
PVC (premature ventricular contraction), 110
Pyrenean-Aquitanian group, depiction of female form by, 8, 9
Pyridostigmine (Mestinon; Regonol), 105, 108
Pyridoxine (B_6), 173
Pythagorean doctrine, 55

Racial differences. *See also* Blacks
in adiposities, 295–298
in female figure, 12
Ranitidine (Zantac), 106
Reconstructive surgery
of breast, 313–315
of face and neck, 320
of foot, 315, 318
of hand and forearm, 309–313, 315–317
lipolysis and, 309, 321
of mandible, 309, 310
of nose, 313
of shoulder and upper arm, 315, 316

Record keeping, risk management and, 89
Recovery period, nutrition and, 173
Recovery room, problems, 112–113
Redo procedures, and billing disputes, 89
Reference pressure, 119
Regonol (Pyridostigmine), 108
Relief phase, 181
Resection-graft, umbilical, 234, 235
Resection-reconstruction, umbilicus, 234–235
Respiratory arrest, 112
Rhenish-Danubian group, depiction of female form in, 9
Rhinoplasty, 192, 194
Rhytidectomy
anesthesia, 202
complications, 194
illustrative cases, 202, 204–209
innovations, 199
lipolysis areas with, 200–201
patient selection, 200
postoperative complications, 202, 203
submental lipolysis, 155, 156
variations, 199
Riding breeches deformity. *See also* Femoral area; Saddlebags
description, 65, 66
removal, 25
treatment, 26–28
Risks, inclusion in consent form, 103
Rubens, portrayal of female, 3, 6
Russia, early cultural depiction of female, 9, 10

Saddlebags, 257–260. *See also* Femoral area; Riding breeches deformity
description, 65, 66
patient positioning during lipolysis of, 157–159
SAFE evaluation, 93, 94
Saliclylates, 88
Satisfaction phase, 181
Scars
abdominal revision, 245, 246
on blacks, 299
dermolipectomy, 19
infraumbilical, 292
nasolabial, 189
surgical, 16, 17, 116
Scopolamine, 106, 112
Secretions, reduction, 106
Sedatives, 106
Self-esteem
body size and, 49
bulimia and, 52
patient evaluation and, 93
Self-image, body weight and, 49
Self-motivation, importance in patient selection, 92
Seromas, postoperative, 20, 34, 115
Serum glutamic oxaloacetic transaminase (SGOT), 170

Serum glutamic pyruvic transaminase (SGPT), 106, 170
Sexual characteristics, secondary, 12, 19
Sexual maturation, body image and, 50
SGOT (serum glutamic oxaloacetic transaminase), 170
SGPT (serum glutamic pyruvic transaminase), 106, 170
Shivering, postoperative, 113
Siberian group, artistic representation of female in, 11, 12
Skin
black, 295
conditions, preoperative, 102
elasticity, 32, 39, 303, 304
evaluation of contraction, 261, 262
excess, 26
flaccidity
with lipodystrophy, 280–285
with no localized lipodystrophy, 292, 293
fold thickness, 61
marking for
abdominal lipolysis, 235, 236
breast lipolysis, 227
facial lipolysis, 187, 188
gynecomastia lipolysis, 219–220
iliac crest lipolysis, 253–254
knee lipolysis, 268
reduction mammoplasty, 227–228
thigh lipolysis, 138–140, 263
tone, 27
Society, body image and, 49–50
Somatotypes, 62
Spare tire. *See* Flank
Spinal block. *See* Central neural block
Square bottom, 65, 66, 263, 264
Staff, informed, 180
Steatomelia, 11, 12
Steatopygia
in blacks, 295–296
in early art, 8–11
as form of beauty, 55
origins, 12
Sternocleidomastoid muscle, 72, 73
Stretch marks, 261
Submandibular area
cannula, 129
lipolysis, 189, 199
clinical results, 191–195
with rhytidectomy, 200–202, 205–209
location of fat, 185, 186
triangle location, 72, 73
Submental area
adiposities, 29, 185, 194, 195
cannula, 129
lipolysis of, 189, 199
candidates, 200
clinical results, 191–193
incisions, 155, 156
preoperative interview, 194–195
results, 196, 197

Submental area, lipolysis of—*Continued*
during rhytidectomy, 200–201, 204, 205, 208, 209
technique, 201
location, 72–73
single midline incision, 195
Succinylcholine, 107, 108
Suction curettage, 20–21
Suction extraction of fat. *See also* Blunt suction lipectomy; Lipolysis; *specific surgical procedure*
instrumentation, 34
movement by air leak, 122, 124
movement by vaporization, 122, 123
terminology, 75
Suction machines
characteristics, 135
high-pressure, 134
pressure of, for facial lipolysis, 185
Suprapatellar fat. *See* Knee(s)
Suprapubic incision, 235, 236
Supratrochanteric incision, 235, 236, 265
Supraumbilical incision, 235, 236
Surital (thiamylal), 106, 107
Swelling, postoperative, 29–30
Symmetry, defined, 60

Tachyarrhythmia, 113
Tachycardia, 153
Tagamet (cimetidine), 106
Teimourian procedure, 122, 124, 125
Temperature, vaporization and, 121
Tensilon (edrophonium), 108, 113
Thiamylal (Surital), 106, 107
Thigh
cannulas, 129, 131, 132
cross section, 147
lipolysis, 38, 39
candidates, 257–260
ideal candidate, 261, 262
incisions, 157
lipodystrophy with skin flaccidity, 283–285
planning of approach, 266, 267

Thigh—*Continued*
lipoplasty, history, 277
medial, 265–266
pinch test, 150, 152
postoperative contour deformities, 305–306
preoperative marking, 138, 139, 140
secondary fatty deformities, 303, 304
slot-like appearance, 266
surgical approaches, 148
upper contour deformities, 301–305
Thiopental (Pentothal), 106, 107, 187
Third party coverage, 104
Thromboembolic phenomena, postoperative, 153
Thrombophlebitis, intravenous diazepam and, 107
Titian, portrayal of female, 3, 5
Torr, 120–121
Touchup procedures
billing disputes, 89
indications, 182
lipolysis, 39
for major irregularities, 153
preoperative understanding about, 102
Toxicity, 110, 111
Tracrium (atracurium), 108
Tranquilizers, 106
Transposition, of umbilicus, 234
Tricyclic antidepressants, 105
Triglycerides
adipose tissue metabolism and, 41–42
fasting and, 47
levels following lipolysis, 170
Trochanteric area
adiposities, in blacks, 298
lipodystrophy with no flabby skin, 280
terminology, 65
Tubocurarine, 108
Tunnel creation
concept, 34
depth, 149, 150

Tunnel creation—*Continued*
prior to suction (pretunneling), 159–161
technique, 22–26, 32, 145, 146

Ultrasound, 176–178, 192
Umbilicus, surgical techniques for, 234, 235
Upper body, nomenclature, 72–73
Urinalysis, 106, 107

Vacuum pumps, 132, 134–135
Valium. *See* Diazepam
Vaporization process, 121
Velazquez, portrayal of female, 3, 5
Venus figurines, 6–11, 55, 56
Verapamil, 113
Violin deformity
description, 65, 66, 68, 69
lipolysis correction, 29
preoperative markings, 140
secondary, 25
surgical selection, 254
variations related to body weight, 257, 259, 260
Vitamin C supplementation, 180
Vitruvius, and diagram of human proportion, 55, 57, 60

Water vapor pressure, 121
Waviness, preexisting, 304, 305
Wydase, 144, 195, 220

X-rays, chest, 106
Xylocaine
effect on hematocrit drop, 116–117
with epinephrine, 116–117, 228
facial lipolysis anesthesia, 187

Zantac (ranitidine), 106
Zinc supplementation, 180
Zyderm injections, 192